BRAIN EDEMA

SPONSORS

Bundesministerium für Unterricht, 1010 Wien, Minoritenplatz 5

Firma Aesca, chem. pharmazeutische Fabrik,Traiskirchen bei Wien, Badnerstrasse 23

Biochemie G.m.b.H. Kundl, Tirol, 1010 Wien, Gluckgasse 1

Firma C. Brady, Erzeugung und Vertrieb chemisch-pharmazeutischer Präparate, 1090 Wien, Hörlgasse 5

Farbwerke Hoechst, Generalvertretung Vedepha G.m.b.H., 1070 Wien, Lindengasse 55

Firma Geigy, Generalvertretung F. Joh. Kwizda, 1010 Wien, Dr. Karl Lueger Ring 6-8

Hoffmann-La Roche G.m.b.H., 1030 Wien, Jaquingasse 16-18

Firma Leitz, Generalvertretung Fa. Optotechnik, 1010 Wien, Dr. Karl Lueger Ring 12

E. Merck A.G. Darmstadt, Vertretung Austro Merck G.m.b.H., 1090 Wien, Mariannengasse 32

Österreichische Stickstoffwerke A.G. Linz, 1030 Wien, Kollergasse 16

Philips G.m.b.H., 1070 Wien, Neubaugasse 11

Sandoz A.G. Basel, Vertretung Schneiderchemie G.m.b.H., 1090 Wien, Spitalgasse 1

Dr. A. Wander G.m.b.H., Pharmazeutische Fabrik, 1010 Wien, Ebendorferstrasse 10

BRAIN EDEMA

Proceedings of the Symposium

September 11-13, 1965, Vienna

Edited by

Igor Klatzo
National Institute of Neurological Diseases and Blindness
National Institutes of Health
Bethesda, Maryland, U.S.A.

and

Franz Seitelberger
Neurologisches Institut der Universität Wien, Austria

SPRINGER-VERLAG • WIEN • NEW YORK • 1967

ISBN-13: 978-3-7091-7547-7 e-ISBN-13: 978-3-7091-7545-3
DOI: 10.1007/978-3-7091-7545-3

Library of Congress Catalog Card Number 67-26445

Title No. 9219

Softcover reprint of the hardcover 1st edition 1967

Contributors

BITO, L., Department of Ophthalmology, College of Physicians and Surgeons, Columbia University, New York, New York, U.S.A.
BLASBERG, R., New York State Research Institute for Neurochemistry and Drug Addiction, Ward's Island, New York, New York, U.S.A.
BRADBURY, M., Cedars Sinai Hospitals, Los Angeles, California, U.S.A.
BRZEZINSKI, J., Department of Neurosurgery, University of Lund, Sweden
BUBIS, J.J., Department of Pathology, Tel-Aviv University Medical School, Tel-Hashomer Government Hospital, Tel-Aviv, Israel
DUFTY, M. L., Department of Pathology, New York Hospital-Cornell Medical Center, New York, New York, U.S.A.
EBELS, E. J., Neurosurgical Clinic, Groningen, Netherlands
ESCOLÁ,*J., Max-Planck-Institut für Hirnforschung, Frankfurt/M.-Niederrad, Germany
FRANKE, H. D., Department of Anatomy and Department of Radiology, University of Hamburg, Germany
FRENCH, L. A., Division of Neurosurgery, University of Minnesota Hospitals, Minneapolis, Minnesota, U.S.A.
GARRO, F., Division of Neuropathology, Armed Forces Institute of Pathology, Washington, D.C., U.S.A.
GIORDANO, P. L., Clinica Psichiatrica Dell' Università di Milano, Italy
GORDON, J. S., Department of Pathology, New York Hospital-Cornell Medical Center, New York, New York, U.S.A.
HARTMANN, J. F., Department of Neurology, Presbyterian-St. Luke's Hospital, Chicago, Illinois, U.S.A.
HASS, G. M., Department of Biochemistry, Presbyterian-St. Luke's Hospital, Chicago, Illinois, U.S.A.
HAYMAKER, W., National Aeronautics and Space Administration, Ames Research Center, Moffett Field, California, U.S.A.
HESS, O., Institute of Pathochemistry and General Neurochemistry, University of Heidelberg, Germany
INVERNIZZI, G., Clinica Psichiatrica Dell'Università di Milano, Italy

*Deceased

KALSBECK, J., Divisions of Neuropathology and Neurosurgery, Indiana University Medical Center, Indianapolis, Indiana, U.S.A.
KARCHER, D., Institut Bunge, Berchem-Anvers, Belgium
KJÄLLQUIST, A., Department of Neurosurgery, University of Lund, Sweden
KLEIHUES, P., Max-Planck-Institute für Hirnforschung Abteilung für Allgemeine Neurologie, Köln-Merheim, Germany
KONDO,Y., Department of Neurosurgery, University of Kyoto, Japan
LAING, I., Department of Biochemistry, Presbyterian-St. Luke's Hospital, Chicago, Illinois, U.S.A.
LEVI, G., Department of Neurology, University of Florence, Italy
LEVINE, S., Laboratory Division, Montefiore Hospital, New York Medical College Center for Chronic Disease, New York, New York, U.S.A.
OZAWA, K., Department of Neurosurgery, University of Kyoto, Japan
PALMEIRO, J. F., Max-Planck-Institut für Hirnforschung Abteilung für Allgemeine Neurologie, Köln-Merheim, Germany
PANDOLFI, S., Department of Biochemistry, Presbyterian-St. Luke's Hospital, Chicago, Illinois, U.S.A.
PEARSON, D., Division of Neurological Surgery, University Clinics, University of Chicago, Illinois, U.S.A.
PONTÉN, U., Department of Neurosurgery, University of Lund, Sweden
RALL, D. P., Laboratory of Chemical Pharmacology, National Cancer Institute, Bethesda, Maryland, U.S.A.
RIVERSON, E., Max-Planck-Institut für Hirnforschung Abteilung für Allgemeine Neurologie, Köln-Merheim, Germany
SCHRÖDER, J. M., Max-Planck-Institut für Hirnforschung Abteilung für Allgemeine Neurologie, Köln-Merheim, Germany
SIESJÖ, B. K., Department of Neurosurgery, University of Lund, Sweden
SKY-PECK, H. H., Department of Biochemistry, Presbyterian-St. Luke's Hospital, Chicago, Illinois, U.S.A.
STREICHER, E., National Institute of Neurological Diseases and Blindness, National Institutes of Health, Bethesda, Maryland, U.S.A.
TER WEEME, C. A., Neurosurgical Clinic, Groningen, Netherlands
TSUJI, H., Department of Neurosurgery, University of Kyoto, Japan
WIŚNIEWSKI, H., Neuropathologisches Institut, Warschau, Poland

Active Participants

ADAMS, R. D., Massachusetts General Hospital, Boston Massachusetts, U.S.A.
BAKAY, L., Edward J. Meyer Memorial Hospital, University of Buffalo, New York, U.S.A.
BEKS, J. W. F., Neurosurgical Clinic, Groningen, Netherlands
BRIGHTMAN, M. W., National Institute of Neurological Diseases and Blindness, National Institutes of Health, Bethesda, Maryland, U.S.A.
BROMAN, T., Department of Neurology, University of Göteborg, Sweden
CAVENESS, W. F., National Institute of Neurological Diseases and Blindness, National Institutes of Health, Bethesda, Maryland, U.S.A.
CAZZULLO, C. L., Clinica Psichiatrica Dell' Universita di Milano, Italy
CERVOS-NAVARRO, J., Institut für Neuropathologie der Universität Bonn, Germany
CLASEN, R. A., Department of Biochemistry, Presbyterian-St. Luke's Hospital, Chicago, Illinois, U.S.A.
COLMANT, H. J., Neuropathologisches Institut der Universität Hamburg, Germany
CUMINGS, J. N., Institute of Neurology, Department of Chemical Pathology, The National Hospital, London, England
DAVSON, H., Department of Physiology, University College, London, England
EVANS, J. P., Division of Neurological Surgery, University Clinics, University of Chicago, Illinois, U.S.A.
FEIGIN, I., New York University Medical Center, New York, New York, U.S.A.
FLEISCHHAUER, K., Abteilung für Neuroanatomie, Anatomisches Institut der Universität Hamburg, Germany
FONCIN, J. F., Laboratoire de Physiologie et Psychologie Neurochirurgicales de l'Ecole Pratique des Hautes Etudes, Hôpital de la Salpêtriere, Paris, France
GLOWACKI, J., Department of Neurosurgery, Academy of Medicine, Cracow, Poland

GRUNER, J. E., 123, Boulevard de port royal, Paris XIV, France
HAGER, H., Abteilung für Neurozytologie, Max-Planck-Institut für Psychiatrie, München, Germany
HIRANO, A., Laboratory Division, Montefiore Hospital and Medical Center, Bronx, New York, U.S.A.
HOFF, H., Psychiatrisch-Neurologische Universitätsklinik, Wien, Austria
HOSSMANN, K. A., Max-Planck-Institute für Hirnforschung, Abteilung für Allgemeine Neurologie, Köln-Merheim, Germany
ISHII, S., Division of Neurological Surgery, University Clinics, University of Chicago, Illinois, U.S.A.
JACOB, H., Universitäts-Nervenklinik, Marburg/Lahn, Germany
JELLINGER, K., Neurologisches Institut d. Univ. Wien, Austria
KATZMAN, R., Department of Neurology, Albert Einstein College of Medicine, Bronx, New York, U.S.A.
KIDD, M., Maida Vale Hospital, London, England
KLATZO, I., National Institute of Neurological Diseases and Blindness, National Institutes of Health, Bethesda, Maryland, U.S.A.
KOLKMANN, F. W., Neuropathologisches Institut Universität Heidelberg, Germany
KRAUS, H., Neurochirurgische Universitäts-Klinik, Wien, Austria
KRÜCKE, W., Max-Planck-Institut für Hirnforschung, Frankfurt/M.-Niederrad, Germany
LAJTHA, A., New York State Research Institute for Neurochemistry and Drug Addiction, Ward's Island, New York, New York, U.S.A.
LAMPERT, P., Division of Neuropathology, Armed Forces Institute of Pathology, Washington, D.C., U.S.A.
LEE, J. C., Buffalo General Hospital, Buffalo, New York, U.S.A.
LIERSE, W., Anatomisches Institut der Universität Hamburg, Germany
LONG, D. M. Department of Surgery, University of Minnesota, Hospitals, Minneapolis, Minnesota, U.S.A.
LOWENTHAL, A., Institut Bunge, Berchem-Anvers, Belgium
McMENEMEY, W. H., Maida Vale Hospital, London, England
MIQUEL, J., National Aeronautics and Space Administration, Ames Research Center, Moffett Field, California, U.S.A.
OPPELT, W., Department of Pharmacology and Therapeutics, University of Florida, Gainesville, Florida, U.S.A.
PAPPIUS, H. M., Donner Laboratory of Experimental Neurochemistry, Montreal Neurological Institute; Department of Neurology and Neurosurgery, McGill University, Montreal, Canada
PENTSCHEW, A., Division of Neuropathology, Armed Forces Institute of Pathology, Washington, D. C., U.S.A.
QUADBECK, G., Institute of Pathochemistry and General Neurochemistry, University of Heidelberg, Germany

SEITELBERGER, F., Neurologisches Institut der Universität Wien, Austria

SLUGA, E., Neurologisches Institut der Universität Wien, Austria

STEINBEREITHNER, K., Institut für Anaesthesiologie, Wien, Austria

STEINWALL, O., Department of Neurology, University of Göteborg, Sweden

TERRY, R., Albert Einstein College of Medicine, Bronx, New York, U.S.A.

THOMAS, E., Max-Planck-Institut für Hirnforschung, Frankfurt/M.-Niederrad, Germany

TORACK, R. M., Department of Pathology, New York Hospital-Cornell Medical Center, New York, New York, U.S.A.

TOWER, D., National Institute of Neurological Diseases and Blindness, National Institutes of Health, Bethesda, Maryland, U.S.A.

ULE, G., Neuropathologisches Institut der Universität Heidelberg, Germany

WALKER, A. E., Division of Neurological Surgery, The Johns Hopkins Hospital, Baltimore, Maryland, U.S.A.

WECHSLER, W., Max-Planck-Institut für Hirnforschung Abteilung für Allgemeine Neurologie, Köln-Merheim, Germany

WOLMAN, M., Department of Pathology, Tel-Aviv University Medical School, Tel-Hashomer Government Hospital, Tel-Aviv, Israel

ZEMAN, W., Divisions of Neuropathology and Neurosurgery, Indiana University Medical Center, Indianapolis, Indiana, U.S.A.

ZIMMERMAN, H. M., Laboratory Division, Montefiore Hospital, The New York Medical College Center for Chronic Disease, New York, New York, U.S.A.

ZÜLCH, K., Max-Planck-Institut für Hirnforschung Abteilung für Allgemeine Neurologie, Köln-Merheim, Germany

Introduction

The Symposium on Brain Edema has been organized by the Österreichische Arbeitsgemeinschaft für Neuropathologie and by the Problem Commission for Neuropathology of the World Federation of Neurology.

We would like to express our thanks to Dr. L. van Bogaert, president of the W.F.N., for his great interest in the design of this conference and for his energetic support.

One of the aims of the Problem Commission for Neuropathology has been to contribute to the advances in various problems which are becoming ripe for elucidation by experts in different fields. The idea of the Symposium on Brain Edema has as its background a compelling necessity to elucidate this subject which is clinically so important and neuropathologically so poorly understood. It was hoped that this could be achieved by a multidisciplinary approach involving a variety of aspects to be discussed and correlated. Brain edema, being an abnormal cerebral condition, belongs basically to the sphere of neuropathology, but to be successful in our endeavors we had to apply neuropathology in its most modern and widest terms. By this we understand that such neuropathology includes the study of all abnormal phenomena in the nervous tissue related to the structural alterations, and by "structural" we mean not only tissual or cellular ones but also changes on ultrastructural and molecular levels. Thus we needed close and integrated cooperation of experts in fields such as neurohistology, histochemistry, electron microscopy, neurochemistry, and neurophysiology.

We fully realized that the sick man suffering from brain edema is the ultimate motive of our undertaking. For this reason we depended greatly on the experience of clinicians who clearly define the clinical problems involved and contribute to the correlation and evaluation of the laboratory data. From morphologists we expected mainly understanding and agreement on histological recognition and definitions of brain edema, a controversial and confused subject in the past. The experts in the neurobiological sciences tackled the complex problems dealing with abnormal accumulation of fluid in the nervous tissue, and by this endeavor they also contributed substantially to the understanding of the basic mechanisms in the normal brain. In the solution of any clinical problem, an experimental model in which many basic aspects can be clearly evaluated is of great importance, and thus the sessions devoted to experimental study on brain edema promised to be most valuable.

In the course of our proceedings, many new observations and facts were demonstrated, but the members of the symposium had not gathered just to present their findings. Our main purpose was the integration of data, and we therefore expected so much from the free and frank discussions to which one whole session had been devoted. What we wanted to achieve was simply this: we wanted to know exactly where we stood and where we should go in this important problem of brain edema.

For the realization of this publication we express our thanks to all co-workers as well as to the authors and the participants in the discussion who kindly supported the edition of the proceedings. We are indebted to Springer-Verlag for the great interest and understanding of the requirements of the present publication.

Franz Seitelberger Igor Klatzo

Contents

*Deceased

I. Clinical Aspects of Brain Edema

Chairman: ***H. Kraus***

HANS HOFF
KURT JELLINGER

BRAIN EDEMA AS A NEUROLOGICAL PROBLEM — I

Brain edema (BE) is still an unsolved problem both pathogenetically and clinico-therapeutically. It is a frequent and dangerous reaction of the brain to various pathogenic noxae and general conditions traversing the field of neurology. Cerebral edema, therefore, becomes one of the most acute problems of clinical medicine as well as basic scientific research. Clinical neurologists most frequently observe symptomatic BE following cranial injuries and in connection with cerebral tumors. Circulatory disorders, inflammatory diseases and intoxications, as well as many other cerebral and general diseases, are often associated with BE. Its importance as a neurological problem lies first in its etiological and biological diversity which is contrasted with a relatively uniform, hardly pathognomonic, clinical syndrome. Secondarily the importance of cerebral edema rests in its severe consequences and complications for function and structure of the central nervous system, and above all in its acute, vital danger by the concurrent increase in intracranial pressure.

COMMON CRITERIA AND PATHOGENIC PROBLEMS

Classical Concepts — Critical Remarks

The concept of BE as a cerebral enlargement due to increased water content was already known by early brain pathologists at the time of Anton (1904). They first accepted the classical definition of edema stated in Virchow's general pathology, i.e., "edema is an accumulation of fluid in the intercellular tissue spaces."

Subsequently, the gross and microscopical characteristics of cerebral edema have been defined. The pathophysiological consequences of increase in brain volume associated with BE and their morphological substrate were studied (Spatz and Stroescu, 1934, Hasenjäger and Spatz, 1937, Riessner and Zülch, 1939). These data were of principal importance for the understanding and interpretation of clinical symptomatology of BE and the explanation of its vital complications. The further delineation of the general anatomical features of cerebral edema were limited by difficulties in direct indentification and study of edema by light microscopy.

Systematic investigations of BE and its morphology revealed several types, differing in regard to their gross localization and expansion as well as to their pathogenesis. Reichardt (1905, 1957) divided cerebral edema into a hemodynamic form and a type caused by disorders of the blood-brain barrier. Whereas hemodynamic BE, e.g., associated with intracranial venous stasis or extracerebral circulatory disorders, is diffusely localized in cortex and white matter of the brain, edema secondary to space-occupying processes (tumors, haemorrhages, etc.), as well as to traumatic cerebral laceration predominantly is perifocally confined to the cerebral gray and white matter. In the brain swollen by inflammatory disease or by generalized anoxia, BE basically concerns the white matter. Similar distribution with perivenous accentuation is found in allergically caused cerebral edema. General poisoning and metabolic-dysenzymatic disturbances (protein deficiency syndromes, crush syndrome, hypoparathyroidism, etc.), may cause diffusely distributed edema in cerebral white and/or gray matter. This demonstration of some gross morphological types of cerebral swelling indicates that Reichardt's classification can only be accepted partially, since in general several factors, e.g., a vascular and a tissue factor, are believed to be engaged in edema formation (Hoff and Jellinger, 1962).

The dualistic concept of Reichardt assuming a principal division of the enlargement of brain volume into brain edema and brain swelling is not generally accepted either. Diffuse cerebral swelling as a comparatively rare type of a "universal" brain reaction (Scheinker, 1938) with increased "intracellular" fluid accumulation without increase of the "free" tissue fluid is seen in acute lethal catatonia, epileptic state, rapidly progressive general paralysis, and certain forms of poisoning (uremia, eclampsia). Biochemically characterized by dehydration of brain tissue and a tendency towards alkalosis (Selbach, 1941, Peters and Selbach, 1943), it has been regarded as the outcome of polymerization and exudative processes designed to neutralize toxic compounds in the cerebral tissue. Though osmotically induced brain swelling (uremia, dialysis) is quite different from trauma induced and other forms of edema, it no longer seems justified to continue drawing a clear-cut distinction between brain "edema" and "swelling," since these two forms are probably different stages of fluid diffusion within the brain tissue.

Modern Concepts – Morphology and Biochemistry

The initial steps in a multi-dimensional and multi-factorial concept of cerebral edema were formed after systematic examinations of its gross and microscopic characteristics. Since definite categories of BE can be established on a morphological basis, we would feel that the burden of proof that these are fundamentally the same rests with those who would uphold the unitarian hypothesis of BE or the proposition that all forms of cerebral edema (and/or swelling) are essentially the same. Though detailed data on various conditions associated with BE have been obtained and some questions concerning ion and water metabolism and their disturbances as well as the nature and function of the blood-brain barrier (BBB) have been solved in the last years, the basic problem of edema formation in the brain remains unclear.

Important progress was achieved by application of modern scientific methods, such as electron microscopy, biochemistry and applied histochemistry.

Recent studies with the electron microscope have shown that edema in cerebral gray matter is characterized by swelling of cellular elements of the neuropil, above all of "clear" glia cells without significant expansion of the extracellular space. These findings clearly indicated an intracellular localization of edema fluid to be considered as a sort of "glial hydrops" in the cerebral gray matter (cf. Ule and Kolkmann, 1962). Since the ultrastructure of the cerebral white matter including the problem of the dimensions and extension of a functional extracellular space are still under discussion, the existence of an extracellular type of edema in the white matter, different from that in the gray, is not yet clear (Hager, 1964, Gonatas, et al., 1963, Aleu, et al., 1964, Tani and Evans, 1965, Herzog, et al., 1965, Lee and Bakay, 1965). The main question unsolved seems to be whether the different data are due to preparatory artifacts or to differing forms of cerebral edema in gray and white matter, as could be suggested in protein-rich forms of cerebral swelling (cf. Schröder and Wechsler, 1965).

Modern biochemistry revealed valuable data concerning the behavior of edema fluid indicating its origin. In various forms of cerebral swelling, e.g., perifocal BE secondary to trauma, tumors, hemorrhages, and inflammatory lesions, edema fluid shows many characteristics of plasma indicating it to be exudate (Cumings, 1961, Herschkowitz, et al., 1965), whereas in other forms it is believed to be more closely related to plasma ultrafiltrate than to whole plasma, as was demonstrated in the model of triethyltin, TET-induced edema (Katzman, et al., 1963, Bakay, 1965). The distribution of electrolytes in this form, however, shows marked deviation from cold-induced edema (Pappius and Gulati, 1963, Bakay and Haque, 1964) and other types of cerebral swelling. Generally speaking, the biochemical basis of BE is not only an increase in water content of the brain tissue, but also, and primarily, an abnormal distribution of fluid and ions in connection with disturbances of ion distribution and transport, particularly with regard to the intra- and extra-cellular sodium/potassium ratio. Oversimplifying the problem, one could characterize BE as a pathological uptake of water and sodium in the cerebral cell. There are exceptions, however, and in TET-induced edema sodium uptake is even lowered (Katzman, et al.).

This simple definition of cerebral edema implicates the question concerning the origin of these substances and the pathomechanisms of their disturbed distribution and transport. These problems are closely connected with our knowledge of nature and function of the blood-brain barrier. Formerly it had been suggested that after a barrier disturbance there would exist a passive sodium influx into the cerebral tissue, causing an equilibrium between brain tissue and serum. Since the substrate of BBB was demonstrated to be composed of the basement membrane of capillaries and the adherent astrocyte membrane without any increase of the extracellular space and without interruption of these barrier membranes, our opinion on the function of BBB had to be revised. Today it is considered a system of cellular membranes with active selective properties and specific mechanisms for the transfer and uptake of certain substances (Hager, 1961, Broman and Steinwall, 1965, Tani and Evans, 1965) or a a combination of active and passive specific barrier phenomena (Cervos-Navarro, 1964). There are data supporting the hypothesis that there exist active, biochemically determined, and energy-assisted transfer and transport mechanisms via the cerebral cellular membrane system as is known in the cells of other organs. The astroglia cells are suggested to play an important role in the further transport of fluid and electrolytes from blood to parenchymal cells.

As is well known, edematous states may occur without any disturbances of the BBB demonstrable with dyes and other tracers. This does not exclude, however, dysfunction of other components of the barrier system, the functions of which are not yet elucidated in all details.

According to present results, one important mode of BE-formation consists of alterations of the active transport phenomena due to disturbances in cellular energy metabolism and a consequent dysfunction of cell membranes. Katzman, et al. (1963), suggested from their findings in TET-induced edema that edema formation results from the inhibition of the "sodium pump" caused by disorders of biochemical barrier-activity. However, it still remains open whether this hypothesis holds for other types of BE, particularly because of the special characteristics of TET-edema. Pathophysiological interpretations gathered from various types of brain swelling can for the time being be transferred to human conditions only with critical reservation. Many facts, however, indicate the basic importance of disturbances of energy-producing metabolic steps at the cellular level for the development of disturbances of water- and ion-transport and distribution (cf. Reulen, et al., 1964).

Problems of Experimental Brain Edema – Models

In order to clarify these problems it is necessary to understand the differences in BE as caused by different types of noxious stimuli. This question studied in a series of experimental edema models, represents a large part of this workshop. The experimental forms of BE show, as is well known, strong differences with regard to chemical composition, localization and ultrastructure, as well as to clinical symptomatology. These facts prove the concept that BE is not a pathogenetically uniform condition or reaction. Furthermore, they stimulate criticism of the present, or classical, concept of BE. The important question still open is whether the experimental forms of BE correspond to the types known in human pathology. First of all, it must be clarified with which human types of cerebral swelling they are compatible.

A number of different experimental BE-models are considered to reproduce the pathological picture in humans, as perhaps cold-induced and other injuries (Klatzo, et al., 1958, Torack, et al., 1959, Bakay and Haque, 1964, Reulen, et al., 1964, Schröder and Wechsler, 1965), increase of intracranial pressure by implanted balloons (Raimondi, et al., 1962, Tani and Evans, 1965), hypercapnic hypoxia (Bakay and Bendixen, 1963), and perifocal edema produced by transplantable tumors (Aleu, et al., 1964, Herzog, et al., 1965), whereas other forms, e.g., the often cited TET-edema, are quite different from them (Aleu, et al., 1963, Katzman, et al., 1963, Bakay, 1965, Lee and

Bakay, 1965). We also know that osmotically induced brain swelling differs from trauma or cold injury induced edema (Pappius).

More systematical and critical studies on a great variety of brain swelling are required before enough data will be obtained to compare these experimental forms and other models with the various types of human BE and to clarify the underlying process. Those studies are also necessary to find out which ideas of the classical concept of cerebral edema should be corrected in order to find out general conditions of this lesion. Moreover, the simultaneous determination of the behavior of all physiological component units of the intracranial spaces — blood, CSF, brain water, cerebral electrolytes, and brain solids — during the course and development of BE is necessary, as all these components are influenced in variable degree in order to maintain the homeostatic mechanisms of intracranial pressure. Though detailed data on different forms of cerebral edema are already available (Katzman, et al., 1963, Rosomoff and Zugibe, 1963, Herzog, et al., 1965), they only give very limited hints at the pathological mechanisms of cerebral swelling.

Cerebral edema should be considered as a collective concept of various regulatory systems, since, up to the present, experimental and clinical BE-research has not solved the basic problem of brain swelling. Until its pathological mechanisms are finally clarified, BE from clinical and practical points of view has to be considered a functional process of the total metabolism, whereby the pathophysiological manifestations following an actual damage are subject to a strict series of biological steps. Their elucidation is one of the main problems which will be solved by basic scientific research rather than by clinical neurology.

Sequelae and Complications of Cerebral Edema

The sequelae of BE in which clinical neurologists are interested concern biochemical, vasocirculatory, and other pathophysiological aspects as well as clinical and morphological problems. Here we would like to point out only some important features of the dangerous circulus vitiosus of cerebral edema.

One of the initial changes in edematous brain tissue is known to be acidosis (Peters and Selbach, 1943) caused by accumulation of lactic acid (Magee, et al., 1957). From recent data on phosphate and lactate metabolism as one probable basis of electrolyte transport mechanisms can be deduced important consequences for the transcellular energy transfer. Energy-assisted disturbances of transcellular ion movement, therefore, are to be considered not only the causes but also immediate sequelae of cerebral swelling.

They are suggested to initiate one step of its circulus vitiosus by increasing the initial disturbances responsible for edema formation.

In early stages acute brain swelling is a reflection of vascular dilation secondary to the impairment of vasomotor tone, which was postulated to result from vascular over-distension and from local oxygen deficiency (Langfitt, et al., 1964). Venous stasis resulting from slowing down of cerebral circulation in increased brain volume may give rise to the above mentioned metabolic disturbances. Venous congestion interferes with the supply of nutritional substances and hence energy to the brain and impedes the removal of metabolites resulting in accumulation of low-molecular products, such as lactic acid, CO_2, acetylcholine, noradrenaline, etc. This causes further impairment of active transport and barrier functions as well as of tissue nutrition, promoting further swelling of brain tissue.

An important complicating factor of BE is cerebral hypoxia resulting from decreased cerebral blood flow and lowered oxygen supply in consequence to increased intracranial pressure. Since the normal counter-regulatory mechanisms (Cushing's phenomenon) break down, the edematous brain takes up less oxygen (Gänshirt, 1957, 1961). Moreover, local energy exchange and transport functions are disturbed because of increase in cerebral volume which in the white matter may be as much as twice its normal size, prolonging the time required to oxygen transport from the capillaries to the nervous parenchyma. They may be complicated by impairment of transport functions of the swollen astrocytes. The disorders of oxygen supply in BE are localized in the edematous tissue itself — a condition referred to as "asphyxial hypoxydosis" — and are complicated by disturbances of cerebral blood supply causing an "ischemic hypoxia." As a result, function and structure of the CNS can be severely affected and further edema formation is promoted.

Edematous increase in cerebral volume leads to rise in intracranial pressure blocking isolated sectors of the intracranial CSF system. Its consequences are those associated with the general picture of elevated intracranial pressure, e.g., impairment of vasopressor response by dynamic axial brain-stem distortion (Thompson and Malina, 1959). It is suggested to play an important role in producing arterial hypertension which by means of flooding the paralyzed cerebrovascular system further increases intracranial pressure. This finally reaches a critical point, where shifting of cerebral substance takes place. The resulting displacement of brain tissue leading to transtentorial herniation and herniation into the foramen occipitale magnum with cerebral compression and incarceration syndromes is less dependent on type and extent of cerebral shifting than on the time factor. The more acute the increase of intracranial pressure, the less favorable is the prognosis.

From these and other complications of cerebral swelling, a further increase of edema and of intracranial pressure with their sequelae result in the circulus vitiosus described.

CLINICAL PROBLEMS OF CEREBRAL EDEMA

The clinical picture of BE is rather uniform and unspecific in comparison to its pathogenic multiplicity postulated from the preceding survey of its experimental and human pathological types. Symptomatology of cerebral swelling in general depends on functional disturbances in connection with localization and tendency of spreading of the fluid accumulation in cerebral tissue, as well as on the degree and rate of intracranial pressure increase.

General Symptomatology

Based on conditions causing temporary impairment of cerebral function, the clinical picture of BE is characterized by a most variable and inconstant course associated with alterations of intracranial pressure. Though no classical syndrome of BE exists, its clinical picture is principally divided into: 1) general symptoms of increased intracranial pressure; 2) various and inconstant focal cerebral signs and lesions; 3) secondary complications such as signs of cerebral herniation.

In spite of its clinical uniformity, a certain differentiation of the various pathogenic forms of BE as well as from other syndromes of increased intracranial pressure might be possible in some cases by exact clinical observations.

The classical syndrome of intracranial pressure increase associated with headache, vertigo, vomiting, papilledema, bradycardia, and impaired conscience is one of the least characteristic neurological pictures. Some differences between the syndrome of increased intracranial pressure by BE and elevated CSF pressure can be observed, however, studying a large number of patients.

In cerebral edema, slight disorders of conscience are frequently the first and most regular signs. Psychotic pictures, such as depressive or delirious states, are rarely observed. Occasionally unconsciousness may occur even without any other manifestations of increased intracranial pressure or other neurological symptoms. This holds primarily for diffuse edema, e.g., following anoxia, poisoning, infections, and general diseases. Among intracranial space-occupying processes malignant gliomas and metastases comparatively often are accompanied by early impairment of consciousness the cause of which is considered to be an acute histotoxic edema. Its rapid expansion may be followed by quantitative disturbances of cerebral function interfering with maintenance of consciousness. On the other hand, intraoperative and angiographic observations show that severe brain swelling with shifting of cerebral substance is not necessarily accompanied by manifest deterioration of consciousness. Therefore, psychopathological dysfunctions in connection with BE are considered as sequelae of cerebral tissue swelling, concommitant cerebral hypoxia, intracranial pressure increase and/or lesions of the brain stem secondary to cerebral herniations. The quantity of organic dysfunctions in brain stem, centrencephalic systems, and cortex could be considered an important factor for the degree of impairment of consciousness. Primarily, however, there seem to be signs of different quality and duration of cerebral dysfunction in variable localizations. Their reversibility is different, also. Therefore, we often are not able to give an exact prognosis during the initial stages of cerebral edema or even in its further course.

In the initial stages of BE, when other neurological symptoms are not yet present, patients may show a positive Edelmann's sign: flexion of the extended leg at the hip-joint (Kernig test) leads to dorsiflexion of the big toe (Hoff and Pateisky, 1958). According to Edelmann this sign indicates a "tendency of the brain towards edema."

Cerebral focal lesions mainly exist in localized BE of varying intensity. Such signs include transitory paralysis, slight hemiparesis, uni- or bilateral pyramidal signs, rarely cerebellar and extrapyramidal symptoms. Furthermore, we can note cerebral fits: Jacksonian and generalized forms, epileptic states and dreamy states.

Intracranial pressure increase accompanied by focal cerebral symptoms frequently gives the impression of other space-occupying processes or of the syndrome of pseudotumor cerebri. These pictures, however, are frequently caused by supratentorial BE of different genesis with more or less progressive course. Besides inflammatory, toxic and allergic noxae, cerebral swelling secondary to venous circulatory disturbances in dextrocardiac failure or sinus thrombosis as well as electrolyte disorders and endocrine or metabolic dysfunctions are to be considered in its pathogenesis.

A dislocation of various parts of the brain into the basal cisterns may occur when the increase in brain volume and intracranial pressure reaches a critical point. Diencephalon, the upper brain stem and medulla oblongata are the areas most sensitive to compressive herniations. The lesion of these critical regions manifests itself by the well known syndromes of acute compression of midbrain and medulla oblongata. Early discovery and treatment with prevention of damage of these critical danger points by increase of intracranial pressure are of vital importance. Therefore, the practical significance of both clinical syndromes should be stressed in the clinical discussion of BE. Though both syndromes often overlap, their differentiation often is of great practical interest, as they may give certain prognostic indications.

Acute compression of midbrain is accompanied by oculomotor lesions (dilatation and fixation of the pupils, etc.), uni- or bilateral pyramidal signs, impaired conscience up to coma, disturbances of tonus up to decerebrate rigidity, and autonomic nervous dysregulation (tachycardia, rise of blood pressure, tachypnea, hyperthermia, etc.).

Acute compression of medullary structures results in stiff neck and opisthotonus, loss of conscience, vomiting, vertigo, bradycardia, hypertonia and "pressure pulse" (Cushing's syndrome), sometimes atonic seizures and areflexia, and prolonged interruptions in respiration which may culminate in respiratory arrest.

These syndromes represent severe brain damage, but today they are no longer regarded as definite signa mali ominis. Their prognosis and reversibility, however, depend on rate, degree and duration of the morphological compression and its complications with regard to function and structure of the vital brain stem centers.

Differential Diagnostic Problems

The rather unspecific syndrome of BE implies serious differential diagnostic difficulties against other space-occupying and brain pressure processes. Careful clinical and anamnestic data are often not able to elucidate the diagnosis and therefore additional examinations are necessary. They, however, can give no specific results.

Registration of CSF-pressure is of less diagnostic than prognostic or therapeutic value. Cell and protein contents of CSF may be normal or elevated.

Electroencephalography often is normal or reveals slight low voltage. In severe cases a nonspecific decrease in frequency and high voltage slow waves can be seen. Generalized delta dysrhythmia and severe general alterations may occur. Localized BE not rarely becomes manifest in obvious focal signs. It should be remembered that high delta waves in brain tumors do not originate in the tumor itself but in its edematous surroundings.

Cranial X-ray in unilateral cerebral edema shows lateral displacement with dislocation of the pineal gland. In bilateral BE the pineal gland is displaced in caudal and occipital direction.

Typical pneumoencephalographic signs of cerebral edema include narrow gyri, narrow lateral ventricles with sharp upright edges, or absence of ventricular shadows.

Angiographically, unilateral BE presents displacement of the anterior cerebral artery. Other typical signs include "marginal edema," "local tumor edema," and "collateral edema" around hemorrhages and areas of cerebral softening. If no displacement is apparent, clinical signs of elevated intracranial pressure may be ascribed to a diffuse edema. In such cases, the vessels frequently follow a hydrocephalic course; alternatively, the three basal cisternae are displaced.

Summarizing, the diagnosis of "cerebral edema" per definitionem comprises the variable clinical signs of increased intracranial pressure, other space-occupying processes being excluded. For this purpose a detailed clinical examination plus all auxiliary investigations, and above all, careful observation of the often fluctuant clinical course (in special cases even exploratory craniotomy) will be necessary.

Clinical Course and Sequelae

Important clinical differences can be noted with regard to the course of BE. They indicate the mentioned pathogenic deviations of various forms of human cerebral swelling. One may speak of acute, subacute and relapsing forms, and of subsequent and residual states of BE.

Acute syndromes with fulminant course are seen after intracranial hemorrhages, rupture of aneurysms, malignant cerebral tumors, inflammatory diseases, circulatory disorders, poisoning and after severe cranio-cerebral injuries. Such events are followed shortly by loss of consciousness and acute signs of cerebral and brain stem compression. In cerebral trauma this course may be obscured by the impaired consciousness due to cerebral concussion. An important point is the influence of obstruction of respiratory passages which may augment these critical syndromes. Whatever the role of anoxia per se on BE, it is clear from clinical experience that an injured brain swells alarmingly with oxygen deprivation. To illustrate its dangerous influences, we may cite the observation of a 19-year-old man who developed morphologically confirmed generalized brain swelling with tentorial and cerebellar herniations 35 minutes after a closed cranial injury without fractures, contusions or hemorrhages secondary to oxygen deficiency following severe aspiration (Hoff and Jellinger, 1963).

Generally, cerebral edema produces a severe clinical syndrome 18-48 hours after the noxious incident, caused by a comlexity of increased intracranial pressure, brain anoxia, swelling, stasis, change in pH, electrolytic imbalances, and various other factors. By contrast, the reactive edema following injuries and cerebral operations is characterized by a certain latency period. Deterioration of the clinical state with impairment of consciousness, increased intracranial pressure and progression of neurological focal lesions does not usually appear until the second or third day, subsequently regressing in about one week.

Subacute forms are associated with progressive signs of increased intracranial pressure and can often hardly be distinguished from cerebral tumors. A typical instance is the pseudotumoral BE in malignant hypertension. A progressive course is also seen following intoxications, e.g., in certain forms of CO poisoning.

Relapsing type of BE causes repeated crises of increased intracranial pressure in brain tumors, traumatic cerebral lesions, cardio-vascular diseases, and late states of starvation dystrophy.

While "pure" BE without complicating cerebral anoxia, metabolic imbalances and circulatory disturbances usually is followed by complete clinical remission, "complicated" forms, including severe reactive and relapsing edema, often lead to diffuse, irreversible damage of the CNS (atrophy, necrosis and sclerosis of the white matter, cortical necroses and vasocirculatory compression necroses etc.). Late neuropathological changes in cerebral edema were stressed by Feigin and Popoff (1963).

The terminal and residual states of BE are clinically characterized by various psycho-organic syndromes, accompanied by focal neurological lesions, seizures, optic atrophy, extrapyramidal syndromes, pathological EEG, and symmetrical or unilateral internal (and external) hydrocephalus. The relations between cerebral edema and atrophy are well known to clinicians and pathologists, especially those revealed in post-traumatic encephalopathies (Rosenhagen, 1956, Peters, 1959, Ule, et al., 1962, Jellinger, et al., 1963, Jellinger, 1965). They also occur as late sequelae of inflammatory, toxic and vascular brain lesions associated with edema. The importance of BE in perinatal brain pathology should be stressed, too.

The establishment of relationships between clinical syndromes of human BE-forms and experimental models with variable symptomatology (cf. Bakay, 1965) as well as the clinical registration of important intra- and extracranial compensatory mechanisms and sequelae of cerebral swelling still represent important problems for clinical BE research. Their elucidation will provide further contributions to the understanding of the alterations of cerebral function secondary to edema.

PROBLEMS OF THERAPY AND PREVENTION

The importance of BE within the field of clinical neurology would be dealt with incompletely if one did not consider the main questions of its prophylaxis and treatment. From our present knowledge concerning the dynamics of cerebral swelling, it is necessary to discover the mechanisms of this complex disorder, in particular the underlying biological reactions. Thus, one could attempt to normalize the metabolic steps involved in BE by direct corrective measures.

One does not treat cerebral edema caused by anemia, reduction of cardiac output, or dysfunction of the lung by measures of dehydration, because unfavorable effects would be obtained. These forms of BE are successfully treated by correction of the basic disturbances.

The treatment of BE is divided into basic etiological and symptomatic measures. At present, the causal therapeutic methods are quite limited. They consist mainly in the treatment of pathological states and conditions causing edema, *e.g.*, in surgical methods of pressure release, cardiac and circulatory management and anti-inflammatory methods as well as prevention of further development of edema. The main methods, however, are still symptomatic ones.

General Treatment of Cerebral Edema

The basis of the therapeutic schedule has to be an elastic one, in order to adapt itself to the complex conditions of metabolism and edema formation. It is based predominantly on experiences with traumatic edema and BE secondary to cerebral tumors.

The general treatment of BE can be divided into three main divisions: 1) acute measures and immediate interventions; 2) general treatment of BE; and 3) continuing maintenance.

According to the urgency we may distinguish: 1) reduction of energy metabolism by treatment against pain as well as by sedation and vegetative suppression, above all by interruption of the acute cerebral herniation and compression syndromes; 2) maintenance of oxygen-supply of brain tissue by keeping the respiratory passages free or by support of the respiration by artificial methods. This requires tracheotomy, intubation, prevention of aspiration and artificial respiration; an unconscious patient in the supine position is subject to obstruction of respiratory passages by tongue and secretion;

in those cases, the prone or lateral position should be adopted; 3) stabilization and regulation of the circulatory system by treatment of shock, regulation of the cardiac output, elimination of venous congestion and exclusion of additional noxae; 4) reduction of energy supply by lowering the basal metabolic rate (supercooling, vegetative suppression, e.g., 1-2 ml of a "lytic cocktail" every 2-4 hours for 12-24 hours); convulsions should be treated with intravenous administration of thiopentone; 5) stabilization of metabolic balance by regulation of the mineral, nitrogen and water metabolism by calculated administration of fluid, electrolytes and protein; furthermore, support of the circulatory and respiratory systems and of all other organ functions; 6) initial dehydration of BE and prevention of further progress in brain swelling by exact control and balancing of water and ion metabolism as well as by additional measures such as administration of drugs increasing vessel impermeability and dilatation.

Problems of Dehydration Therapy

Up to now only the removal of water entering the brain tissue at the time of the break-down of the barrier was attempted. This dehydration therapy is based on the concept of removing the pathological surplus of fluid in cerebral tissue by changing the osmotic balance (cf. Rosomoff, 1961). Cerebral swelling or edema, however, appears to be more a disorder of water distribution than merely surplus. As long as we do not know the basic mechanisms involved, the initial dehydration of the brain is justified as a vital measure. Any further dehydration without control of water and ion metabolism, however, is dangerous.

The obviously contradictory reports on success and failure in BE therapy by application of hypertonic solutions, drugs sealing the BBB and therefore decreasing vessel permeability, diuretics and tonics for the circulatory system show that all these agents only have a positive effect when being applied at the moment when they act as a real substitution in a distinct stage of the pathophysiological reactions of BE.

If dehydration therapy of BE is indicated, it should be carried out as early as possible. There are several methods. 1) Osmotherapy, using intravenous administration of hypertonic solutions based on a dehydrating effect by osmotically withdrawing water from the brain. The electron microscopically proved effect is predominantly restricted to cerebral cortex, but even there, only slight effects are often to be seen (Struck and Umbach, 1964, Nemecek-Gansler, et al., 1964). Moreover, several of these solutions have severe and undesirable side effects. Infusions of 300-400 ml of 33% dextrose solution or 40-80 ml of 40% laevulose solutions are still sometimes given. Good results were reported after administration of hypertonic sorbitol and mannitol solutions (Hemmer, 1961). Another useful measure, though not dramatic in its effects, is administration of human albumin in doses up to 100 ml.

Among all dehydrating substances only hypertonic urea solutions, freshly prepared and given intravenously, have met our clinical demands, providing a comparatively safe method for clinicians to reduce intracranial swelling (Javid and Settlage, 1956). As shown by recent experimental data, this efficiency is considered to be based on dehydration of the intact brain tissue, whereas withdrawal of water and electrolytes from the edematous tissue may happen later on and in a comparatively moderate extent (Clasen, et al., 1965, Pappius and Dayes, 1965). Swelling of astrocytes as an important morphological substrate of BE in the gray matter is not influenced or only slightly influenced by urea (Levy, et al., 1965). Decrease of CSF pressure seen after intravenous administration of hypertonic urea does not necessarily reflect a decrease in cerebral edema but also can be caused by extraction of fluid from intact parts of the brain. The prompt and significant reduction of augmented brain volume in intracranial hypertension, however, provides an urgent and life-saving intervention. Hypertonic urea, usually given as 30% urea-invert sugar solutions in slow infusion (dosage 1-1.5 g/kg body weight) is indicated for preoperative cerebral decompression and for prevention and interruption of acute shifting and incarceration syndromes. Since the use of intravenous hypertonic urea to shrink the brain in neurological procedures has recently become commonplace, and since this method is also being used to treat certain non-surgical neurological conditions, it should be emphasized again that its administration is not entirely harmless, because of the known rebound effect with excessive excretion of fluid and electrolytes. In severe intracranial hemorrhages urea application is dangerous, too. The use of intravenous hypertonic urea therefore requires highest caution by the clinical therapist.

Among diuretics, preference is given to those drugs which provide increased water and sodium excretion. This holds for the group of carbonic anhydrase inhibitors (so-called saluretica). As electrolyte imbalance, primarily sodium retention, is considered to be of basic importance for the development of cerebral swelling, one could speak of a physiological correction, if those substances directly influenced the sodium/potassium transport and balance mechanisms. Their effect is, however, primarily restricted to a reduction of the extracellular sodium surplus. It is considered to be based above all upon the partially outdated "extracellular" concept of BE. French authors, therefore, recommended diuretics to be used in the treatment of cerebral swelling secondary to hypertonia (cf. Lazorthes and Campan, 1963). Personally, we still often use "Esidrex" or "Esidrex K" (50 mg 2-3 times daily) or "Chlotride" (500 mg 1-2 times daily), alternating with "Diamox" (250 mg 1-2 times a day), each in series of about four days. A good initial dehydration effect by water and sodium diuresis, almost comparable to hypertonic urea was reported after administration of "Lasix" (40 mg) which we could confirm from personal experience. Its protracted administration, however, is followed by undesirable electrolyte imbalances (Kramer, 1964). Like "Esidrex" and "Chlotride," it may lead to hypokalemic alkalosis by excessive potassium diuresis, whereas administration of "Diamox" is combined with hypochloremic acidosis. Loss of potassium can be reduced by use of spironolactone (aldosterone antagonist), the dehydrating effect of which to the brain itself seems to be without significance.

Principally any dehydration treatment of BE has to follow the schedule of equilibrated metabolic balance. We, therefore, should intervene only in order to correct those imbalances which can be assumed immediately following acute cranio-cerebral injuries consisting of an intracrebral increase of water and sodium secondary to various physical and biochemical changes. In those instances, among other corrective procedures, an initial dehydration often will be necessary. It may lead, however, to a decrease of excretion of water and electrolytes as volume regulation after withdrawal of fluid. Its determination results from routine calculations of water and ion metabolism — ionogram, haematrocrit, fluid balance, alkali reserve, non-protein nitrogen, and blood sugar, as well as from dermal turgor and clinical picture. The extent of further fluid and electrolyte supply by infusion will depend on these data. In equilibrated balances dehydration therapy will not be necessary. Its further application only should be restricted for finer corrections of this equilibrium.

As Jefferson (1951) stressed years ago, the days are over when dehydration was a routine measure in the treatment of BE. From our knowledge of disturbances of water and ion metabolism, a serious warning must be uttered against any blind, rule-of-thumb administration of dehydrating substances. Any physico-chemically induced withdrawal of fluid and electrolytes has to be based on a stable and compensated circulatory system. Dehydration therapy in each individual case has to be controlled and regulated following the schedule of equilibrated metabolic balances. Any indiscriminate use of such methods involves the risk of setting up undesirable counter-regulatory mechanisms. Moreover, in cases of circulatory and/or renal dysfunction, they even may place a severe load on the organism as a whole.

Administration of corticosteroids and ACTH is still an eagerly discussed point in BE therapy. Their short-time application is considered to prevent intracellular water and potassium retention in cerebral tissue. They are recommended after hypophysectomy and for preparing neurosurgical intervention in malignant gliomas and metastases (B. Weill). These effects were supported by encouraging results in certain experimental edema models (Taylor, et al., 1965), whereas Facon and Schwartz (1964) reported fairly good effects of corticosteroid treatment of BE following cerebro-vascular accidents. We are still very cautious in using corticosteroids in edema therapy, as they may lead to water and sodium retention, which are believed to augment edema formation. After prolonged administration of corticosteroids, even pseudotumoral cerebral swelling may develop (Walker and Adamkiewicz, 1964).

Possibilities of Causal Treatment

From our present knowledge of causes and basic conditions of BE, we must say that etiologically-based measures of therapy are very scarce. Indications for an etiologically-based edema treatment may appear, for instance, from the reduction of fluid and sodium from brain tissue after application of "Complamin" in experimental traumatic cerebral swelling. Its effect on the pathophysiological process of BE probably depends more on an activation of the disturbed energy dependent active transport of cations than on an increase of the cerebral circulation or diuresis. This effect is probably caused by the active component of nicotinic acid which is introduced into hydrogen transferring pyridine-nucleotides (Reulen, et al., 1964). Any further development of causal treatment of BE, therefore, is connected with the elucidation of the etiological and pathophysiological backgrounds and mechanisms of cerebral swelling.

Despite the great variety of therapeutic measures available, there is still no satisfactory causal therapy of BE, once the fateful chain reaction has become manifest. The need for effective prevention of cerebral edema is therefore all the more essential.

Prophylactic Measures

A successful prophylaxis of BE can be expected only from rapid and immediate elimination of the most relevant causal factors and their insidious effects on the central nervous system.

Prophylaxis of cerebral edema is based upon: 1) assurance of sufficient oxygen supply to the brain by providing for optimal respiration and eliminating respiratory disorders; 2) control of heart and circulatory functions; 3) control of water and electrolyte metabolism; 4) prevention of metabolic and enzymatic disturbances of the energy-dependent water- and ion transport functions of the CNS. Simply put, prevention of cerebral edema still must be regarded as the best therapy.

FINAL REMARKS

To talk about the importance of BE as a neurological problem is like adding water to a swollen brain. Here, only some major problems were pointed out which appear of utmost importance for clinical and practical medicine. Today we are able to treat increase of brain volume successfully up to certain stages of its development, since we know something about its nature and course. Moreover, we are acquainted with symptoms that may announce the onset of cerebral edema and its dangerous development associated with increase of intracranial pressure. The danger that medical help is too late may occur, however, when the clinical syndrome of BE is already well advanced, when the brain is more or less saturated with fluid or irreversible imbalances of water and ion transport are manifest. Sometimes this occurs within a very short period and leads to severe, even irreparable, damage of the CNS and to death.

The actual task of theoretical and practical medicine as well as of basic sciences is, therefore, to elucidate those links of the pathogenic chain of processes responsible for the formation of BE and to clarify its causes and underlying processes. Only then will we be able to attempt corrections of the pathological processes with all available measures. We hope that the knowledge gained at this workshop will give an important and valuable contribution to this aim and will permit us a certain optimism with regard to the solution of the neurological and general medical and scientific problems of cerebral swelling and edema.

TRADE AND GENERIC OR CHEMICAL NAMES OF DRUGS AND MANUFACTURERS

Chlotride	(MERCK, SHARP & DOME) — 6-chlor-7-sulfanyl-1,2,4-benzothiadizin-1,1-dioxide
Complamin	(WÜLFING, Düsseldorf) — 7-(2-hydroxy-3-(N-2-hydroxy-ethyl-N-methylamino)propyl)-1,3-dimethylxanthin-pyridin-3-carboxylate
Diamox	Azetazolamide (LEDERLE)
Esidrex	(CIBA) — 6-chloro-7-sulfanyl-3,4-dihydro-1,2,4-benzo-thiadizin-1-1-dioxide
Lasix	(HOECHST) — Furosemide

REFERENCES

Aleu, F. P., F. H. Edelman, R. Katzman and H. C. Scheinberg: Ultrastructural and biochemical analysis in cerebral edema associated with experimental mouse glioma, J. Neuropath. Exp. Neurol., 23, 253-263 (1964).

_____, R. Katzman and R. T. Terry: Fine structure and electrolyte analysis of cerebral edema induced by alkyl tin intoxication, Ibid., 22, 403-413 (1963).

Anton, G.: Gehirnödem, in: Hdb. path. Anat. d. Nervensystems, Vol. I. Berlin: Springer, pp. 396-467 (1904).

Bakay, L.: Morphological and chemical studies in cerebral edema: Triethyl tin-induced edema, J. Neurol. Sci., 2, 52-67 (1965).

_____ and H. H. Bendixen: Central nervous system vulnerability in hypoxic states: Isotope uptake studies, in: Selective Vulnerability of the Central Nervous System in Hypoxaemia (ed. by W. H. McMenemy and J. F. Schadé). Oxford: Blackwell, pp. 63-78 (1963).

_____ and I. Haque: Morphological and chemical studies in cerebral edema, I: Cold induced edema, J. Neuropath. Exp. Neurol., 23, 393-418 (1964).

Broman, T. and O. Steinwall: Model of the blood-brain barrier system, Proc. Symp. on Brain Edema. (ed. by I. Klatzo and F. Seitelberger). Springer-Verlag New York (1967).

Cervos-Navarro, J.: Elektronenmikroskopische Befunde an den Capillaren des Kaninchengehirns nach der Einwirkung ionisierender Strahlen, Arch. Psychiat. Z. Neur., 205, 204-222 (1964).

_____: Die Bedeutung der Elektronenmikroskopie für die Lehre vom Stoffaustausch zwischen dem Zentralnervensystem und dem übrigen Körper, Dtsch. Z. Nervenheilk., 186, 209-237 (1964).

Clasen, R. A., P. M. Cook, S. Pandolfi, G. Carnecki and G. Bryar: Hypertonic urea in experimental cerebral edema, Arch. Neurol. (Chicago) 12, 424-434 (1965).

Cumings, J. N.: Soluble cerebral proteins in normal and oedematous brain, J. Clin. Path., 14, 289-294 (1961).

Facon, E. and B. Schwartz: Le traitement hormonal de l'oedème cérébral dans les accidents cérébro-vasculaires, Presse méd., 72, 2377-2379 (1964).

Feigin, I. and N. Popoff: Neuropathological changes late in cerebral edema: The relationship to trauma, hypertensive disease, and Binswanger's encephalopathy, J. Neuropath. Exp. Neurol, 22, 500-511 (1963).

Gänshirt, H.: Die Sauerstoffversorgung des Gehirns und ihre Störung bei der Liquordrucksteigerung und beim Hirnödem. Berlin-Göttingen-Heidelberg: Springer (1957).

Gonatas, N. K., H. M. Zimmerman and S. Levine: Ultrastructure of inflammations with edema in the rat brain, Amer. J. Path., 42, 455-469 (1963).
Hager, H.: Elektronenmikroskopische Untersuchungen über die Feinstruktur der Blutgefässe und perivaskulären Räume im Säugetierhirn, Acta Neuropath. (Berlin), 1, 9-33 (1961).
_____: Die feinere Cytologie und Cytopathologie des Nervensystems. Veröff. aus der morphol. Pathologie, H. 67, Stuttgart: G. Fischer (1964).
Hasenjäger, T. and H. Spatz: Über örtliche Veränderungen der Konfiguration des Gehirns bei Hirndruck, Arch. Psychiatr., 107, 193-222 (1938).
Hemmer, R.: Vergleichende Untersuchungen über medikamentöse Hirndrucksenkungen, Med. Klin., 56, 105-108 (1961).
Herschkowitz, N., B. B. MacGillivray and J. N. Cumings: Biochemical and electrophysiological studies in experimental cerebral edema, Brain, 88, 557-584 (1965).
Herzog, I., N. A. Levy and R. P. Scheinberg: Biochemical and morphological studies on cerebral edema associated with intracerebral tumors in rabbits, J. Neuropath. Exp. Neurol., 24, 244-255 (1965).
Hoff, H. and K. Jellinger: Das Hirnödem, Wien. Z. Nervenheilk, 19, 305-341 (1962).
_____ and _____: Cerebral Oedema, Ciba Symposium, 11, 64-72 (1963).
_____ and K. Pateisky: Die Dekompensation bei den Alterspsychosen und ihre Behandlung mit Diamox, Wien. klin. Wschr., 70, 571-575 (1958).
Javid, M. and P. Settlage: Effect of urea on cerebrospinal fluid pressure in human subjects, J. Amer. Med. Assn., 169, 943-949 (1956).
Jefferson, G.: The balance of life and death in cerebral lesions, Surg. Gyn. Obstetr., 93, 444 (1951).
Jellinger, K.: Protrahierte Formen der posttraumatischen Encephalopathie. Zur Morphologie und Pathogenese cerebraler Läsionen nach gedecktem Schädel-Hirntrauma mit langdauernden Komazuständen, Beitr. gerichtl. Med., 23, 65-118 (1965).
_____, F. Gerstenbrand and K. Pateisky: Die protrahierte Form der posttraumatischen Encephalopathie, Nervenarzt, 34, 145-159 (1963).
Katzman, R., F. Aleu and C. Wilson: Further observations on Triethyl-tin edema, Arch. Neurol., (Chicago), 9, 178-187 (1963).
Klatzo, I., A. Piraux and E. J. Laskowski: The relationship between edema, blood-brain barrier and tissue elements in a local brain injury, J. Neuropath. Exp. Neurol., 17, 548-564 (1958).

Kramer, G.: Zur medikamentösen Regulierung des Wasserhaushaltes beim Hirnödem, Med. Welt, 2238-2244 (1964).
Langfitt, T. W., J. D. Weinstein and N. F. Kassel: Cerebral vasomotor paralysis produced by intracranial hypertension, Trans. Amer. Neurol. Assn., 214-215 (1964).
Lazorthes, G. and L. Campan: L'oedème cérébral. Paris: Masson et Cie. (1963).
Lee, J. C. and L. Bakay: Ultrastructural changes in the edematous central nervous system, 1: Triethyltin edema, Arch. Neurol. (Chicago), 13, 48-57 (1965).
Levy, W. A., J. M. Taylor, I. Herzog and L. C. Scheinberg: The effect of hypertonic urea on cerebral edema in the rabbit induced by triethyl tin sulfate, Arch. Neurol. (Chicago), 13, 58-64 (1965).
Magee, P. N., H. B. Stoner and J. M. Barnes: Experimental production of oedema in the central nervous system of the rat by triethyltin compounds, J. Path. Bact., 73, 107-124 (1957).
Nemetschek-Gansler, H., F. Loew and H. R. Plogsties: Phasenkontrast und elektronenoptische Untersuchungen zur Wirkung des Harnstoffes auf das Gehirn, Acta Neurochir. (Wien), 11, 663-675 (1964).
Pappius, H. M. and D. R. Gulati: Water and electrolyte content of cerebral tissues in experimentally induced edema, Acta Neuropath. (Berlin), 2, 451-460 (1963).
_____ and L. A. Dayes: Hypertonic urea. Its effect on the distribution of water and electrolytes in normal and edematous brain tissues. Arch. Neurol. (Chicago), 13, 395-402 (1965).
Peters, G.: Die Veränderungen an Gehirn und Hirnhäuten bei chronischen traumatischen Störungen, Verh. dtsch. Ges. Path., 43, 103-120 (1959).
_____ and H. Selbach: Über die Neutralisationsfähigkeit des Hirngewebes und ihre Beziehung zu den histopathologischen Vorgängen nach experimentellen Hirncontusionen, Arch. Psychiatr., 116, 531 (1943).
Raimondi, A. J., J. P. Evans and S. Mullan: Studies of cerebral edema. III. Alterations in the white matter, Acta Neuropath. (Berlin), 2, 177-197 (1962).
Reichardt, M.: Zur Entstehung des Hirndrucks, Dtsch. Z. Nervenheilk, 28, 306-355 (1905).
_____: Das Hirnödem, Anhang: Die Hirnschwellung, in: Hdb. spez. path. Anat. Histol., Vol. XIII/1B. Berlin-Göttingen-Heidelberg: Springer (1957).
Reulen, H. J., H. F. Hofmann and A. Baethmann: Die Beeinflussung des experimentellen traumatischen Hirnödems bei der Ratte mit einer Nicotinsäuretheophyllin-Verbindung, Zschr. ges. exp. Med. 138, 246-256 (1964).

Riessner, D. and K. J. Zülch: Über die Formveränderungen des Gehirns bei raumfordernden Prozessen, Dtsch. Zschr. Chir., 25: 1-61 (1940).

Rosenhagen, H.: Encephalographie bei hirnatrophischen Prozessen nach gedeckten Schädelhirnverletzungen, in: Das Hirntrauma (ed. by E. Rehwald). Stuttgart: G. Thieme (1956).

Rosomoff, H. L.: Distribution of intracranial contents after hypertonic urea, J. Neurosurg., 19, 859-864 (1962).

_____: Effect of hypothermia and hypertonic urea on distribution of intracranial contents, Ibid., 18, 753-759 (1961).

_____ and F. T. Zugibe: Distribution of intracranial contents in experimental edema, Arch. Neurol. (Chicago), 9, 26-34 (1963).

Selbach, H.: Physikalisch-chemische Untersuchungen zur Frage der Hirnvolumenvermehrung, Arch. Psychiatr., 112, 409-440 (1940).

Scheinker, I. M.: Histopathologie von Ödem und Schwellung bei Hirı geschwülsten, Dtsch. Z. Nervenheilk, 147, 137-262 (1938).

Schröder, J. M. and W. Wechsler: Ödem und Nekrose in der grauen und weissen Substanz beim experimentellen Hirntrauma, Acta Neuropath (Berlin).

Spatz, H. and G. J. Stroescu: Zur Anatomie und Pathologie der äusseren Liquorräume des Gehirns, Nervenarzt, 7, 425-437, 481-498 (1934).

Struck, G. and W. Umbach: Vergleichende elektronenoptische Untersuchungen an der menschlichen Hirnrinde vor und nach Ödemtherapie, Virchows Arch. path. Anat., 337, 317-327 (1964).

_____ and _____: Das elektronenmikroskopische Bild in Rinde und Mark beim gleichen Patienten vor und nach Dehydrierung, Neurochir. (Stuttgart), 7, 64-77 (1964).

Tani, E. and J. P. Evans: Electron microscopic studies of cerebral swelling, I: Studies of the permeability of brain capillaries, Acta Neuropath. (Berlin), 4, 507-526 (1965).

_____ and _____: Electron microscopic studies of cerebral swelling, II: Alterations of myelinated nerve fibers, Ibid., 604-623 (1965).

_____ and _____: Electron microscopic studies of cerebral swelling, III: Alterations in the neuroglia and the blood vessels of the white matter, Ibid., 624-639 (1965).

Taylor, Y. M., W. A. Levy, I. Herzog and L. C. Scheinberg: Prevention of experimental cerebral edema by corticosteroids, Neurology (Minnesota), 15, 667-674 (1965).

Thompson, R. K. and S. Malina: Dynamic axial brain-stem distortion as a mechanism explaining the cardio-respiratory changes in increased intracranial pressure, J. Neurosurg., 16, 664-674 (1959).

Torack, R. M., R. D. Terry, and H. M. Zimmerman: The fine structure of cerebral fluid accumulation, I: Swelling secondary to cold injury, Amer. J. Path., 35, 1135-1147 (1959).

_____, _____ and _____: The fine structure of cerebral fluid accumulation, II: Swelling produced by triethyltin poisoning and its comparison with that in the human brain, Ibid., 36, 273-287 (1960).

Ule, G., W. Döhner and E. Bues: Ausgedehnte Hemisphärenmarkschädigung nach gedecktem Hirntrauma mit apallischem Syndrom und partieller Spätrehabilitation, Arch. Psychiatr. Z. Neur., 202, 155-176 (1961).

_____ and F. W. Kolkmann: Zur Ultrastruktur des perifokalen und histotoxischen Hirnödems bei der Ratte, Acta Neuropath. (Berlin), 1, 519-526 (1962).

Walker, E. A. and J. J. Adamkiewicz: Pseudotumor cerebri associated with prolonged corticosteroid therapy, J. Amer. Med. Assn. 188, 779-784 (1964).

A. EARL WALKER

BRAIN EDEMA AS A NEUROLOGICAL PROBLEM—II

Brain edema resulting from local involvement as the result of trauma, surgical procedures, vascular accidents, tumors or inflammation of the brain has been recognized for some time. It is not quite so well appreciated that cerebral edema occurs from generalized systemic disorders, one of which follows the discontinuance of cortico-steroid therapy in children. Patients who have been treated for nephrosis, asthma, eczema, etc., for some period of time, upon the elimination or decrease in cortico-steroid therapy may develop within a few days or weeks, headaches, vomiting, diplopia, drowsiness and/or stupor. The primary condition for which the steroid was administered does not seem to be a significant or determining factor, although the majority of the reported cases suffered from the chronic afflictions mentioned above. Males seem to be involved more frequently than females, but the difference does not attain statistical significance at even a 5% level. The age of such patients between five and ten is about the same for both sexes, but the condition is rarely, if ever, found in adults, in which pseudotumor syndromes from other causes are much more commonly seen.

The clinical history and findings are quite similar in all cases. The patient has been treated with cortico-steroids, the most popular being prednisone and triamcinolone, for some months or even longer, in the cases reported for an average of $2\frac{1}{2}$ years. Often as a result of this therapy, the patient has developed some signs of Cushing's syndrome: moon-face, obesity, abdominal stria, osteoporosis, etc., and may be stunted in growth. Within days or weeks after a change in the dosage or type of steroid, sometimes associated with an intercurrent infection, the patient complains of headache often accompanied by vomiting, diplopia due to paresis of the sixth cranial nerve and occasionally drowsiness or stupor. Examination of the eye grounds in practically all cases reveals a bilateral low grade papillodema usually without hemorrhages. The remainder of the neurological examination is normal. The electroencephalograms are abnormal by reason of generalized slow waves and diffuse or focal spikes. Roentgengrams of the skull usually show a diastasis of the cranial sutures. In pneumoencephalograms, however, the ventricles are normal in position and size or somewhat small. The spinal fluid pressure is usually increased but may be within normal limits. The total protein of the spinal fluid is normal as are the other chemical constituents.

The pathogenesis of the condition is not known. In practically all cases the syndrome developed as the steroid therapy was modified by a decrease in quantity or a change to another compound. In the few cases in which 17 ketosteroids have been examined, they have been found to be subnormal, suggesting a suppression of adrenal activity. Since the syndrome developed after or during treatment with several steroid preparations, it seems that the condition is not caused by a specific factor, but the more general effect of adrenal suppression. Possibly vitamin A metabolism may be impaired so that its degradation products increase. It is known that vitamin A intoxication can produce a pseudotumor syndrome. Whatever the mechanism, it does seem that an edema of the brain develops as may be demonstrated in pneumoencephalograms by the small ventricular system. However, the amount of water retained is relatively small, probably not more than 25 or 30 cc's if calculations upon the relative volumes of the brain and intracranial cavity are reliable.

The treatment of the condition at present is largely empirical. Temporarily increasing the cortico-steroid therapy and then slowly reducing it to levels just sufficient to control the primary disturbance usually has relieved the pseudotumor syndrome. Whether diagnostic and repeated spinal punctures are of value is difficult to determine. For patients who run a more fulminating course and are seen in stupor or coma, the use of urea or manitol in addition to cortico-steroid therapy may be advisable to improve immediately the condition and decrease the intracranial pressure.

REFERENCE

Walker, A. E. and J. J. Adamkiewicz: Pseudotumor cerebri associated with prolonged corticosteroid therapy, J. A. M. A., 188, 779-784 (June 1, 1964).

W. F. CAVENESS

BRAIN EDEMA AS A NEUROLOGICAL PROBLEM—III

Professor Hoff has presented the clinical effects of cerebral edema from various causes. I will augment his comments regarding trauma as an etiological factor. We may begin by reminding ourselves of the forces at play in head injury.

When the head is struck, the brain, in its semirigid, uneven housing, is subjected to varying degrees of acceleration, deceleration, rotation, compression, expansion, and swirling motions about its attachments. As a result, there may be diffuse neuronal injury, contusion, laceration, or all three. When the dura is penetrated, brain structure can be ruptured by indriven bone fragments or the agent of injury. If the agent is a missile traveling at high velocity, radial force is added to the direct trauma. As major vessels are torn, ventricles traversed, or the brain stem encroached upon, the gravity and complexity of the injury is accentuated.

Following the impact, and depending roughly on the site and extent of the injury, secondary physical and biochemical changes, local or general, extend the brain damage. The more apparent changes include brain anoxia, swelling, stasis, change in pH, and electrolytic imbalance. These may be augmented by subsequent hemorrhage or sepsis. General changes in respiration, circulation, endocrine function, and temperature can take place from impaired regulatory centers and wound products. Concurrent injuries elsewhere in the body can add to these adverse influences.

From the preceding, it is apparent that brain swelling, or edema, may be only a part of a very complex picture. In an attempt to sort out the clinical reflection of this aspect of the reaction to injury, three cases will be presented.

Case #1: A 32-year old male was thrown from an overturned

horse-drawn carriage. There was nothing to indicate a head injury other than road dirt in his hair. Within half an hour he became listless and vomited. An X-ray at a provincial hospital indicated a 6 cm linear fracture of the right parietal bone extending toward the base. Within two hours he was somnolent but occasionally restless. The right pupil was larger than the left but both reacted to light. It was decided to transfer him to a municipal neurosurgical unit, a six-hour trip by ambulance. En route he was allowed to remain on his back with little attention to maintaining a free airway. Upon arrival, the patient was comatose, both pupils were dilated and fixed, breathing was irregular and gasping in type. Pulse ranged between 60 and 50 per minute. Blood pressure was 160/80. Within the hour, there was decompensation, with a precipitous elevation in pulse, drop in blood pressure, and prolonged interruptions in respiration. He expired fourteen hours after injury.

Post-mortem examination revealed, grossly, a swollen brain with flattened gyri and obliterated sulci, small ventricles, and herniations at the incisura and the foramen magnum. This case exemplifies two points. In closed head injuries, with generalized edema, the signs and symptoms reflect the increasing intracranial pressure with the trapping of the third cranial nerve and local compression of the diencephalon by the herniation of the medial aspects of the temporal lobe (or lobes) through the tentorium, and the compression of medullary structures by the herniation of the cerebellar tonsils through the foramen magnum. The second point is the influence of an impaired airway on brain edema. An unconscious patient in the supine position is subject to obstruction of respiratory passages by the tongue and secretions. Whatever the role of anoxia <u>per se</u> on brain edema, it is clear from clinical experience that an injured brain swells alarmingly with oxygen deprivation. Further, impairment of regulatory centers, through medullary compression, accentuates the difficulty.

Case #2: A 21-year-old U. S. Marine in the Korean conflict was struck by a fragment of an exploding landmine. The missile entered the left malar region, traversed the orbit, and lodged in the tip of the left frontal lobe. There was no loss in consciousness. Three hours after injury he was transferred by helicopter to the hospital ship. Alert and oriented, the patient recalled precise details of the accident. The right foot was partially amputated by the explosion, and there were generalized hyperactive deep tendon reflexes. Seven and one-half hours after injury he became profane and combative. Craniotomy, eight hours after injury, revealed local swelling around fragments of metal and bone in the anterior portion of the left frontal lobe. With a wedge resection, 25% of the lobe was removed, in a manner that permitted complete pial cover of the external surface of the resected area, and closure effected in layers. Recovery was prompt. Two days after injury the patient was alert and rational, with no neurological deficit and no apparent defect in mental function.

Comment: This illustrates limited edema developing around a focal injury. It is of interest that the clinical expression, irrational and explosive behavior, came on with abruptness seven and one-half hours after injury. After removal of the foreign bodies and surrounding neural tissue, there were no further symptoms. Such behavioral changes, transient, are not uncommon after lesions in the frontal or temporal lobes.

Case #3: A 21-year-old U. S. Marine received a tangential wound of the scalp in the left temporal region from schrapnel. Immediately unconscious, within thirty minutes the patient was irritable and writhing. The pulse was forceful, irregular at about 60 per minute. Blood pressure, 160/80. The left pupil was 4 mm, the right 2 mm. All limbs were in decerebrate posture. Deep tendon reflexes were hyperactive throughout with clonus at the ankles. Plantar response was flexion, bilaterally. There were occasional rhythmic movements in the right face. A burr hole was made in the left temporal bone. When the dura was opened, a large subdural clot was evacuated, following which the brain was seen to be pulsating. A similar finding followed trephination of the left parietal bone. Additional burr holes were placed in the left occipital and the right temporal and occipital areas without evidence of other hemorrhage. Two days after injury, the patient was semicomatose, with almost continuous right facial seizures. Other signs were unchanged. Within eight days he had become more responsive. Twenty-one days after injury, he was able to feed himself and walk about the ward. He had difficulty with speech, a right homonomous visual field defect, and cortical sensory loss on the right side of the body. Hyperreflexia and plantar flexion persisted on the left. A pneumoencephalogram fifty-four days after injury showed a dilated ventricle on the left, without shift.

Comment: In this case, the brain damage may be attributed to the lateral force of the high velocity missile, the rapid compression from the subdural hematoma, and the brain swelling from the latter. Under these circumstances, it is probable that the swelling was greater in the white than in the grey matter. Of especial clinical interest is the slow time course of partial recovery, even though the hematoma was removed within an hour of injury.

Therapeutic efforts consist of supportive measures, including the maintenance of an adequate airway and gas exchange, attention to fluid and electrolyte balance, nutrition, and, where indicated, skilled surgical repair. Steroids and hypothermia are thought to be of value in retardation of developing edema, and urea and mannitol are often effective in the reduction of brain volume. While these methods represent improved understanding over the past two decades, the enigma that remains and the area in which the next advance must be made is that of the processes that take place after the moment of impact. What are the fundamental functional and/or structural alterations? Is one of these loss in membrane transport energy? If so, how is this brought about? How can the continuing destruction of neurons, glia, and blood vessels be reversed? Those things that you will discuss at this symposium are at the heart of the matter and will be attended by clinicians with the greatest of interest.

SHOZO ISHII
HIROSHI TSUJI
KAZUE OZAWA
YUSHI KONDO
JOSEPH P. EVANS

BRAIN EDEMA

*SOME CLINICAL AND EXPERIMENTAL CORRELATIONS**

INTRODUCTION

When the neurological surgeon has occasion to expose the brain in the presence of increased intracranial pressure, he indeed opens a Pandora's box. Cushing in his Cameron Lectures of 1925 succinctly summarized his understanding of the problems of cerebrospinal fluid circulation as he and his contemporaries faced them (1). In the intervening forty years, particularly with the advent of more elaborate physiological recording techniques, with the development of experimental models simulating clinical conditions, and with the introduction of the electron microscope, a fuller, though even yet an incomplete, understanding of pressure problems has evolved.

The individual responses and various interactions of the four intracranial elements participating in intracranial pressure variations have now been extensively studied. These elements are: the brain substance itself, the circulating blood volume at any particular moment, the cerebrospinal fluid with reference both to its volume and to its circulation, and the nature, variability in size, and

*Aided in part by a grant from the U. S. Public Health Service, No. NB 04683-02, and in part by the Junior Auxiliary of the University of Chicago Cancer Research Foundation.

rate of formation of a particular lesion. At the time Cushing wrote his 1925 monograph, it was not appreciated that there were wide variations in intracranial pressure from those seen under the relatively normal circumstances of well conducted anesthesia to the wide fluctuations that may be seen in association with intracranial neoplasms. Nor was it fully appreciated that asymmetrical lesions, because of mechanical shifts through the various septal and bony openings of the intracranial cavity, were often of greater importance than elevations of intracranial pressure.

The first full-scale effort to understand alterations in intracranial pressure was carried out by Ryder and his associates and was reported in a series of papers (2, 3). Confirmation of the essential findings has since come from a number of laboratories (4, 5, 6). The Ryder formula, $V_{ic} = V_{br} + V_{bl} + V_{csf} + V_l$ expresses in simple terms the interrelationships of the four primary elements* (Fig. 1). Volume changes in brain substance, which occur particularly in the white matter, are of relatively slow development. Volume changes in the circulating blood are extremely rapid and may occur within fractions of a second. Volume changes in the cerebrospinal fluid may be relatively abrupt and measured in minutes, or may be extremely slow in their development, occuring over months and even years. The volume change of the lesion may be abrupt as that seen in the pulped, hemorrhagic brain following a gunshot wound or the slightly less abrupt development of a clot in extradural bleeding, and then ranging through the slow development of a relatively benign intracranial neoplasm to the possibly even slower development of hydrocephalus when the volume of the cerebrospinal fluid, increased by low grade obstruction, becomes of itself the volume of a lesion. The interactions among the elements in the formula may in themselves bring about very abrupt alterations because of the influence of one factor upon another. Thus, for example, the gradually expanding volume of a chronic subdural hematoma (V_l) may eventually produce alterations in V_{bl} which may be very abrupt, indeed, leading in some instances to a wholly unexpected denouement.

It is clear that if a reasonable understanding of these various factors is to be achieved, use must be made of an experimental model which can guarantee fairly reproducible results and which is subject to experimental control. The model, in order to have clinical applicability, should approximate closely a clinical situation. Such an experimental model has been developed by Ishii and his coworkers and has been a source of information that has helped to

*V_{ic} = Intracranial volume
V_{br} = Brain volume
V_{bl} = Blood volume
V_{csf} = Cerebrospinal fluid volume
V_l = Lesion volume

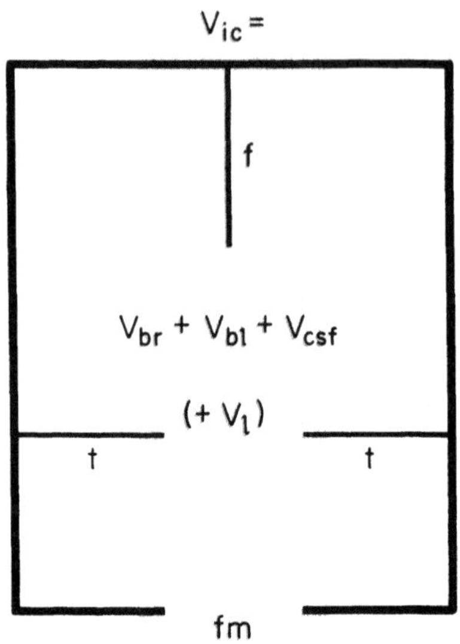

Fig. 1. The normal intracranial volume is made up of the volume of the brain (V_{br}), plus the volume of the circulating blood (V_{bl}) at any particular moment, plus the volume of cerebrospinal fluid (V_{csf}). To these volumes may be added the volume of a lesion (V_l). These three (or four) elements are contained in a "closed box," subdivided by partitions, the falx (f) and tentorium (t) within which subdivisions mechanical shifts of the cerebral elements may occur. The foramen magnum is indicated by "fm." Herniations may occur under the falx, through the tentorial opening and through the foramen magnum.

elucidate some of the problems with which the clinical neurosurgeon has to deal (7, 8, 9, 10, 11).

Attention must be drawn to the considerable confusion that has existed in relation to the term "brain edema." The present situation has been well summarized in this conference by Zülch (12) and elsewhere by his co-workers, Schröder and Wechsler (13). It is evident that the differentiation between brain swelling and brain edema has led to genuine semantic difficulty. The surgeon might wish to reserve the term "brain swelling" to denote any form of fullness of the brain which he notes during its exposure. Since, however, the term has already been appropriated by the neuropathologist, the neurosurgeon must coin a new phrase, such as "brain fullness," and then attempt to analyze it in terms of the Ryder formula.

The work to be reported here deals with observations designed to simulate experimentally the human condition of epidural hematoma with its accompanying alterations in the brain. From these experimental studies two sets of observations have evolved, each dealing primarily with one of the four factors in the Ryder equation. We shall first record some observations and conclusions related to changes in the intracranial blood volume (V_{bl}) and, secondly, report associated alterations in brain volume (V_{br}).

I. CIRCULATORY ALTERATIONS (i.e., Changes in V_{bl})

When a rubber balloon placed in the epidural space of a lightly anesthetized dog is slowly inflated by the addition of increments of .2 cc. of saline, an immediate response in intracranial pressure is noted, followed by an almost equally prompt return of the pressure towards normal. With successive increments of fluid, however, the baseline of pressure is gradually elevated, and when the intracranial pressure approximates 1200 mm. of water, the blood pressure begins to rise in order to ensure a sufficiency of circulation. If such an inflation is carried out slowly and over a period of only ten to fifteen minutes, deflation of the balloon may result in the return of the pressure to wholly normal limits. If, however, balloon inflation is maintained for a longer period of time and emptying of the balloon is delayed for thirty minutes, there occurs a fall, but shortly thereafter, over the next twenty to thirty minutes, one may observe a steadily rising baseline of pressure (Fig. 2).

If the critical compression is continued longer, e.g., for sixty to ninety minutes, the rebounding rise in intracranial pressure after the deflation is more marked and it appears within a shorter period (Fig. 3). The intracranial pressure sometimes assumes the pre-deflation level or rises even higher. Animals that have been subjected to this type of compression usually die within a couple of hours. It is this type of swelling, or "brain fullness," we believe, with which the neurosurgeon is confronted at operation when the brain suddenly and mercilessly starts marching out under pressure.

What is the nature of the mechanism underlying this form of acute cerebral swelling? As shown in Figure 4, when the secondary rise of intracranial pressure has developed, the therapeutic effect of dehydrating agents is not obvious. Even with repeated administration of hypertonic urea solution, the overall tendency to continuous rise of intracranial pressure cannot be aborted and only a transient fall is noted during and after each injection. The pressure then quickly returns to the original level or mounts even higher. Another interesting fact is that each injection of urea solution is associated with a marked increase in the amplitude of intracranial arterial pressure, suggesting a rapid expansion of the vascular bed to fill the space left by the withdrawal through osmotic action of the tissue fluids of

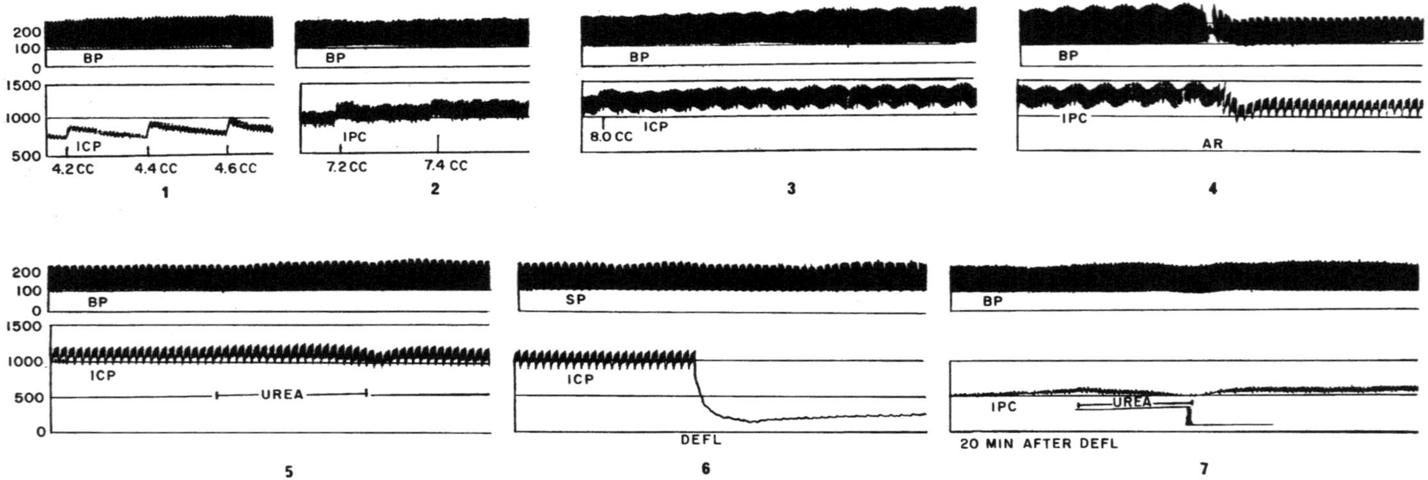

Fig. 2. Changes in blood pressure (BP) and intracranial pressure (ICP) during and after cerebral compression. In 1, in the early stages of balloon inflation, there is an immediate rise in intracranial pressure, followed by a prompt return. With further increments, as in 2, the tendency of ICP to return to normal following an increment becomes less obvious. In 3, after further compression, ICP continues to rise with the blood pressure. In 4, a moderate decrease in ICP and BP are seen after the initiation of controlled respiration (AR) and, in 5, after administration of a dehydrating agent. In 6, the balloon is deflated, and in 7, there is to be noted the secondary rise in ICP occurring twenty minutes after deflation.

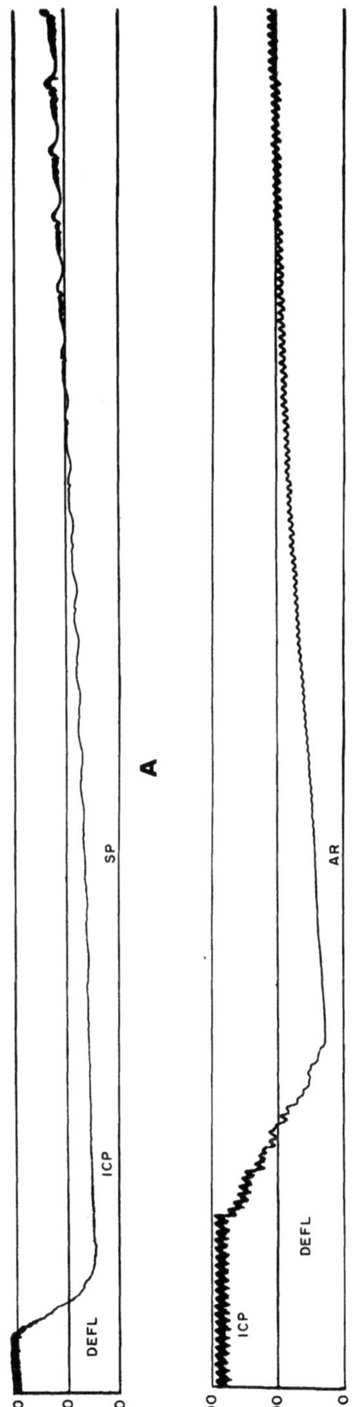

Fig. 3. Rebounding rise in intracranial pressure (ICP) after the deflation of the balloon. A. Spontaneous respiration. B. Controlled positive-negative respirations. The rebound is somewhat less in B.

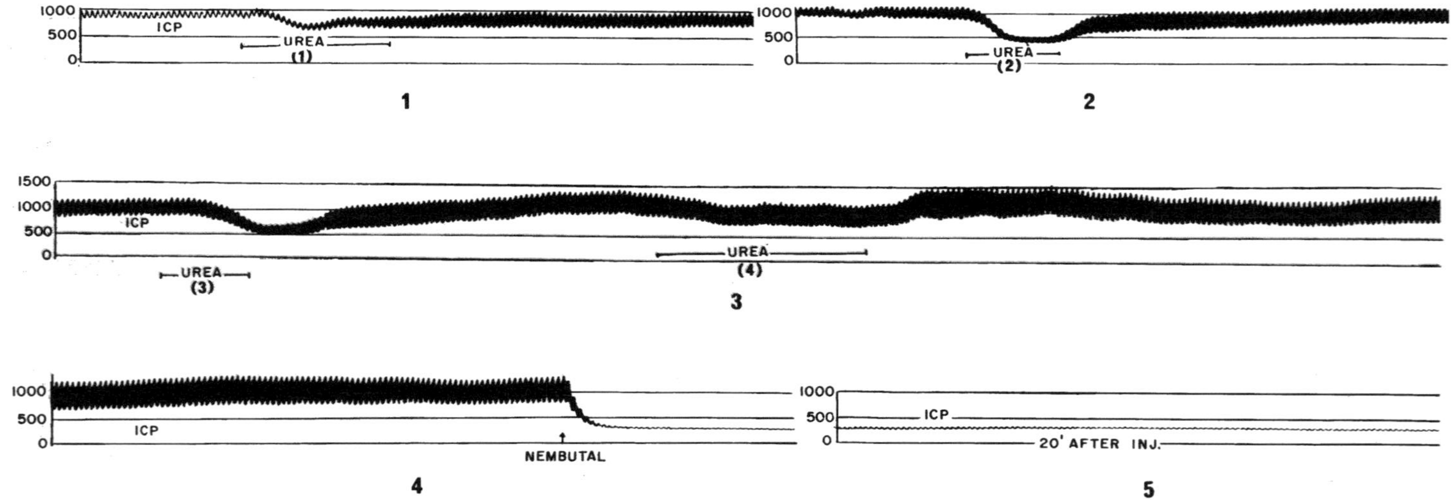

Fig. 4. The effects of hypertonic urea and of a barbiturate upon the elevated intracranial pressure (ICP) after the deflation of the balloon. One to 3 show only transient drop of ICP and marked increase in the amplitude of the cerebral arterial pulsation following each injection. Section 4 shows a rapid drop of ICP following the intravenous injection of Nembutal and Section 5 shows the persistent lowering of ICP twenty minutes after the injection.

of the brain. Langfitt has attributed this phenomenon to paralysis of vasomotor tone (14).

On the other hand, it was found that the administration of barbiturates caused a prolonged fall of intracranial pressure, even after acute swelling had fully developed. This response is indicated in the last tracing in Figure 4. It seems most unlikely that barbiturates could offset the vasomotor paralysis and consequent cerebral vascular distention; nor is the fall in intracranial pressure that is produced by barbiturates a mere reflection in the fall in systemic blood pressure. The lower row of Figure 5 demonstrates a typical Cushing effect, for when the intracranial pressure rises to a certain level after the deflation of the balloon, a progressive rise in systemic blood pressure is associated with marked slowing in the pulse rate. Administration of a barbiturate at this stage causes an immediate increase in the pulse rate and a normalization of blood pressure, which, though not depicted in this tracing, is associated with a fall in the intracranial pressure. This effect is clearly due to the anesthetic effect of the barbiturate on the vasopressor center.

The reduction in systemic blood pressure and the return to normal of the pulse rate that follow balloon deflation when compression has been but briefly maintained is, then, the result of removal of the pressure effect of the balloon upon the medullary vasopressor center (upper row, Fig. 5).

Thus, the mechanism of this form of acute brain swelling appears to be the following: If the extradural balloon is evacuated after a period of critical compression and at the point when cerebrovascular tonus has been seriously impaired, the intracranial pressure may at once return to a normal level. Soon, however, because of a sudden decrease in cerebrovascular resistance, blood flows into the intracranial cavity to fill the flaccid vascular tree, replacing space previously occupied by the balloon and thus causing some increase again in intracranial pressure. When the intracranial pressure rises to that sufficient to activate the vasopressor mechanism, the resultant increase in systemic blood pressure in turn augments the inflow of blood into the brain, raising the intracranial pressure again, thus leading to another vasomotor response. In this vicious cycle, intracranial pressure and blood pressure continue to rise together.

But why the impairment of vascular tone in the cerebral blood vessels? Wolff and Forbes (15), had found that pial arteries and veins, observed through a skull window, dilated when intracranial pressure was increased. Scheinker and one of us (JPE) (16), on histological grounds, following the lead of Reichardt (17) had sup-

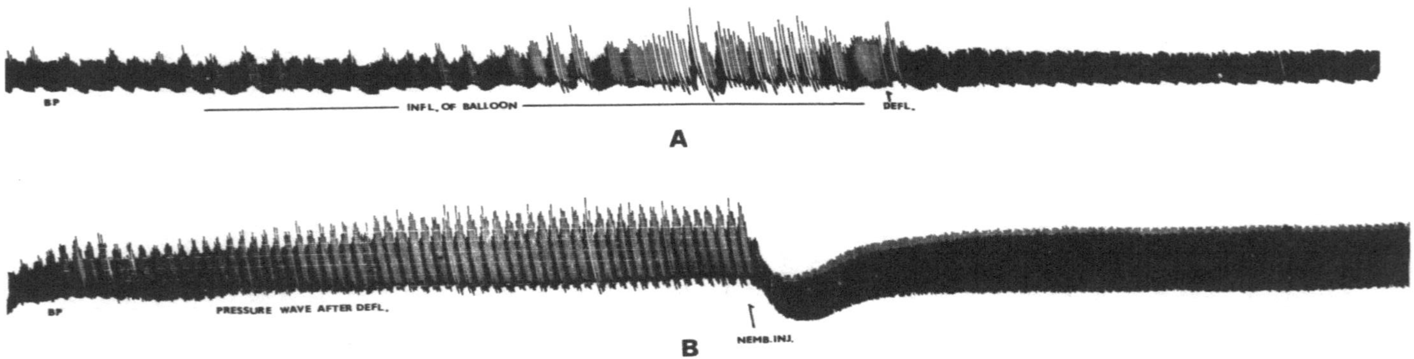

Fig. 5. Systemic blood pressure (BP) in intracranial hypertension. A. demonstrates BP changes during and after brief cerebral compression. B. demonstrates the blood pressure alterations occurring after the cessation of prolonged cerebral compression during the period of a rebounding rise in intracranial pressure up to 1200 mm. of water, the sharp drop following directly after the administration of a barbiturate. In both instances, the Cushing phenomenon is well-demonstrated, there being in addition to the arterial hypertension a high pulse pressure and a bradycardia. In A, immediate normalization of blood pressure and pulse rate follow the removal of the indirect pressure effect on the vasopressor center. In B, normalization follows the anesthetic action of the barbiturate upon the vasopressor center.

ported the concept of "vasoparalysis" as playing an important role in the clinical picture of patients who had suffered head injury. Langfitt also noted the development of vasomotor paralysis during his studies of experimental cerebral compression (14).

In an attempt to find a higher center of vasomotor control – one postulated by LeBeau (18) and sought futilely by one of us (JPE) in the frontal and temporal lobes nearly twenty years ago (19) – our present team has explored stereotactically the hypothalamus. Here, in the region of the dorsomedial nucleus (Fig. 6) has been found an

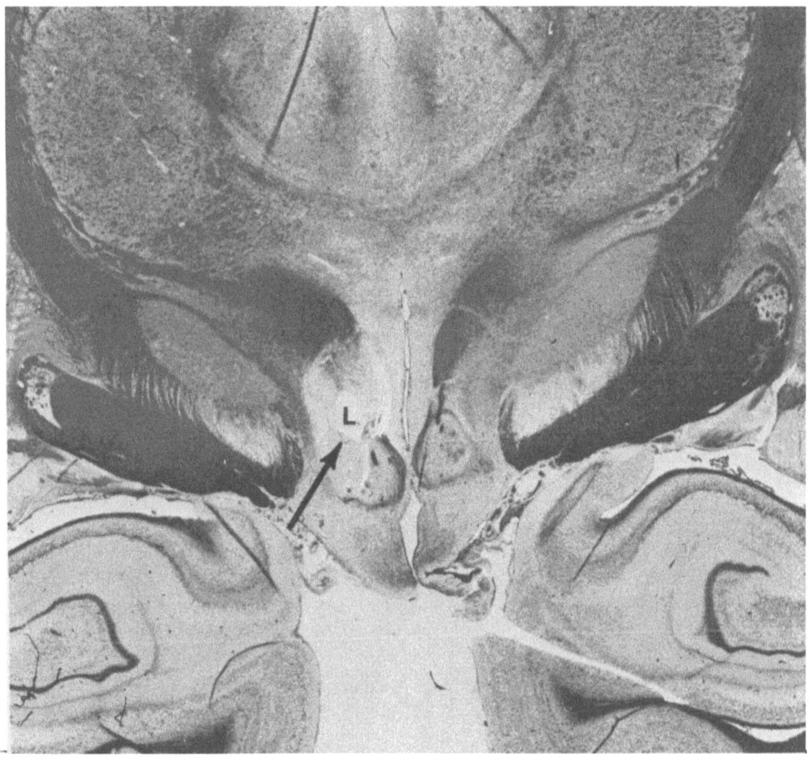

Fig. 6. L indicates the focus of the possible higher center of cerebral vasomotor control in the hypothalamus. The lesion (L) is in the dorsomedial nucleus rostral to the mammillary body (A 12.5, L 1.0, H +2).

isolated neural center which actively controls the cerebral vascular bed and the consequential change in the intracranial pressure (monkey).

As shown in Figure 7a, if this area of the hypothalamus is punctured with a needle, a considerable rise in intracranial pressure

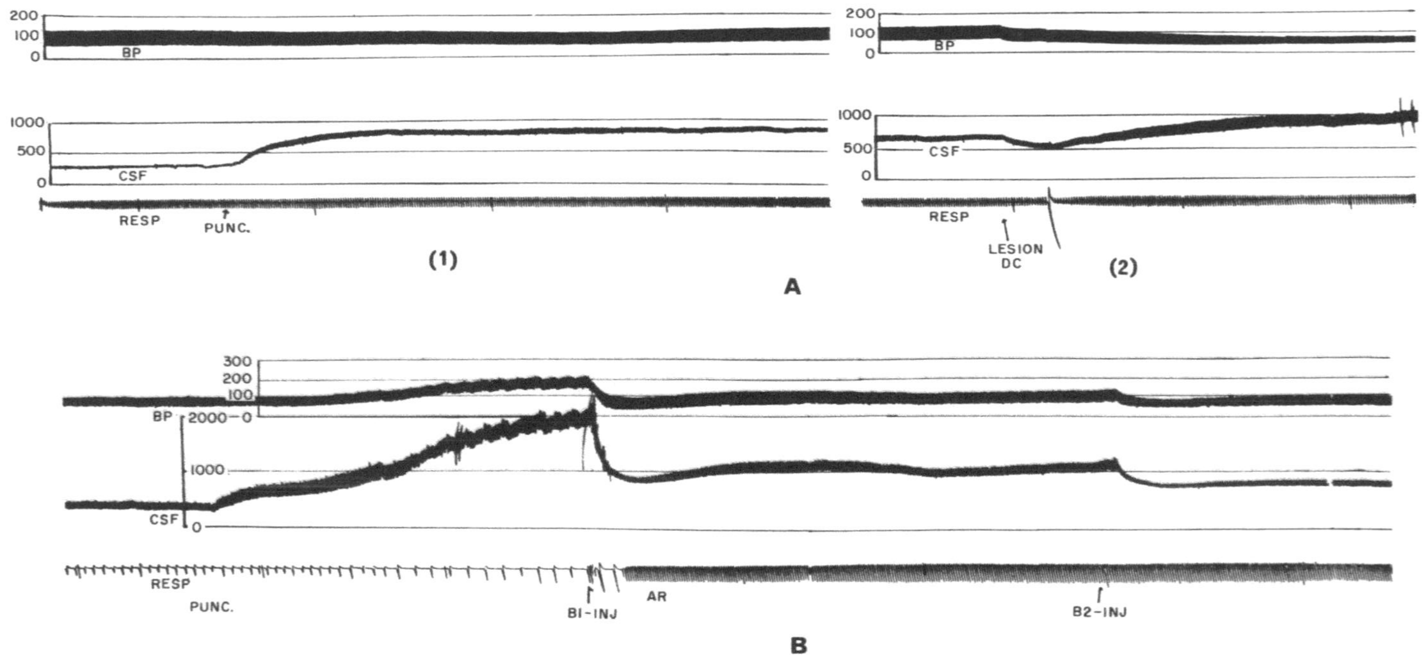

Fig. 7. A (1) and A (2) show the changes in blood pressure (BP), intracranial pressure (CSF) and respiration seen after puncture and coagulation of the hypothalamus respectively. Puncture (Punc.) in A (1) is followed by a striking rise in intracranial pressure unaccompanied by blood pressure change. A (2) shows a further rise in intracranial pressure after D.C. coagulation (D.C. Lesion). In B, as the intracranial pressure rises to approximate the diastolic blood pressure, the blood pressure is seen to increase, demonstrating the effect of rising intracranial pressure on the vasopressor threshold.

occurs. When a small lesion is produced by DC current at this point, a further increase in intracranial pressure results (Fig. 7B). Considering the rapidity of the pressure change together with the absence of increase in blood pressure, we can safely conclude that this neurally induced intracranial hypertension is due to expansion of the cerebral vascular bed. If the needle puncture in this area produces an increase in intracranial pressure high enough to reach the level of the vasomotor threshold, secondary increase in systemic pressure takes place, then the two pressures rise together, demonstrating the typical picture of acute brain swelling due to vascular engorgement. When two intermittent administrations of thiopental sodium are made at this stage, normalization of blood pressure and a considerable fall in intracranial pressure result (Fig. 7B). We assume that functional damage of this area may occur in response to mechanical distortion of the balloon or as a result of impaired blood supply to the hypothalamus in association with an acutely expanding intracranial lesion, as suggested by Johnson and Yates (20). This functional alteration is postulated to result in diminution of vasomotor tone in the cerebral vessels.

Thompson and Malina (21) have adduced evidence to indicate that "dynamic axial brain-stem distortion" occurring at the incisura tentorii heightens the systemic vasopressor response. Deep anesthesia or profound damage to the brain stem decreases the responsiveness of the systemic vasopressor system (4). Ranson and his co-workers (22) concluded that blood pressure was controlled by a dual mechanism, inhibitory stimuli being derived from the more rostral part of the brain and the facilitatory control from the more caudal portion. It seems reasonable to assume that the caudal facilitatory center located in the relatively resistent hind brain, remaining relatively intact, might be released from the rostral inhibitory control because of functional interruption of neural pathways in the upper mid-brain. If these postulates be correct, the seemingly lowered vasopressor threshold and the obvious effect of barbiturate upon the blood pressure during acute swelling can be easily explained.

Thus, it is our belief that this form of acute swelling appears to be due to a "release phenomenon," comparable physiologically to the development of decerebrate rigidity following brain stem transsection.

In any event, as suggested in Figure 8, the best therapeutic results in the experimental animal appear to be derived from: 1) eliminating the vicious cycle of concomitant rises in intracranial pressure and systemic blood pressure through the action of barbiturates, 2) conteracting cerebrovascular dilation by adequate oxygen supply with controlled positive-negative respiration as pointed out by Langfitt (14), and 3) reducing the intracranial pressure, when possible, by

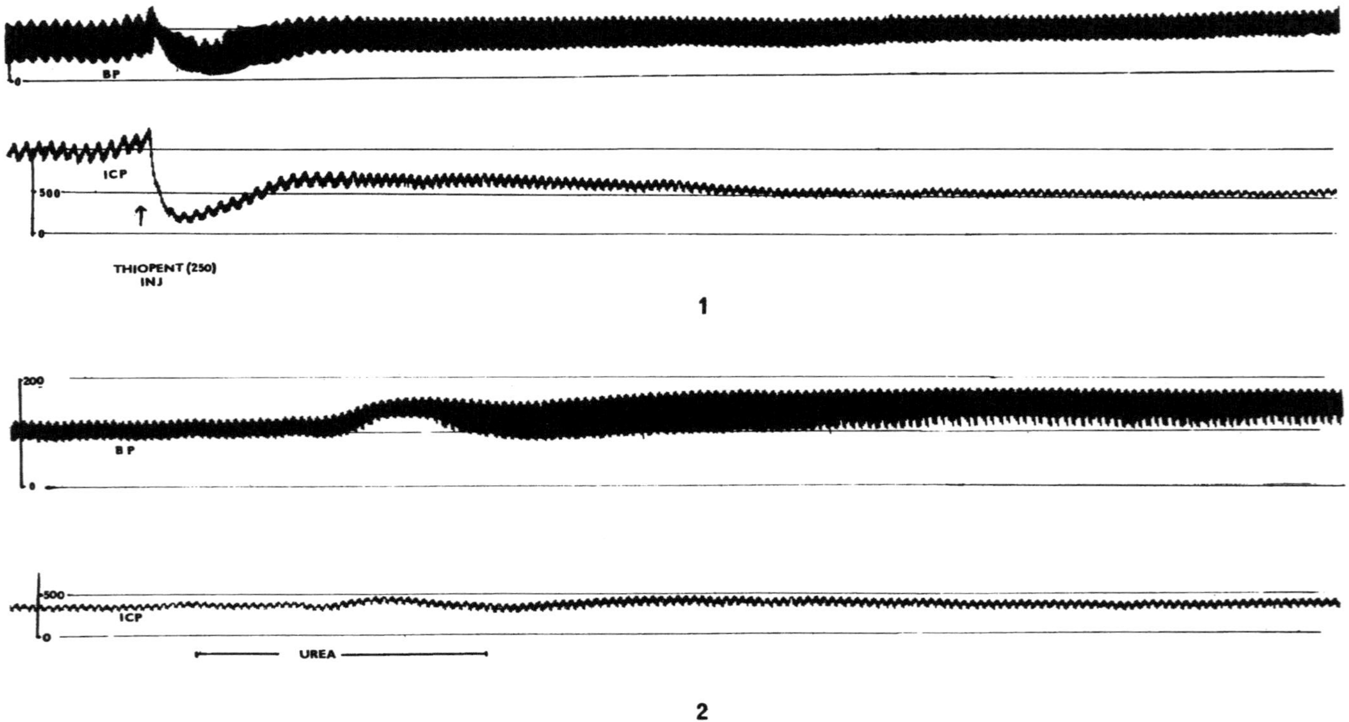

Fig. 8. Records demonstrating the effect upon blood pressure and intracranial pressure of barbiturate administration and controlled positive-negative respiration, followed by urea. After injection of a barbiturate (arrow), intracranial pressure (ICP) and blood pressure (BP) fall, and a further fall in ICP is to be noted independent of blood pressure alteration. The amplitude of BP is gradually reduced during controlled respiration (Section 1). In Section 2, the administration of urea fails to reduce the intracranial pressure.

the use of dehydrating agents. It should be noted that even when the intracranial pressure is not reduced, as in the last line, the cardiac stroke volume, and therefore cardiac efficiency were benefited. This tends to compensate for any lowering of the blood pressure.

We have developed at length these vasomotor aspects because we believe these responses, productive of cerebral "fullness," must be clearly differentiated from those changes developing in brain tissue itself, properly referred to as brain edema.

II. EXPERIMENTAL CEREBRAL EDEMA (i.e., Alterations in V_{br})

Applying the same technique of epidural balloon compression described in detail in the papers of Ishii and his co-workers (7, 8, 9, 10, 11), an experimental model can be produced which appears to mirror accurately the edema seen in the human who has sustained an epidural hematoma. By more prolonged and less severe balloon compression, monitored by observation of EEG changes, one can demonstrate, by sacrificing animals at different time intervals, a spectrum of edema. The ultrastructural changes in these brains have been reported by us in a series of papers (7, 8, 9, 10, 11, 23). In this presentation we propose to indicate briefly changes noted in cerebral lipids at different chronological stages.

It has been known for some time that the regulation of water and the proper distribution of electrolytes in cells is dependent upon energy produced by cellular metabolism. The cellular components of the brain are no exception. A continuous supply of metabolically produced energy is required for the maintenance of normal glial structure and for the support of proper cellular hydration through active transport of water and ions. It has recently become clear that the cerebral lipids act not as inert structural constituents of the nervous system but are intimately related to the cellular activities of the brain. For example, lecithin is one of the essential constituents of the intracellular membrane system (24, 25), and it is known that its deprivation from the mitochondrial membrane results in defective ATP synthesis and cellular restoration. Biochemical approaches suggest, then, a new understanding of cerebral edema.

Phospholipids fractionated by Schneider's method (26) show a decrease in lipid content after the brain has been compressed. The most remarkable decrease is seen when the animal's symptoms are worst and the level gradually returns toward normal as the animal's condition improves (Fig. 9). Further fractionation of phospholipids is made according to Lowry's method (27). No significant change in any fraction of phospholipids is found in the gray matter. In the white matter, however, where maximal swelling if found, lecithin is markedly decreased on the compressed side compared to the non-

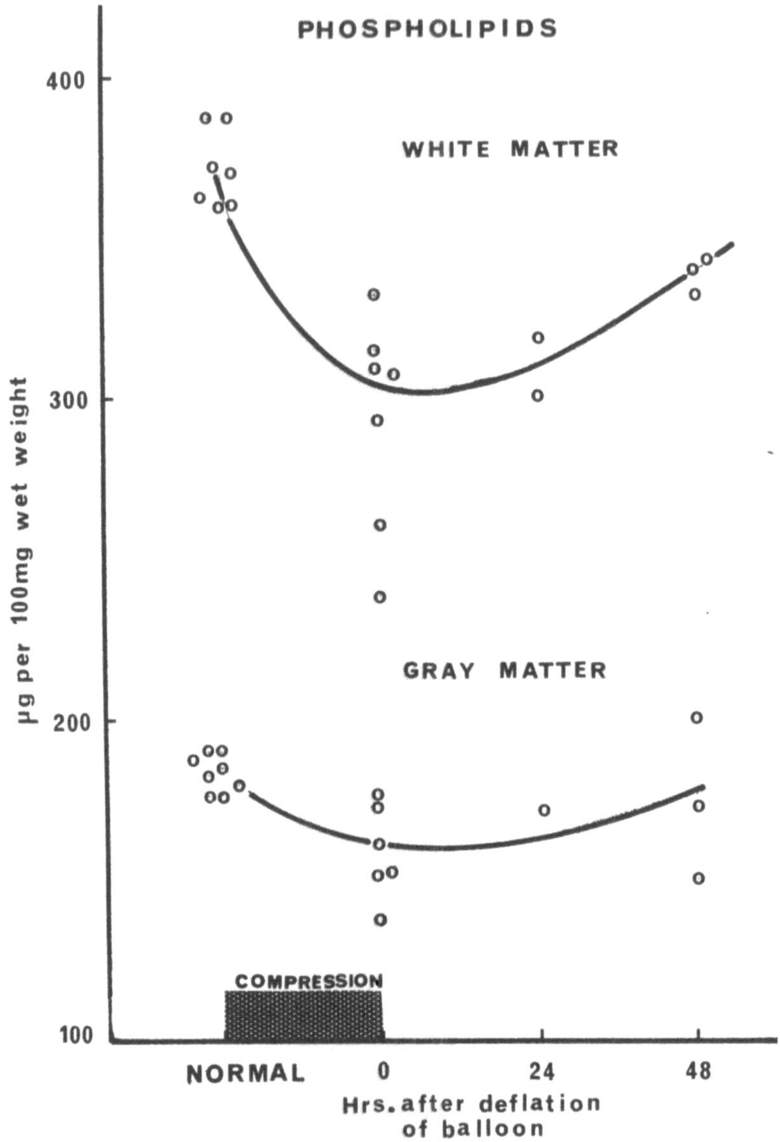

Fig. 9. The change in phospholipid content of the brain after cerebral compression of 24 hours duration. The maximum decrease noted in the white matter corresponds with the maximum deterioration in the animal's condition

compressed side. No significant difference is found between the two hemispheres in either cephalin or sphingomyelin (Fig. 10). In simi-

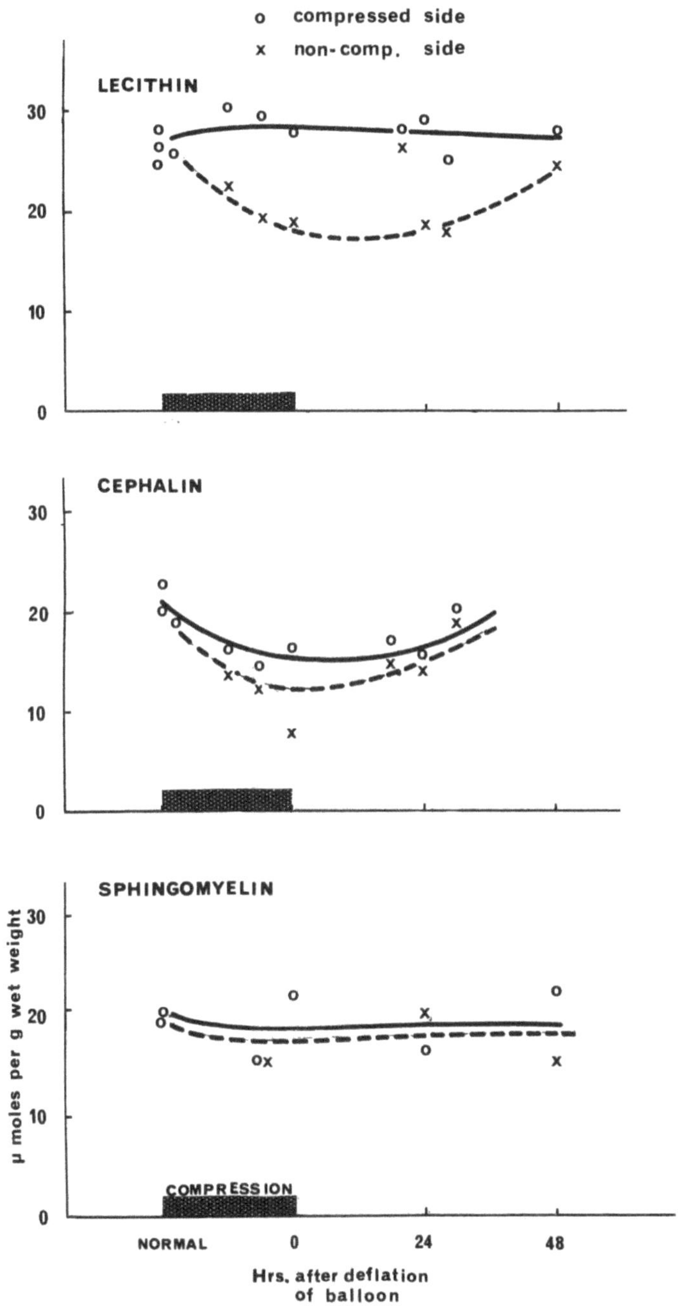

Fig. 10. Changes in the content of lecithin, cephalin and sphingomyelin in the white matter after 24 hours of cerebral compression. The marked reduction in lecithin on the compressed side contrasts with the absence of marked change in cephalin and sphingomyelin.

lar studies dealing with metabolism of cerebral glycolipids, (28, 29, 30), marked reduction in ganglioside, which is found only in the gray matter is noted after cerebral compression (Fig. 11). Again,

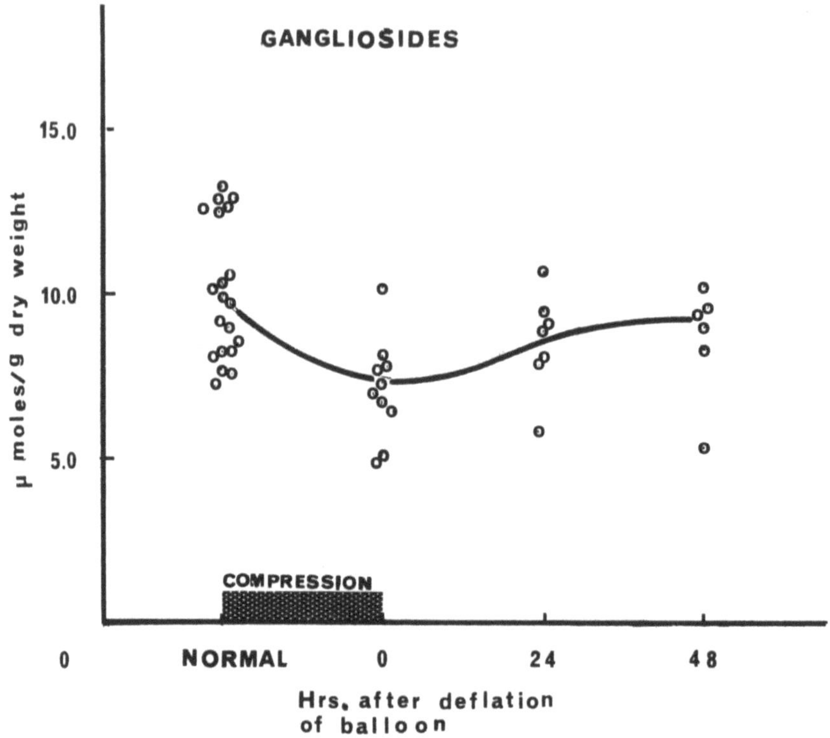

Fig. 11. The reduction in ganglioside content is maximal after 24 hours of compression. The depression in cerebral activity follows a roughly comparable course.

the change is roughly proportional to the deterioration of the animal's condition. There is no obvious change in cerebroside content in either the white matter or in the brain stem.

Gangliosides are known to be related not only to the excitability of the cerebral tissue, but they are also involved in the energy-assisted ion movement across the cell membrane (31, 32, 33, 34).

It has been proved that the cytidine nucleotides, especially CDP-choline (cytidine-diphosphate-choline) play a key role in the biosynthesis of lecithin (35). Thus, to offset the metabolic disturbance in lecithin, the synthesis intermediate of CDP-choline was tested. When the nucleotide is injected intravenously, the beneficial effect on the animal's condition is quite obvious, and on occasion even dramatic, as judged by conscious level and EEG pattern (Fig. 12).

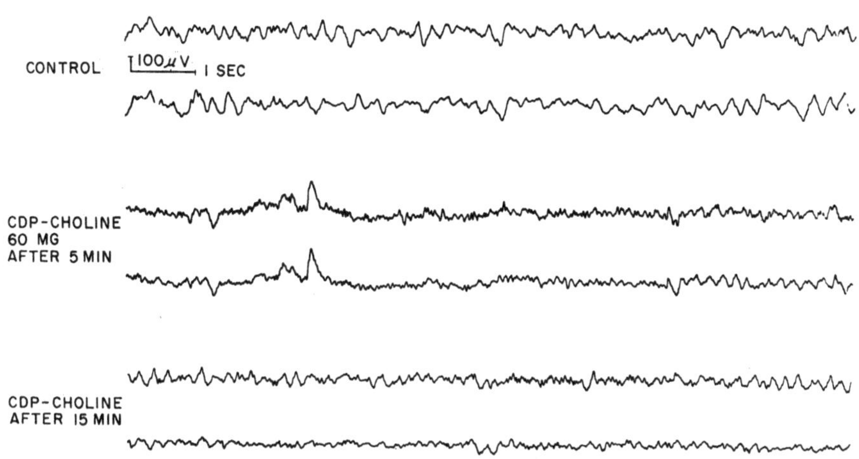

Fig. 12. Sixty mg. of CDP-choline are administered to a cat made drowsy by cerebral compression. The EEG marked "control" is that of the animal immediately before injection. Within five minutes of the administration, increased motor activity was noted and the abnormal high voltage, slow EEG returns toward normal. The beneficial effects upon the animal's condition and the EEG persisted for approximately fifty minutes.

Since it has been known that UDP-glucose (uridine-diphosphate-glucose) may serve as the glucose donor in the synthesis of gangliosides (36), it was thought worthwhile to try the administration of uridine nucleotides in the effort to restore cerebral activity. These uridine derivatives proved less effective than the intravenous injection of uridine itself, which in reproducible fashion, tended to eliminate high voltage slow waves and restore nearly normal alpha EEG activity (Fig. 13). Visible improvement in the animal's symptoms, however, is less obvious than is the case with the administration of cytidine nucleotides.*

*These drugs have been used by Dr. Ishii, during an interlude in Japan, on more than fifty patients. The results will be reported at a subsequent date.

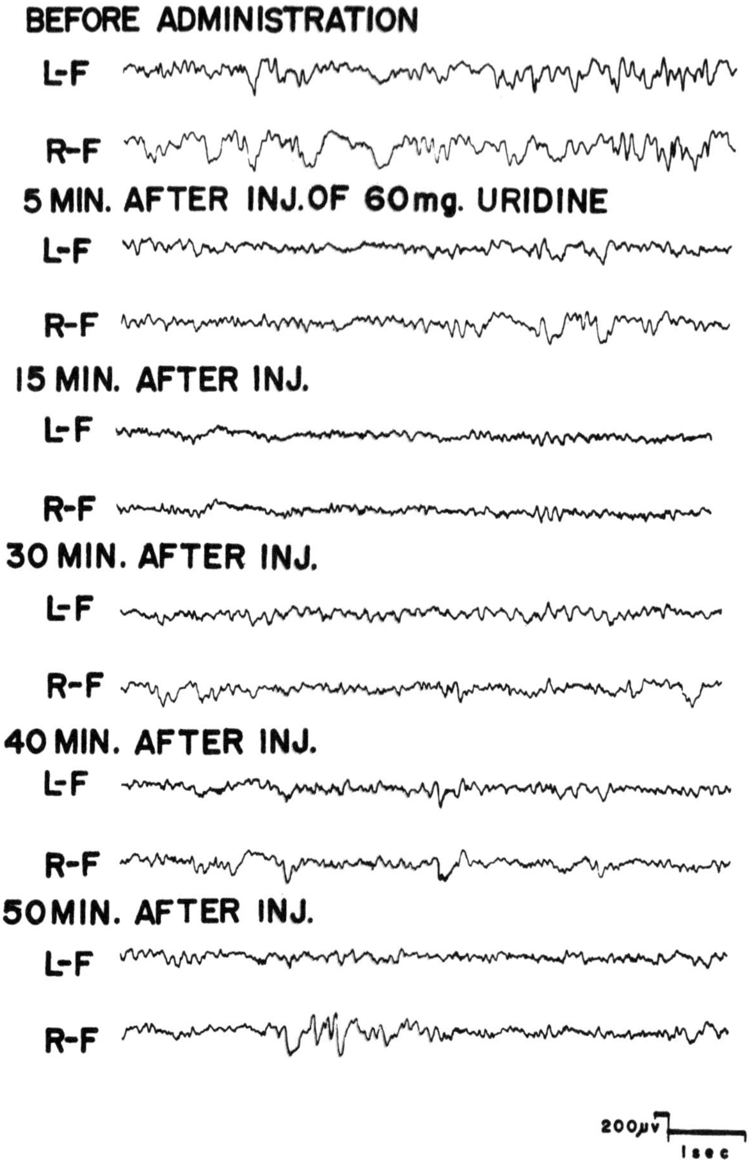

Fig. 13. The effect of uridine (60 mg. IV) upon the EEG of a cat following cerebral compression. The beneficial action evidenced by the elimination of high voltage slow waves in both hemispheres and the restoration of a normal aplha pattern persisted for forty minutes.

III. IN VITRO STUDIES
(Further observations relevant to changes in V_{br})

An in vitro method has been employed in the effort to gain greater insight into the relationships between ultrastructure and the metabolic changes associated with cerebral swelling.

Adult albino rats have been used. Brain slices of 0.4 mm thickness have been made from the cortex and then quickly transferred to the various kinds of media to be employed. They are incubated at either 30°C or 37°C in the metabolic shaking incubator under aerobic conditions. At various periods of incubation, they are removed from the incubator and fixed in osmium tetroxide. Electron microscopic studies of the brain slices incubated at 30° and 37° revealed morphological changes proceeding in the same direction. However, at the higher temperature, the alterations develop more rapidly and to a greater degree. Only the ultrastructural findings of slices incubated at 30° C will be shown.

Figure 14 demonstrates the appearance of normal rat brain cortex, whereas Figure 15 of the same magnification shows maximal swelling of the cell body and processes of astrocytes incubated for 20 minutes in Krebs-Ringer solution. There will be noted alterations of virtually all the cytoplasmic organelles of which, however, the mitochondria seem to be most sensitive. Swollen mitochondria with a pale matrix devoid of granules are seen (Fig. 16). These changes are identical with those seen following the in vivo production of edema by brain compression or by middle cerebral artery ligation. The incubation changes could not be effectively prevented by adding substrates such as glucose or glutamate, a result somewhat at variance with the findings of Elliot (37).

As a next step, since the most obvious changes associated with swelling are the various regressive alterations noted in the mitochondria, the biological functions of the mitochondria associated with cerebral edema were examined. From edematous brain produced in vivo by experimental compression, the mitochondrial fraction has been isolated by differential centrifugation, and the function of oxydative phosphorylation has been examined. Figure 17 demonstrates the marked narrowing of mitochondrial activity both in ATP formation and in respiration.

With this determined, return was made to the in vitro experiment and 2 mM of ATP were added to the glucose-Krebs-Ringer solution and the slices incubated. After 20 minutes, there was little swelling of the glial cells and the cellular ultrastructure remained virtually unaltered with relatively little mitochondrial change (Fig. 18). It was found, however, that ATP is not able to restore glial swelling that has once developed. Furthermore, when DNP (2-4-

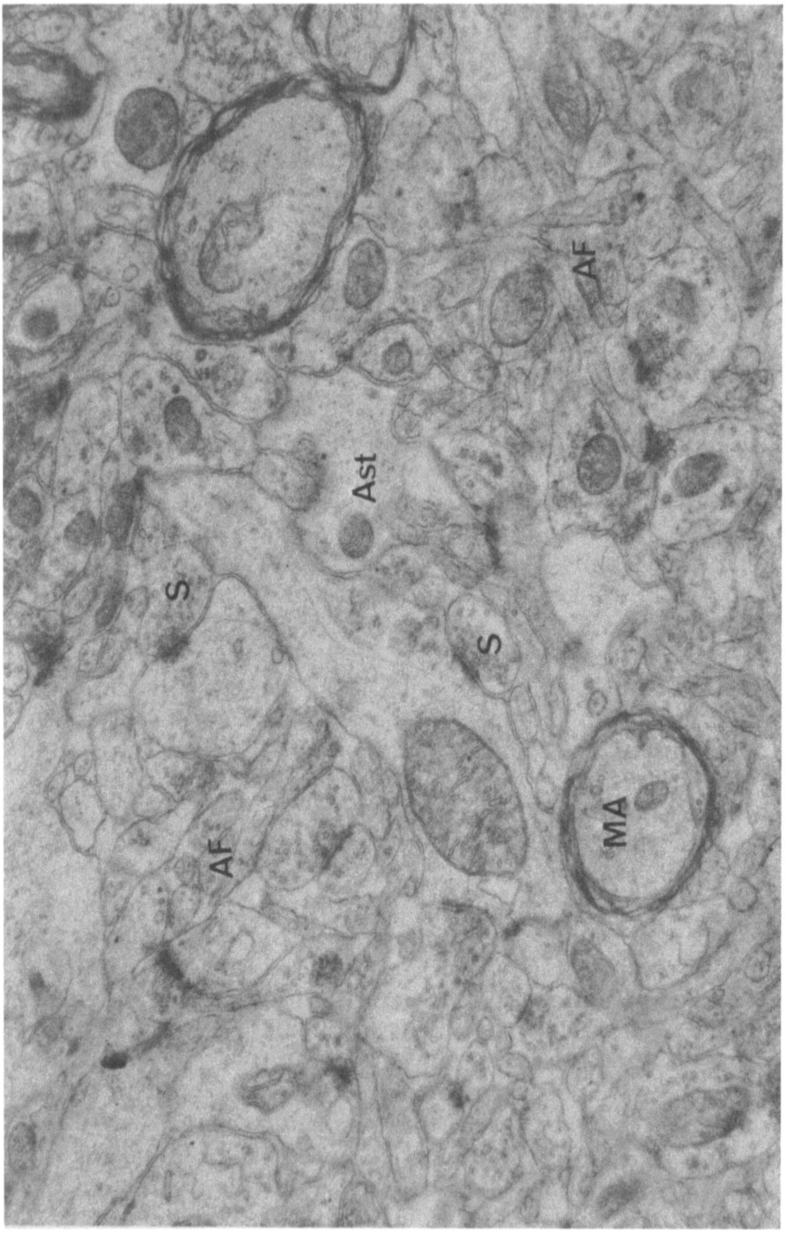

Fig. 14. Normal cortex of the cat. There are shown astrocytic processes (Ast) with a few inclusions, myelinated axon (MA) and axon fields (AF) and presynaptic terminals (S). The neuropil is closely packed with minimal extracellular space.

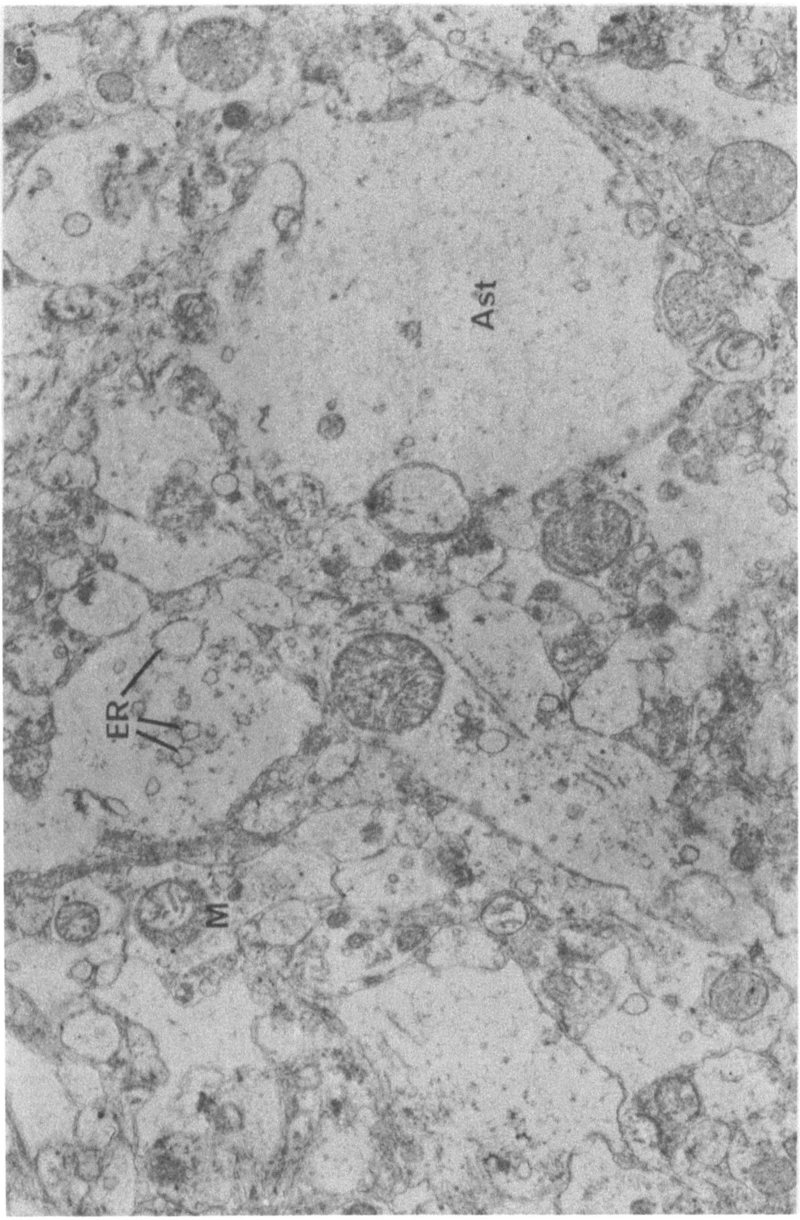

Fig. 15. A cortex slice incubated for twenty minutes in isotonic Krebs-Ringer solution, to be contrasted with Figure 14. There is marked astrocytic swelling (Ast) and the endoplasmic reticulum (ER) shows distention. Mitochondrial alteration (M) is to be noted.

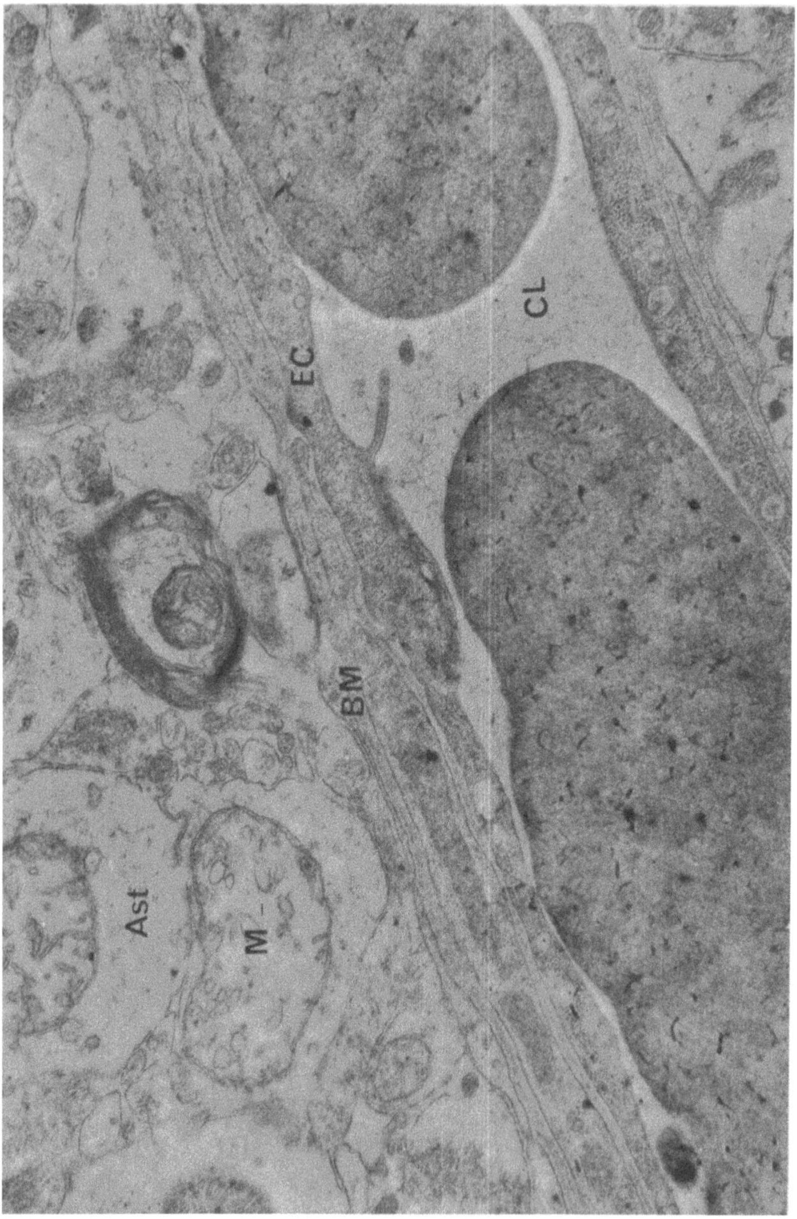

Fig. 16. Cortex incubated in isotonic Krebs-Ringer solution for twenty minutes. The capillary lumen (CL) is bounded by an endothelial cell (EC) enveloped in turn by the basement membrane (BM). An adjacent astrocyte (Ast) is greatly swollen

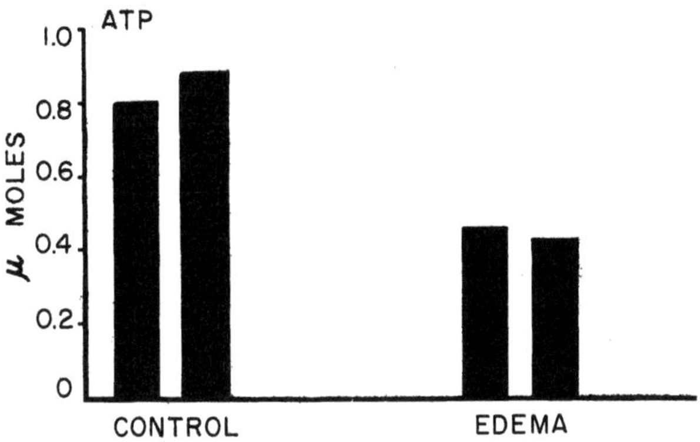

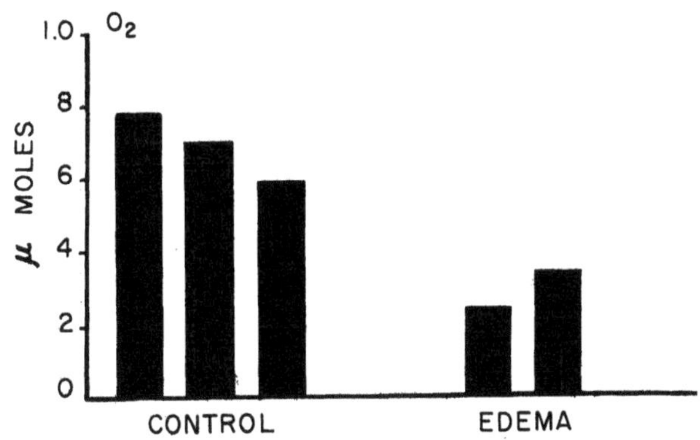

Fig. 17. Determinations of the oxydative phosphorylating function of the isolated mitochondrial fraction of normal and of edematous brain (edema produced in vivo; see text). There is marked reduction in the biological activity of the mitochondria of the edematous brain tissue, manifested both in ATP formation and in reduced respiration.

dinitrophenol), an uncoupler which inhibits ATP formation, is added to ATP reinforced medium, considerable swelling in the astrocytes is noticed after 20 minutes of incubation (Fig. 19). These findings seem to indicate that if metabolically produced cellular ATP is com-

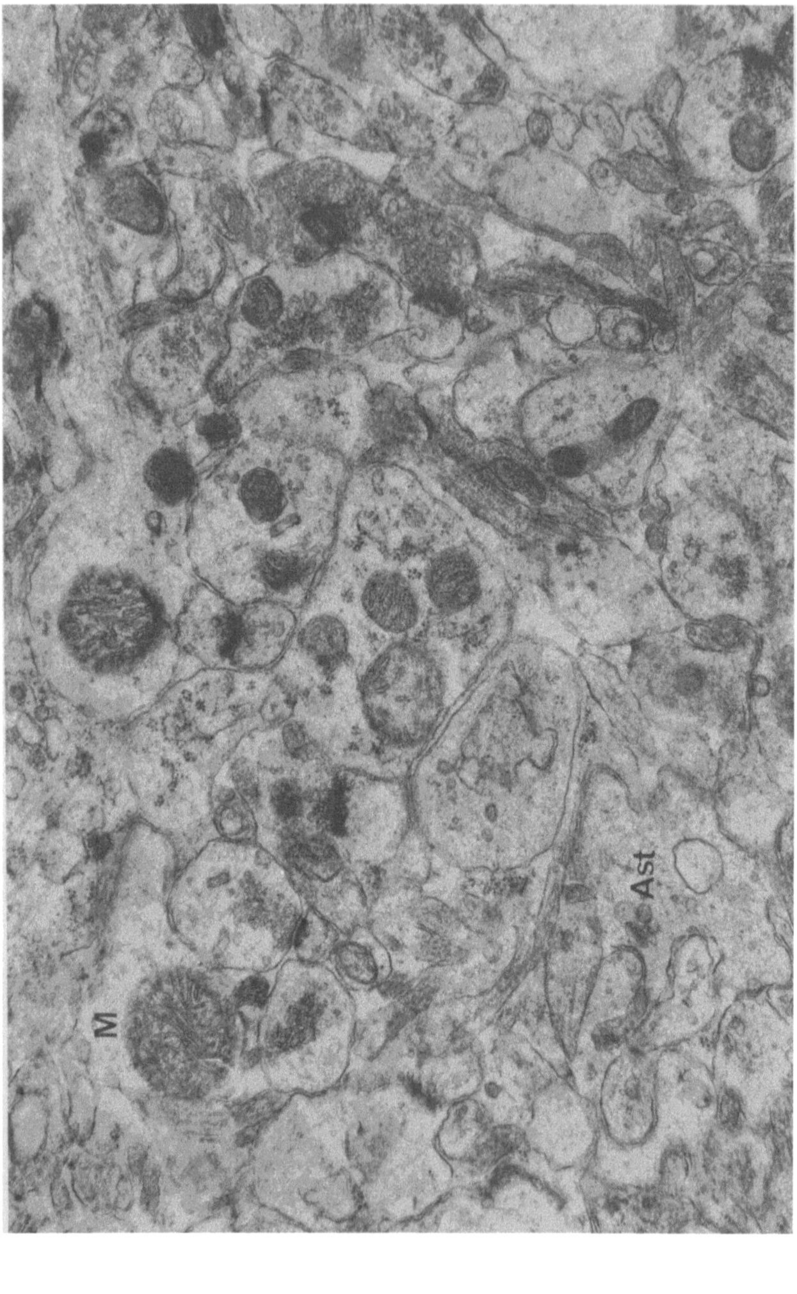

Fig. 18. Section taken from a brain slice incubated for twenty minutes in glucose-Krebs-Ringer solution that has been reinforced with ATP. The section has been taken from an area comparable to those employed in Figures 14 and 15. Note that the astrocytic swelling (Ast) is less obvious and that there is relatively little alteration in the mitochondria (M).

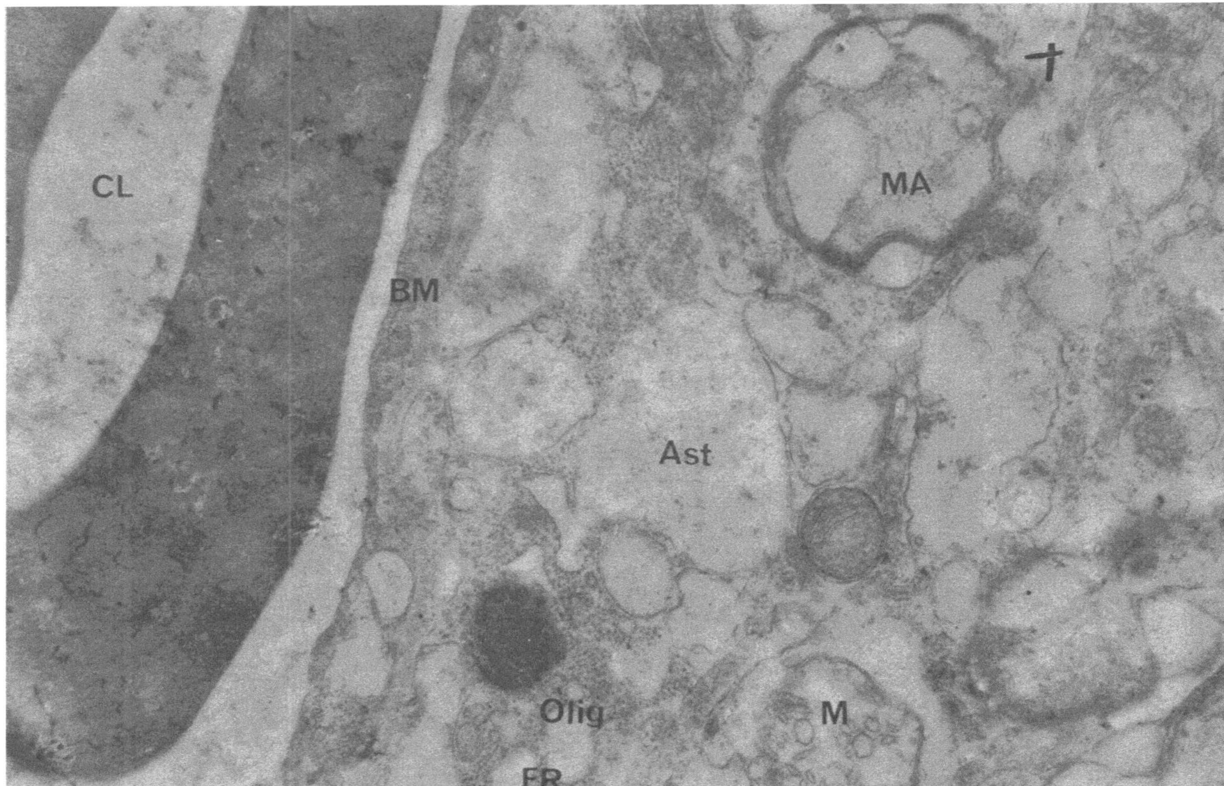

Fig. 19. Section from a brain slice incubated for twenty minutes in glucose-Krebs-Ringer solution, reinforced with ATP but to which has been added DNP. The pericapillary astrocytes (Ast) and the mitochondria (M) show regressive changes comparable to those seen in Figure 16. The endoplasmic reticulum (ER) of an oligodendrocyte (Olig) shows distention, and vacuolated changes are to be seen in a myelinated axon (MA). Capillary lumen (CL) and basement membrane (BM) are also seen, the basement membrane being significantly swollen.

pletely exhausted, exogenous ATP added to the medium cannot provide sufficient energy to maintain normal glial structure.

When slices incubated in glucose-Krebs-Ringer solution for 10 minutes are transferred to a medium reinforced with ATP and 2mM of caffein, the volume of the glial cytoplasm which was once swollen in the initial incubation approaches normal (Fig. 20). According to Polis (38), caffein and its related compounds appear to stimulate lowered oxydative phosphorylation, although the mechanism of this stimulation was not fully understood by them. One may theorize that caffein accelerates intrinsic ATP formation, liberating energy for membrane function and intracellular fluid control. It was found that the increase in weight in the slices incubated in ATP reinforced medium is less than that occurring in tissues incubated in isotonic Krebs-Ringer solution or glucose-Krebs-Ringer solution. On the other hand, when there was added to the Krebs-Ringer solution an azide or DNP, an oxydative phosphorylation inhibitor or uncoupler, the weight gain of the incubated slices was significant (Fig. 21).

Determination of the protein content in the incubation medium proved illuminating. Since the protein in the medium is evidently derived from the cell, possibly with other soluble cellular constituents, it is possible that protein accumulation may be a function of the degree of membrane damage. The protein content in the Krebs-Ringer solution in which the slices were incubated showed a steady increase while protein in the incubation medium was found to be decreased in the ATP reinforced fluid. These findings suggest the protective action of ATP on the cellular membrane (Fig. 21).

DISCUSSION

Any discussion of the fullness of the brain seen by the surgeon at operation, by the experimentalist in the laboratory, or by the pathologist at necropsy is immediately plagued by semantic problems. Unhappily, the term "cerebral swelling" has been used by various authors, ourselves included, to define a pathological entity.

We would now urge that the term "cerebral swelling" be applied to that fullness of the brain seen under all the above circumstances, and that it be recognized simply as a descriptive term. We shall use it henceforth in that sense.

Ryder has proposed the formula $V_{ic} = V_{br} + V_{bl} + V_{csf} + V_{l}$ to express the interrelationships among the various factors playing a role in cerebral swelling. In the present contribution, we have isolated for study, so far as we have found it possible to isolate them, two of the four factors in the equation. Alterations in these two fac-

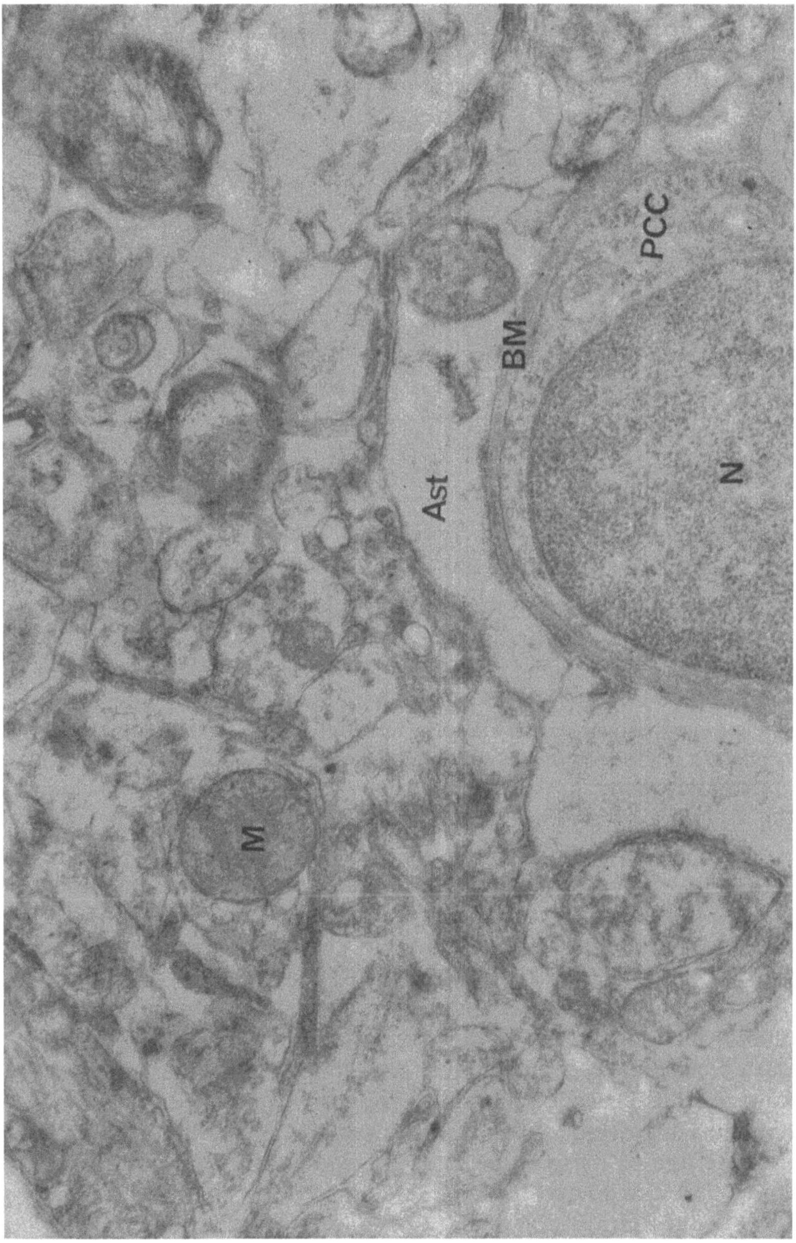

Fig. 20. Cortex incubated for ten minutes in glucose-Krebs-Ringer solution subsequently transferred for ten minutes to a medium reinforced with ATP and caffein. The regression changes may be noted to be somewhat less severe. Nucleus (N) of pericapillary cell (PCC) whose basement membrane is marked BM. The neuropil shows a less swollen astrocyte (Ast), numerous mitochondria (M) show only moderate changes.

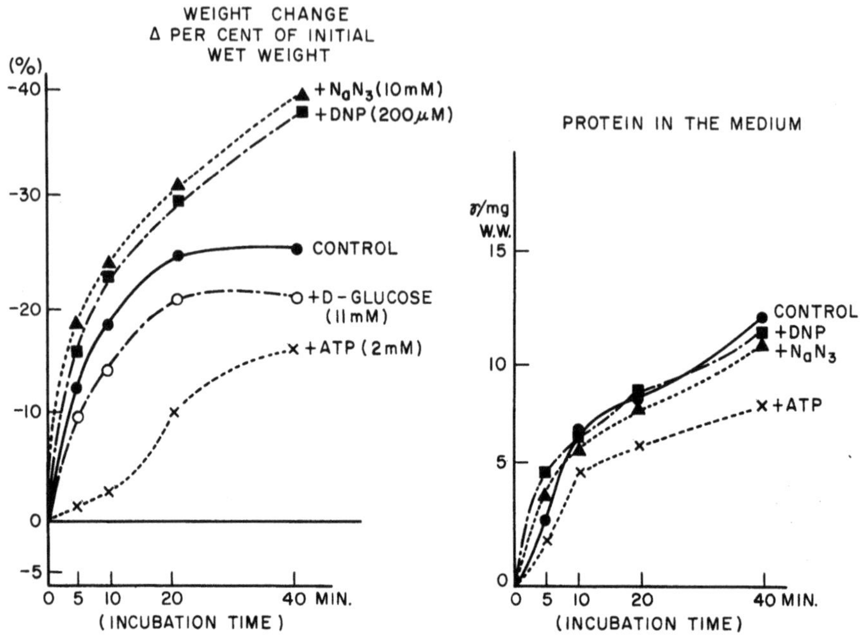

Fig. 21. Weight changes of brain slices incubated in various incubation media (left) and protein content alterations in the incubation medium in which the slices have been incubated (right). The weight increase is less in slices incubated in the ATP reinforced medium. The addition of DNP or azide to the medium causes a further gain in weight. In ATP reinforced media the protein content is less than that in the other media in which there is virtually no alteration.

tors have been produced by the inflation in dogs, cats and monkeys of an epidural balloon. By controlled inflation and deflation, it has been possible to produce, in successive animals, a spectrum of brain swelling.

On the basis of our experimental data, we are able to confirm the conclusion of Langfitt that in its early stages acute swelling is a reflection of vascular engorgement secondary to the loss of vasomotor tone. As did Langfitt, we too have found increased oxygen saturation and controlled ventilation to be of benefit, whereas hypertonic solutions are of little help. Langfitt demonstrated again in his experiments that successive increments in blood pressure develop in the face of increasing intracranial pressure, presumably nature's effort to offset the resultant ischemia, the Cushing phenomenon. This has long been looked upon as a salutory mechanism.

We concur in Langfitt's belief that there at least two factors operating in the development of acute swelling: 1) impairment of cerebrovascular tone and 2) vasopressor responses dependent upon an intact medullary mechanism.

Questions need to be asked concerning both of these factors.

1. Vasomotor Tone. Why should there be an impairment of vasomotor tone in the cerebrovascular tree? Langfitt has postulated that this results from vascular over-distention and from local oxygen want. We have adduced evidence for an additional explanation. We have been able to demonstrate in the hypothalamus a specific center which on puncture or coagulation produces what we interpret as a neural form of vasoparalysis, productive of distention of the vascular bed and of concomitant rise in intracranial pressure. We believe further that it is possible that mechanical distortion of the hypothalamic area as the result of displacemnt by balloon distention evokes a similar response and, through the resultant vasoparalysis, leads to an acute increase in intracranial pressure: a form of cerebral swelling.

The therapeutic maneuvers to offset the deleterious effect of vasodilatation, whether of peripheral origin as postulated by Langfitt or of central origin as suggested by us, appear to be twofold: controlled ventilation with abundant oxygen, supplemented by control of arterial hypertension which floods the distended vascular tree, causing a recurrent rise of intracranial pressure. We now wish to consider this second aspect.

2. Vasopressor Response. What is the nature of the vasopressor response that occurs during acute cerebral compression? Is there evidence to suggest that the responsiveness of the vasopressor system is abnormally heightened during acute cerebral swelling? Various authors, including Langfitt and Thompson and Malina, have given reasons for believing that the vasopressor threshold is lowered in the face of rapidly expanding asymmetric lesions, the production of "dynamic axial distortion of the brain stem." Lightening of anesthesia may also allow greater vasopressor response.

In the experiments reported above, we have shown that the administration of barbiturates, by normalizing blood pressure in animals subjected to acute brain swelling, results in the restoration of intracranial pressure toward normal. This confirms the role played by arterial hypertension in flooding the paralyzed vascular tree, thereby increasing the intracranial pressure. With controlled respiration and increased oxygen saturation, peripheral ischemia appears to be corrected. Therefore, we believe on experimental grounds that judicious use of the barbiturates clinically is warranted, and we are subjecting this thesis to controlled observations. But it should be emphasized that if the vasopressor mechanism is to be eliminated clinically, it is imperative that controlled respiration and adequate oxygen saturation be employed concurrently.

Our second area of concern has dealt with the changes in cerebral metabolism that occur in subacute cerebral swelling. We have studied the metabolic alterations in various lipids and we have tried to correlate these with the cerebral activity of the animals and the ultrastructural changes in the brain tissue. The experimental material has been produced by balloon inflation to a sub-critical level maintained for longer periods than in the case of acute swelling.

Of the phospholipids contained in the white matter, lecithin is found to be markedly decreased on the compressed side. The changes are roughly proportional to the deterioration in the animal's condition No marked change has been noted in the content of either cephalin or sphingomyelin. Studies of the glycolipids in the cortex have shown a marked reduction in gangliosides of the compressed hemisphere. Again, the changes are roughly proportional to the animal's condition, the most remarkable decrease being noted when the cerebral activity of the animal is lowest and when maximal swelling of the astrocytes is seen electron microscopically.

Because cytidine nucleotides, particularly CDP-choline, play an important role in the biosynthesis of lecithin, the effect of intravenous injections of CDP-choline was tested. Marked beneficial effects were found. When uridine derivatives were employed in the effort to restore ganglioside metabolism, less clear-cut effects were noted upon the animal's condition, though EEG abnormalities were largely eliminated.

The findings, coupled with the increased understanding of the biochemical nature of membrane activity, suggest the very important role played by the cerebral lipids of the central nervous system.

There is reported in the last section of this paper an in vitro study of cerebral swelling under circumstances that permit altering of the composition of the medium at will, thus producing reproducible and rigidly controlled experimental conditions.

Brain slices of normal rat cortex that have been incubated in an isotonic Krebs-Ringer solution always swell. The ultrastructural alterations seen in such slices are fairly comparable to those that have been noted in experimentally produced in vivo swelling. Substrates added to the medium do not alter the incubation changes.

When ATP is added to the glucose-Krebs-Ringer solution, swelling of the glial cells is delayed and the ultrastructure has remained unaltered, but once the swelling has developed, ATP is ineffective in reversing it.

On the other hand, caffein or xanthine, which are believed to stimulate lowered oxydative phosphorylation in mitochondria, does reverse to some extent the swelling once it has developed.

Further, it has been observed that the weight gain in slices incubated in isotonic Krebs-Ringer solution is reduced when ATP is added to the medium but is increased when DNP, an uncoupler of oxydative phosphorylation which inhibits the ATP formation in mitochondria, is added to the medium.

The protective action of ATP on membrane function is also demonstrated by the determination of the protein content in the incubation medium.

Great theoretical importance in the demonstration that the addition of ATP to the medium prevents glial swelling rests in the fact that in brain slices the blood-brain-barrier is not functioning.

It is clear, then, that a continuous supply of metabolically produced energy is required for the support of normal glial structure and function. We believe that more emphasis should be put on metabolic studies in order to understand better the nature of those alterations in the volume of brain substance (V_{br}) which we customarily refer to as cerebral edema.

SUMMARY

This contribution has dealt with two of the four factors that may play a role in the occurrence of cerebral swelling.

We have first given attention to the alterations in the volume of circulating blood (V_{bl}) within the intracranial cavity and have discussed their mechanism, and means of influencing them favorably, with special attention to vasomotor and vasopressor effects. Next, we have considered the alterations in cerebral lipids that occur in association with alterations in brain substance (V_{br}) produced in the experimental animal.

These studies have been interpreted further in terms of in vitro observations on the cortex under circumstances where the medium could be varied at will.

In the discussion, the implications of these observations have been considered.

REFERENCES

1. Cushing, H.: The third circulation and its channels: Studies in intracranial physiology, London: Oxford University Press, pp. 1-51.
2. Ryder, H. W., F. F. Espey, F. D. Kimball, E. J. Penka, A. Rosenauer, B. Podolsky and J. P. Evans: The mechanism of the change in cerebrospinal fluid pressure following an induced change in the

volume of the fluid space, J. Lab. and Clin. Med., 41, 428-435 (1953).
3. Evans, J. P., F. F. Espey, F. D. Kristoff, F. D. Kimball and H. W. Ryder: Experimental and clinical observation on rising intracranial pressure, Arch. Surg., 63, 107-114 (1951).
4. Weinstein, J. D., T. W. Langfitt and N. F. Kassel: Vasopressor response to increased intracranial pressure, Neurology, 14, 1118-1131 (1964).
5. Lundberg, N., H. Troop and H. Lorin: Continuous recording of the ventricular fluid pressure in patients with severe acute traumatic brain injury, J. of Neurosurg., 22, 581-591 (1965).
6. Langfitt, T. W.: Possible mechanisms of action of hypertonic urea in reducing intracranial pressure, Neurology, 11, 196-209, (1961).
7. Ishii, S., R. Hayner, W. A. Kelly and J. P. Evans: Studies of cerebral swelling, II: Experimental cerebral swelling produced by supra-tentorial extra-dural compression, J. Neurosurg., 16, 152-166 (1959).
8. _____ and E. Tani: Electron microscope studies in blood-brain barrier in cerebral swelling, Acta Neuropath. (Berlin), 1, 474-488 (1962).
9. Tani, E. and J. P. Evans: Electron microscope studies of cerebral swelling, I: Studies on the permeability of brain capillaries using ferritin molecules as tracers, Acta Neuropath., 4, 507-526 (1965).
10. _____ and _____: Electron microscope studies of cerebral swelling, II: Alterations of myelinated nerve fibers, Ibid., 604-623.
11. _____ and _____: Electron microscope studies of cerebral swelling, III: Alterations in the neuroglia and the blood vessels of the white matter, Ibid., 624-639.
12. Zülch, K.: Proc. Symp. on Brain Edema (ed. by I. Klatzo and F. Seitelberger). Springer-Verlag New York (1967).
13. Schroeder, J. M. and W. Wechsler: Ödem und Nekrose in der grauen und weissen Substanz beim experimentällen Hirntrauma (Licht-und elekronen microskopische Üntersuchungen), Acta Neuropath., 5, 82-111 (1965).
14. Langfitt, T. W., J. D. Weinstein and N. F. Kassel: Cerebral vasomotor paralysis produced by intracranial hypertension, Transact. of Am. Neurol. Assoc., pp. 214-215 (1964).
15. Wolff, H. G. and H. S. Forbes: The cerebral circulation, V: Observations of the pial circulation during changes in intracranial pressure, Arch. Neurol. Psychiat., 20, 1035-1047 (1928).
16. Evans, J. P. and I. M. Scheinker: Histologic studies of the brain following head trauma. VI: Posttraumatic central ner-

vous system changes interpreted in terms of circulatory disturbances, Research Publ., J. Nerv. and Ment. Diseases, 24, 254-273 (1945).
17. Reichard, M.: Das Hirnödem (appendix section Die Hirnschwellung), in the series: "Handbuch der Speziellen pathologischen Anatomie und Histologie," Vol. 13, Part 1B, p. 1229. Berlin, Göttingen, Heidelberg: Springer-Verlag (1957).
18. Lebeau, J.: L'oedeme aigu du cerveau par lesiones experimentales du tronc cerebral: Ses rapports avec l'hypertension arterielle, Rev. Canadienne de Biol., 7, 254-293 (1948).
19. Evans, J. P. and F. F. Espey: Unpublished observations from the Laboratory of Physiology, Yale University (1948).
20. Johnson, R. T. and P. O. Yates: Brain stem hemorrhages in expanding supratentorial conditions, Acta Radiologica (Stockholm), 46, 250-256 (1956).
21. Thompson, R. K. and S. Malina: Dynamic axial brain-stem distortion as a mechanism explaining the cardio-respiratory changes in increased intracranial pressure, J. Neurosurg., 16, 664-667 (1959).
22. Kabat, H., H. W. Magoun and S. W. Ranson: Electrical stimulation of points in the forebrain and midbrain, Arch of Neurol. and Psychiat., 34, 931-955 (1935).
23. Raimondi, A. J., J. P. Evans and S. Mullan: Studies of cerebral edema, III: Alterations in the white matter: An electron microscopic study using ferritin as a labelling compound, Acta Neuropath. (Berlin), 2, 177-197 (1962).
24. Basford, R. E. and D. E. Green: Studies on the terminal electron transport system, XXI: On the properties of a soluable lipoprotein dissociated from succinic dehydrogenase complex, Biochem. Biophys. Acta, 33, 185-194 (1959).
25. Basford, R. E.: Studies on the terminal electron transport system, XXII: The lipid composition of coenzyme Q lipoprotein, Ibid., 195-201 (1959).
26. Schneider, W. C.: Phosphorus compounds in animal tissue: extraction and estimation of desoxypentose nucleic acid and of pentose nucleic acid, J. Biol. Chem., 161, 293-303 (1945).
27. Lowry, O. H. and E. J. Robins: Micro determinations of phospholipids and sphingolipids in brain, Ibid., 220, 661-675 (1956).
28. Folch, J., M. Lees and G. H. Sloane Stanley: A simple method for the isolation and purification of total lipids from animal tissue, Ibid., 226, 497-509 (1957).
29. Dische, Z.: Über charakteristische Farbreaktionen der Milchsäure, des Methylglyoxals und der Kohlehydrate mit Carbazol und Schwefelsäure, Biochem. Zeitschrift., 189, 77-80 (1927).

30. Warren, L. J.: The thiobarbituric acid assay of sialic acids, J. Biol. Chem., 234, 1971-1975 (1959).
31. McIlwain, H.: Characterization of naturally occurring materials which restore excitability to isolated cerebral tissue, Biochem., J. 78, 24-32 (1961).
32. Wolf, L. S. and H. McIlwain: Migration of histones from the nuclei of isolated cerebral tissues kept in cold media, Ibid., 33-40 (1961).
33. Thompson, C. G. and H. McIlwain: An attachment of protamine to cerebral tissue, studied in relation to gangliosides, suramin and tissue excitability, Ibid., 79, 342-347 (1961).
34. Deul, D. H. and H. McIlwain: Activation and inhibition of adenosine triphosphatase of subcellular particles from the brain, J. Neurochem., 8, 246-256 (1961).
35. Kennedy, E. P.: Biosynthesis of Phospholipids, Fed. Proc., 16, 847-853 (1957).
36. Burton, R. M.: Uridine nucleotides and the metabilism of nerve tissue, in: The Neurochemistry of Nucleotides and Amino Acids (ed. by R. O. Brady and D. B. Tower). New York, London: John Wiley & Sons, Inc., pp. 51-69 (1960).
37. Elliot, K. A. C.: Measurement of experimentally induced brain swelling and shrinkage, Am. J. Physiol., 157, 122-129 (1949).
38. Polis, B. D.: Studies on rate controlling factors in oxydative phosphorylation, Regional Neurochemistry, Pergamon Press, pp. 37-48 (1961).

K. STEINBEREITHNER

HYPOXIA AND BRAIN EDEMA

SOME ANESTHESIOLOGICAL CORRELATIONS

One of the main tasks confronting the anesthesiologist at all times is to prevent hypoxemia or, in other words, to continuously safeguard adequate oxygenation of all organs, above all the brain, as is expressed in the well-known slogan: "Give blood to the heart and oxygen to the brain!". In doing so he finds himself in a peculiar situation: he treats acute and chronic hypoxia of varying degrees and many times he can ascertain the correctness of his treatment only on the basis of the clinical success without having at his disposal verified experimental data. In spite of extensive research it is, for instance, still a matter of controversy whether or not there is a close causal interrelationship between hypoxia and cerebral edema. Experimental data on the morphological relationships are still scanty and partly contradictory.

Nolens volens the anesthesiologist is thus forced to act the part of the clinical experimenter, the so-called "clinical impression" constituting a major criterion for him. But perhaps, where other methods of the experimental researcher fail, he is able to contribute to the solution of some of the problems of cerebral edema. The following is an attempt to examine the complex questions of acute and chronic hypoxic cerebral lesions from this aspect.

ACUTE HYPOXIA

The most dramatic episode that gives rise to severe hypoxia is undoubtedly cardiac arrest occurring, according to international statistics, about once in every 2,500 to 3,000 cases of anesthesia independently of the technique used and the surgical procedure (with the exception of heart and brain operations that are particularly difficult from the technical point of view). Outside the operating room cardiac arrest is not rare, either.

This illustrates a rather extraordinary observation from the recent past. A 60-year-old retired man under treatment for chronic lues at a Clinic for Skin Diseases, had a fatal collapse a few minutes after having received a penicillin shot. Immediate extrathoracic cardiac massage was performed, followed by artificial respiration. The ECG revealed ventricular fibrillation. After external defibrillation had been performed eight times, normal sinus-rhythm recurred; circulation was satisfactory, but there was jerky respiration. Neurologically there were extensor spasms and signs of brain-stem incarceration. Following immediate dehydration by means of mannitol, fursemid, and human albumin, there was improvement of spontaneous respiration; signs of brain-stem incarceration, however, remained. Twice ventricular fibrillation recurred and was relieved immediately by means of double electroshock.* For four months now the patient has been without major complaints. The cause of cardiac arrest has remained obscure.

Provided neurological symptoms are not disguised by deep anesthesia, cardiac arrest thus produces typical manifestations of acute cerebral edema similar to those accompanying cranial trauma, tumors, and intracranial hematomas. These are extensor spasms, convulsions, signs of brain-stem incarceration and, in case of irreversibility, transition to "coma dépassé," according to Mollaret and Goulon (1959).

It is of secondary importance whether one assumes an "early" edema like Edström and Essex or, in the light of the experiments of Loenhning, et al. (1962), ascribes the immediate elevation of intracranial pressure to a hypoxic increase in blood supply (in the case of cardiac arrest the latter does not seem to be of any importance) and considers brain edema a secondary manifestation.

As Harley (1964) has pointed out recently, there is no consensus as to whether or not severe hypoxia causes a clinically significant increase in brain volume. The majority of authors (Williams and Spencer (1958); Ehrenhaft, et al. (1961), and others) have come out in favor of this assumption, whereas Brierley (1963), among others, has not found any evidence of brain swelling in patients who succumbe after heart surgery (with or without cardiac arrest) exhibiting signs of cerebral lesions.

In view of comprehensive clinical evidence, there is no doubt

*Under continued dehydration, complete reversal of all symptoms took place within 24 hours.

that hypoxia, as is so convincingly demonstraded by Argent and Cope (1956), triggers off a vicious circle which, according to Hoff and Jellinger (1962), leads to "mixed" cerebral edema with disturbances in the blood-brain barrier and a hemodynamic ischemic component; this is accompanied by asphyxial tissue hypoxydosis in the terms of investigations carried out by Gänshirt (1957).

How can we account for this discrepancy in the points of view? It is a startling fact that so far hardly any investigations have been made into the ultrastructural cerebral changes following hypoxia (Harley, 1964). Two reasons seem to be responsible for this. On the one hand, most authors (Altmann and Schubothe, 1942; Büchner, 1942; Opitz and Thorn, 1949) are of the opinion that moderate chronic hypoxia does not produce irreversible cerebral lesions and even the manifest histologic lesions are considered to be potentially reversible by some authors (Buzzard and Greenfield). On the other hand, as we have stated earlier (Kucher and Steinbereithner, 1952), an interval of hours is required for the morphological lesions to become manifest in the brain after hypoxia. This interval is referred to as "manifestation time." Thus acute fatal hypoxia seems to remain inaccessible to morphological investigations.

We encounter a similar ambiguous situation when dealing with the problem of the therapy of hypoxic cerebral edema. Osmotic dehydration is often criticized on the grounds that its effectiveness is dependent on an intact blood-brain barrier (Stubbs and Pennybaker, et al., 1960), which does not hold true in hypoxic brain damage (Harley, 1964) and after a trauma (Klatzo and Miquel). This view seems to be untenable for several reasons. The results of Rosomoff (1965) show that hypertonic solutions (contrary to the opinions held by Clasen, et al., 1957), markedly lower the water content of the brain. This loss of fluids temporarily exceeds the compensatory increase in vessel and spinal-fluid compartments. This temporary invalidity of the Munro-Kellie hypothesis often suffices to bring about a decompression of the brainstem (Lévy, 1961; author's experience) and a normalization of blood supply to the brain (Schmidt, 1963; Steinbereithner, 1963). The abrupt onset of cerebral dehydration due to the actions of diuretics acting solely on the kidneys also casts doubt upon the barrier concept held so far (Hofmann and Reulen, 1963).

Varied experience has shown that acute hypoxic edema responds well to dehydration measures, provided the revival time of the brain has not been surpassed. An optimum effect is achieved by the combination of several agents: Fursemid (Lasix) for rapid induction (Kramer, 1964), Mannitol 25% (Vourch, 1964; Krayenbühl and Bühlmann, 1963), or urea (Rosomoff, 1965; Gött, et al., 1962). Mannito in our view, deserves preference because of the lack of the "rebound-effect" (Shenkin, et al., 1962), and other side effects. Human albumin 20% (Steinbereithner, 1954; Bozza-Marrubini, 1965) is valuable as well as highly concentrated sugar solutions for prolonged therapy.

HYPOXIA IN SEVERE CRANIAL TRAUMA

Our interest is not focused on the acute changes caused by mechanical or central hypoventilation (L'Allemand, 1962), or respiratory disturbances and circulatory failure (Hoff and Jellinger, 1962). With the exception of focal manifestations, they fully correspond to the syndrome discussed above. We rather wish to touch upon a disturbance that has only recently been discussed in greater detail, chronic hypoxia after cranial trauma.

As can be seen in Table 1, patients with cranial trauma as a rule exhibit a considerable reduction in the arterial oxygen tension down to values that correspond to degrees of hypoxia II-III, according to the classification of Lindenschmidt (1953). One case (S. V.), in par ticular, indicates the extent of a period after trauma during which hypoxemia may persist. Attention has been called to general hypoxidosis following cranial trauma especially by Frowein, et al. (1962). In more recent investigations, these authors have arrived at the conclusion that 70 mm mercury is to be considered the critical level of arterial oxygen tension. If pO_2 does not increase with oxygen administration, permanent survival according to our experience cannot be expected (see Table 1; Steinbereithner, 1966).

Closely associated with this syndrome is a phenomenon which we might refer to as "central neurogenic hyperventilation" in accordance with Plum and Swanson (1959). Frowein (1963) made special reference to this polypnea in patients with cranial trauma; almost at the same time, Huange, et al., (1963), were able to show, on the basis of a fairly large series of neurologic trauma cases, that hyperventilation was present in almost all unconscious patients.

TABLE 1

VALUES OF ARTERIAL pO_2 IN CASES OF SEVERE BRAIN TRAUMA

(Intensive Care Unit, I. chirurgische Univ. Klinik Wien)

Patient	Age	Diagnosis	Time of determination (days after trauma)	pO_2 (mmHg)	Oxygen (Tracheotomy + O_2)	Remarks
S. I.	66	Conquassatio cerebri	3	46	+	died
H. A.	17	Conquassatio cerebri	2	62	+	died
E. B.	62	Conquassatio cerebri Diabetes	4	58	+	died
T. H.	52	Conquassation frontal pole	2	61		
Z. T.	68	Contusio cerebri	2, 8, 9, 10	55, 50, 61, 55	+	died
H. R.	25	Subdural haematoma	8, 9, 12, 38, 40, 43	77, 83, 104, 77, 83, 106	+	
D. N.	20	Contusio cerebri, open tibial fracture	2, 3, 8, 10	37, 69, 88, 86	+	in rehabilitation
S. V.	36	Contusio cerebri	2 months	75	+	in rehabilitation
P. C.	20	Meningitis uraemic acidosis		67	+	died

Table 2 compiled from our own patients reveals that hyperventilation alkalosis occurs regularly in cranial trauma and may persist for weeks. As we have been able to show elsewhere (Steinbereithner, 1964) this chronic hyperventilation may occasionally lead to severe metabolic disturbances, the so-called "hyperventilation syndrome," which has a fatal outcome in the majority of cases; (we cannot go into detail here concerning this problem).

Let us now try to discover the causes of this symptom complex. It is known that a lowering of oxygen tension below 80 mm/Hg produces hypoxic hyperventilation. To make aspiration, bronchopneumonia, pre-edema of the lung and atelectasis primarily respon-

TABLE 2

HYPERVENTILATION-ALKALOSIS IN CEREBRAL TRAUMA

(Astrup-analyses: capillary blood ear lobe)

Patient	pH	pCO_2 (mmHg)	Standard-Bicarbonate (mval/l)	Remarks
L. I.	7.47	28.6	22.6	
A. C.	7.49	24.7	21	
K. A.	7.51	26.2	24.6	
L. U.	7.44	31	22.7	
L. V.	7.43	32	23.4	
F. L.	7.45	28	22	
S. V.	7.44	30.2	22.2	2 months after trauma
S. T.	7.44	34.5	23.6	
H. O.	7.44	34.2	23.4	

sible for a decrease in the pO_2 (Frowein, et al., 1964; Maciver, et al., 1958), seems to us an unjustified simplification, since experimental pulmonary edema is invariably associated with hypercapnia (Said, et al., 1964). It seems to be a fact, as we have also been able to show by our own studies, that the cause of hypoxemia lies in the increased admixture of insufficiently arterialized, shunted blood. This shunting in the lungs is favored by anemia (Freeman and Nunn) of central genesis in cranial trauma and also by the pathological type of breathing which is referred to as "machine breathing" (Frowein, 1962), the controlling element of deep breathing being lost (Laver, et al., 1964). Finally, hyperventilation leads to a considerable increase in airway-resistance (Newhouse, et al., 1964).

This brings us again to the hyperventilation phenomenon. Cohen (1964) infers from his investigations that in the region of the posterior diencephalon and superior mesencephalon, those parts of the brain which are mainly involved in an edematous swelling, there is located a control system which increases the frequency of breathing. It is conceivable that hyperventilation should serve to reduce intracranial pressure by diminishing the blood flow through the brain (Lundberg, et al., 1959). This assumption opens up new vistas. It is well known that deficient oxygenation leads to a significant increase in the cerebral blood flow. According to recent investigations, this occurs only at rather low oxygen tension (Harper, 1965). Hypoxemia and brain edema would thus be interrelated. Hyperventilation would then have to be interpreted as the attempt to normalize the cerebral blood flow which was elevated due to oxygen shortage.

These interrelationships, however, seem to be more complicated since, according to Honda, et al. (1963), the decisive impulse for breathing seems to emanate from carbon dioxide even in acute hypoxia (see Harper, 1965) and hypoxemia seems to break the constrictive effect of reduced carbon dioxide tension on the cerebral vessels.

These considerations are only of theoretical interest as long as we know too little of the effects of such changes on the brain itself.

We have tried to come closer to the real situation by determining oxygen tension and acid-base changes not only in the arterial blood but also in the cerebro-spinal fluid. (A nomogram elaborated by Swanson and Rosengren (1962) makes possible the application of the Astrup technique to CSF tests.) In order to be able to draw conclusions as to the intracerebral conditions, we examined, by the method of Gleichmann, et al. (1965), the intracellular acid-base balance on the model of the erythrocyte.

Table 3 was compiled on the basis of hitherto unpublished studies carried out jointly with Wagner and gives two examples of such measurements.

TABLE 3

DETERMINATION OF ACID-BASE-PARAMETERS AND pO_2 IN "CENTRAL" HYPERVENTILATION

Patient		Acid-base-parameters Femoral artery	Erythrocytes	CSF	pO_2 Femoral artery	CSF
D. N.	pH	7.43	7.275	7.31	80	40
	pCO_2	34.3	34.3	38.7		
	St. B.	23	17	18.3		
Z. D.	pH	7.50	7.285	7.35	63	27
	pCO_2	28.5	28.5	36.7		
	St. B.	23.5	16.3	18.8		

With regard to oxygen tension, we found that oxygen tension in the CSF does not diminish below critical values in spite of arterial hypoxemia. Since, according to Bloor, et al. (1961), the pO_2 of the CSF is in balance with the brain, the oxygen content in the brain seems to be adequate. Cater, et al. (1963), found comparable results by direct pO_2 measurements in the gray matter. The hypocapnic shift of the oxygen dissociation curve apparently causes an improvement in the oxygenation of cerebral blood. We must not forget, however, that the Bohr-effect impairs the conditions for the transfer of oxygen to the tissues.

When examining the acid-base balance, we recognize that the carbon dioxide tension of the CSF is diminished but still higher than that of the blood and that, owing to the reduction of bicarbonate, the pH of the CSF is virtually within the normal range. The content in bicarbonate decreases to a level below that of blood, a change which Semple (1965), among others, has pointed out. It is striking that the CSF values (except pCO_2) closely approach the intracellular readings, which suggest an indirect conclusion as to the intracerebral conditions. Summarizing, we may say that in spite of inadequate oxygen saturation and hypocapnia, acidity in the CSF (and probably also in the brain) is maintained at rather constant levels.

Our observations are in agreement with the results of Mitchell, et al. (1965), who found comparable conditions in altitude hypoxia. Pauli (1964) has shown that after altitude stress, even when breathing oxygen, considerable residual hyperventilation persists. A further interesting parallel has emerged from the studies of Kreuzer, et al. (1964); altitude stress in mountain inhabitants leads to increased shunting in the lung and thus to hypoxemia, rather than to improved adjustment of respiration. This has brought us back to the point of departure in our considerations.

We are led to assume that post-traumatic cerebral edema produces acute respiratory changes similar to those of the altitude test but of still obscure genesis. Their manifestations are oxygen deficit in the blood and hyperventilation alkalosis. Since, in spite of this severe aberration, the conditions in the cerebrospinal fluid (and probably also in the brain) are normalized antagonistically, a new hypoxic-hypocapnic state of balance seems to develop. This shift of a central regulating system may persist for weeks and to date has not been amenable to therapy.

It is true that the anesthesiologist may occasionally be able to intervene successfully in acute hypoxia. In severe cranial trauma, however, he often plays a role which Marrubini (1963) has described as "modeste, monotone et peu brillant." We are far from having a satisfactory insight into the patho-physiological relationships, and it will require comprehensive clinico-experimental investigations in order to open up new therapeutic possibilities.

SUMMARY

Since morphological evidence of causal interrelationships between hypoxia and brain edema is rather scanty, the anesthesiologist, by treating acute or chronic hypoxia, finds himself in a situation where clinical results are the only proof of taken measures. But these clinical observations still might contribute to the knowledge of patho-physiologic states inaccessible to experimental procedures.

Referring to symptoms and treatment in a recently observed case of recurring cardiac standstill, the question of acute hypoxic edema is discussed; in spite of contradictory reports in the literature, the existence of this clinical entity is beyond any doubt. The theoretical and clinical problems of dehydration treatment are briefly outlined.

Chronic cerebral hypoxia most regularly is encountered in cerebral trauma; this is not attributable to pulmonary hypoventilation, since in almost every case hyperventilation with respiratory alkalosis ensues. Investigations on acid-base-balance, pCO_2 and pO_2 in blood, erythrocytes and CSF are presented. The prognostic value of these observations is discussed. As to the meaning of the results, some working hypotheses are given. In this type of chronic brain edema, a new hypoxic-hypocapnic steady-state might develop which can outlast the acute lesion for a long time.

REFERENCES

Altmann H. W. and H. Schubothe: Funktionelle und organische Schädigungen des Zentralnervensystems der Katze im Unterdruckexperiment, Beitr. path. Anat, 107, 3-116 (1942).

Argent, D. E. and D. H. P. Cope: Cerebral hypoxia: aetiology and treatment, Brit. Med. J., 1, 593-598 (1956).

Bloor, B. M., J. Fricker, F. R. Hellinger, H. Nishioka and J. J. McCutchen: A study of cerebrospinal fluid oxygen tension, Arch. Neurol., 4, 37-46 (1961).

Bozza-Marrubini, M. L.: Les possibilités actuelles de la réanimation dans les comas consécutifs aux traumatismes craniens, Cah. D'Anesth. 11, 5-29 (1963).

_____: General Anaesthesia for Intracranial Surgery, Brit. J. Anaesth., 37, 268-287 (1965).

Brierley, J. B.: Neuropathological findings in patients dying after open-heart surgery, Thorax, 18, 291-304 (1963).

Büchner, F.: Die pathogenetische Wirkung des allgemeinen Sauerstoffmangels, insbesondere bei der Höhenkrankheit und beim Höhentode, Klin. Wschr. 21, 721-725 (1942).

Buzzard, E. F. and J. G. Greenfield: Quoted by Lucas and Strangeways.

Cater, D. B., D. W. Hill, P. J. Lindop, J. F. Nunn and I. A. Silver: Oxygen washout studies in the anesthetized dog, J. Appl. Physiol., 18, 888-894 (1963).

Clasen, R. A., R. R. Prouty, W. G. Bingham, F. A. Martin and G. M. Hass: Treatment of experimental cerebral oedema with hypertonic glucose, albumin and dextran, Surg. Gyn. Obst., 104, 591-606 (1957).

Cohen, M. I.: Respiratory periodicity in the paralyzed, vagotomized cat: hypocapnic polypnea, Amer. J. Physiol., 206, 845-854 (1964).

Edström, R. F. S. and H. E. Essex: Quoted by Loehning, et al.

Ehrenhaft, J. L., M. A. Claman, J. M. Layton and G. R. Zimmerman: Cerebral complications of open heart surgery: further observations, J. Thorac. Surg., 42, 514-526 (1961).

Freeman, J. and J. F. Nunn: Quoted by Hart.

Frowein, R. A.: Zentrale Atemstörungen bei Schädel-Hirnverletzungen und bei Hirntumoren, Monographien aus dem Gesamtgebiete der Neurologie und Psychiatrie, No. 101, Berlin-Göttingen-Heidelberg: Springer-Verlag (1963).

_____, A. Karinmi and K. H. Euler: Hypoxydose nach schweren Schädel-Hirntraumen, Zbl. Neurochir., 23, 3-11 (1962).

Frowein, R. A., K. H. Euler and A. Karimi-Nejad: Grenzen der Wiederbelebung bei schweren Hirntraumen, Langenb. Arch., 308, 276-281 (1964).

Ganshirt, H.: Die Sauerstoffversorgung des Gehirns und ihre Störung bei Liquordrucksteigerung und Hirnoedem. Berlin-Göttingen-Heidelberg: Springer-Verlag (1957).

Gleichmann, U., H. v. Stuckrad and M. Zindler: Methode zur Bestimmung des intracellulären Säurebasenhaushaltes (pH, pCO_2, Standardbicarbonat, Basenüberschuss) im Erythrocyten, Pflügers Arch., 283, 43-55 (1965).

Gött, U., W. Grte and R. Wüllenweber: Erfahrungen mit Harnstoff als hirndrucksenkender Substanz in der Neurochirugie, Langenb. Arch. 299, 413-422 (1962).

Harley, J. R. S.: The use of hypothermia and dehydration in the treatment of severe cerebral hypoxia, Brit. J. Anaesth., 36, 581-590 (1964).

Harper, A. M.: Physiology of Cerebral Bloodflow, Brit. J. Anaesth., 37, 225-235 (1965).

Hart, S. M.: The anaesthetist and the early management of acute head injuries, Brit. J. Anaesth., 37, 189-198 (1965).

Hoff, H. and K. Jellinger: Das Hirnoedem. Öesterr. Arztezeitg., 17, 207-217 (1962).

Hofmann, H. F. and J. Reulen: Untersuchungen über Wasser- und Elektrolyt-störungen beim experimentellen traumatischen Hirnoedem, Langenb. Arch., 302, 151-158 (1963).

Honda, Y., T. Natsui, N. Hasumura and K. Nakamura: Threshold pCO_2 for respiratory system in acute hypoxia of dogs, J. Appl. Physiol., 18, 1053-1056 (1963).

Huang, C. T., A. W. Cook and H. A. Lyons: Severe Craniocerebral Trauma and Respiratory Abnormalities, Arch. Neurol., 9, 545-554 (1963).

Klatzo, I. and J. Miquel: Quoted by Harley.

Kramer, G.: Zur medikamentösen Regulierung des Wasserhaushaltes beim Hirnoedem, Med. Welt, 1964, 2238-2244 (1964).

Krayenbühl, H. and A. Bühlmann: Le facteurs osmotiques et l'osmothérapie, in: L'Odème Cérébral (ed. by G. Lazorthes and L. Campan). Paris: Masson, pp. 146-154 (1963).

Kreuzer, F., S. M. Tenney, J. C. Mithoefer and J. Remmers: Alveolar-arterial oxygen gradient in Andean natives at high altitude, J. Appl. Physiol., 19, 13-16 (1964).

Kucher, R. and K. Steinbereithner: Zur Frage der intra- und postoperativen Hirnanoxie, Brun's Beitr. Klin. Chir., 185, 207-225 (1952).

L'Allemand, H.: Pathophysiologie, Klinik and Therapie der postop. Ateminsuffizienz. Fortbildungskurse 1. Europ. Kongr. Anaesth., German Section 3, Wien (1962).

Laver, M. B., J. Morgan, H. H. Bendixen and E. P. Radford: Lung volume, compliance and arterial oxygen tensions during controlled ventilation, J. Appl. Physiol., 19, 725-733 (1964).

Lévy, A.: Zur Therapie der akuten zerebralen Einklemmung. Dtsch. Med. Wschr., 86, 2280-2283 (1961).

Lindenschmidt, T. O.: Der Sauerstoffpartialdruck des arteriellen Blutes bei chirurgischen Lungenerkrankungen, Thoraxchir., 1, 65-74 (1953).

Loehning, R. W., H. Ueyama and I. Ueda: Brain volume studies in animals: Effects of Hypercardia, hypoxia and intravenous urea, Anaesth. Analg. Curr. Res., 41, 529-537 (1962).

Lucas, B. G. B. and D. H. Strangeways: The effect of intermittent anoxia on the brain. J. Path. Bact., 64, 265-271 (1952).

Lundberg, N., A. Kjällquist and C. Bien: Reduction of Increased Intercranial Pressure by Hyperventilation, Acta Psychiat. Scand. 34, (Suppl. 139), 5-57 (1959).

Maciver, I. N., I. J. C. Frew and J. G. Matheson: The Role of Respiratory Insufficiency in the Mortality of Severe Head Injuries, Lancet, 1, 390-393 (1958).

Mitchell, R. A., C. T. Carman, J. W. Severinghaus, B. W. Richardson, M. M. Singer and S. Shinder: Stability of cerebrospinal fluid pH in chronic acid-base disturbances in blood, J. Appl. Physiol., 20, 443-452 (1965).

Mollaret, P. and M. Goulon: Le coma dépassé (Mémoire préliminaire), Rev. Neurol., 101, 3-15 (1959).

Newhouse, M. T., M. R. Becklake, P. T. Macklem and M. McGregor:

Effect of alterations in end-tidal CO_2 - tension on flow resistance, J. Appl. Physiol., 19, 745-749 (1964).
Opitz, E. and W. Thorn: Überlebenszeit und Erholungszeit des Warmblütergehirns unter dem Einfluss der Höhenanpassung, Pflüg. Arch. 251, 369-387 (1949).
Pauli, H. G.: Die respiratorische Säure-Basen-Regulation in Physiologie und Klinik, Basel-Stuttgart: Schwabe (1964).
Plum, F. and A. G. Swanson: Central neurogenic hyperventilation in man, Arch. Neurol. Psychiat., 81, 535-549 (1959).
Rosomoff, H. L.: Adjuncts to neurosurgical anaesthesia, Brit. J. Anaesth., 37, 246-261 (1965).
Said, S. I., J. W. Longacher, R. K. Davis, C. M. Banerjee, W. M. Davis and W. J. Wooddell: Pulmonary gas exchange during induction of pulmonary edema in anesthetized dogs, J. Appl. Physiol., 19, 403-407 (1964).
Schmidt, K.: Zur Wirkung einiger Osmotherapeutica, Anaesthesist, 12, 216-222 (1963).
Semple, S. J. G.: Respiration and the cerebrospinal fluid, Brit. J. Anaesth., 37, 262-267 (1965).
Shenkin, H. A., B. Goluboff and H. Haft: The use of Mannitol for the reduction of intracranial pressure in intracranial surgery, J. Neurosurg., 19, 897-900 (1962).
Swanson, A. G. and H. Rosengren: Cerebrospinal fluid buffering during acute experimental respiratory acidosis, J. Appl. Physiol. 17, 812-814 (1962).
Steinbereithner, K.: Neue Möglichkeiten parenteraler Eiweisstherapie, Wien Klin. Wschr., 66, 406-408 (1954).
_____: Die Bedeutung der Anaesthesiologie bei Schädel-Hirntraumen, Wien. Klin. Wschr., 75, 457-460 (1963).
_____: Probleme des Stoffwechselgleichgewichtes bei Intensiv-Pflegepatienten (Vortr. Sitzg. Ges. D. Arzte in Wien), Wien. Klin. Wschr. (4.12. 1964), 77, 967-969 (1965).
_____: Blutgasanalysen in der täglichen Anaesthesiepraxis, Proc. 2nd Postgrad. Course Clin. Anaesth., pp. 103-142 (Wien) (28.5-3. 6. 1965).
_____: Zur Überwachung und Bilanzierung von Intensiv-Pflegepatienten, Klin. Med., 21, 410-413 (1966).
Stubbs, J. and J. Pennybacker: Reduction of intracranial pressure with hypertonic urea, Lancet, 1, 1094-1097 (1960).
Vourc'h G.: Utilisation des solutés de mannitol à 25 p.100 en clinique, Acta d'Anesthésiologie, 13, 113-147 (1964).
Williams, G. R. and F. C. Spencer: The clinical use of hypothermia following cardiac arrest, Ann. Surg. 148, 462-466 (1958).

JAN GLOWACKI

BRAIN EDEMA AS THE ANATOMICAL SUBSTRATE OF SUPRATENTORIAL CEREBRAL PSEUDOTUMORS

The clinical syndrome of intracranial hypertension which simulates brain tumor was initially described by Nonne in 1904. Nonne (23) at first assumed it to be a neurological entity of an unknown origin. A few months after the publication of Nonne's article, however, Reichardt (29) introduced the concept that "Hirnschwellung" or "brain-swelling" which could well explain the symptoms of intracranial hypertension in so-called cerebral pseudotumor. For the next twenty years numerous papers appeared in which the authors searched for the anatomical substrate suggested by Nonne (30, 13, 43, 36, 27, 38, 2, 12, 25).

During the last sixty years the concept of "pseudotumor cerebri" has evolved through serous meningitis (26, 8), otitic hydrocephalus (37), toxic hydrocephalus (21), sinus thrombosis (28), to reach the current name "brain swelling of unknown causes" (31, 32). This terminological confusion was chiefly caused by the lack of objective diagnostic criteria. The application of ventriculography proved a turning-point in this field. Vincent's observation (40) in 1933 that in cases of pseudotumor the cerebral ventricles are smaller than average, without displacement or deformation is still valid. In cases showing clinical pseudotumor symptoms, he found anatomically "large, heavy brains with small ventricles," which in neuropathological terms indicates a generalized cerebral edema.

In 1937, Dandy, in a series of 22 cases of cerebral pseudotumors examined by ventriculography and treated by decompression, assumed brain edema or changes in the cerebral vascular bed with a background of vasomotor disturbances to be the alternative causes of intracranial hypertension. Since Dandy's (11) publication, most of those interested in the problem of cerebral pseudotumors have assumed that the symptoms of intracranial hypertension simulating brain tumor are caused by brain edema (15, 31, 4, 41, 32, 7, 3, 34, 24, 6, 16, 18). It is also known that intracranial events of establishe(origin, such as thrombi of the cerebral arteries, veins, and venous sinuses, or the appearnce of symptoms of intracranial hypertension in obese women with hormonal disturbances are caused by brain ede ma (22, 14, 24, 44, 33, 19). This has been confirmed at operation and histopathologically. In some cases of cerebral pseudotumor recently described in the course of treatment with corticosteroids (9, 35, 42) or with hyper-vitaminosis A, and also in connection with "Stalinon" (organic tin compound) poisoning affair which occurred a few years ago in France, symptoms of intracranial hypertension caused by brain edema were manifested. In these cases edema was the only pathological finding (1, 10).

With regard to this problem, I have examined fourteen anatomically verified cases with a clinical picture of cerebral pseudotumor in the Neuropathological Institute, Antwerp, Belgium.

In 3 cases operated on for symptoms of cerebral tumor brain edema was found at operation, while at post-mortem concentric multiple sclerosis of the Baló type was shown. Histopathological examinations also showed features of brain edema in these cases (Figs. 1, 2).

Ten cases verified at post-mortem as van Bogaert's leucoencephalitis sclerotisans subacuta (LESS) were examined. They had clinical course characterized by headache, vomiting, papilledema; the cerebrospinal fluid showed no signs of inflammation but the pres sure was increased. These cases showed the complex of symptoms which is usually regarded as characteristic of the cerebral pseudotumor syndrome.

This material also includes van Bogaert and de Busscher's (39) "cas princeps" of LESS in 1937 in which at first a glioma of the parietal lobe was clinically suspected. An exploratory craniotomy was performed to make certain, but this showed only a marked degree of brain edema (Fig. 3).

Histopathologically, brain edema was found in each of these cases. It varied in intensity, the degree of which depended on the stage of the disease at which the brain was examined post-mortem (Figs. 3-5). In one case in which death occurred after two and a half years, diffuse atrophy as a sequel to edema was found at the time of post-mortem examination. The correlation between this condition and the clinical picture was shown by the regression of the symptoms of intracranial hypertension and the transition to papilledema with atrophy of the optic disc.

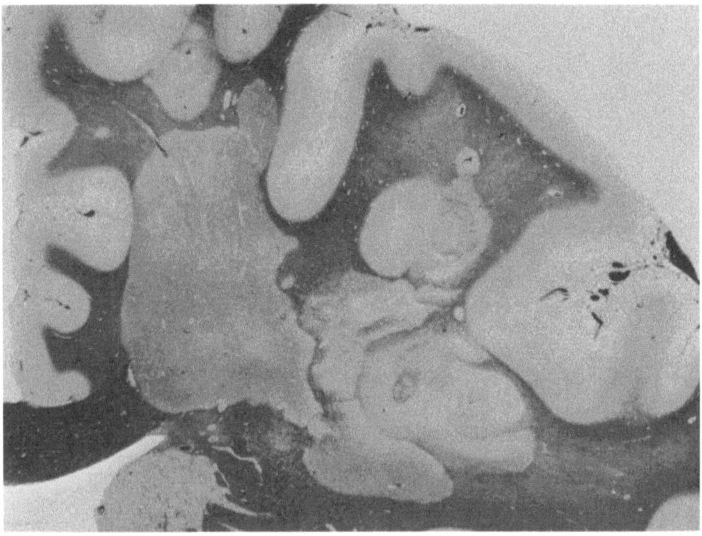

Fig. 1. Case No. 3 of concentric sclerosis of Baló type. Diffuse brain edema. Demyelinisation with aspect of "transsection oi agathe," "en tranche d'agathe." Celloidin, met. Woelke-Heidenhain.

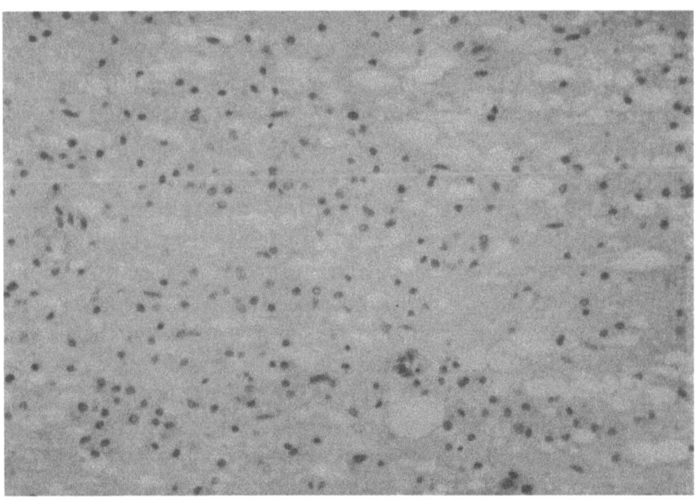

Fig. 2. Microspongiotic aspect of the white matter. Paraff., Hemat. Eosin.

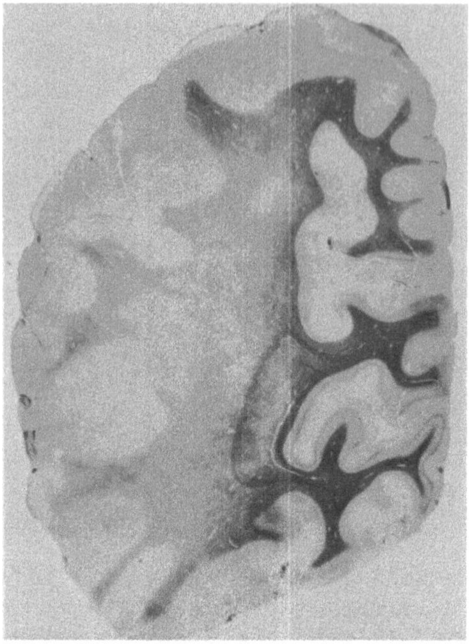

Fig. 3. "Cas princeps of LESS," van Bogaert et de Busscher. Diffuse brain edema. Celloidin, met. Woelke-Heidenhain.

In a group of endocrinogenic pseudotumors, one case of hypoparathyroidism was observed. This developed a year after an operation on the thyroid and was manifested by intracranial hypertension among other symptoms. Death ensued from subtentorial herniation and the herniation of the cerebellar tonsils into the vertebral canal; diffuse edema of the cerebral hemispheres was revealed at post-mortem.

These observations are in complete agreement with those of the authors mentioned: the symptoms of intracranial hypertension simulating a supratentorial cerebral tumor are caused by brain edema independently of the provoking cause.

It should be emphasized that there are distinct differences between supratentorial cerebral pseudotumors, characterized by small ventricles compressed by diffuse edema, and subtentorial pseudotumors, which on the contrary are manifested by internal hydrocephalus caused not by edema of the cerebellum but most frequently by adhesions around the cisterns at the base of the brain, the Dandy-Walker syndrome, sometimes by subarachnoidal cysts, etc.

The name "pseudotumor cerebri" introduced by Nonne has often been criticized (17, 4, 20, 16). This criticism seems to be only

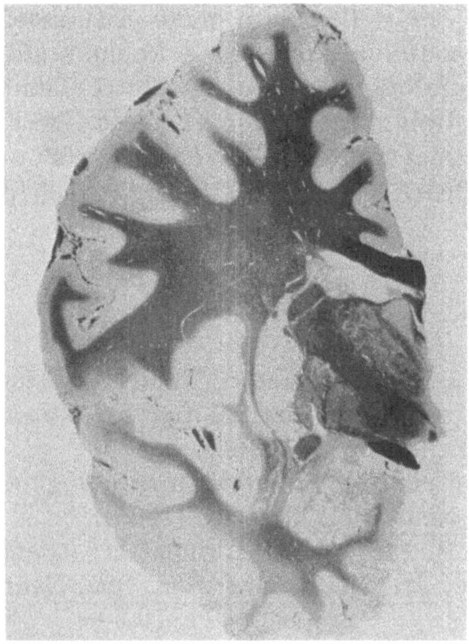

Fig. 4. Case No. 9 of LESS. Diffuse brain edema. Cell., met. Woelke-Heidenhain.

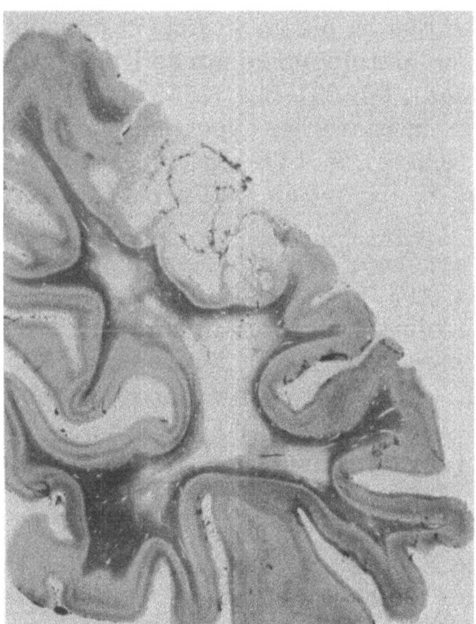

Fig. 5. Case No. 10 of LESS. Diffuse brain atrophy following edema. Necrotic fibers in centrum of Meynert are better preserved. Freezing, met. Spielmeyer.

partially justified, but if I were to make still another attempt at nomenclature, it would only be to give Nonne's old name a new twist emphasizing the etiological role of cerebral edema as an anatomical substrate of this clinical syndrome. I would like to propose for the group of cases of supratentorial cerebral pseudotumors the new name, OEDEMA CEREBRI PSEUDOTUMORALE (pseudotumoral brain edema).

REFERENCES

1. Alajouanine Th., Dérobert and S. Thieffry: Étude clinique d'ensemble de 210 cas d'intoxications par les sels organiques d'étain, Rev. Neurol., 98, 85-96 (1958).
2. Bailey, P.: Contribution to the histopathology of pseudotumor cerebri, Arch. Neur., 43, 401-416 (1920).
3. Belloni, G. B., P. Frugoni, G. Campailla: L'encephalopatia pseudotumorale, Atti XIII Congr. Soz. Ital. Neurol., Messina, 559-596 (1959).
4. Caesar, K. G.: Über Erkankungen, die unter dem Bilde einer Hirngeschwülst verlaufen, mit besonderer Berücksichtigung des sog: pseudotumor cerebri, Arch. Psychiat., 113, 655-676 (1941).
5. Chavany, J. A. and R. Messimy: L'hemiplegie recidivante in situ dans la sclerose en plaques. Aspect pseudofocal de la maladie. Vérifications histologiques après l'intervention exploratrice, Presse Méd., 66, 531-534 (1958).
6. Capriles, L. F.: Intracranial hypertension and iron deficiency anemia, Arch. Neurol., 9, 147-153 (1963).
7. Cardona, F. and F. Barontini: Sul problema dello pseudotumore cerebrale, Riv. Patol. Nerv. Ment., 78, 875-888 (1957).
8. Claude, H.: L'arachnoido – piermerite sereuse cérébrale, Rev. Neurol., 40, 824 (1933).
9. Cohn, G.: Pseudotumor cerebri in children secondary to administration of adrenal steroids, J. Neurosurg., 20, 784-786 (1963).
10. Cossa, P. et al.: Encéphalopathies toxiques au Stalinon, Rev. Neuröl., 98, 97-108 (1958).
11. Dandy, W.: Intracranial pressure without brain tumor, Ann. Surg., 106, 492-513 (1937).
12. Fairbanks: 1922, cited by Puusepp (1926).
13. Finkelnburg and Eschbaum: Zur Kenntnis der sog. Pseudotumor cerebri mit anatomischen Befund, D. Zeit. Nervenheilk., 38, 35-67 (1910).
14. Foley, J.: Benign form of intracranial hypertension, Brain, 78, 1-41 (1955).
15. Ford, F. R. and E. L. Murphy: Increased intracranial pressure. Clinical analysis of the causes and characteristics of several

types, Bull. J. Hopkins Hosp., 64, 369-398 (1939).
16. Frick, E.: Pseudotumor cerebri mit Stauungspapille, Münch. Med. Wchschr., 105, 493-498 (1963).
17. Glettenberg, O.: Pseudotumor of the cerebrum, Zbltt. f. Neurochir., 2, 357 (1937).
18. Goebell, H.: Die Stauungspapille unklarer Genese. Ein Beitrag zum Bild des "Pseudotumor cerebri," Fort. Neurol. Psych., 32, 265-279 (1964).
19. Joynt, R. J. and A. L. Sahs: Endocrine studies in Pseudotumor cerebri, Tr. Am. Neurol. Ass., 87, 10-13 (1962).
20. Kehrer, F.: Zur Frage des "Pseudotumor cerebri," D. Zeit. Nervenheilk., 160, 1-9 (1949).
21. McAlpine, D.: Toxic hydrocephalus, Brain, 60, 180 (1937).
22. McCullagh, E. P.: Menstrual edema with intracranial hypertension (pseudotumor cerebri), Clev. Clin. Quart., 8, 202-212
23. Nonne, M.: Über Fälle vom Symptomenkomplex "Tumor cerebri" mit Ausgang in Heilung (Pseudotumor cerebri): Uber letal verlaufene Fälle von "Pseudotumor cerebri" mit Sektionsbefund, D. Zeit. Nervenheilk., 27, 169-216 (1904).
24. Paterson, Ruth, N. De Pasquale and S. Mann: Pseudotumor cerebri, Medicine, Baltimore, 40, 85-99 (1961).
25. Puusepp, L.: Pseudo-tumoren des Gehirns, Fol. Neuropath. Eston., 6, 31-48 (1926).
26. Quinke, H.: Uber meningitis serosa, D. Zeit. Nervenheilk., 9, 149 (1897).
27. Ranke and Nissl: cited by Bailey (1920).
28. Ray, B. S. and H. S. Dunbar: Thrombosis of dural venous sinuses as cause of "pseudotumor cerebri," Ann. Surg., 134, 376-386 (1951).
29. Reihardt, M.: Zur Entstehung des Hirndrucks bei Hirngeschwülsten und anderen Hirnkrankheiten und über eine bei diesen zu beobachtende besondere art von Hirnschwellung, D. Zeit. Nervenheilk., 28, 306-355 (1905).
30. Rosenthal, St.: Histologische Befunde beim sog. Pseudotumor cerebri, Zeit. f. ges. Neurol. Psych., 7, 162-178 (1911).
31. Sahs, A. L. and O. R. Hyndman: Intracranial hypertension of unknown cause: cerebral edema, Arch. Surg., 38, 428 (1939).
32. Sahs, A. L. and R. J. Joynt: Brain swelling of unknown cause, Neurology, 6, 791-803 (1956).
33. Sànchez, Juan J., et al.: Seudotumores cerebrales con obesidad "Z" (sindrome de Zondek), Rev. Clin. Españ., 67, 92-101 (1957).
34. Sluga-Gasser, E., W. Sluga and H. Tschabitscher: H. Über Pseudotumor cerebri, Wien. Zeit. Nervenheilk., 17, 398-409 (1960).
35. Songo, N.: Pseudotumor cerebri associated with corticosteroid administration, Exc. Med. Neur. Psych., ref. no. 5657 (1963).

36. Spielmeyer: cited by Bailey (1920).
37. Symmonds, C. P.: Otitic Hydrocephalus, Brain, 54, 55-71 (1931).
38. Urechia, C. I.: Pseudo-tumeur par intumescence aiguë du cerveau, Rev. Neur., 36, 1185-1190 (1920).
39. Van Bogaert, L. and J. De Busscher: Sur la sclérose inflammatoire de la substance blance des hémispheres (Spielmeyer). Contribution à l'étude scléroses diffuses non familiales, Rev. Neurol 71, 679-701 (1939).
40. Vincent, C., M. David and P. Puech: Sur la ventriculographie dans certaines pseudotumeurs du cerveau, Rev. Neurol., 40, 1060-1069 (1933).
41. Wagener, H. P.: Pseudotumor cerebri, Am. J. Med. Sci., 227, 214-225 (1954).
42. Walker, A. E. and J. J. Adamkiewicz: Pseudotumor cerebri associated with prolonged corticosteroid therapy, J. A. M. A., 188, 779-784 (1964).
43. Yamakawa: (1913), cited by Bailey (1920).
44. Zondek: (1955), cited by Sanchez-Juan (1957).

DISCUSSION

EVANS: Has Dr. Glowacki's enthusiasm for neurosurgical treatment diminished on the basis of his studies? In other words, what does he now suggest as a neurosurgical approach to pseudotumors?

GLOWACKI: The extensive repertory of diagnostic methods now used in neurosurgery enables an earlier and more accurate diagnosis of cerebral tumors and the necessity of surgical treatment can be eliminated in cases of cerebral pseudotumors. We are in an incomparably better situation than our colleagues of half a century ago, who treated such cases (sometimes with good results) with mercury and iodine ointments. In spite of this progress, however, some cases of cerebral pseudotumor still present a specific diagnostic and therapeutic problem. Even today, in spite of all our diagnostic resources, we are sometimes forced to open the skull for fear of overlooking a tumor. I remember a case described in 1958 by Chavany and Messimy of Paris, in which three diagnostic methods (angiography, EEG and gamma-encephalography) all indicated a parietal tumor. In this situation fractional encephalography was not even performed, for the site and the nature of the disturbance seemed obvious. An exploratory craniotomy was performed, and the pathology was found to be multiple sclerosis which had been clinically suspected.

Exploratory craniotomy remains the method of choice in the final decision for doubtful cases or palliative treatment. Naturally, this should only be performed in cases of cerebral pseudotumor when such means as osmotically active drugs for combating brain edema have failed, or when the use of such drugs is impossible and decompression becomes a vital necessity.

KRAUS: Dr. Glowacki, what type of decompression are you doing? What procedure?

GLOWACKI: In cases of pseudotumoral brain edema which cannot be effectively treated by modern osmotically active drugs, and especially in urgent cases with imminent cerebral herniation we perform a decompressive craniotomy: a large osteoplastic flap on the right site, with large opening of the dura mater, and sometimes, if necessary, with removal of the bone flap.

STEINBEREITHNER: Concerning the interesting cases Dr. Earl Walker talked about, namely brain edema after corticosteroid therapy, I would like to ask a question. If one treats adults with corticosteroids for a prolonged period, there is a fall in serum potassium. It has not been stressed that hypopotassaemia produces a rather severe metabolic alkalosis and the mechanism by which this is corrected normally is respiratory acidosis, i.e., by use of the pCO_2. Elevated pCO_2, of course, dilates the brain vessels and that could be one cause of brain edema in those children. Secondly, the potassium pool in children is lower than in the adult; therefore the ion-pumps, especially in the cerebral cells, could become deranged. Were there any investigations done in this respect?

KATZMAN: I would like to ask an additional question of Dr. Walker as to whether there could be an element of water intoxication in these children with the somewhat high normal sodium during steroid therapy, and then a low, perhaps slightly subnormal, sodium after steroid therapy. This would still result in quite a difference in the total osmolarity of the serum before and after the steroid therapy.

DAVSON: Could I just ask is the condition of edema is proved in this case or is it merely a case of raised intracranial tension?

GRASHCHENKOV: Unfortunately I had no opportunity to prepare any slides for demonstration, but my laboratory investigated brain edema with several biochemical methods. For instance, we studied, during closed traumatic lesions of the brain, adrenalin-like substances, epinephrine, norepinephrine and the level of histamine, acetylcholine, as well as some dynamic 17-keto-steroids, potassium, and sodium; these studies gave us some information and some results concerning the pathogenesis of the brain edema, and some hints for the therapy which we use in such conditions. I would like to stress only one point: biochemical methods will be very useful in the study of the mechanism of brain edema and in the evaluation of therapeutic measures against this disorder.

WALKER: First I would like to express my appreciation to the discussors for raising these interesting problems. I think it is possible that a factor of alkalosis might be responsible for some of the cases of increased pressure which we have seen in children. However, the values of potassium and sodium have been within normal limits. The same is true of the pCO_2. The question as to whether there is truly a cerebral edema in these cases or simply an increased intracranial pressure is one which is difficult to answer absolutely. If one does a pneumoencephalogram these cases do show a decrease in the size of the ventricular system, and if one estimates the amount of intracranial fluids, spinal fluid and ventricular fluid, it seemed to us that there was approximately 20 cc less space occupied by these fluids than under normal circumstances, and we assumed that this was due to cerebral swelling, but the exact nature of this is not clear. However, it does seem that the volume of the brain is greater than normal.

FONCIN: With reference to brain hypoxia and especially hypoxic brain swelling: I think that many electron microcopists, like myself, do have such pictures, but they do not like to show them, because they are not pretty at all, and too similar to artefacts due to delayed fixation.

LOWENTHAL: I would like to put a question to Dr. Glowacki. In his case of pseudotumor with hypoparathyroidism, had he also calcification in the basal ganglia, and could he comment on the 3 or 4 cases found in the literature of papilledema and calcification of the basal ganglia?

GLOWACKI: Yes, Doctor Lowenthal, in our case of hypoparathyroidism with pseudotumoral clinical picture (papilledema, highly increased CSF pressure), there were only fine calcifications around small vessels of the basal ganglia bilaterally, and not the picture as seen in Fahr's disease.

LEE: I would like to make a comment on Dr. Steinbereithner's interesting paper on hypoxic edema. In our experience, hypoxia alone does not produce brain edema, but a combination of hypoxia and hypercapnia does. Since Dr. Steinbereithner did not present any histological slide or electron micrograph to substantiate the presence of edematous changes, I wonder if his criterion of brain edema might indicate an increase in the intracranial pressure caused by factors other than a real cerebral edema.

BAKAY: We did a number of experiments in animals to study various parameters of hypoxia with particular relation to hypoxic swelling of the brain, and whatever animal we used under whatever circumstances, we found that pure anoxia, i.e., a decrease in oxygenization of brain tissue with normal CO_2 elimination and no venous congestion, did not result in cerebral edema as defined by increased water content and increased volume of the brain. This occured only when hypoxia was combined with hypercapnia. With the combination of these two factors, true cerebral edema occurred, which again did not occur on CO_2 inhalation alone unless an enormous inhalation of CO_2 took place, e.g., if an animal is given 50% of CO_2. Under 10 or 20% of CO_2 inhalation we found venous congestion, an increase of intracranial pressure due to venous congestion, but not true cerebral edema.

HOFF: I am quite certain that hypoxia of the brain alone does not produce cerebral edema, otherwise many more people would suffer from brain edema. Hypoxia is just one important component in the syndrome causing brain edema. For the development of traumatic and posttraumatic edema, but not of all the other types of brain edema, systemic blood pressure must be lowered and there must be a combination of circulatory and metabolic disturbances. If these factors combine, brain edema develops, but not only as the result of hypoxia alone. I think that this holds only for traumatic brain edema, and I am sure that there are other kinds of cerebral edema, because I believe what we call toxic edema is something different. Therefore, I think that our findings in traumatic brain edema cannot be transferred to toxic brain edema as well.

KRAUS: Are there any further questions on Dr. Steinbereithner's paper?

WOLMAN: I would like to ask one question. Almost all speakers, including the author of the paper we are discussing, have assumed that brain edema is the cause of the clinical symptoms. Now, we know one mechanism by which edema can cause various clinical symptoms and that is by various herniations. For all other cases I wonder whether brain edema is the cause or the effect of damage which has been done. I don't know whether there is any evidence that compression, increased pressure per se will cause damage. As a matter of fact, we can bring people down to 5 atmospheres of pressure in a bell, and if the relation between the gases is correct they do not suffer any damage, although increased pressure is also acting on the nerve cells, the white matter, etc. So my question is this. Is there any clinical evidence that brain edema per se is a damaging agent in a short experiment?

ZIMMERMAN: In view of what Dr. Wolman just said, I would like to cite the experiments that we had done quite a number of years ago. These apply to what Dr. Steinbereithner had mentioned in relation to the deleterious effect of the barbiturates on the system that you have described. In experiments with hypoglycemia that we had done years ago in animals, no cerebral edema was produced, but the lowering of the blood sugar levels below critical points produced extensive cerebral destruction. We found that barbiturates on top of lowered hypoglycemic states had a marked deleterious effect. Evidently the suppression of respiration and the alteration of the oxygen-CO_2 ratio produced further depression of cerebral metabolism to the point of affecting deleteriously the ganglion cell structure in the nervous system. And edema, as far as we were able to determine at that time, played no role in this state of affairs.

KRAUS: Somebody else? Dr. Steinbereithner, would you answer, please?

STEINBEREITHNER: First to Dr. Lee. I quite agree that this is the main point of the whole problem. I think at least one group of investigators tried to solve this question, namely Loehning, et al. (1962), in the USA; These anaesthetists made the following experiments: they cannulated the third ventricle in order to abolish a rise in cerebrospinal-fluid pressure. Secondly, they sealed off the spinal cord with paraffin to avoid the pressure increase in the vertebral vessels and filled also the cisternae with paraffin. Then they exposed the animals to anoxia. There is an initial rise in intracerebral pressure, which is mainly attributable to increased filling of the brain vessels. But after a delay of about 15-20 minutes, when hypoxia had ceased and the animals were breathing oxygen, "real" brain swelling ensued, as they think, and from a clinical point of view I should also say that it was brain swelling or brain edema, whatever you might call it. In our clinical situation it is of no great importance which of the 3 components of the Monroe-Kellie hypothesis is involved. That brings me to Professor Wolman's question, that brain edema might not only be a sequel but also a cause of cerebral hypoxia. In the cases of brain-stem herniation, we encountered what I think was, beyond any doubt, an acute post-hypoxic edema. May I also thank Professor Hoff for his kind assistance in this respect?

May I then answer Professor Zimmerman? The German school of aviation medicine has abandoned the term "hypoxia" and accepted instead the term "hypoxidosis." Hypoxidosis does not only mean oxygen deficit but also hypoglycemia. (Kety and Smith have shown a long time ago that this depresses cerebral metabolism.) Also the ischemic component which ensues in cardiac standstill is not only "hypoxia" as we use that word in a slogan-like way, but rather and more correctly "hypoxidosis."

Now to Professor Bakay: I would have preferred to discuss this question after his paper because his results and ours are rather contradictory in this respect. If I am informed correctly, Professor Bakay uses RIHSA for demonstrating penetration of proteins in brain edema. He states that not only lowered pO_2 but also raised pCO_2 is necessary to increase penetration. May I now show 2 slides which might contradict his opinion? There is a rather severe post-operative hypoxemia after simple operations such as cholecystectomy. Figure 1 (adapted from a paper of Nunn and Payne) shows that after such operations, for about 24 hours pO_2 is rather low, almost at critical levels, whereas pCO_2, the main point in which we differ from Professor Bakay, is almost normal. The same values have been found by the group of Gordh, et al., in Stockholm and by Rodewald in Hamburg.

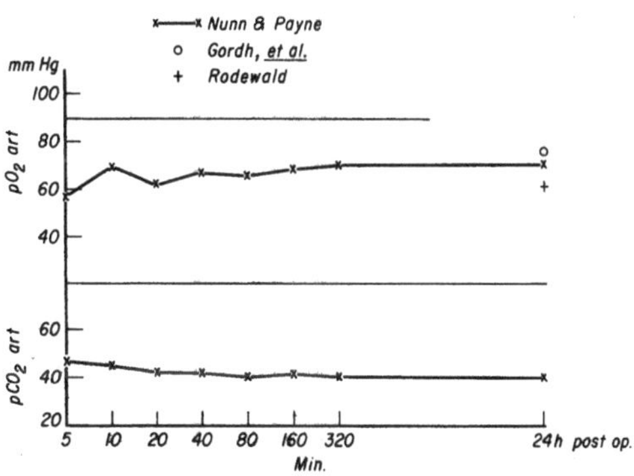

Fig. 1. Postoperative arterial blood-gas values.

We tried now to evaluate whether giving oxygen in those circumstances is of any value by measuring the disappearance rate of iodinated human albumin. (Fig. 2.) Preoperatively there is a loss from the intravascular space of about 8% after 1 hour. After surgery without oxygen disappearance rate rises above 18%. Under oxygen the loss is much lower, about 12% which is near normal. Although pCO_2 is not elevated in these cases, capillary permeability (and this permits us to draw conclusions as to the conditions in the brain) may seriously be impaired by hypoxia alone.

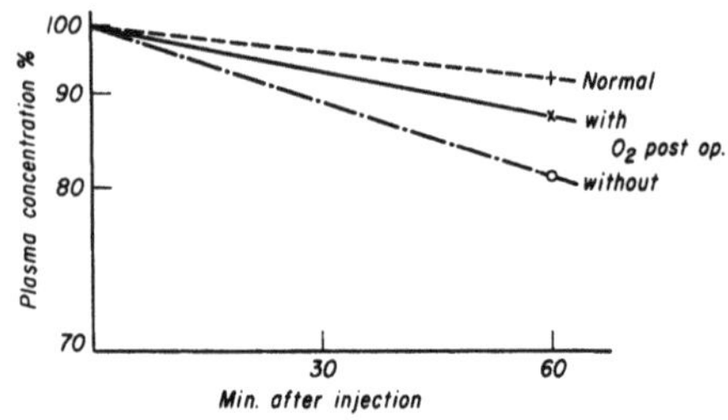

Fig. 2. Decrease of tracer-activity in the circulation (% of initial value) according to Boehmig, et al.

REFERENCES

Boehmig, H. J., G. Fraundorfer, and K. Steinbereithner: Wien, Klin. Wschr. 1964, 172.

Gordh, T., H. Linderholm, and O. Norlander: Acta anaesth. Scand. 2, 15 (1958).

Loehning, R. W., H. Ueyama, and I. Ueda: Anesth. Analg. Curr. Res. 41, 529 (1962).

Rodewald, G.: Langenb. Arch. klin. Chir. 301, 532 (1962)

II. Brain Edema in Human Pathology

Chairman: ***W. H. McMenemey***

K. J. ZÜLCH

NEUROPATHOLOGICAL ASPECTS AND HISTOLOGICAL CRITERIA OF BRAIN EDEMA AND BRAIN SWELLING

SOME OBSERVATIONS ON EXPERIMENTAL MODELS OF BRAIN EDEMA

In the beginning of my talk I would like to recall the names of three men: first, Martin Reichardt, who in his 91st year spiritually plays a great part in our discussion and has in particular inspired the discussion of our subject by his separation of primary brain swelling from brain edema. Reichardt, in measuring skull capacity and weighing brains and thus formulating the skull-brain-index, came to the conclusion that there must be an increase of volume other than that produced by brain edema and apart from tumor, or hemorrhage which could easily be excluded. He recognized the brain edema when free fluid came from the slices of a recently cut brain, when there was a subsequent loss of weight of brain slices and when the bleeding points on the wet surface were obscured. In other cases when the brain appeared dry, without loss of fluid and with preservation of bleeding points, he spoke of brain swelling. I shall come back to his distinction of brain swelling and brain edema later on.

Secondly, speaking here in Vienna I would like to mention the name of the anatomist Obersteiner, the founder and first director of the "Anatomisches Institut." His description of the pericellular and pericapillary spaces has up to now given rise to discussion about their pathogenesis. His figures of the glia sheaths around the capillaries in 1896 can hardly be surpassed by modern impregnations of the astroglia. Lastly, we should mention the late professor of internal medicine, Hans Eppinger, whose books on "Seröse Enzündung" and "Permeabilitätspathologie" are still relevant to us because in spite of the special characteristics dependent upon the blood-brain barrier, brain edema is only a local example of abnormal permability.

HISTORICAL DEVELOPMENT OF THE PROBLEM OF EDEMA AND SWELLING

At the commencement of our discussion it is necessary to have a precise definition based on concepts familiar to all of us. Otherwise, our discourse must inevitably remain full of misunderstandings. If we cannot agree with a contemporary definition of edema, we must adopt a new terminology, because otherwise we will have misunderstanding. I, therefore, must first emphasize here what the general pathologist understands by "brain edema." It is to him "a saturation of the tissues with water which has penetrated into the tissue spaces from within the vessels."

Edema in the brain was well described by Anton and by Schmauss at the end of the last century. They were even able to describe histologically the transudate around the veins (Anton). In contrast to this brain edema so clearly defined and described in neuropathology, Reichardt in 1905 introduced the concept of brain swelling in which there was an increase in the volume of the brain, but with a "dry" cut surface. Brain swelling according to him was predominantly localized to the white matter. Histologically it was not possible to demonstrate a free perivascular fluid. Reichardt had shown that primary brain swelling was particularly likely to occur in psychiatric disorders as, for example, in catatonic schizophrenia and also in intoxications.

I will refrain from going into detail on the later historical development of our knowledge of the process in the human brain during the last century and will mention only the work of Alzheimer and Rosenthal, Jaburek, Schaltenbrand and Bailey, Spatz, Scheinker, Schürmann, Jacob, Scholz, Stämmler and co-workers, Greenfield, Alajouanine and Hornet and the groups working with Tönnis (for references, see Zülch, 1943, 1953, 1957).

In discussing the pathogenesis the German neuropathologists in particular came to the conclusion that in brain swelling there was an intra-cellular increase in volume, whereas in brain edema there was an inter-cellular accumulation of fluid, and thus an increase of volume (Fig. 1).

This distinction between brain swelling and brain edema remained through several decades a problem solely of German neuropathology. Only in the 1930's did the schools of other countries begin to occupy themselves with the distinction between brain edema

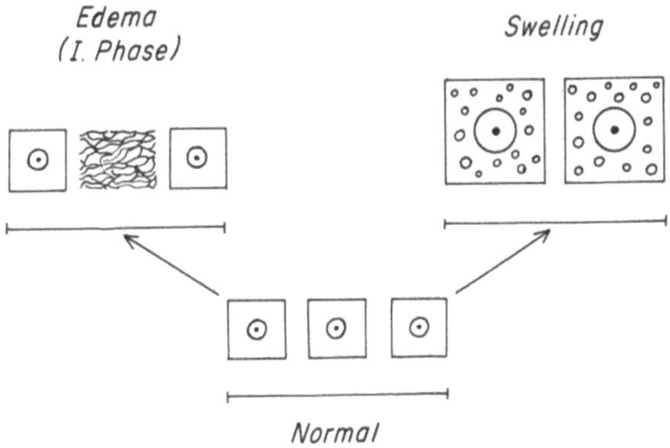

Fig. 1. Drawing showing increase in volume from "edema" (intercellular accumulation of fluid) or "swelling" (intracellular increase in fluid or protein).

and brain swelling, and even then the dominating concept remained that of brain edema. Only a few references were made to brain swelling. Greenfield in his report in 1952 in Rome said that in burns of the brain he had observed that the brain was swollen though histologically he had not been able to detect any changes. He spoke only of a "necrosis edema" and did not go deeply into the question of brain swelling. The French school has not concerned itself with this concept of brain swelling either.

The simplest way to clarify these questions of the existence of two forms of increase in volume would be by experimentation. It would appear to be academic hair splitting to distinguish between the two processes if it were not that the treatment of the two conditions could well be different.

I must summarize here the further discussion by referring to the literature and my own studies from 1940-1953 reported at the German Neurosurgical and Neurological Congress in Hamburg, 1953. In this report I said that I believed that one should distinguish with Reichardt between brain edema and brain swelling, because they seemed to be pathogenetically different processes. Primary brain swelling in the definition of Reichardt was particularly found in cases of catatonic schizophrenia or in intoxications as in certain forms of uremia and other exogenous and endogenous intoxications. Macroscopically the white matter (Fig. 2) appeared to be swollen while the cortex was hardly affected, and the cut surface was dry. Histologically, the myelin sheaths appeared swollen as were also the

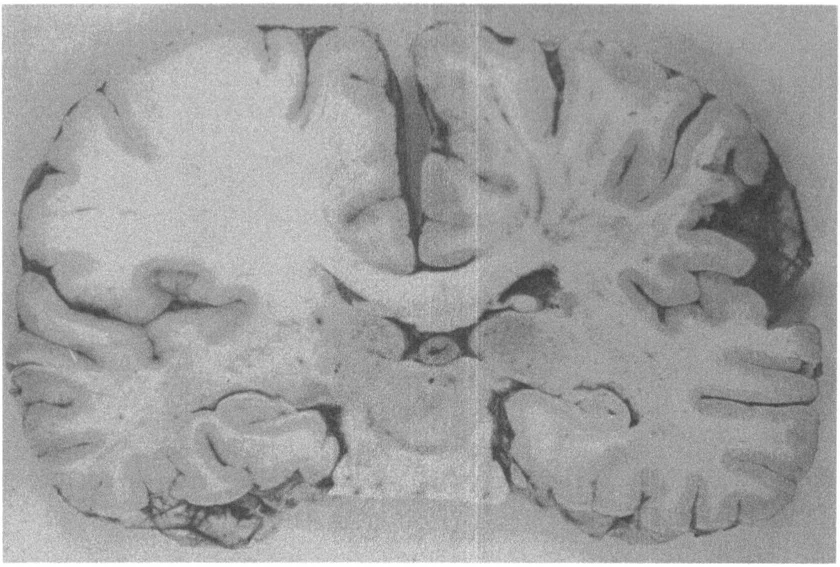

Fig. 2. Marked swelling in a parietal glioblastoma.

oligodendroglia and macroglia, and there was clasmatodendrosis. The whole white matter in myelin stains appeared broader and paler. The changes in the myelin sheaths and axons were particularly characteristic. They were permeated by very small vacuoles, so that in places they looked like bunches of grapes (Fig. 3). This applied to the white matter diffusely throughout a whole hemisphere or even the whole brain. This vacuolated swelling of the myelin sheath was often seen in relation to small oligodendroglia cells. We had seen in a few cases apart from the regressive changes in the glia also progressive changes as, for example, mitotic increase in oligodendroglia. Sometimes also a secondary acidophilic swelling of oligodendroglia was seen; many of the cells resembled the Alzheimer ameboid glia. With the various staining techniques, in particularly the Masson-method, no edema fluid could be demonstrated in the tissue spaces around the vessels. The astroglia was usually swollen and clasmatodendrotic.

With regard to primary brain swelling, I sought to establish the pathogenesis in the following words (1943, 1953): "If one accepts that the blood-brain barrier is situated at two levels, namely in the endothelium and in the glial membrane, then one must with Held, Schaltenbrand and Bailey and Roussy-Oberling envisage the astroglia as being more than a supporting tissue of the brain and postulate for it a nutritive function. It must then be regarded as a highly developed participant in tissue metabolism and, in comparison with the vascular endothelium, at least an equally active collaborator in

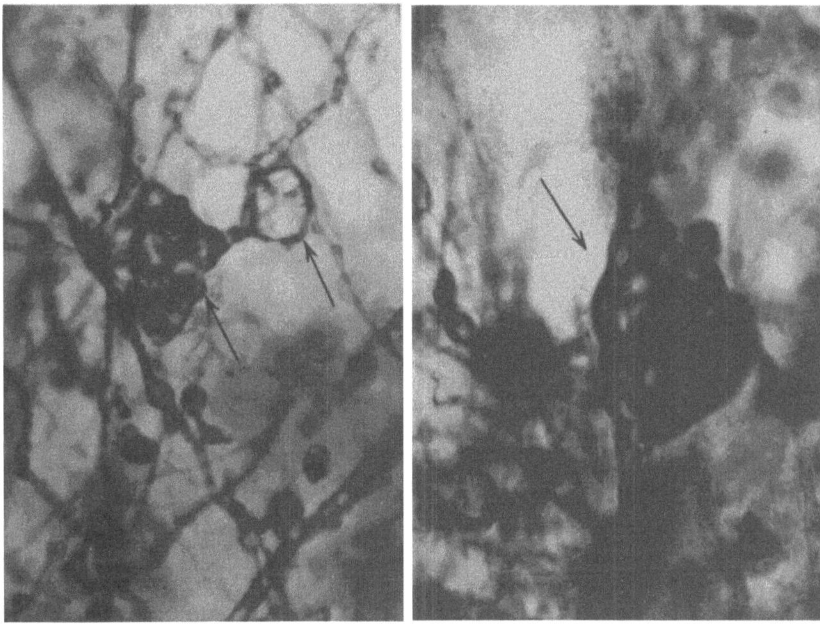

Fig. 3. Vacuolated swelling of myelin sheaths (partly "like a bunch of grapes"). Primary brain swelling.

the formation of the blood-brain barrier. The whole metabolism must, therefore, be orientated around the astrocytes and on that side of the external membrane would begin the milieu peculiar to the brain." One could, therefore, believe that a disturbance of the metabolic exchange through the astrocytes (Fig. 4) could lead to the increase in size of myelin sheaths and thus dry swelling could occur. So much for the concept of the pathogenesis of brain swelling at that time.

We will now concern ourselves with the light microscopic pictures in the different forms of brain edema. We saw with Masson's Trichrome-method a diffuse edema positively stained at the border of an abscess, starting perivascularly. It was so intense that it seeped through the entire white matter of a hemisphere (Fig. 5) from the temporal to the occipital lobe, as we had often seen in traumatic abscesses. Lesser in degree was the edema at the border of a massive hemorrhage where infection was absent. This was not rich in albumin though it could also be made clearly visible by the blue

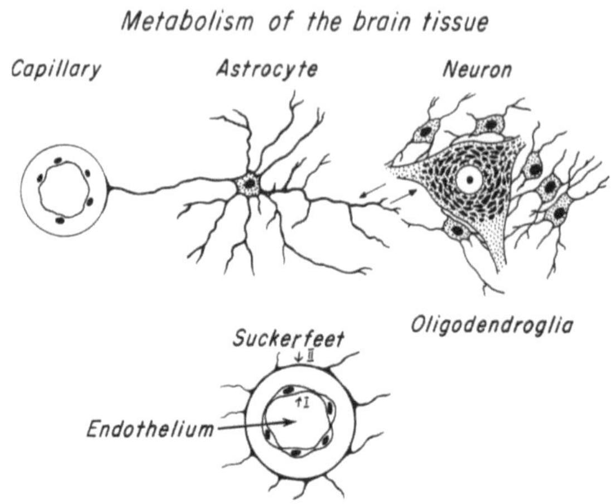

Fig. 4. Blood-brain barrier has to be presumed at two levels: 1) at the endothelial, 2) at the glial barrier (sucker feet of astroglia).

staining. Still lesser in extent, as a rule, was the edema at the border of a brain contusion. In these cases the edema appeared to be due to the exudation of fluid, particularly around the small veins (Fig. 6) and capillaries. A perivenous edema was also seen in human pathology in the so-called perivenous encephalitis and can be produced today experimentally with the help of the Freund adjuvant method. Purely hemodynamic edema, a transudate, was seen in occlusion of the venous drainage as it classically occurs in sinus thrombosis. In summary, brain edema was easily demonstrated by staining of the fluid by the Masson's method in the white matter.

Usually no fluid could be demonstrated in the cortex by the same method. Here we could only expect to find an "equivalent" in Nissl's sense and indeed this we could see in the broadening of the perivascular and pericapillary spaces and in the spongy loosening of the tissues around the capillaries and veins.

This increase of the perineuronal and periglial spaces (Fig. 7) in the cortex was the predominant feature in cases of either local venous obstruction or in the brains of children dying from dystrophy (Zülch, 1953). The white matter, in contrast, was very little affected in the latter cases. We believed that this broadening of the pericellu-

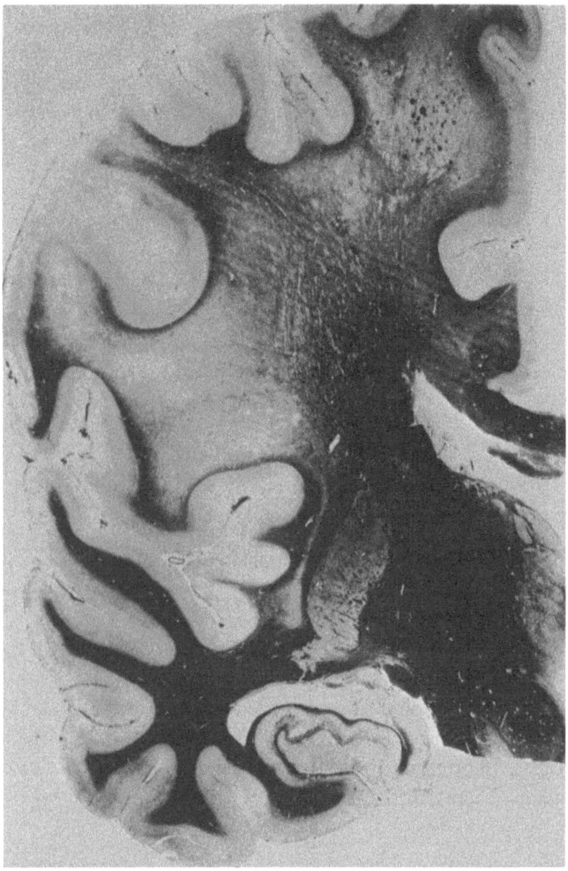

Fig. 5. Plasmatic edema near infected gun shot wound after trephining. Edema has been advancing along the internal capsule to the island of Reil, but is arrested in the temporal lobe. U-fibers well preserved. Death after 25 days.

lar and pericapillary spaces, or the "microspongy" change around the vessels, could be explained on the basis that the intercellular edema fluid of the grey matter was extremely rapidly absorbed because of the enormous surface areas of the cell membranes already available at the very moment when the transudation was occurring, so that the fine network of the neuropil absorbed the fluid and became swollen. Thus we interpreted the equivalent picture of the cortex pathogentically as a sort of secondary swelling of tissue elements after primary brain edema.

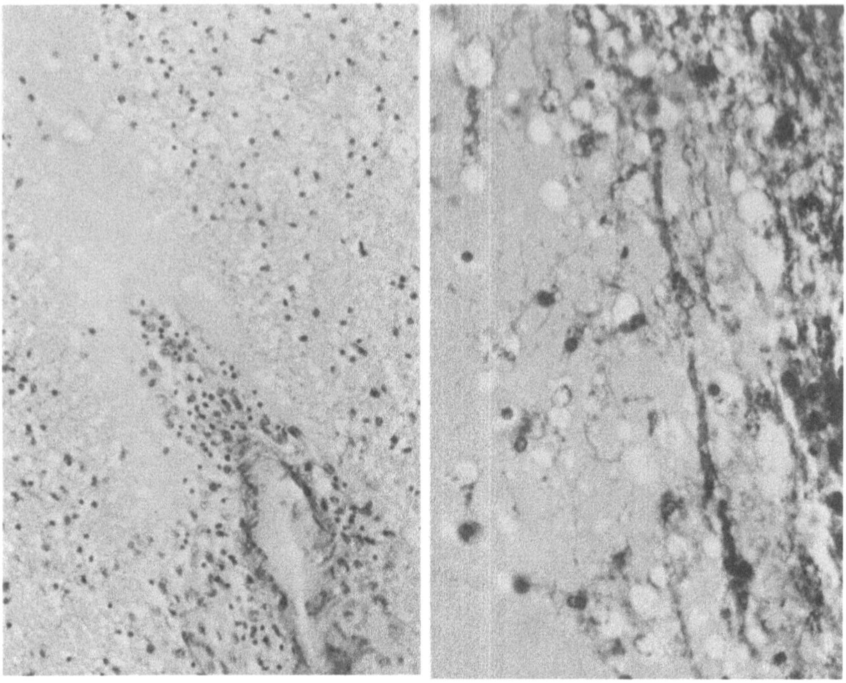

Fig. 6. Left: Perivenous edema with cellular exudation. Vacuolar disintegration after paraffin embedding. H. and E., X160.
Right: Secondary swelling of the myelin sheath in edema, fluid rich in protein. Paraffin, Masson stain, X200.

Although brain edema exhibited a feature common to all varieties, namely an increase in fluid, the various appearances in the different pathogenetic states could be distinguished from one another by their finer topography, the amount of protein, and finally by their effect on the tissue (Table 1).

According to Schmauss, Schürmann, Jacob, Greenfield and our own investigations, the damaging effects could be shown occasionally after a short time. As an example, I may mention a case of an edema very rich in proteins in the case of an infected gunshot wound, where we have observed the almost total destruction of the white matter after 4 days at a 5-8 cm distance from the abscess.

In addition to this primary myelolytic effect of the brain edema there is also the hypoxic damage described by Eppinger and Scholz. This description of brain edema and swelling was summarized in the "Handbuch der Neurochirurgie" (Olivecrona; Tönnis, 1959).

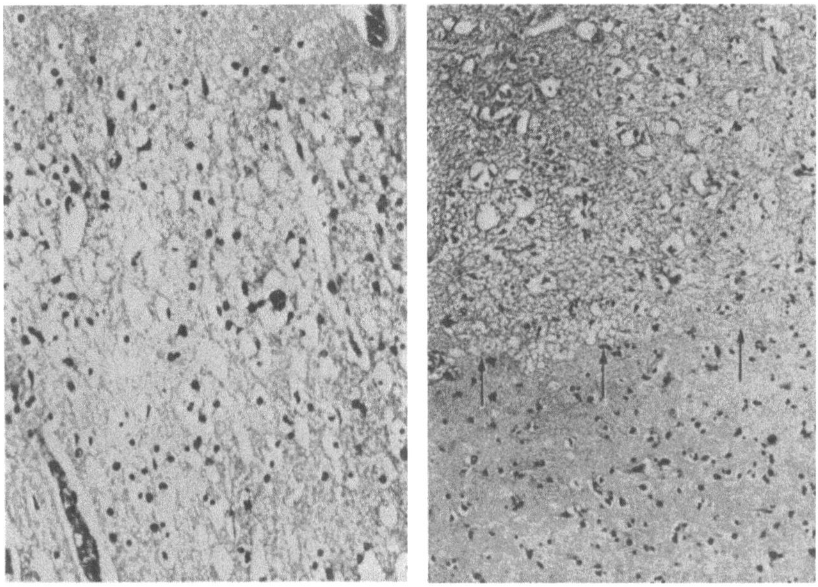

Fig. 7. Left: Enlargement of perineuronal, periglial and perivascular spaces in the cortex. "Equivalent" of edema in the sense of Nissl. H. and E, X164.

Right: Sharply demarcated zone of so-called "edema" of the cortex (see left), H. and E, X96.

This was the state of our knowledge as I reviewed it in 1953, but I had to admit that the interpretation of other authors differed very markedly from my own. I concluded my report by saying that we now had reached an end to the discussion of the findings available up to that time. Only new methods and findings could again give us the possibility of a new understanding of the pathogenesis.

These methods did not have to be awaited long. Electron microscopy made it possible to bring the tissue into a state of fixation which seemed to correspond more closely with that which was present in life, fixation artefacts being reduced to a minimum.

One could recognize with the electron microscope changes at an early stage that could not be detected with the light microscope.

The demonstration of fine structure, particularly of the cell membranes, made it possible to localize the swelling and/or fluid accurately within or outside the cell.

The first electron microscopic investigations of what the authors called brain edema were concerned particularly with the gray matter. An accumulation of fluid in the extracellular space could

TABLE 1
TYPES OF "BRAIN EDEMA" ACCORDING TO PATHOGENESIS AND LOCALIZATION

Pathogenesis	Lesion in man	Localization
A: chemico-toxic	1) mass hemorrhage 2) infarct 3) traumatic necrosis 4) toxic { necrosis / necrobiosis 5) infections: purulent abscess encephalitis, etc. 6) blastoma	perifocal — cortex / white matter
B: allergic (?)	perivenous encephalitis (postvaccin.-postinfectious), etc.	white matter: perivenous
C: hemodynamic 1) vaso-motor (?)	post-concussional state	white matter (perivenous?)
2) arteriolar/ capillary blockage	fat embolism	white matter, perivenous!
3) venous obstruction (with collat. circul.)	ligation / thrombosis } of sinuses	white matter > cortex perivenous pericapillary
4) compression	extra/subdural hematoma extracerebral tumor	white matter > cortex

not be established. Only an intracellular increase in volume could be shown within the astrocytes or neurons. Thus it came about that all previous concepts on the different forms of cerebral edema had to be abolished, perhaps somewhat prematurely, and brain edema was redefined as an increase in volume principally on the part of the astroglia.

Personally, I was somewhat astonished to see that the concepts of a multiple pathogenesis (Table 1) and varied histological features in brain edema were converged into this monistic concept. This was particularly difficult to accept since we had always convincingly seen edema fluid with the light microscope flowing between the myelin sheaths which convinced us that it must lie in the extracellular space.

In the meantime we have carried out in our institute (Gabryel) phase-contrast-microscopic investigation in which we were able to examine the brains of experimental animals within 10 minutes after death. This enabled us to avoid the objection that the changes were post-mortem artefacts. The observations were presented by Gabryel (1962) at the International Neuropathological Congress in Munich. I would also mention Pinto (1953) who reported some light-microscopic findings.

NEW EXPERIMENTAL INVESTIGATIONS ON BRAIN EDEMA

In the second part of my paper I shall now report on the first results of investigations on five large models of brain edema and the paper of Dr. Wechsler will give you further details (Table 2). 1) Trauma by needle stab wound in the mouse brain (Schröder/Wechsler); 2) Local subacute increase in brain pressure by introduction of a laminaria slither (Riverson); 3) Venous stasis by ligation of the sagittal sinus or simultaneous ligature of both jugular

TABLE 2
EXPERIMENTS

Pathogenesis	Animal
1) Trauma	mouse
2) Compression	cat
3) Circulatory lesions	
a) venous	cat, monkey
b) arteriolar (microembolism)	cat
4) Intoxication (diphtheric)	guinea-pig cat

veins (Palmeiro/Hossmann); 4) Increased intracerebral administration of diphtheria toxin; here the initial series of experiments by Gabryel have been carried farther by Kleihues. 5) Experimental microemboli into the carotid artery by plastic globules, 30-37 microns in diameter, which I have studied with Tzonos.

An acute focal brain trauma is produced by stabbing the mouse brain with a needle. The traumatization of the tissues can be clearly recognized from the disturbance of the blood-brain barrier with regard to Evans blue. Histologically, there is a microspongy loosening of the tissues at a distance from the trauma both in the cortex and also in the white matter. No edema fluid can be demonstrated by means of Masson staining. With the electron microscope the spongy loosening in the cortex can be recognized by the swelling of astrocytes and in the white matter through the accumulation of edema fluid in an intercellular position between the myelin sheaths. Further experiments are now being carried out on cats, because in human pathology a Masson stainable edema fluid can be seen and we have not been able to demonstrate it in the mouse. In addition we are studying closed head injuries because of the importance of the therapeutic problems posed by brain edema for the neurosurgeon.

In the next model we have produced a subacute circumscribed cerebral compression corresponding to an epidural or acute subdural hematoma and to a certain extent also to the conditions produced by extracerebral tumors. A very small slither of laminaria is introduced extradurally and this swells during the next few days. The investigation period is from four hours to the end of the fifth day. The expected lateral shift of structures occurs (Fig. 8) and

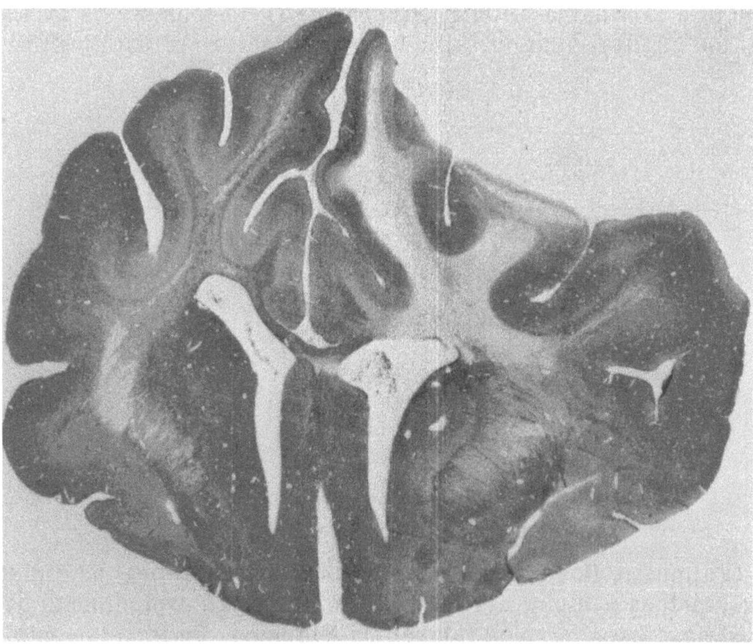

Fig. 8. Local moulding of cerebral hemisphere of a cat after extradural implantation of laminaria slither. Enlargement of white matter from accumulation of edema fluid T 738, H. and E.

the effects upon the blood-brain barrier can be shown particularly well with Evans blue in the white matter. From the first day there is an escape of Masson-positive plasmatic edema fluid, predominantly in the white matter, which swells and then by the third day the blue fluid disappears.

By means of this model we can clarify a fundamental question for the pathology of edema: does the swelling of the myelin (especially in the white matter) which is encountered in extracerebral brain tumors and many other compressions result from swelling of myelin sheaths and axons and in part also of the glia, or does it result from an infiltration by unstainable extracellularly situated edema fluid?

The electron microscope shows that the factor principally responsible for the increase in volume in this experiment is a fluid lying outside and between the cells. This is particularly clear when you see that the normal 200 Å-space is here increased up to 10 microns or more. This constitutes a thousand-fold increase of this space in terms of its surface and correspondingly also in volume. Naturally there is a massive swelling of axons and myelin sheaths in the finely vacuolar form we have described earlier, together with a swelling of the glia. But the electron microscope shows that these are not the factors mainly responsible for the volumetric increment.

The sagittal sinus or the sagittal and transverse sinuses and both jugular veins are ligated in cats, a model of the situation often encountered after thrombosis in man. According to our present knowledge, disturbance of the venous drainage is also the most frequent cause of the so-called "pseudotumor cerebri" and the clinical syndrome of "otitic hydrocephalus" of Symonds. We find already in the first day a very plasma-rich, Masson-positive edema fluid in the white matter of the parasagittal region on both sides (Fig. 9). Around the capillaries we see the typical ring hemorrhages seen in human pathology. The plasmatic edema fluid disappears in the course of two days, though it can still be recognized in the cortical region and is scarcely to be seen by the third day. Then again the white matter is enlarged but a Masson-positive edema can no longer be demonstrated. The glia is particularly active and we find numerous mitoses, probably in oligodendroglia. The myelin sheaths show vacuolar swelling, which is seen with the electron microscope. Furthermore, I can also show you the plasmatic edema fluid in the white matter. One can already demonstrate in the markedly broadened extracellular spaces an osmiophilic amorphous, darkly stained, material (Fig. 10) among which the swollen astrocytic processes stand out as light structures. In later stages the electron microscope shows the ultrastructure of the so-called eosinophilic oligodendroglia which I mentioned above (Fig. 11).

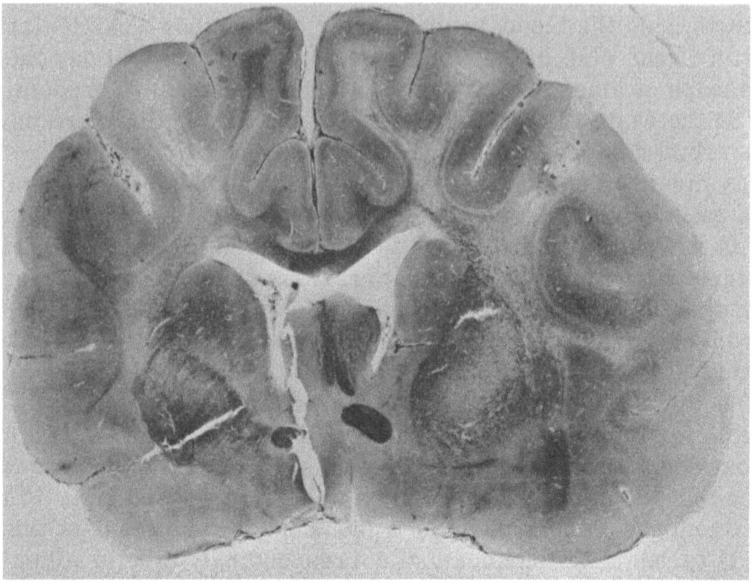

Fig. 9. Enlargement of white matter after accumulation of edema fluid in the upper parts of the brain on both sides of the midline in the parasagittal region. Ligature of sagittal sinus. T 699, Masson's stain.

Repeating the earlier experiments of German pathologists, Gabryel in our institute has studied the necrotizing effects of intracerebral diptheria toxin injections which he reported to the International Congress in Munich, 1961. His investigations have been continued with variations in the technique by Kleihues in mice, guinea pigs, and cats. In these experiments one finds at the site of injection a severe, necrotizing, hemorrhagic focus. In the surroundings there is a very wide zone of edema which one can demonstrate with the light microscope partly as consisting of Masson-positive "plasmatic" edema fluid and partly as swelling of tissue elements and partly also as a "serous"edema. The spread is not confined to the perifocal zone as can be demonstrated with the Evans blue experiments, but edema fluid in the cat seeps through almost the whole hemisphere. With the electron microscope a very extensive, predominantly plasmatic, though partly serous intercellular edema can be demonstrated in the white matter (Fig. 12). This is less pronounced in the cortex but there is also extracellular edema there. (The names of "serous" or "plasmatic" edema are related to the content of proteins in the edema fluid). In this case the toxic effects of the plasmatic edema are so strong that we must assume that we are dealing with a destructive form of edema with resultant primary damage to the neurons, particularly the myelin sheath and the axon,

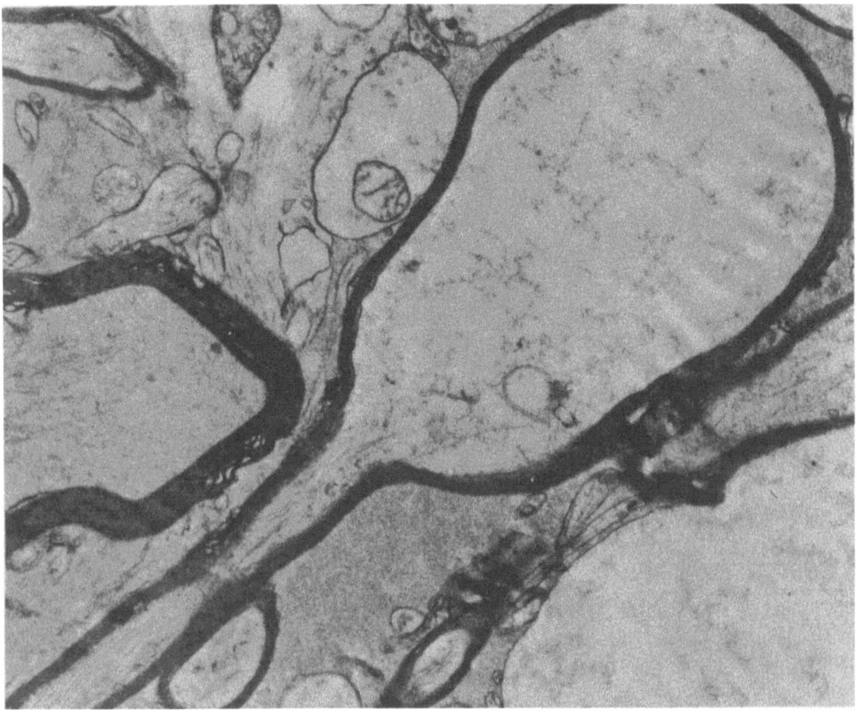

Fig. 10. White matter of cat's brain. Ligature of sagittal sinus. Marked enlargement of extracellular space filled with osmiophilic exsudate. Focal swelling of axon, beginning at Ranvier's ring, X15,000.

at the same time as there is destruction of the nutritive glia.

This model with formation of a toxic necrosis apparently constitutes a very severe insult to the integrity of the brain tissue. We have, therefore, chosen further models; for example, injection of blood into the same site in order to imitate the process of edema in the spontaneous massive hemorrhage of hypertensive patients.

Microemboli of a standard size of 30-37 microns are injected into the carotid artery of a cat and the findings studied between half an hour and four weeks. The details have already been reported (Zülch and Tzonos). Fat embolism in man can be studied by such a model.

Morphologically fat embolism in the human brain produces a very characteristic picture. In the cortex, numerous capillaries, very rarely arterioles, are blocked by fat emboli, but the histological changes in the cortex are surprisingly slight or they may not even be visible. Genuine microinfarcts are certainly a rarity. In

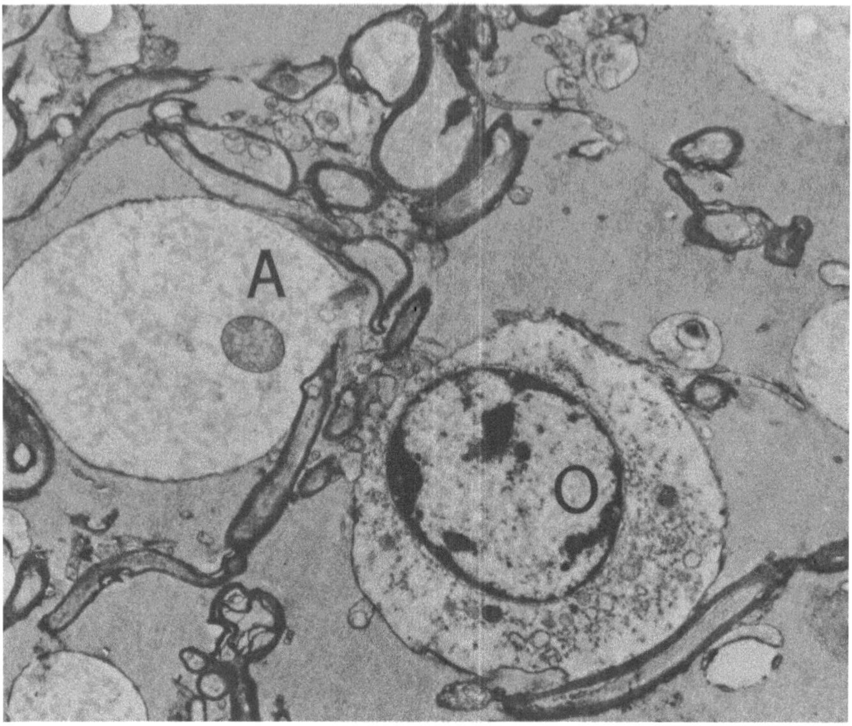

Fig. 11. White matter of cat's brain. Marked enlargement of extracellular space which is filled with osmiophilic substance. Swelling of astrocytic processes (A), swelling of oligodendroglia cell (O). Only minimal changes in the axons, X6,300.

contrast, the deep white matter is the part most severely affected and shows an extensive "flea-bite encephalitis" with gross edema. Histologically the first change is a perivascular accumulation of fluid with ring hemorrhages around veins and venules; then a granuloma is formed, and later a severe demyelination occurs as a result of the edema.

The pathogenesis of this damage has not been sufficiently discussed and clarified, and particularly the characteristic discrepancy in severity of damage between cortex and white matter which is not explicable on hemodynamic grounds. One may emphasize the paradox by pointing to the fact that while the obstructive emboli lie mostl in the cortical capillaries, the morphological damage is in the white matter. Only animal experiments can give us insight into the pathological mechanism.

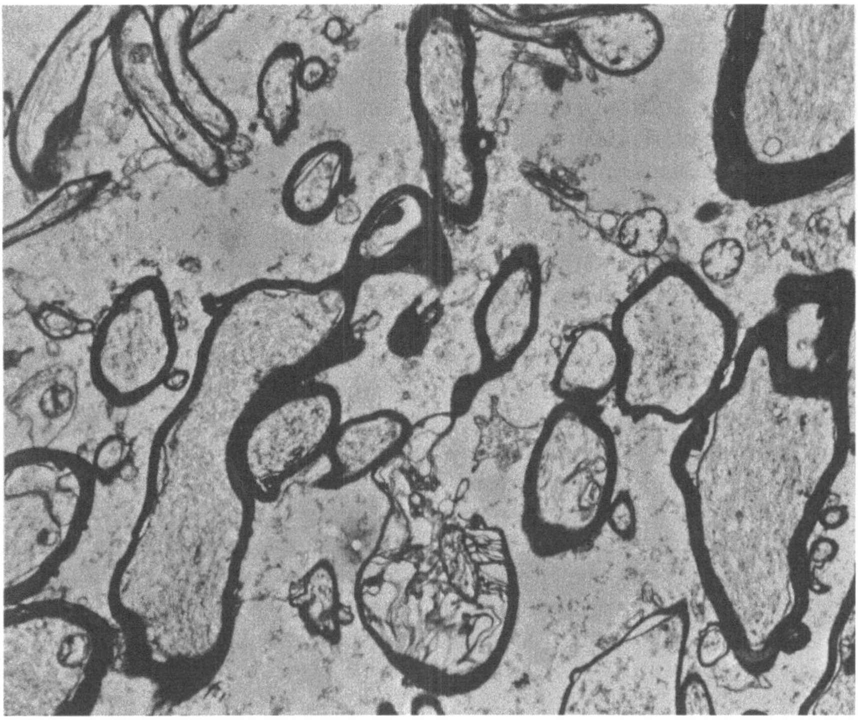

Fig. 12. Local intoxication by diphtheria. The edema zone of the white matter shows marked enlargement of extracellular spaces filled with osmiophilic precipitates. Dissociation of axons, but only minimal changes. Swelling of myelin sheath near Ranvier's ring, X6,600.

Artificial embolism of the brain has often been attempted in animal experiments in the last century. The results of these experiments are very difficult to compare because the emboli used varied in their type, size, and quantity. A standardization of emboli by size and number should be the starting point for any precise model experiment in which it is desired to obtain insight into the pathogenesis of the lesions produced and influence on them by pharmacological agents. In modern plastic materials we possess an ideal experimental material for embolism; for example, the Hostalen PP-granules which are 30-37 microns in diameter. With this material we have produced emboli via the carotid arteries in cats with amounts of 20, 10, 5 and finally 2ml (dissolved in 5 milliliters of a colloidal solution). Tzonos has already reported in detail on the technique. The mortality of the cats receiving injections of more than 5 ml was always 100%. Therefore, the experiments were usually carried out with only 5 ml, in which case the post-operative loss of animals was only 40%, while with 2 ml it was 25%. The period of observation was between 15 minutes and 28 days.

The morphological investigations were carried out with the methods of conventional histology. In addition, the brain was examined through a glass window in the living state after trephining. As a result of the injection, a few arterioles and small arteries in the cortex were blocked with plastic emboli at the level of the second to third cell layers of the cortex. In the regions related to the vessels, there were microinfarcts. Only in a few cases did we find primary infarcts also in the white matter. These changes were easy to understand hemodynamically, but the results of this embolism in the white matter were unexpected. In this situation from the fourth hour on, there were dense rings of an albumin-rich (staining "positively" with Masson's Trichrome-stain) edema around the venules and veins. This became more marked during the course of hours and days. Later, a diffuse edema from the vessels occurred in the white matter and seeped through it. In more severe cortical embolism, there was a veritable lake of edema. The result of the edema was a marked demyelination with focal complete softenings. The softened white matter then liquefied and was broken down to the fat granule stage. Finally, after three to four weeks, a large part of the white matter was destroyed. Cysts were present which were filled with fat granule cells or had already been emptied and the scavenger cells transported to the vessels. There was a corresponding hydrocephalus ex vacuo of the neighboring part of the ventricle.

How should we explain these secondary phenomena in the white matter far away from the blockage? I have the following working hypothesis to offer. Because of the embolic blockage in a large region of the cortical tissue, the flow of blood to the veins draining from the depths into the cortex is quantitatively reduced so that there is a slowing of the circulation since it is not possible for veins to contract. This is the first phenomenon which we can deduce from the hemodynamics and which we have also seen on the cortex with intra vitam observations of the veins reaching the leptomeninges from the depths. A second phenomenon is very likely present. The extent of the actually infarcted regions is smaller than would correspond to the irrigation area of the embolized arteries. The border zone is, as in man, collaterally supplied with blood by neighboring arteries and capillary network. Thus a large extent of the cortical tissue is not nourished by its own vessels but by diffusion from the neighborhood. In this way the oxygen and glucose utilization of the blood reaching the veins in the depths is greater than normal. This is possible because normally there is a very considerable oxygen reserve in the venous cerebral blood. The so-called arterio-venous difference lies between 6 and 8 volumes per cent. The vein wall is normally nourished and oxygenated by the blood.

If, however, the oxygen content of the venous blood falls, endogenous damage occurs which leads to increased permeability (dyshoria in the sense of Schürmann), and diapedesis of serum with perivenous escape of edema fluid. An alternative nutrition of the vein wall from the blood apparently occurs in the cortex with its dense capillary network. One might have thought that this could occur in the white matter through diffusion from the richly nourished tissues in the neighborhood, but the capillary system of the white matter is poorly developed. There is probably no difference between the quantitative reduction of flow associated with qualitative reduction of oxygen and glucose which follows embolization of the arterioles (as in the experiments) and that caused by blockage of the capillaries by fat emboli (as in human pathology). In cats we have microinfarcts; in man anoxic changes are prevented because the tissue of the "infarcted" Krogh-cylinders can be nourished by the adjacent Krogh-cylinders. In either of the two examples, the border zones will be collaterally supplied by the vasculature of the undamaged neighboring tissues.

In this way the pathogenesis of the processes which occur in microembolism in animal experiments and in human pathology can to a large extent be understood. These transudation phenomena are the expression of a new "effect" which is not caused by vasomotor or hormonal factors. Changes in the blood itself are introducing these grave alterations. We cannot explain why the perivenous hemorrhages occur in man. In animals we have never seen them round the veins and very rarely in the proximal parts of cortical infarcts.

Can these processes of a secondary "perivenous edema" ("perivenous syndrome," Zülch, 1953) also explain other neuropathological findings? They may well operate as a localizing factor in the so-called perivenous encephalitis which is also called postinfectious or postvaccinal and can be produced experimentally by an allergic mechanism. Even in disseminated sclerosis perivenous demyelination can, as we know from Rindfleisch, Borst, Fog, and Courville, occur in up to 80% of the foci as proven by serial sections.

I suggest that this mechanism of formation of a primary perivenous edema plays an active role in most of the models of edema of the white matter. But this has to be proven by careful electron microscopical investigations.

One must put forward the question whether in some neurological states obstructions or impedance to the arterial and/or capillary circulation may not be a pathoplastic factor. This interesting perivenous effect may, therefore, influence the basic pattern of many neuropathological entities. If our working hypothesis is correct, we have to note that the transudation phenomena are an expression of a new transmitting "effect" of the blood itself.

Further investigations on our models should clarify the pathogenesis of the formation of edema and test our concept that the edema fluid is not formed in the cortex and then runs down into the white matter; it is a perivenous transudation resulting from the lesions in the cortex.

According to our views, it would be better in the future if only models in which a close pathogentic relationship with human pathology exists were used for the investigation of edema.

REFERENCES

Alajouanine, Th. and Hornet: L'oedème cérébral généralisé (Etude anatomique), Ann. anat. path., 16 (1939).

Alzheimer, A.: NISSLs Arbeiten 1910, III.

Anton, G. Gehirnoedem und Compression, in: Handbuch der Pathologischen Anatomie des Nervensystems, Vol. I, (ed by S. Karger), pp. 396-467, Berlin (1904).

Eppinger, H.: Die seröse Entzündung. Wien: J. Springer (1935).

Gabryel, P.: Morphologische Veränderungen im Hirngewebe beim experimentellen Ödem. Phasenkontrast- und elektronenmikroskopische Untersuchungen, IV. Int. Kongr. für Neuropath. Vol. 3, Georg Thieme, Stuttgart: pp. 173-176 (1962).

Greenfield, J. G.: The histology of cerebral oedema associated with intracranial tumors. Brain, 62, 129 (1939).

_____: Oedème cérébral en neurochirgurgie, Rev. Neurol., 79, 280-283 (1947).

_____: Spontaneous Diseases Associated with Demyelination in Man and Animals, Proc. of the 1. Int. Congr. of Neuropath., Vol. 1, 107-120 Rome (1952).

Held: Die Entwicklung des Nervengewebes bei den Wirbeltieren, Leipzig: Barth (1909).

Hossmann, K. A., M. Schröder and W. Wechsler: Das morphologische Substrat der Bluthirnschranke unter physiologischen und pathologischen Bedingungen, Verh. Dtsch. Ges. Path., 49, 350-356 (1965).

Jaburek, L.: Hirnödem und Hirnschwellung bei Hirngeschwülsten, Arch. Psychiatr. Nervenkrankh., 104, 518-547 (1936).

_____: Über das Gewebslückensystem des Grosshirns und seine Bedeutung für die Ausbreitung verschiedener pathologischer Prozesse (Ödeme, Blutungen, Abscesse, Geschwülste und Entmark-

ungskrankheiten), Ibid., 105, 121 (1936).
Jacob, H.: Zur histopathologischen Diagnose des akuten und chronischen rezidivierenden Hirnödems, Ibid., 179, 158 (1947).
Pinto, F.: Sobre o problema do edema e da tumefacao cerebral, Med. Cirurg. Farm., 208, 337-353 (1953).
Reichardt, M.: Zur Entstehung des Hirndrucks, Dtsch. Zschr. Nervenhk., 28, 306 (1905).
_____: Hirnschwellung, Allg. Z. Psych., 75, 34-103 (1919).
_____: Das Hirnödem, Anhang: Die Hirnschwellung, in: Handb. der spez. path. Anat. u. Histol. Vol. XIII, 1B, Berlin-Göttingen-Heidelberg: Springer-Verlag, 1229 ff. (1957).
Riebeling, C.: Das Problem der Hirnschwellung, Dtsch. Med. Wschr., 63, 1440-1442 (1937).
_____: Eine chemische Untersuchung der Hirnschwellung, Z. Neur., 166, 149 (1939).
_____: Zur Frage der Hirnschwellung, Dtsch. Z. Nervenhk., 170, 209-236 (1953).
Rosenthal: Histologische Befunde beim sog. Pseudotumor cerebri. Z. Neur., 7, 163 (1911).
Roussy, G., J. Lhermitte and C. Oberling: La névrologie et ses réactions pathologiques. Rev. Neurol., 37, 878 (1930).
Schaltenbrand, G. u. P. Bailey: Die perivaskuläre Piagliamembran des Gehirns, J. Psychol. Neurol., 35, 199-278 (1928).
Scheinker, I. M.: Zur Histopathologie des Hirnödems und der Hirnschwellung bei Tumoren des Gehirns, Dtsch. Zschr. Nervenhk., 147, 137-162 (1938).
_____: Cerebral swelling. Histopathology, classification and clinical significance of brain edema, J. Neurosurg., 4, 255-275 (1947).
_____: Clinical significance, histopathology and classification of cerebral swelling, Neurology (Minneapolis), 2, 177-194 (1952).
Schmaus, H.: Vorlesungen über die pathologische Anatomie des Rückenmarks. Wiesbaden: Verlag von J. F. Bergmann (1901).
Scholz, W.: Histologische und topische Veränderungen und Vulnerabilitätsverhältnisse im menschlichen Gehirn bei Sauerstoffmangel, Ödem und plasmatischen Infiltrationen. I. Problemstellung und feingewebliche Situation, Arch. Psychiatr. Nervenkr., 181, 621-665 (1949).
Schröder, M. and W. Wechsler: Zur Frage unterschiedlicher Adhäsionskräfte zwischen den Zellmembranen in der grauen und weissen Substanz des Gehirns, Naturwissenschaften, 52, 86-87 (1965).
Schürmann: Hirnschwellung Veröff. Heeressan. Wes., No. 105 (1938); Vern. Path. Ges. (1936).
Selbach, H.: Physikalisch-chemische Untersuchungen zur Frage der Hirnvolumenvermehrung (Hirnschwellung und Hirn-Ödem), Arch. Psychiatr. Nervenkr., 112, 409-440 (1940).
Spatz, H.: Die Bedeutung der "symptomatischen Hirnschwellung" für die Hirntumoren und andere raumbeengende Prozesse in der Schädelgrube, Ibid., 88, 790 (1929); 101, 280-292 (1933).

Staemmler: see Panofsky and Stämmler, Frankf. Z. Path. 26, 519-549 (1922).

Steinmann, H. W.: Hirnelektrische tierexperimentelle Untersuchungen zum Problem des Hirnödems, Zbl. ges. Neurol. Psychiatr. 122, 10 (1953).

Tzonos, T.: Über eine neue Methode zur Erzeugung von stereotyper Mikroembolien im Gehirn der Katze, Acta Neuropath., 3, 392-397 (1964).

Wechsler, W.: Ödem und Nekrose in der grauen und weissen Substanz beim experimentellen Hirntrauma, (Licht- und elektronenmikroskopische Untersuchungen), Ibid., 4, (1965).

Zülch, K. J.: Morphologische Befunde bei Hirnschwellung, Zbl. Neurochir., 5, 166-175 (1940).

_____: Die Entstehung des Hirndruckes, insbesondere des Prolapses bei der Hirnwunde und ihren Folgezuständen, Ibid., 6, 212-232 (1941).

_____: Hirnödem und Hirnschwellung, Virch. Arch., 310, 1-58 (1943 Os Traumatismos Cranianos Fechados, J. Brasil. Neurol. II, 31-51 (1950); Hirnödem, Hirnschwellung, Hirndruck. Zbl. Neurochir. 11, 350-355 (1951), Ibid., 12, 174-186 (1952). Ibid., 365-372 (1952).

_____: Hirnschwellung und Hirnödem, Dtsch. Zschr. Nervenhk., 170 179-208 (1953).

_____: Neuropathological observations on the cerebrospinal fluid pathway. Ciba Foundation Symposium on the cerebrospinal Fluid, pp. 230-242, London: J. & A. Churchill Ltd. (1958).

_____: What do we actually know about brain edema and brain swelling?, Annual Meeting of the Association of British Neuropathologists, Bristol (1962).

_____: Neurologische Diagnostik bei endokraniellen Komplikationen von otorhinologischen Erkrankungen, Arch. Ohren- Nasen- u. Kehlkopfhk., 183, 1-78 (1964); 79-85 (1964).

_____:Edema ehinchazon cerebral. Rev. Espan. Oto-Neuro-Ofthal. Neurocirugia,24, 280-293 (1965).

_____ and T. Tzonos: Transsudationsphänomene an den tiefen Hirnvenen nach Blockade von Arteriolen oder Kapillaren der Rinde durch Mikroembolien, Naturwissenschaften, 51, 539-540 (1964).

_____: Transudation Phenomena at the Deep Veins after Blockage of Arterioles and Capillaries by Micro-Emboli, III Europ. Conf. Microcirculation, Jerusalem (1964); Bibl. anat., Vol. 7. Basel, New York: S. Karger, pp. 279-284 (1965).

HANS JACOB

COURSE AND SEQUELAE OF BRAIN EDEMA

General and focal swelling of brain substance can be found in different pathological syndromes. Some histopathological characteristics of such "tissue swelling syndromes" are fairly typical. Similar regressive and progressive alterations, however, may sometimes be found in unswollen parts of tissue. We are, therefore, not able to decide from the histopathological picture, whether it is related to a pathologically increased tissue turgor or to some lesion with characteristics of brain edema and brain swelling. Initial swelling of encephalomalacic tissue cannot be merely explained by regressive and progressive changes of the tissue elements. It often is not clear if swelling of tissue caused the tissue damage or only accompanied or followed it. This may sometimes be applied to the problem of the generalized "primary" or "secondary" brain edema or brain swelling.

Special, pathogenetically clear conditions, however, allow comparatively reliable conclusions. This was demonstrated by Scholz (1949) in cortical lesions near hemorrhagic infarcts caused by emboli and sinus thromboses. In these cases we often have to differentiate between "Erbleichungsherde" (paling foci) of acute circulatory disturbance and the areas of edema, serous transudation or hemorrhage. In most instances the cortical "Erbleichungen" go beyond the edematous area and enclose them entirely. The serous tissue transudation or the hemorrhages take place in parts already damaged by hypoxidosis. Similar lesions can be seen in cuneiform "paling areas" of cortex and white matter with central demyelination foci (Jacob, 1942). Similar conditions may sometimes be found in perifocal edema of the white matter in tumors. Here an accumulation of acutely swollen oligodendroglia with homogenization of nuclei can be observed in the not yet demyelinated border zone, whereas in the regions of central myelin necrosis additional clasmatodendrosis is recognizable (Jacob, 1964). From a different point of view we may regard the "Randzentrum-Phaenomene" (border-center phenomena) as they occur in the swollen medullary substance in purpura cerebri. Here the multiple foci of purpura and plasmatic exudation often appear in the areas of a diffuse myelin pallor with diffuse swelling of oligodendroglia. The same phenomenon we find in perivenous encephalitis.

Besides these pathogenetically ambiguous pictures we are also interested in the histopathological characteristics of the tissue swelling syndromes. Concerning cortical edema, Scholz distinguished two different tissue syndromes: 1) cortical lesions with pronounced loosening of tissue, progressive astroglia, and regressive oligodendroglia associated with remarkable resistance of the nerve cells, whereas myelin sheaths are more vulnerable to edema; 2) alterations in areas showing protein-rich edema with severe ballooning of nuclei and pericarya, tigro- and dendrolysis and vacuolar lesions of nerve cells, as well as disintegration of myelin sheaths with intense glial reaction. Contrary to the hypoxidotic "Rindenerbleichung with mostly intact myelin sheaths, the myelin radiation of the cortex seems specially susceptible to edema. Scholz (1960) considered the pure cortical demyelination foci within loose progressive astrocytic network containing intact nerve cells, which he observed in gas emboli, to be edematous lesions. According to my own observations, the cortical edema, contrary to edema of the white matter, often is characterized by a granular diffuse or reticular disintegration of myelin sheaths. In the molecular layer of the edematous cerebellar cortex, besides an edematous appearance of the Purkinje cell layer, swelling may also involve the Purkinje dendrites and the processes of the Fañanas cells which become stained with hematoxylin in myelin preparations (Figs. 2a, 2b). In purpura cerebelli, besides the hemorrhages, focal areas with swelling of dendrites are obvious (Figs. 1a, 1b). In such acute stages the glia is inactive. Here, therefore, the swelling of Purkinje dendrites precedes the glial reaction.

The tissue swelling syndromes of the white matter are histopathologically different in appearance. This depends upon the relation of the regressive symptoms in axon and myelin sheaths and progressive-regressive reactions in the glia. Our findings agree with Scheinker's (1947). The acute swelling of oligodendroglia in areas of diffuse myelin pallor seems to indicate early edematous lesions. The significance of homogenizing swelling of nuclei has been discussed elsewhere. There is a different kind of acute oligodendroglial alteration, where a network of wide empty meshes develops in swollen and rounded cytoplasm. Thus myelin sheaths and

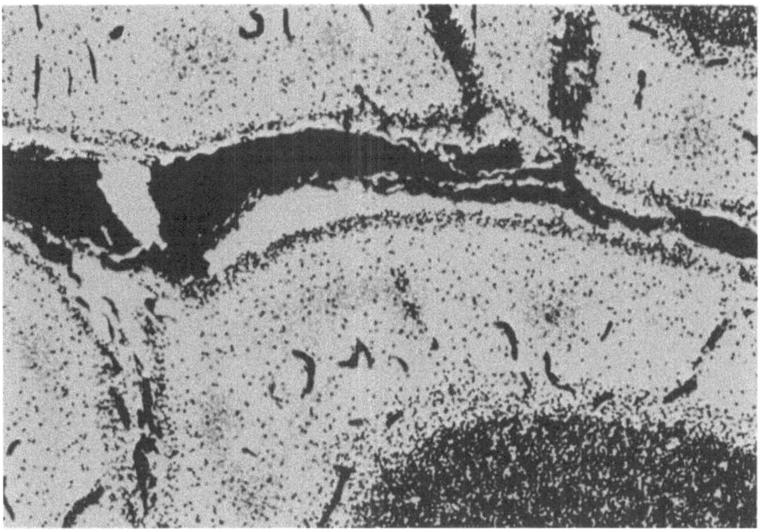

Fig. 1a. Mü. 13 months (22a/55). Purpura cerebelli. Edematous swelling of dendrites of Purkinje cells which show hematoxylin affinity (Heidenhein-Woelcke).

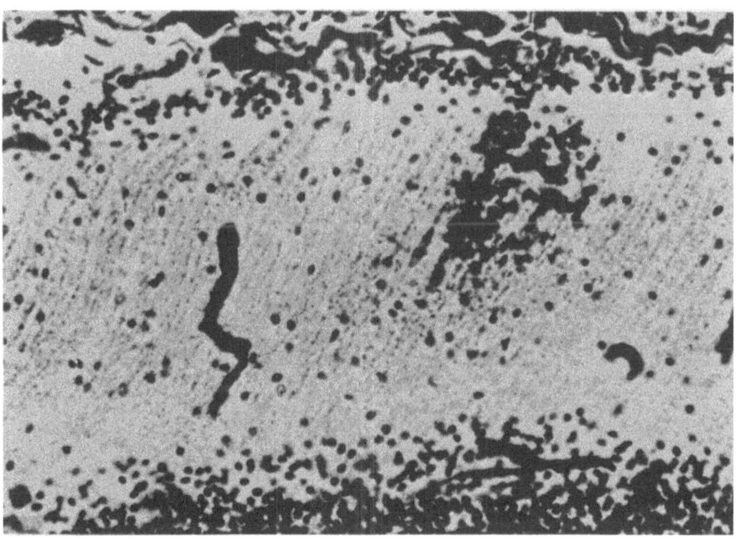

Fig. 1b. Mü. 13 months (22a/55). Purpura cerebelli. Edematous swelling of dendrites of Purkinje cells (Heidenhein-Woelcke).

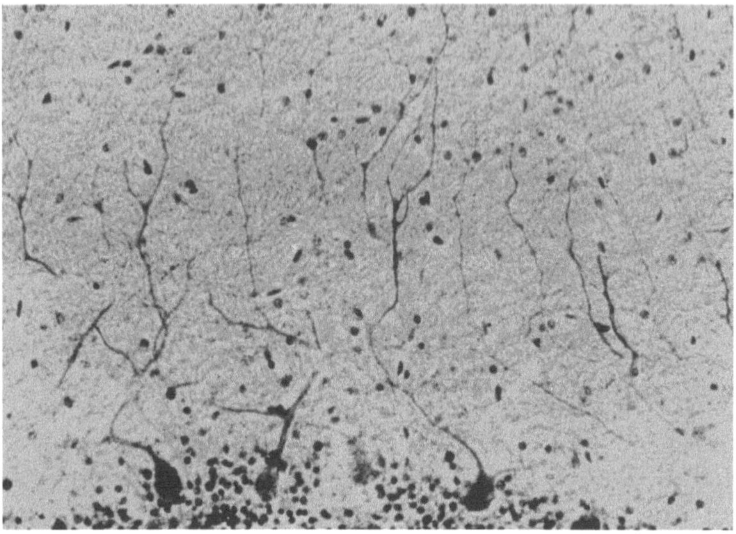

Fig. 2a. Ra. 42 years ♀ (82a/57). Death 24 hours after strangulation. Diffuse edematous necrosis of the white matter of the brain with erythro-and plasma diapedesis. Necrosis and liquefaction of Purkinje cells. Swelling of dendrites of Purkinje cells (Heidenhein-Woelcke).

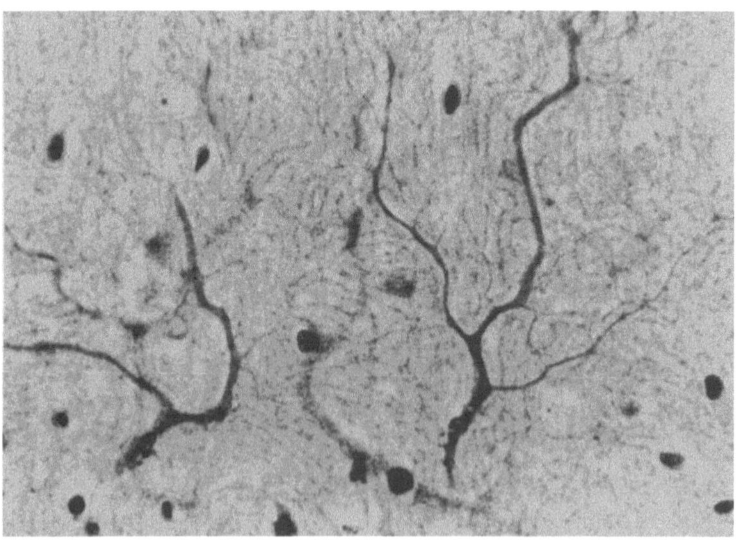

Fig. 2b. Ra. (82a/57). See Fig. 2a.

axons are separated, causing a kind of "pseudo-spongy state." Contrary to acute swelling of oligodendroglia with homogenizing swelling of nuclei, we see oligodendrocytes with protoplasmic girders and with normal nuclei. Plasmatic swellings of astroglia, pre-amoeboid glia and clasmatodendrosis we usually find in the areas with severe damage of myelin sheaths such as cluster formation, ballooning, hyperimpregnation. But there are also exceptions. The extent of swelling of myelin sheaths usually is greater than that of axonal swellings. Here, as well as in the cortex, the greater inclination to edema of glia and myelin sheaths compared to more edema-resistant nerve cells and axons is obvious.

Tissue holes in myelin preparation can be explained by the proliferated plasmatic swollen macroglia or swelling of oligodendroglia with pushing aside of myelin sheaths. Tissue holes in hematoxylin-eosin preparations may be produced by ballooning and clustering of myelin sheaths. In the first case the edematous lesion is characterized by glial swelling and density, in the second by swelling of myelin sheaths. Amoeboid glia, swelling of oligodendroglia, and clasmatodendrosis do not cause a spongy tissue disintegration in the early stages of acute edema of the white matter. The products of disintegration, primarily the swollen homogenizing nuclei of oligodendroglia, remain as amorphous substances for some time in the tissue. It is well known that swollen myelin tissue may also appear as "spongy" alteration because circumscribed ballooned axons have a displacing effect (i.e., Borst's "Lückenherde"). All these cases only represent a "pseudo-spongy state," caused by progressive astroglial swelling, oligodendroglial swelling, ballooning of myelin or swelling of axons. Otherwise, there is definitely a true "spongy state" in myelin caused by dissolution. Some swelling of white matter merely shows a fine network of narrowed and pallid myelin sheaths and axons. Here the glia shows practically no proliferation; glial cell cytoplasm is not altered in a progressive or regressive fashion; glial cell nuclei appear intact. The lesion is recognizable merely in a narrowing of fibers with pallor of myelin sheaths and axonal disintegration. We were able to observe this in a case of post-narcotic death. After a 4-day survival period, there was a pronounced swelling of hemispheres and severe hypoxic lesions of the gray matter. In cortical edema, however, the frequent spongy deterioration of tissue in the upper layers and in the area of the "Demarkationszonen" (Spatz, Jacob, 1941) may be explained by glial insufficiency. This is even more obvious in the coarse cystic disintegration in collequation necrosis.

Of special interest are tissue reactions in subacute, chronic or chronic relapsing tissue swelling in slowly developing tumors. In such cases proliferation of substituting astrocytic fibers and mesenchymal proliferation in the progressively dilating Virchow-Robin's spaces are found (Jacob, 1947). In obviously rarer instances the plasmatic fibrillary astroglia in the myelin swelling may, in quantity and quality, reach an extent that is far more than normal. In this case the excessively proliferating plasmatic fibrillary astrocytes permeate the almost completely demyelinated tissue with formation of giant glia (Figs. 3-6). Affected by the clasmatodendrotic disintegration of this obviously insufficient glia, a spongy lesion within the still intact glial fibrous network is possible. We were able to observe this twice in obvious chronic swelling of the white matter

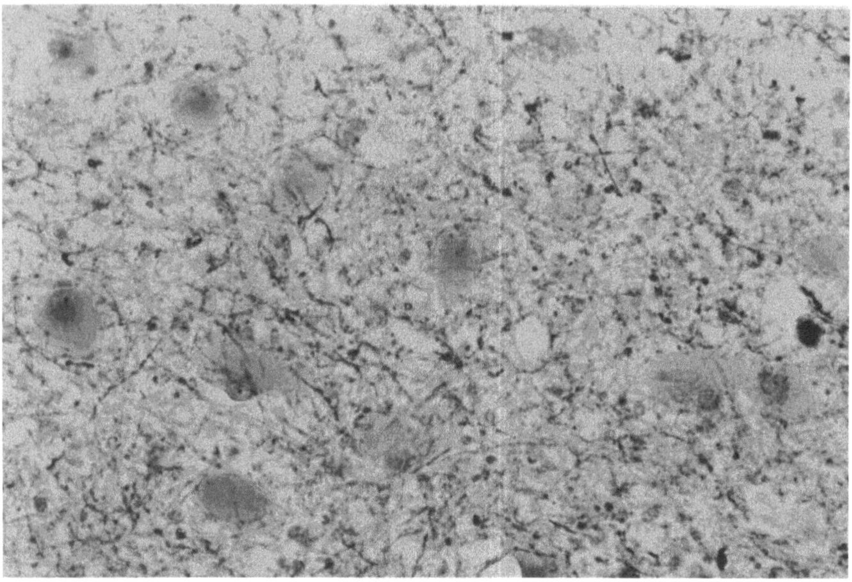

Fig. 3. Lo. (19/60). Edema cerebri maligna in meningioma. Enormous plasma-swelling of giant astrocytes, demyelination with hyperchromatosis (Klüver-Barrera).

in meningiomas. Such processes give a picture of a progressive disintegration, so that we may speak of a malignant tissue swelling, and of malignant edema of the white matter. The development of the meningioma strikes us as a more benign process than that in the chronically swollen peritumerous myelin tissue. The resulting diffuse isomorphous fibrous gliosis appears completely different from sequelae of transient myelin edema that basically affects the oligodendroglia (Fig. 7). Therefore, we may observe fibrous gliosis in cases where the myelin sheaths have remained intact, i.e., the dissociation glio-myelinique of van Bogaert. Another syndrome in ad-

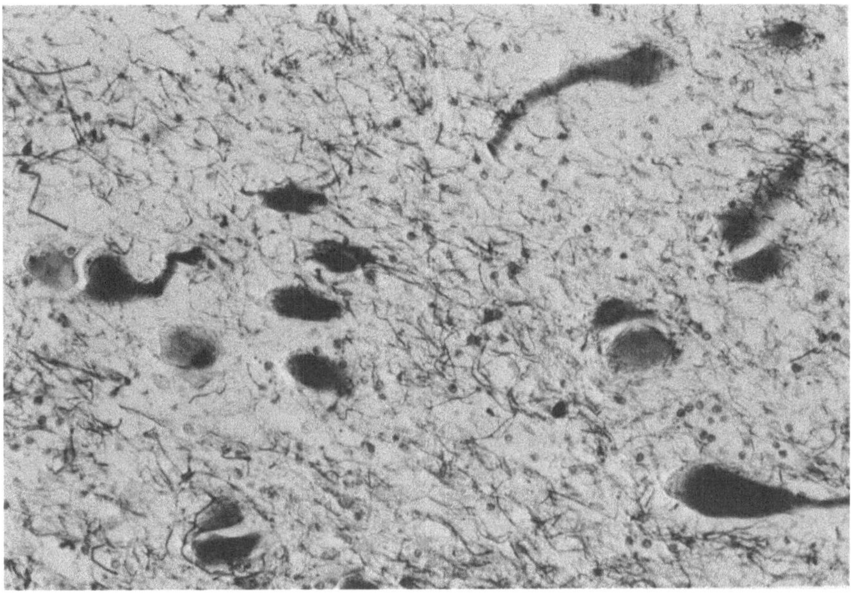

Fig. 4. Lo. (19/60). See Fig. 5 (Kanzler).

vanced states of tissue swelling is characterized by tissue liquefaction of variable genesis. Scheinker (1947) called such tissue destruction "cerebral liquefaction" or the third stage of cerebral swelling. Scheinker and Segerberg (1948) stressed the importance of vascular, mostly vaso-paralytic disturbances for such cystic formations in post-traumatic brain swelling. My former collaborator, Bonhoff (1952), undertook detailed comparative neuropathological study of transudative formation of cysts and serous "Massenergüsse" in perifocal myelin swelling and development of edema. He discovered that the contents of the cysts resemble the perivascular transudations and blend into surrounding tissue with regard to the tinctorial characteristics. Rosenhagen (1956) described the development of such traumatic brain cysts from comparative clinical aspects. Under special circumstances these serous "Massenergüsse" in the primarily damaged tissue are of clinical significance, because the progressive pressure in the cysts may lead to displacement symptoms. The question arises whether there is relation between such progressive liquefactions and serous "Massenergüsse" in the swollen myelin tissue and those cavities in the white matter that were encephalographically and neuropathologically observed after pre-frontal leucotomy. This seems of importance as leucotomy doubtlessly

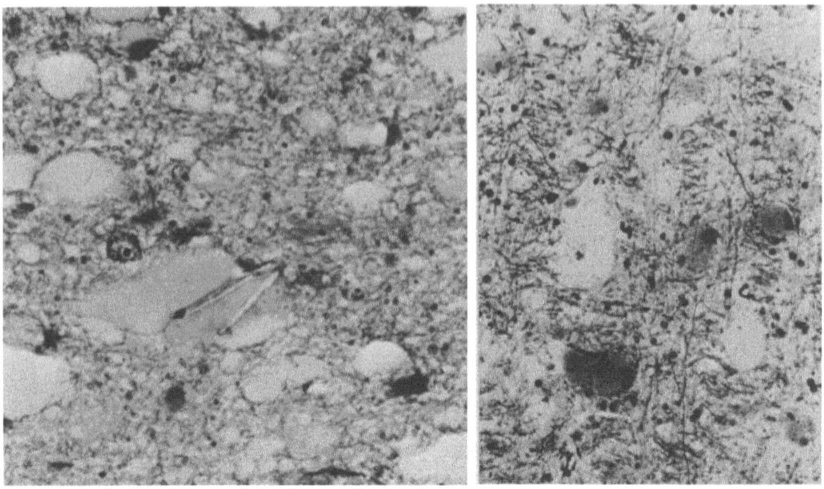

Fig. 5. Gro. 60 years ♀ (26a/55) Edema cerebri maligna in falxmeningioma. Enormous plasmatic swelling of giant astrocytes, vacuolation in astrocytes. Left: Klüver-Barrera. Right: Bodian.

causes a severe disorder in the liquid exchange of the whole hemispheric medullary matter (cf. Yokoi, 1957).

Such serous "Massenergüsse" and transudative cystic formations in the peri-tumorous or post-traumatic swollen myelin tissue belong, as progressive processes, to the malignant forms of tissue swelling in connection with brain edema and brain swelling.

SUMMARY

Swelling of the gray and white matter can develop under various pathogenic conditions. In hemorrhagic infarcts with initial tissue swelling caused by emboli or sinus thromboses, often the serous transudation and hemorrhage take place into an already primarily hypoxically damaged tissue which is still recognizable at the border zones. Such "border-center-phenomena" can also be observed in a different pathogentic form if brain purpura and serous plasmatic foci develop on the background of a diffuse myelin pallor with diffuse swelling of oligodendroglia. The same thing can be seen in edematous perivenous encephalitides where the perivenous foci of demyelination stand out from diffuse myelin pallor of the white matter. Among different histopathological features of the tissue swelling, a nun ber of easily characterized swelling syndromes can be recognized. To

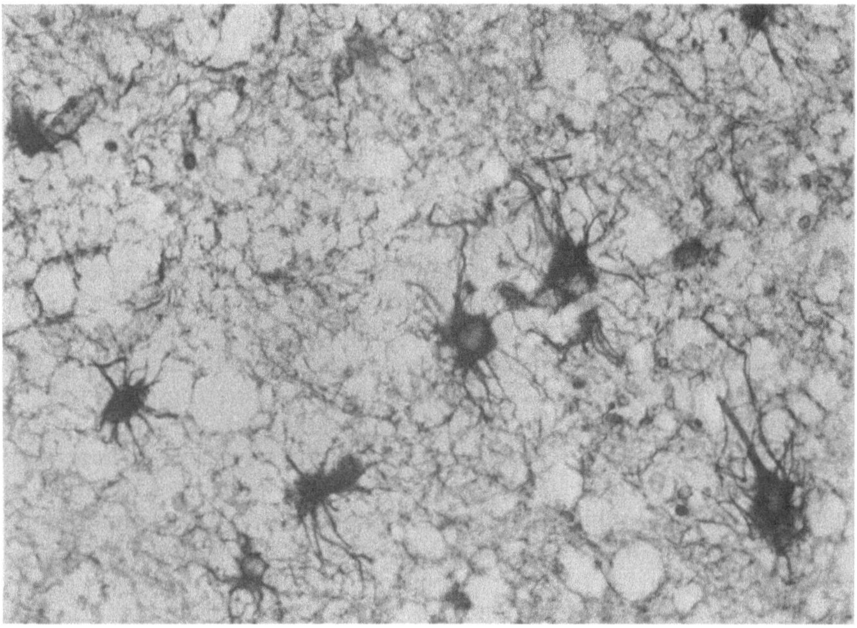

Fig. 6. Gro. (26a/55) See Fig. 5, Cajal-impregnation.

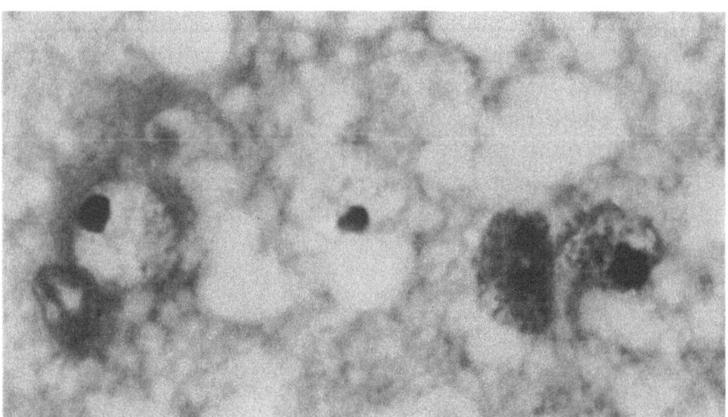

Fig. 7. Po. 43 years ♀ (60a/54). Metastatic carcinoma uteri. Edema of the cerebellar white matter. Oligodendrocytes with protoplasmatic girders and status spongiosus (PAS).

the various types of edematous lesions in cortex and white matter analyzed by Scholz must be added the syndrome of focal and diffuse swelling of dendrites in the molecular layer of the cerebellum and that of fine granular reticular disintegration of myelin sheaths in cerebral cortex. Acute swelling of oligodendroglia with homogenizing swelling of nuclei is a good indicator of early edematous lesions which may be restituted in the manner of the "dissociation glio-myélinique" with diffuse glioses, the structure of myelin sheath being preserved.

Residual formation of "tissue holes" often appears as the pseuc spongy state. Protoplasmatic astroglia, swelling of oligodendroglia, oligodendro-girder cells and ballooning of myelin sheaths or swelling of axons can simulate a spongy disintegration. In such case we are dealing with an infiltrating process (by swelling of cells, ballooning of axons or swelling of myelin sheaths). Besides this, a true spongy state in the swollen tissue of cortex and white matter exists, caused by glial insufficiency or by dissolution of axons or myelin sheaths. In this case the alteration may regress, leaving a general thinning of fibers with pallor of myelin sheaths and axon disintegration.

A special form represents the coarse cystic disintegration in colliquation necroses. The tissue process in subacute, chronic or chronic-relapsing tissue swellings can sometimes consist of merely mesenchymal proliferation within the progressively dilating Virchow Robin spaces or replacing astocytic proliferation. In some instances, especially in meningiomas, a malignant swelling of myelin tissue with formation of disintegrating, insufficient, giant glia cells takes place. A second form of malignant tissue swelling may develop from cerebral liquefaction, transudative formation of cysts, and serous "Massenergüssen" within the posttraumatic swelling of the white matter (Scheinker, Bonhoff). The term "malignant cerebral edema-resp. cerebral swelling" is applied to special processes within chronically or intermittently swollen tissue areas. In such cases, the development of edema may show a more malignant course than the original tumor.

REFERENCES

Bonhoff, G.: Über serösen Massenerguss und transsudative Zystenentstehung, Dtsch. Zschr. f. Nhlk., 168, 441 (1952).

Greenfield, J. G.: Criteria of cerebral edema, Proc. Roy. Soc. Med., 35, 525 (1942).

____: The histology of cerebral edema associated with intracranial tumors (with special reference to changes in the nerve fibres of the centrum ovale), Brain, 62, 2 (1939).

Jacob, H.: Über die Herdentwicklung bei Transsudationsschäden des Gehirns, Arch. f. Psych. u. Zschr. Neur., 186, 327 (1951).

_____: Über die Lückenherdbildung im "Nekrosenstadium" der Hirnerweichung. Zschr. f. d. ges. Neur. u. Psych., 172, 483 (1941).

_____: Zur Gruppierung der entzündlichen Erkrankungen des Nervensystems (insbesondere zur Frage der sog. "Entmarkungsencephalitiden" und der "serösen Entzündung"), Allg. Zschr. f. Psych. u. i Grenzgebiete, 121, 83 (1942).

_____: Die Kernhomogenisierungen der akut geschwollenen Oligodendroglia und der prae-amöboiden Glia beim Hirnödem, Arch. f. Psych. u. Zschr. f. d. ges. Neur., 206, 690 (1965).

_____: Zur histopathologischen Diagnose des akuten und chronisch rezidivierenden Hirnödems, Arch. f. Psychiat. u. Zschr. f. Neur., 179, 158 (1947).

_____: Über die diffuse Markdestruktion im Gefolge eines Hirnödems, Zschr. f. d. ges. Neur. Psychiat., 168, 382 (194).

_____: Zentralnervöse Gewebsschäden und Funktionsstörungen nach Erstickungvorgängen (Obstruktionshypoxydosen), Dtsch. Zschr. d. ges. gerichtl. Medizin 51, 3, 352 (1960).

_____; G. Mumme and H. Solcher: Entmarkung bei cerebralen Ödemschäden (Strangulationsmyelopathie), Arch. f. Psych. u. Zschr. f. d. ges. Neur., 203, 311 (1962).

Rosenhagen, K.: Über traumatische Hirnzysten, Dtsch. Zschr. f. Nhlk., 174, 541 (1956).

Scheinker, I. M.: Posttraumatic cerebral swelling resulting in cyst formation, J. Neuropath. and Exp. Neurol., 7, 321 (1948).

_____: Cerebral swelling and edema associated with tumor, Arch. Neurol., 45, 117 (1941).

_____: Cerebral swelling, Histopathology, Classification and clinical Significance of brain edema, J. Neurosurg., IV, No. 3, 255 (1947).

Scholz, W.: Histologische und topische Veränderungen und Vulnerabilitätsverhältnisse im menschlichen Gehirn bei Sauerstoffmangel, Ödem und plasmatischen Infiltrationen, Arch. f. Psych., 181, 621 (1949).

_____ and W. Wechsler: Nekrotisierende und Entmarkungsvorgänge bei cerebraler Gasembolie, Acta Neuropathologica, 1, 85 (1961).

Yokoi, S.: Neuropathological study of prefrontal lobotomy, J. Neuropath. and Exp. Neur., 16, 251 (1957).

Zülch, K. J.: Morphologische Befunde bei Hirnschwellung, Zbl. f. Neurochirurgie, 5, 4, 166 (1940).

IRWIN FEIGIN

SEQUENCE OF PATHOLOGICAL CHANGES IN BRAIN EDEMA

This paper will describe observations on the characteristics, course and sequelae of cerebral edema in man, and will attempt to draw some inferences from these observations as to the nature of the process and the mechanisms involved. In general, these observations are in accord with many earlier reports (Greenfield, Perret and Kernohan; Scheinker) and the interpretations drawn are classical, including that which considers cerebral edema to be an increment of fluid in an extracellular space, as is true in other organs.

Nearly all of our observations have been made on the human brain, and much of these have already been reported in detail (Feigin & Popoff, 1962, 1963). Edema was present as a consequence of trauma, both accidental and operative, of the presence of primary or metastatic neoplasms, of inflammatory processes such as abscesses, of vascular insults including infarcts and hemorrhages, and of hypertensive disease. Of these, neoplasms were probably the single most common causative lesion in our studies of acute edema, and trauma and hypertensive disease the most common in our studies on the late effects of cerebral edema. No essential differences were recognized in the edema observed in these differing situations. Others (Zülch; Zimmerman) emphasize basic distinctions among a variety of forms of edema which they hold to be fundamentally different, and which are characteristic of some and not others of the edema producing conditions listed above. The descriptions in this paper, however, should be considered applicable to the edema in all of these circumstances.

*This study was supported in part by Research Grant HE 02872 from the National Heart Institute of the United States Public Health Service and forms part of a study of cerebrovascular diseases at Bellevue Hospital by the Cornell-New York University Study Group on cerebrovascular diseases.

The brains were fixed in formalin, generally 20% with 1% acetic acid, occasionally 10% formalin. Histologic studies were performed exclusively on paraffin embedded sections. These were stained with hematoxylin and eosin (H & E), the Luxol blue-periodic acid Schiff (LBPAS) technique, with gold sublimate impregnations as modified for staining astrocytes in paraffin sections (Naoumenko & Feigin, 1961), with silver carbonate impregnations as modified for staining microglia in paraffin sections (Naoumenko & Feigin, 1963), the Romanes stain for axons, the phosphotungstic acid-hematoxylin (PTAH) stain, and occasionally with other stains as indicated. Of these, the LBPAS and the gold sublimate stains were most informative.

OBSERVATIONS

The Acute Phase (Feigin & Popoff, 1962)

Grossly, the edematous portions of the brain appeared swollen, the gyri flattened and the sulci narrowed. Cingulate and uncal herniations were sometimes present. On section, swelling was present predominantly in the white matter with the overlying cortex and adjacent basal gray structures showing virtually no grossly evident intrinsic change. The affected white matter, however, was enlarged, moist, slightly more translucent than normal and occasionally, of a very slightly yellow tinge (Fig. 1). In jaundiced individuals, however, and sometimes in edematous tissues adjacent to hemorrhage, the yellow or brown pigmentation was more intense, and served more clearly to indicate the gross normality of the overlying cortical gray matter. In some such instances, it was also apparent that the arcuate zone of the white matter just beneath the cortex, was relatively spared, remaining white in color in contrast to the discoloration of the deeper white matter (Fig. 2). This partial preservation followed the intricate folds of the gyral pattern, as if the arcuate zone served as a barrier to the spread of edema fluid.

Microscopically, the acutely edematous white matter stained more palely than did normal white matter with most stains. The axons were intrinsically normal, with only minimal morphological irregularities in caliber, but were separated from each other to a greater than normal degree. The same was true of the myelin sheaths, though slightly greater intrinsic morphological changes in the form of focal areas of slight swelling, were noted. The pallor of the edematous tissues appeared to result from the separation of the myelinated fibers, rather than any intrinsic change within them. No change in the microglial cells were recognized, and no phagocytes were present in the acute stages. In most instances, the oligodendroglia were also normal in appearance. On occasion, some of their nuclei assumed a homogeneous purple color and chromatin detail was obscured. The oligodendroglial cytoplasm was usually unstainec but in some severe cases, an enlarged perinuclear halo was present, and in rare instances, a small quantity of eosinophilic cytoplasm sur rounded cells thought to be oligodendroglia.

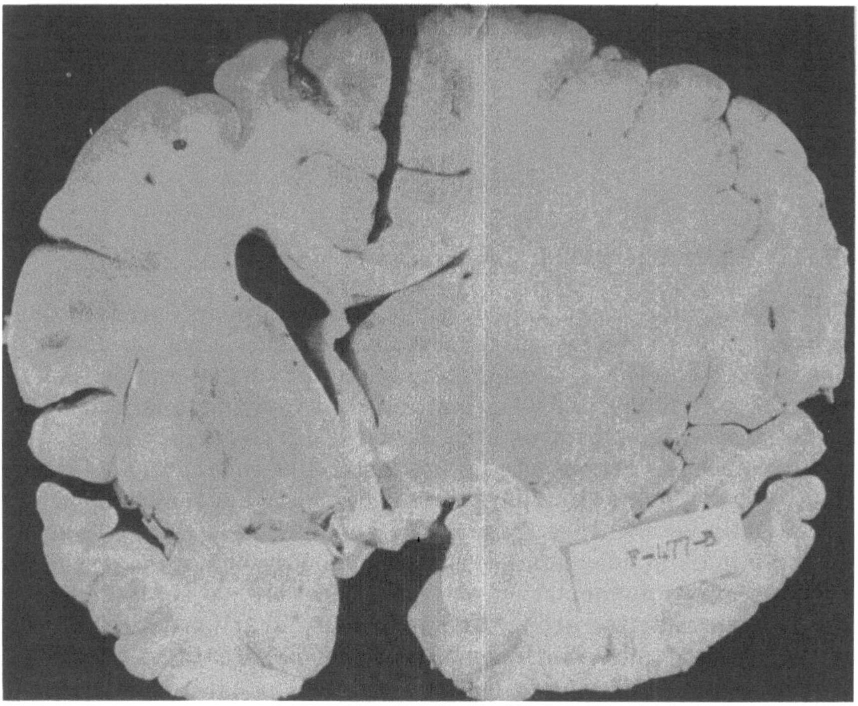

Fig. 1. Acute edema of right hemisphere due to metastatic carcinoma, X1.

The nuclei of most astrocytes were normal or slightly enlargec The astrocyte cytoplasm was unstained with H&E or PTAH technique in areas affected mildly for a short period of time. In areas affected more severely and for longer periods, the cell bodies of a few, clearl a small minority of astrocytes, were stained, and these cells appear enlarged. With gold sublimate stains, relatively severe and widespread regressive changes in the cell bodies and processes of a great majority of the astrocytes, were demonstrated (Figs. 3a, b). Some cells stained poorly. Some were rounded with only a few short stubby proces

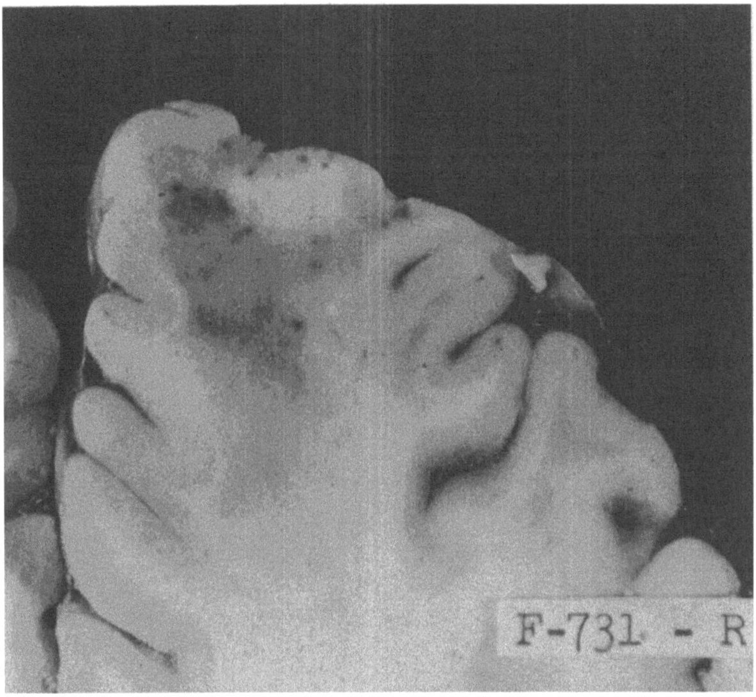

Fig. 2. Acute edema due to trauma in jaundiced individual. The edematous tissues deep in the white matter are colored yellow, while the arcuate zone remains white, X2.

In some, processes were fragmented, though retaining normal contour and depth of staining (Fig. 3b), while in others, the processes were lost (Fig. 3a). A few appeared enlarged with well-stained processes.

In instances in which the edema was relatively severe, lakes of stained materials were present within the neural tissues of the affected white matter, and in the perivascular spaces. With each stain, these materials appeared the same as materials within the lumen of blood vessels, and were pink with H&E, blue with the azocarmine stain, tan with the PTAH stain, and red with the LBPAS stain. The materials were most often smooth and homogeneous, rarely slightly granular, and occasionally contained vacuoles (Fig. 4). The LBPAS stain was optimum for their demonstration, the red color of these materials contrasting sharply with the blue-green of the myelinated fibers. The quantity of these stained materials was often very great, at times greater than the sum of all other histologic elements, and these materials passed through the tissues for considerable distances. These materials are interpreted as repre-

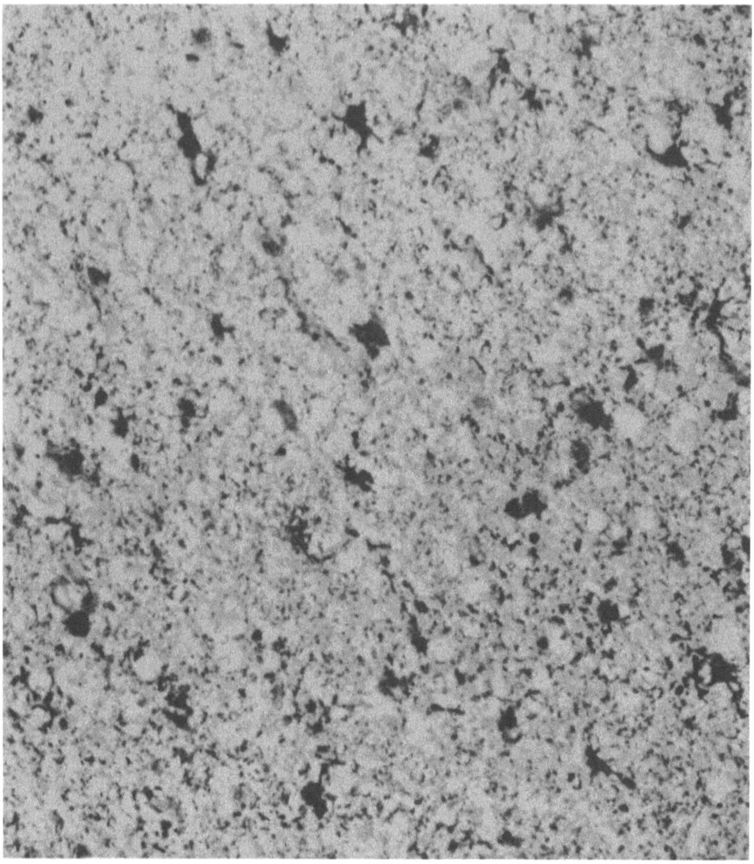

Fig. 3a. Acute edema due to malignant astrocytoma. The deep white matter. The astrocytes show severe regressive changes. Paraffin gold sublimate X225.

senting components of blood plasma and of the edema fluid derived from plasma, and may be protein in nature.

The severity of edema as indicated by the quantity of these stained materials, did not necessarily parallel the severity of the regressive changes in astrocytes as visualized with gold stains. In cases of severe diffuse edema of very short duration, the astrocytic changes were sometimes of lesser severity, though generally with focal areas of accentuation. In older cases in which the edema had receded, the astrocytic changes were often of great severity, and probably permanent.

In many instances, the arcuate zone appeared less affected than the deeper white matter. It was darker in color, particularly

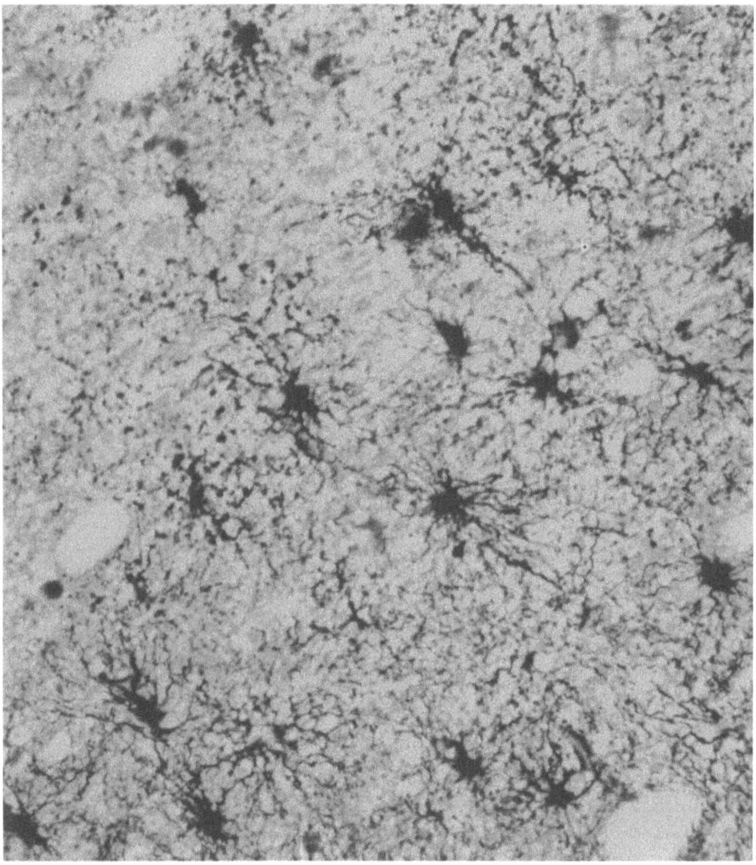

Fig. 3b. Acute edema due to malignant astrocytoma, thought to be of short duration. Some of the astrocytes are hypertrophied, while others show marked regressive changes. Paraffin gold sublimate X225.

with myelin stains, apparently because the myelinated fibers were less widely separated. Lakes of stained fluid in the deeper tissues often failed to penetrate into the arcuate zone. With gold sublimate stains, the astrocytes in the arcuate zone often appeared normal or nearly normal, although those in the deeper white matter showed severe changes like those described above.

Water Content of Normal and Acutely Edematous Brain

The readily volatile water contents of brain tissues were determined in a series of edematous and normal human brains fixed in

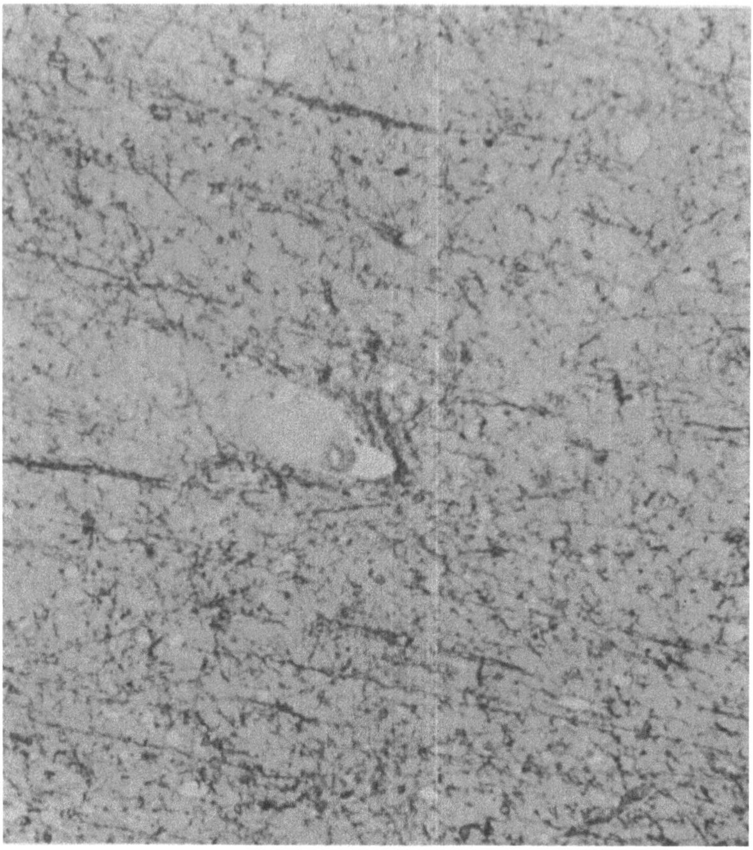

Fig. 4. Acute edema due to malignant astrocytoma, same block as Figs. 3a, b, and 5. The extracellular spaces are permeated by lakes of pink stained materials among the myelinated fibers. The latter are widely separated. Luxol blue-periodic acid Schiff X225.

20% formalin with 1% acetic acid (Feigin & Popoff, 1962). The sample was excised, blotted dry, weighed, and placed in an incubator at 67°C. The weight decreased reaching a constant value in 100 hours. The decrement of weight, expressed as a percentage of original wet weight, is considered to represent the readily volatile water. The water content of edematous white matter was 72% adjacent to an abscess; 74% adjacent to a focal hemorrhage; 79% in lead intoxication; 81% adjacent to an anaplastic astrocytoma; 83% adjacent to a fresh infarct; and 85%, 86%, 90% and 92% adjacent to metastatic carcinomatous nodules (four different brains). In 7 of these 9 cases, the water content of the contralateral apparently normal hemisphere, was determined, and with one exception (60%), ranged from 66%-

72%. In 5 additional normal cases, the water content of white matter ranged from 66%-74%.

In a second study (Adachi & Feigin) the water content of gray matter, arcuate white matter, deep white matter and corpus callosum was determined in a series of 9 normal human brains fixed in 20% formalin-1% acetic acid for 1-2 weeks. The determinations were in duplicate, but taken serially, so that the second sample of each tissue was not taken until the first samples of all tissues had been taken. Values for cortex ranged from 84% to 88% (average 85.4%); for deep white matter 68% to 74% (average 71.2%); for arcuate white matter 77% to 81% (average 79.0%); for corpus callosum 70% to 77% (average 73.3%). The difference between the water content of normal arcuate and normal deep white matter is highly significant ($P < 0.01$); between normal corpus callosum and deep white matter, barely significant ($P < 0.1$). In a supplementary study performed on samples of two fresh (unfixed) brains, arcuate white matter was found to contain 76.7% and 78.5% water (average 77.6%) in instances in which the deep white matter contained 70.7% and 71.4% (average 71.2%) water, respectively. The cortex contained 84.2% and 87.4% (average 85.8%), respectively.

This latter study had been suggested by the observation (Adachi & Feigin) that in coronal sections of formalin fixed human brains permitted to dry at room temperatures, the deeper white matter often assumed a gray-brown discoloration at a time when the arcuate zone remained normally white in color. This distinction became apparent after approximately four hours, beyond which observations became difficult.

A series of 21 brains were weighed at autopsy, and weighed again after fixation in 20% formalin-1% acetic acid for 7 to 14 days. This reproduced the parameters of fixation used in the studies described above. The change in weight, expressed as percentage of original weight, was +15.4, +12.4, +7.5, +5.8, +5.0, +4.2, +2.3, +1.5, +1.4, +0.8, +0.7, 0, 0, −0.7, −1.0, −1.9, −2.6, −6.1, −6.7, −7.7. −8.1, respectively (Adachi & Feigin). The median value was +0.7%. When small samples of normal unfixed brain tissues were fixed for a like period in the same medium, the change in weight was considerably greater, ranging from +14% to +47%. Samples approximately 100 mgs. in weight swelled more than those approximately 1 gram in weight, and white matter swelled more than gray.

The Late Effects of Cerebral Edema (Feigin & Popoff, 1963)

The description which follows is based initially on observations on formalin fixed human brains following accidental trauma, operative trauma and a few cases of persistent metastatic carcinoma.

These are situations in which antecedent edema may be postulated with a reasonable degree of certainty.

The changes attributable to edema consisted essentially of a degeneration of the white matter. This degeneration was often severe and extensive, spreading from a focus of traumatic cortical injury or tumor to involve a major portion of the deeper white matter (Fig. 5). In the course of this spread, the degeneration undermined large segments of cortex and often, large segments of arcuate white matter (Fig. 6). The cortex and arcuate zones generally showed only minimal changes, their preservation contrasting sharply with the severe degeneration of the deeper white matter.

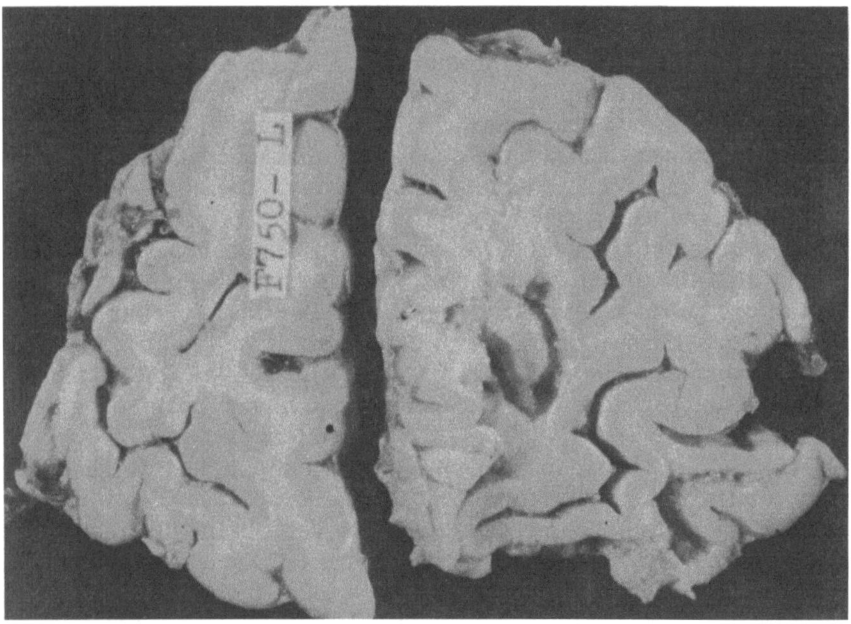

Fig. 5. Degeneration of white matter extending upwards from zone of old trauma in orbital gyri, X2.

Grossly, the degenerated white matter appeared softened, somewhat retracted on cut section, slightly gray in color, and, occasionally, markedly rarefied and even cystic (Fig. 7a). Microscopically, the affected tissues were pale and rarefied with most stains, and particularly with myelin stains. The loss of myelin sheaths was variable, and was often very severe, though not total. A few myelinated fibers were generally preserved except in the totally cystic areas, and there was little intrinsic change in the per-

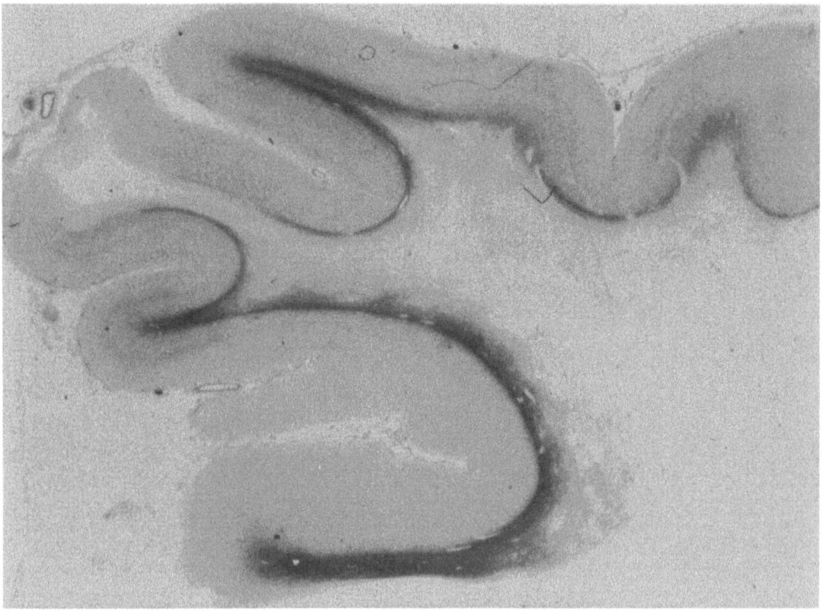

Fig. 6. Degeneration of white matter, extending from focus of old traumatic contusion on left. The arcuate zone is relatively preserved. Mahon stain for myelin X6.

sistent myelin sheaths, though focal swellings and globule formation were noted in the subacute cases. The axons were also decreased in number, but generally the myelin loss was very much greater than the axon loss. In cases of cystic degeneration, the axon loss was also total. The oligodendroglial cells were decreased in number, approximately in proportion to the myelin loss. With H&E, and PTAH stains, the cell bodies of some astrocytes appeared swollen, though a proliferation of glial fibers was not prominent. With gold sublimate stains, the astrocytes tended to be poorly stained, the cell bodies swollen, the processes decreased in number, shortened, thickened, and poorly formed. (Fig. 7b). In most instances, only a rare microglial phagocyte was present, even in cases in which myelin loss was profound. In cases in which the process was still active, however, many activated microglial cells were demonstrable (Fig. 8). The walls of some of the small blood vessels were thickened and hyalinized.

In sharp contrast, microscopic changes in the preserved arcuate zone of the white matter were minimal. The number of myelinated fibers and their appearance, were normal or almost normal.

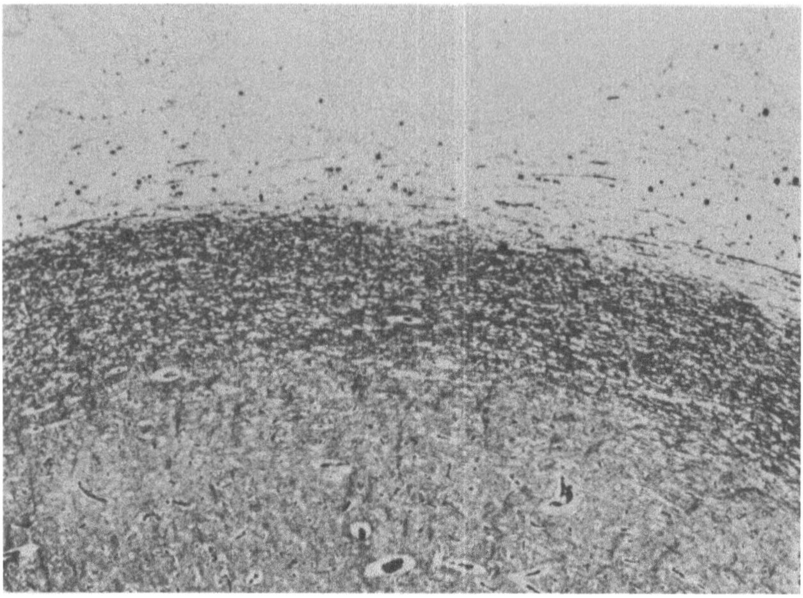

Fig. 7a. Loss of myelin in degenerated white matter (top) adjacent to white matter infarct in hypertensive individual. The arcuate zone (central transverse band) is relatively preserved. The cortex (bottom) is normal. Luxol blue-periodic acid Schiff X40.

With gold stains, the astrocytes tended to be normal, though some appeared hypertrophied and some slight regressive changes were also noted.

A similar pattern of pathological change was observed in the brains of individuals in circumstances in which antecedent trauma or neoplasm was not present. In most such cases, the presence of antecedent or coexistent hypertensive disease was established clinically or by pathological examination of the heart and kidneys. A direct relationship between the intensity of the cerebral changes and the height of the blood pressure, was not evident. Frequently, the white matter degeneration spread from a focus of tissue destruction with the characteristics of an infarct. It is our experience that infarcts affecting the white matter occur more frequently in hypertensive than in normotensive individuals, and parenthetically, are more likely to induce a collagenous reaction. Occasionally, the pattern of degeneration in the white matter appeared to spread from a lesion resembling an old focal hemorrhage (Fig. 9). In a few cases, the degeneration was diffuse, widespread and bilateral, and antecedent focal lesions were not recognized. The small cavitations some-

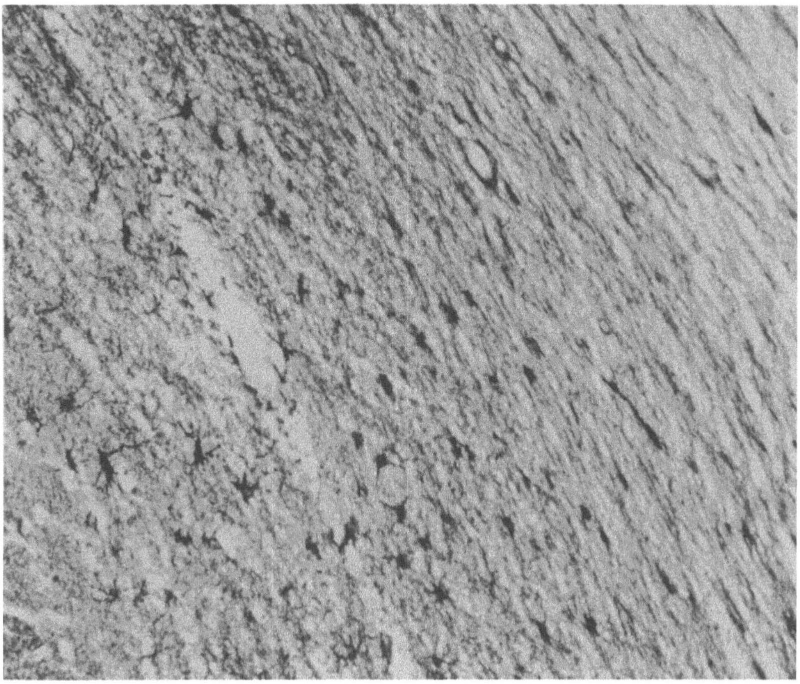

Fig. 7b. Same block. The astrocytes in the deep white matter (right) are unstained, while some in the arcuate zone (left) are better preserved. Paraffin gold sublimate X225.

times present in such tissues did not resemble infarcts, but were like similar areas in the traumatic cases, in which the degeneration was particularly severe. It is these cases which are pertinent to the problem of Binswanger's encephalopathy as discussed below.

The Gray Matter in Edema

In most instances in which the white matter showed severe changes like those described above, the overlying or adjacent gray matter showed almost no significant changes on gross inspection or by histologic studies. Enlarged paraneuronal or paragliocytic spaces were not generally present. With acute trauma or infarction, necrosis of gray matter was present and this was often associated with lakes of stainable fluid like those seen in acutely edematous white matter. These were not seen in the absence of acute necrosis. Necrotic astrocytes in such lesions were unstained with gold sublimate.

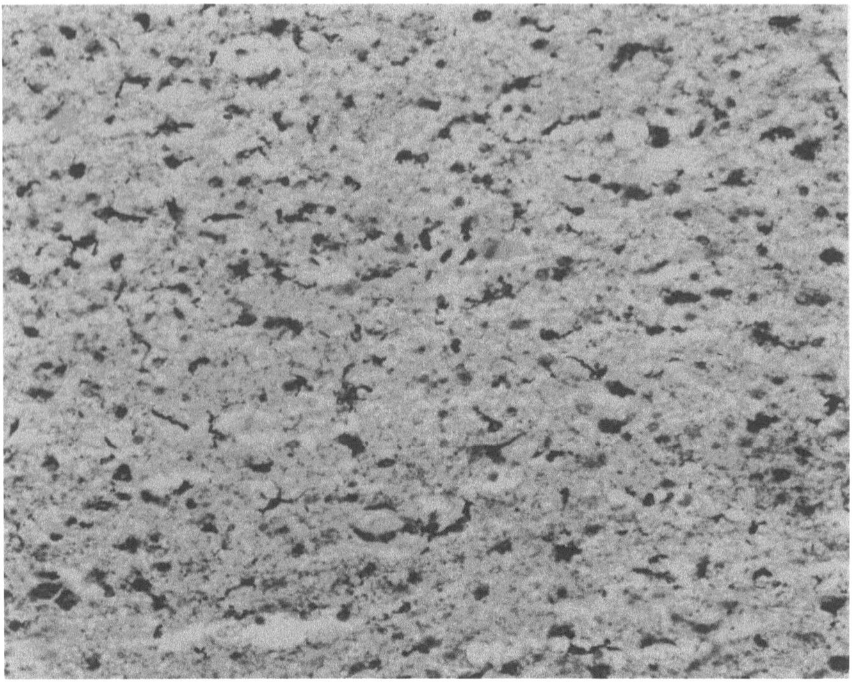

Fig. 8. Edema due to malignant astrocytoma. Area of subacute change showing microglial proliferation. Paraffin silver carbonate X225.

In instances in which an individual survived such trauma or infarction, the affected gray matter showed a loss of neurons and of other neural elements. The underlying white matter often showed a far more extensive lesion, which centered beneath the cortical scar but extended widely so as to undermine apparently normal cortex lateral to the lesion. This white matter degeneration is described above. The normality of the overlying cortex, lateral to the cortical scar, was quite striking even in instances in which there was appreciable axon loss in the subjacent tissues. The neurons were almost normal in number and appearance. The astrocytes were generally normal, though sometimes they appeared somewhat enlarged with gold sublimate stains, and their processes better defined A slight increase in microglial cells was sometimes noted.

"Spongy" Edema

In a small number of cases of edema, portions of the affected tissues contained relatively large rounded cavities resulting in a "spongy" appearance. Some of these cavities contained PAS stained materials like those characteristic of edema, and the astrocytes in the septae showed changes like those seen in edema. The sponge cavities were very much larger than the astrocyte cell bodies or processes, and did not appear to lie within them. There was no relationship between the PAS stained material and the astrocytic processes.

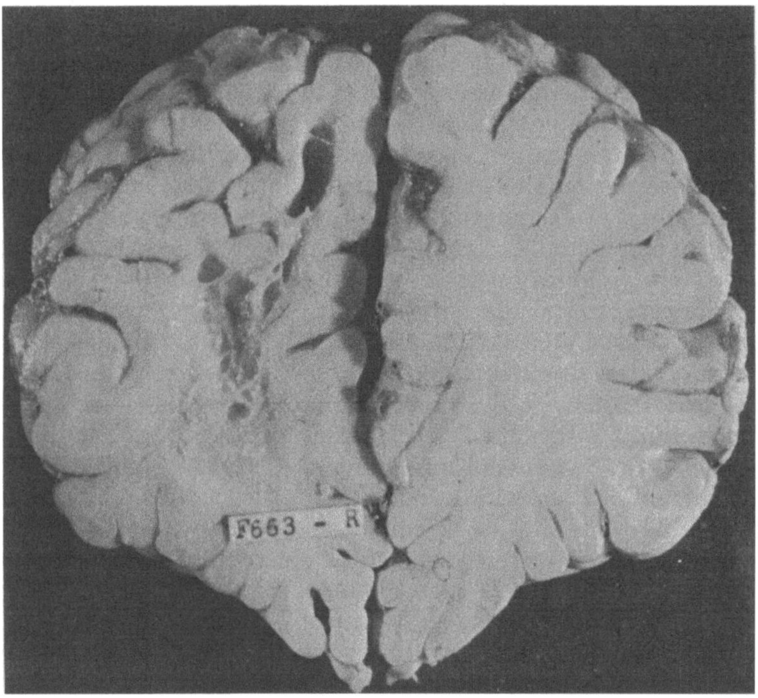

Fig. 9. Severe degeneration of white matter in hypertensive individual. There was no evidence of trauma or of neoplasm, X1.2.

The precise nature of the spongy change is not clear. In some instances, it appears to be artifact. It is evident, however, that this change is not identical to edema, but the two processes may be associated.

COMMENTS

Our first concern is the failure to appreciate a distinction in our studies between "cerebral swelling" and "cerebral edema." The concept that these represent two fundamentally distinct processes has been supported by many eminent pathologists (Zülch; Zimmerman) and rejected by others of equal distinction (Greenfield; Perret and Kernohan; Scheinker). "Cerebral swelling" is said to result from the presence in the brain of primary or metastatic neoplasms, and in other circumstances. Such material is particularly well represented in our studies of the acute process. These edematous tissues appear to us to be quite wet, not dry as has been described. In this feature, and indeed in all aspects, the edema with neoplasms appears identical to the "cerebral edema" of trauma and in some other circumstances, which some would consider a separate entity.

The suggestion has been made that "cerebral swelling" like that associated with neoplasms, is characterized by an increment in the intracellular water content (Zülch) or of fluid accumulation in intramyelinic vacuoles (Zimmerman); in either case, the presence of an increment of extracellular fluid is excluded. Some earlier electron microscopic studies, which in retrospect, may have been performed entirely on gray matter, appeared to support the thesis that the fluid accumulation was entirely intracellular. These described a marked swelling of the cytoplasm of "clear glial processes" variously interpreted as those of astrocytes (Gershenfeld, et al.; Torack et al., 1959; Torack, et al., 1960) or oligodendroglia (Luse & Harris) and it was implied that the traditional concept of an extracellular increment of fluid in edema was untenable (Torack, et al., 1959). The increment of fluid within intramyelinic vacuoles has been described in the white matter of animals poisoned with triethyl tin; while at first, these were thought to be extracellular in location (Aleu, et al., 1963a), more recent interpretation did not consider them to be so located (Aleu, et al., 1963b). We are not aware of any report in which these intramyelinic vacuoles were the essential change in human edema, or in experimental edema of other origin. The relevance of tin intoxication to human edema remains to be clarified. In any case, the weight of evidence seemed so overwhelming, that the editors of an annual review in this field were constraine to say (Mackay): "The recent electron microscopic denial of extracellular space and restriction of edema to intracellular and especially intraglial water and electrolytes is now all but established, though the light microscopists... find some evidence for extracellular edema."

In contrast, the classical concept of cerebral edema has held that an extracellular accumulation of fluid was characteristic, either of all of the conditions under consideration, or at least of those characterized as "cerebral edema" in contradistinction to "cerebral swelling." Our own studies performed when the denial of extracellular fluid was "all but established," led to the inference that in all of the conditions being considered, (both "edema" and "swelling" in our view) acute edema is in fact characterized by an extracellular accumulation of fluid (Feigin & Popoff, 1962). The inference was based on the presence of stainable materials interspersed among the myelinated fibers in an obviously extracellular location, the astrocytic changes demonstrable with gold stains which did not support the intracellular concept, and the very magnitude of the fluid increment calculated to be as much as 2.5G water to each 1G of normal white matter. More recent electron microscopic studies have provided clear evidence that an extracellular accumulation of fluid may occur in both animals (Raimondi, et al.; Gonatas, et al.) and humans (Long & Hartmann). In these circumstances, light microscopists may choose to remain confident of the validity of their findings, even when these seem to be contradicted by electron microscopic studies, though some reports continue to disparage the contributions of light microscopic studies in this field (Zimmerman; Hirano, et al.).

Cerebral edema of white matter is very often focal, being more severe in the immediate vicinity of a local edema producing lesion such as a carcinomatous nodule, and becoming progressively less severe in a centrifugal fashion. The appearance suggests that the edema fluid is produced locally, and then diffuses outwards through the extracellular spaces of the white matter. If this be true, there may not be any primary alteration in the vessels of the edematous areas peripheral to the central source of fluid in this circumstance. The concentration of fluid in the perivascular spaces so often observed, may simply reflect the fact that these spaces permit the diffusion of fluid to an even greater degree than the tissue spaces.

Of equal interest is the tendency for some portions of the white matter to be spared by the edema which may be very severe in adjacent areas. This is most striking with respect to the arcuate zone of the white matter, but some sparing of the corpus callosum and internal capsule has also been described. Histologically, these tissues appear very much like the deeper central white matter in which severe edema is so often noted. The tangential direction of fibers in the arcuate zone might serve as a barrier, but no such factor is evident in regard to the corpus callosum or the internal capsule. No significant difference is recognized with respect to the astrocytes of these tissues.

A significant factor may be the water content of these tissues in the normal state (Adachi & Feigin). Compared to the deep white matter with a water content of 71.2%, the high water content of normal arcuate tissues (79%) is associated with a high degree of immunity to edema, and the moderate water content of the corpus callosum (73.3%) with a moderate degree of immunity. Stewart-Wallace reported an even higher water content in the normal corpus callosum,

75.7%. The mechanisms involved in the relative preservation of the arcuate zone and the other tissues in edema, are not clear, but the sparing of the arcuate zone is so striking that it may well be considered an attribute of edema and an aid in its recognition.

Our quantitative data on water content has been challenged because they were obtained from formalin fixed tissues. Our studies are so designed that our analysis consists of a comparison of tissue derived from the same fixed brain. If, for example, the arcuate and deeper white matter were truly identical, identical values would be obtained for these tissues in an individual brain even if fixation had distorted such values. Actually, no distortion of the water values in our fixed brains are observed for those tissues for which comparable values are available for fresh unfixed tissues. Thus, the values for cortex and deep white matter in our fixed brains are well within the normal values established for these tissues in fresh material (Folch-Pi & LeBaron). Our arcuate values, however, are much higher, in both fixed tissues and in two samples obtained from unfixed brains.

We do not imply that a marked swelling of brain tissue never occurs with formalin fixation, but only that it does not occur in the circumstances employed by us. There is evidence that such swelling is less with high concentrations of formalin than with low (Flata Hrdlicka; Lagerlof & Torgersrund; Bahr, et al.; Adachi & Feigin). It is less in acid than in neutral or alkaline media (Gross & Lohans Lagerlof & Torgersrund; Adachi & Feigin). It is less in the large brains of higher species of animals, than those of lower species (Hrdlicka). It is less if a whole brain is fixed than if a small sample of a similar brain is fixed (Adachi & Feigin), and this impression is reinforced if one surveys the other references cited in this paragraph, though no other observer has specifically compared whole brains and small samples. With respect to all of these factor the conditions employed in our studies would minimize the swelling anticipated. An estimate of the degree of swelling actually present in human brains fixed in 20% formalin-1% acetic acid for 1-2 weeks was determined in a separate group of brains from our laboratory. The median value for an increment of weight due to fixation was +0.7%, with 19 of 21 brains showing less than a ±10% change. The effect of such change, if it had occured, on the observed water content of the white matter, is also quite small. If the increment were 10% and uniformly distributed, a brain containing 70% water in the white matter, an average figure, would contain 72.7% water after fixation. This latter value is still well within normal limits. It can be calculated that a swelling of 26.9% uniformly distributed, would be required to increase the water content of the white matter of a brain from the lower limit of normal, 67%, to the upper limit of normal, 74%. For these reasons, the high value for the water content of normal arcuate white matter, 79%, should not be attributed to fixation swelling.

Edema of the gray matter is certainly present in the human brain in cases of traumatic contusion, in infarction, and possibly in other circumstances. In contusion and infarction, the tissues appear necrotic, and the increment of fluid is seen to be extracellular. This may be manifest in the form of lakes of stained materials like those seen in edema involving the white matter. The astrocytes are also necrotic and do not stain with gold.

Another pattern of gray matter change has been described as "edema" in some reports (Zimmerman). This consists essentially of the presence of enlarged clear paraneuronal, paragliocytic, and perivascular spaces. Such changes can readily be reproduced in normal, non-edematous tissues, by too rapid processing of the tissues in preparing histologic sections, and possibly by other errors in processing (Fig. 10a,b). These changes are absent in the gray

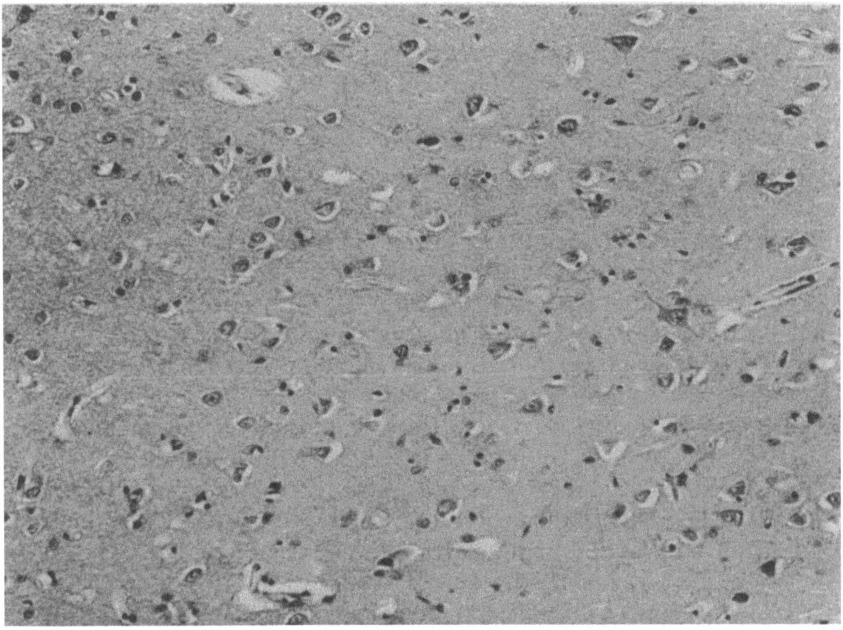

Fig. 10a. Normal cortex. Hematoxylin and eosin X225.

matter adjacent to severely edematous white matter. For these reasons, we consider such changes to be artifacts unless error in processing can clearly be excluded.

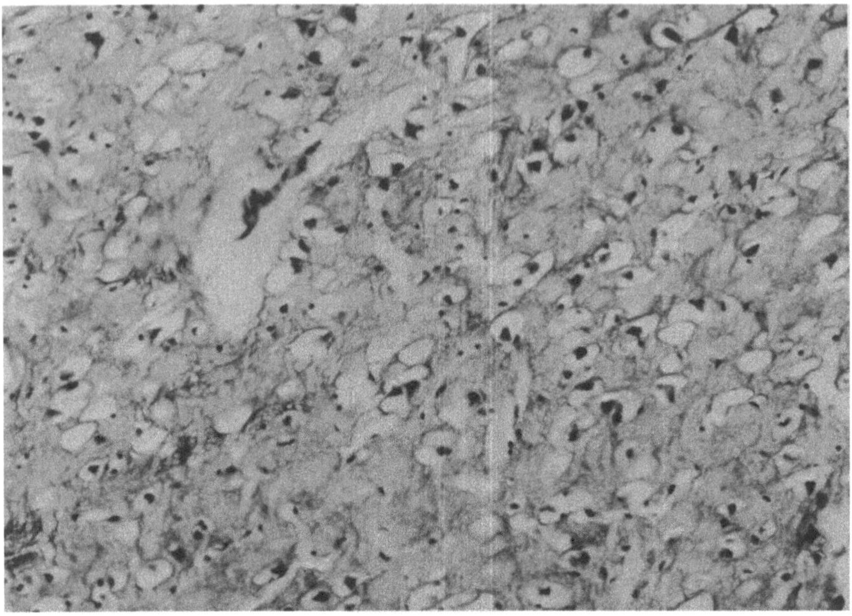

Fig. 10b. Normal cortex. These tissues had been dehydrated rapidly before embedding. The enlarged paraneuronal, paragliocytic and perivascular spaces had been artifactually induced. Hematoxylin and eosin X225.

With the electron microscope, studies on gray matter have revealed a fluid accumulation within the processes of clear glial cells (astrocytes) in tissues adjacent to neoplasms, with no extracellular fluid component (Torack, et al., 1960). This intracellular form of "edema" of the gray matter is like that originally postulated for the brain as a whole. In gray matter showing such changes, the water content was not considered significantly increased, as compared to normal gray, in a study of rabbit brain containing a transplanted tumor (Herzog, et al.), or injured by triethyl tin intoxication (Taylor, et al.) The highest value for an increment of water in gray matter, to our knowledge, is that reported by Aleu, et al. (1964), associated with a glioma in mouse brain, in which the water content rose from 79.5% to 82.6%, representing an increment of 0.236 G of water for each 1G of original brain tissue. Such increments contrast with those reported for white matter, which are appreciably greater. The highest increment of water in white matter of which we are aware, occurred in the white matter of a human brain with a metastatic carcinoma, in which the water in edematous tissues was 92%, while the contralateral normal white matter was 71%, representing an increment of 2.549G of water for each 1G of original tissue (Feigin & Popoff, 1962). Our failure to recognize such intracytoplasmic fluid accumulation in non-necrotic gray matter of the human brain, does not exclude its occurrence, but this does suggest that it is a far less significant phenomenon than is the edema of white matter.

Some of the characteristics of the tissue changes which remain after an episode of cerebral edema has receded, could have been predicted from our knowledge of the acute changes. These include the paramount localization to the white matter, the relative preservation of the arcuate zone, and the marked regressive changes in the astrocytes, which are apparently permanent. The edema fluid itself, manifest by the presence of stained material in the acute stage, is no longer visible, but the water content of these tissues is generally quite high. This is probably a relative, not an absolute increase in water, reflecting a loss of tissue elements. The loss of tissue in the post-edematous white matter is very great and includes an unexpectedly severe loss of myelin. It will be recalled that only minor intrinsic changes in myelin are recognized in the acute state, though these fibers are widely separated from each other. In the rare instances in which the edema is though to be in an intermediate stage of evolution, more severe myelin changes are noted, associated with an appreciable microglial proliferation. Such cases are uncommon; most individuals will either die during the acute phase of cerebral edema, if this be sufficiently severe, or will survive for a long enough time to permit the process to become obsolete. It is in this latter stage that the severity of the myelin loss is best appreciated. The relative preservation of axons in the demyelinated area is noteworthy.

As the pattern of tissue change characteristic of the post-edema state was established in cases of accidental and operative trauma, and in some cases of neoplasm, it became apparent that this same pattern was present in association with hypertensive disease. This relationship warrants emphasis and further study. In the tissues surrounding hemorrhages in hypertensive individuals, fresh edema may be noted about fresh hemorrhages, and the pattern of post-edema degeneration is noted about old hemorrhages. Infarcts are most numerous in gray matter, but infarcts in white matter occur with a disproportionately high frequence among hypertensive individuals, and parenthetically, are more likely to contain collagen, than is true of normotensive individuals. The tissues surrounding such lesions often show the stigmata of antecedent edema.

Of even greater interest is the occasional occurrence in hypertensive individuals, of broad diffuse zones of tissues altered in this fashion without any focal lesion being present to which the edema might have been a consequence. Such tissues often contain numerous thick walled, hyalinized blood vessels, so that the appearance comes to resemble Binswanger's encephalopathy. We suggest that this condition is in fact, the end result of antecedent cerebral edema associated with hypertensive disease, and that the vascular changes are secondary to hypertension and to the tissue changes, and are not the cause of the tissue changes (Feigin & Popoff, 1963). It may be noted that the cases originally reported by Binswanger were described as having arteriosclerotic, atrophic kidneys, some with enlarged hearts and that the relationship to hypertension had been recognized earlier by Blackwood.

The severity of the hypertension, and even its persistence, are not major factors related to this edema. Indeed, in some cases, the presence of hypertensive disease is best inferred from pathological studies of the kidneys and heart, since clinical confirmation may be inconclusive and even absent. It will be recalled that Byron describe cerebral edema in animals in which hypertension had been experimentally induced.

Utilizing the histologic criteria for the recognition of edema as outlined above, the occurrence of edema may be suspected in a great variety of pathological conditions. These include phenylketonuria, maple syrup urine disease, hepato-cerebral degeneration, cystic infantile encephalomalacia, multiple sclerosis, diffuse cerebral sclero sis, and possibly syringomyelia. Each of these must be separately evaluated with material adequate for this purpose, pending which, the implication of edema as one pathogenetic factor must be held in abeyance.

SUMMARY AND CONCLUSIONS

1) The tissue changes noted in brains rendered edematous by trauma, the presence of neoplasms, by inflammatory processes, by vascular lesions and by hypertensive disease, are described in the acute stage, and in the obsolete, postedematous state.

2) It is suggested that the edema is essentially the same in all of these circumstances, and that a distinction between "cerebral edema" and "cerebral swelling" is not warranted.

3) The process is thought to consist essentially of a fluid accumulation in the extracellular spaces of the white matter, with a relative sparing of the arcuate zones. The latter may be related to the normally high water content of this tissue. The gray matter also shows a lesser degree of involvement, except when necrotic.

4) Hypertensive individuals have a significant predisposition to cerebral edema. Edema may be an important pathogenetic factor in a variety of other pathologic conditions.

REFERENCES

Adachi, M. and I. Feigin: Cerebral edema and the water content of normal white matter, J.Neurol.Neurosurg.Psychiat., 29, 446 (1966).

Aleu, F. P., R. Katzman and R. D. Terry: Fine structure and electrolyte analyses of cerebral edema induced by alkyl tin intoxication, J. Neuropath. Exper. Neurol., 22, 344 (1963a).

_____, _____ and _____: Fine structure and electrolyte analyses of cerebral edema induced by alkyl tin intoxication, Ibid., 403-413 (1963b).

Bahr, G. F., G. Bloom and V. Friberg: Volume changes of tissues in physiological fluids during fixation in osmium tetroxide or formaldehyde and during subsequent treatment, Exper. Cell Res., 12, 342-355 (1957).

Blackwood, W.: in Greenfield's Neuropathology, 2nd ed., Baltimore: Williams & Wilkins Co., 126 (1963).

Binswanger, O.: Die Abgrenzung der allgemeinen progressiven Paralyse. Berl. Klin. Wschr., 31, 1103-1105, 1137-1139, 1180-1186 (1894).

Byrom, F. B.: The pathogenesis of hypertensive encephalopathy and its relation to the malignant phase of hypertension: Experimental evidence from the hypertensive rat, Lancet, 2, 201-211 (1954).

Feigin, I. and N. Popoff: Neuropathological observations on cerebral edema: The acute phase, Arch. Neurol., 6, 151-160 (1962).

_____ and _____: Neuropathological changes late in cerebral edema: The relationship to trauma, hypertensive disease and Binswanger's encephalopathy, J. Neuropath. Exper. Neurol., 22, 500-511 (1963).

Flatau, E.: Beitrag zur technischen Bearbeitung des Centralnervensystems, Anat. Anzeiger, 13, 323-329 (1897).

Folchi-Pi, J. and F. N. LeBaron: Chemical composition of the mammalian nervous system, in: Metabolism of the nervous system (ed. by D. Richter). New York: Pergamon Press, 68 (1957).

Gerschenfeld, H. M., F. Wald, J. A. Zadunaisky and E. P. D. De Robertis: Function of astroglia in the water-ion metabolism of the central nervous system, Neurology, 9, 412-425 (1959).

Gonatas, N. K., H. M. Zimmerman, and S. Levine: Ultrastructure of inflammation with edema in the rat brain, Am. J. Path., 42, 455-469 (1963).

Greenfield, J. G.: The histology of cerebral edema associated with intracranial tumors (with special reference to changes in the nerve fibers of the centrum ovale), Brain, 62, 129-152 (1939).

Gross, W. and H. Lohaus: Untersuchungen über die Wirkung von Härtungsflüssigkeiten auf tierische Gewebe, Ztchr. f. Wiss. Mikroskop., 49, 168-190 (1932).

Herzog, I., W. A. Levy and L. C. Scheinberg: Biochemical and morphologic studies of cerebral edema associated with intracerebral tumors in rabbits, J. Neuropath. Exper. Neurol., 24, 244-255 (1965).

Hirano, A., H. M. Zimmerman and S. Levine: The fine structure of cerebral fluid accumulation. III. Extracellular spread of cryptococcal polysaccharides in the acute stage, Amer. J. Path., 45, 1-19 (1964).

Hrdlicka, A.: Brains and brain preservatives. Part I. Physical changes in human and other brains collected under different conditions and preserved in various formalin preparations, Proc. U. S. Nat'l. Museum, 30, 245-276 (1906).

Lagerlof, H. and T. Torgersrund: Zur Kenntnis der Gewichts — und Volumen Veranderungen bei Formalin Fixation von Gehirngewebe und der Einwirkung von NaCl-Zusatz darauf, J. f. Psychol. u. Neurol., 46, 178-188 (1934).

Long, D. M. and J. F. Hartmann: The ultrastructure of human cerebral edema, J. Neuropath. Exper. Neurol., 24, 150-151 (1965).

Luse, S. A. and B. Harris: Electron microscopy of the brain in experimental edema, J. Neurosurg., 17, 439-446 (1960).

Mackay, R. P.: Year Book of Neurology, Psychiatry and Neurosurgery, 1962-1963, Chicago Year Book Publishing Co., p. 7.

Naoumenko, J. and I. Feigin: A modification for paraffin sections of the Cajal gold-sublimate stain for astrocytes, J. Neuropath. Exper. Neurol., 20, 602-604 (1961).

_____ and _____: A modification for paraffin section of silver carbonate impregnation for microglia, Acta Neuropath., 2, 402-406 (1963).

Perret, G. E. and J. W. Kernohan: Histopathologic changes of the brain caused by intracranial tumors (so-called edema or swelling of the brain), J. Neuropath. Exper. Neurol., 2, 341-352 (1943).

Raimondi, A. J., J. P. Evans and S. Mullan: Studies of cerebral edema, III, Alterations in the white matter: An electron microscopic study using Ferritin as a labeling compound, Acta Neuropath., 2, 177-197 (1962).

Scheinker, I. M.: Cerebral swelling: Histopathology, classification and clinical significance of brain edema, J. Neurosurg., 4, 255-275 (1947).

Stewart—Wallace, A. M.: A biochemical study of cerebral tissue and the changes in cerebral oedema, Brain, 62, 426-438 (1939).

Taylor, J. M., W. A. Levy, I. Herzog and L. C. Scheinberg: Prevention of experimental cerebral edema by cortico-steroids. Biochemical and ultrastructural studies, Neurology (Minn.), 15, 667-674 (1965).

Torack, R. M., R. D. Terry and H. M. Zimmerman: The fine structure of cerebral fluid accumulation: I. Swelling secondary to cold injury, Amer. J. Path., 35, 1135-1147 (1959).

_____, _____ and _____: The fine structure of cerebral fluid accumalation, II: Swelling produced by triethyl tin poisoning and its comparison with that in the human brain, Amer. J. Path., 36: 273-287 (1960).

Zimmerman, H. M.: Some contributions of electron microscopy to problems in pathology, The 24th Middleton Goldsmith Lecture, Bull. N. Y. Acad. Med., 40, 831-862 (1964).

Zülch, K. J.: Hirnödem und Hirnschwellung, Virchow Archiv Path. Anat., 310, 1-58 (1943).

FRANZ SEITELBERGER

THE PROBLEM OF STATUS SPONGIOSUS

The term "status spongiosus" (STSP) means an alteration of the central nervous tissue in the form of a spongy loosening, presenting a three-dimensional network of fibrillar tissue constituents and appearing as a system of vesicular cavities filled with fluid. This alteration can be defined as partial necrosis, which appears in the gray as well as in the white matter. It can be present in small patches and may consist of an aggregation of a few fluid-containing vesicles; the alteration can also be more extensive, sometimes affecting the griseum as a whole in pseudocyst-like distribution, or affecting laminar areas of the cortices and of the cortico-subcortical border zones; further, it can appear in large continuous areas of the central white matter. The status spongiosus is not caused by one specific lesion. Pathogenetically it has not been defined. Various types of lesions can cause this state, and therefore it is not a disease and not a neuropathological entity. It is a histopathological syndrome that is neither dependent on a single endogenous nor an exogenous condition. It is found in connection with degenerative, inflammatory, and circulatory syndromes or diseases.

Histopathological analysis reveals several different types of STSP which pathogenetically deviate from one another. They show different types of development and indicate different origins. The intention of this paper is to describe the lesions of STSP, stressing the differential pathogenesis and to try to design the histopathological differential diagnosis of various types of STSP, and finally to derive a morphologically-based classification.

The central nervous tissue mainly consists of three separable constituents: 1) nerve cells with dendrites and neurites, 2) glial cells and processes, and 3) the intracerebral vascular network. These three types of nervous tissue components are arranged three-dimensionally and intertwined with each other. In the gray matter the space between the distant perikarya of the nervous and glial cells is filled with a felt of neuronal and glial processes. This neuropil is interlaced with a comparatively tightly meshed capillary network. In the white matter the densely packed myelinated processes of the nerve cells are interspersed with a sparse arrangement of glial cells and processes and with a broad-meshed vascular network. Status spongiosus will occur, if one of these three tissue components mentioned is lost, no matter for what reason. In a similar way a fabric woven from three different threads would become transparent, or "spongy," as it were, if one of the threads were extracted. The main types of STSP, therefore, consist of selective partial necrosis of single nervous tissue components. Thus, we would theoretically expect the following types of STSP: I) Selective type: 1) Neurogenic STSP caused by loss of a) pericarya and dendrites, b) axons and neurites; 2) Gliogenic STSP due to loss of a) astroglia, b) oligodendroglia; and 3) Mesenchymogenic STSP caused by loss of vascular structures (non-existent); II) Non-Selective type: spongio-necrosis of brain tissue; representative: spongio-necrosis due to inflammatory changes.

It is obvious that these hypothetical basic types cannot exist in a pure form, for the complete lack of one of the three tissue constituents cannot be without effect on the other components. Especially, a mesenchymogenic STSP in the sense of a selective partial necrosis cannot exist, because the elimination of the vascular system immediately causes a total necrosis of the affected area. Nevertheless this classification is of heuristic value and, therefore, we can accept it as a basis for the following discussion.

1) NEUROGENIC TYPE OF STSP

a) In the gray substance of the brain, a quantitatively important selective loss of neuronal elements causing an STSP can be of endogenous or exogenous origin. As a matter of fact, even a partial loss of nerve cells and processes should bring about a loosening of the neuropil (Grundgewebestruktur). Usually this is not the case, for the loss of substance is substituted by a proportional proliferation of macroglial cells and fibers (reparative or substitutive glial proliferation), and the remaining tissue elements draw closer. If the loss of neurons is high enough or if the reparative potency of the macroglia is lacking, disintegration of cerebral tissue will become manifest in the form of STSP.

Neurogenic STSP is found in different types of neuronal dystrophy (following the classification of Seitelberger). In connection with Pick's disease (localized cortical atrophy), neurogenic STSP in the cortex is caused by neuronal dystrophy (Fig. 1); in the so-called

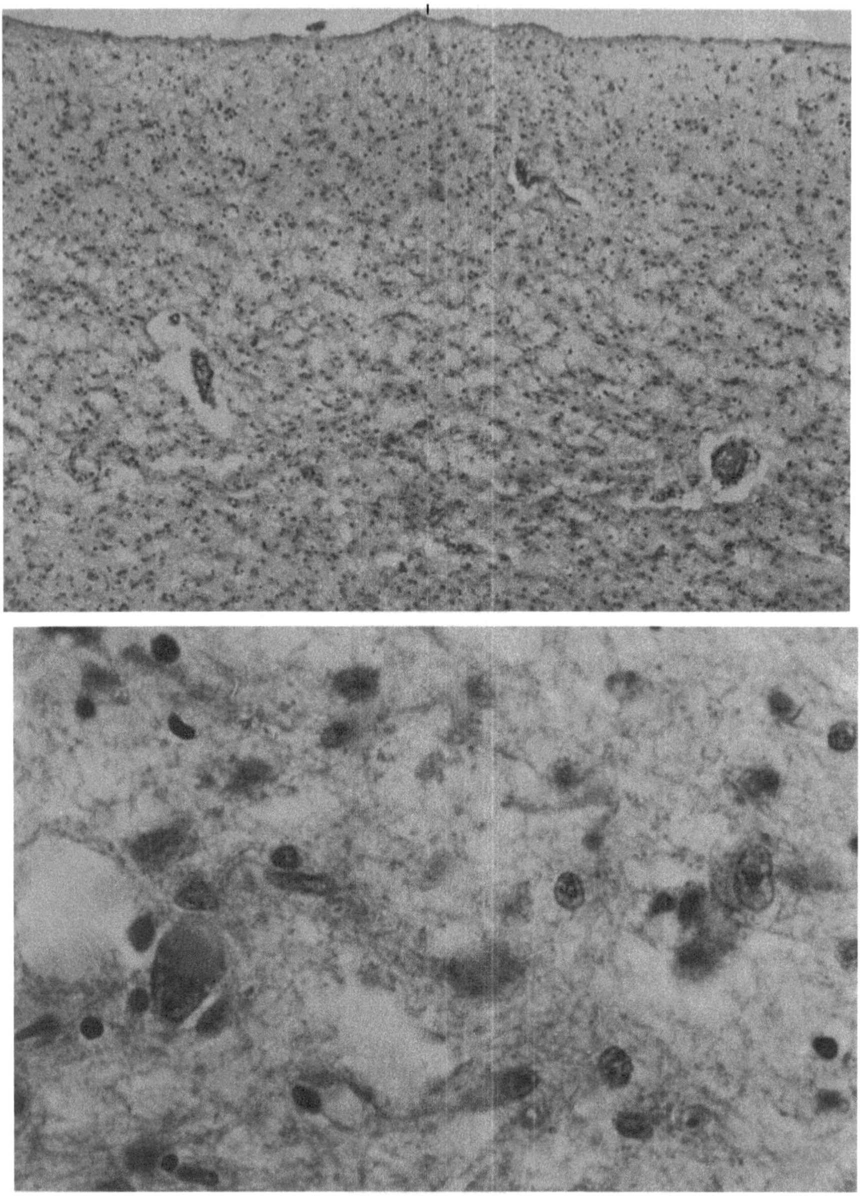

Fig. 1. Neurogenic status spongiosus; Pick disease; Cortex temporalis; Formalin, paraffin, H & E; Top: X87; Spongy alteration of the middle cortical layers due to almost complete loss of nerve cells; Bottom: X700; In the spongy area 2 residual nerve cells, one with a distinct cytoplasmic inclusion body ("Silberkugel") can be seen. Between plasmatic and fibrillary astrocytes the spongy cavities are established.

parenchymal type of Alzheimer's presenile dementia (Seitelberger & Jellinger), it is caused by a massive synaeretic neuronal dystrophy; it also occurs in a special type of amaurotic idiocy dependent on severe storage dystrophy (Fig. 2), (myoclonic type of cerebral lipidosis; Seitelberger; Seitelberger, et al.), as well as in Hallervorden-Spatz disease or in infantile neuro-axonal dystrophy in regions heavily affected by neuro-axonal dystrophy (Seitelberger). Because of the pathoclitic pattern of the degenerative diseases mentioned above, STSP can appear in laminar distribution in the cortex corresponding to certain nerve cell layers or to the architectonics of dendrites. As an exogenous cause of STSP in the gray substance, we may consider intense "elective parenchymal necrosis" according to Scholz, caused by ischemia in the form of a pseudo-laminar STSP of the cerebral cortex (Crompton). In most cases, however, the macroglia is also affected or even lost because of the intensity of the responsible vaso-circulatory disturbance. Therefore, we cannot speak of a selective, but rather of a partial parenchymal necrosis, comprising several tissue elements.

b) In the white matter the neurogenic STSP is not often found. It can develop with a massive loss of axons in connection with neuro-axonal dystrophy of endogenous or exogenous origin. On account of the relative stability of the axonal degenerative products (Schollen, spheroids), STSP is slight and appears late. As examples can be listed infantile neuro-axonal dystrophy, late infantile Hallervorden-Spatz disease (cerebellar white matter) (Seitelberger & Gross, Seitelberger, et al.), and the small foci (Lückenherde) in funicular myelopathy. If there is a great loss of myelinated neurites and oligodendroglia in connection with leucodystrophy and in demyelinating diseases, in most cases a substitution of the defect is established by strong astroglial proliferation. There are exceptions in the large foci of Schilder's disease and in inflammatory demyelinating disease (subacute sclerosing leucoencephalitis). Examples for leucoencephalitic STSP are found in the author's observations concerning a child (Seitelberger & Jellinger) and in a case recently published by Schubert (Fig. 3). The loss of neurites may also lead to a partial necrosis comprising several components of tissue including oligodendroglia.

2) GLIOGENIC TYPE OF STSP

a) The astroglial type of STSP is the most frequent manifestation of the STSP and may be of endogenous as well as of exogenous origin. Its substrate is the selective loss of the astrocytic tissue element, which, as far as we know at present, serves the transport of metabolites from the vessel to the nerve cell. Regressive changes of this tissue element ("glial dystrophies"), therefore, are called in

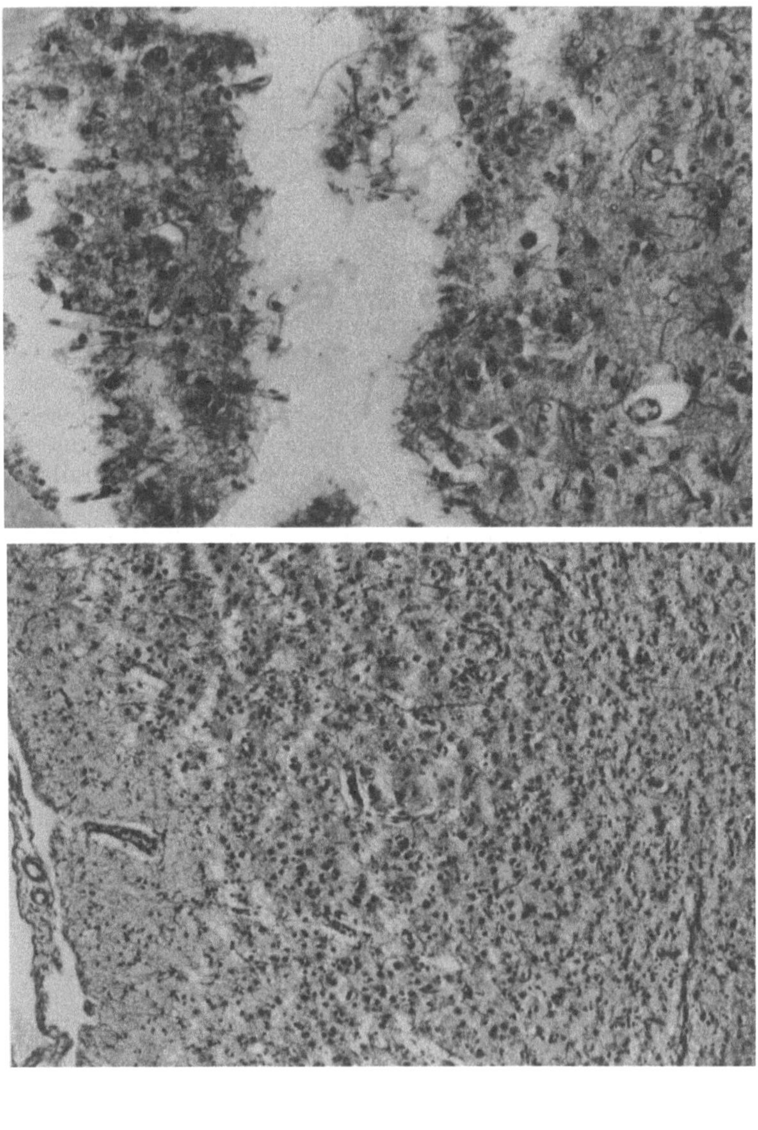

Fig. 2. Neurogenic STSP; Myoclonic type of cerebral lipidosis; Cortex frontalis; Formalin, paraffin, Bodian; Left: X87; Diffuse spongy alteration due to massive loss of nerve cells; Right: X220; Artificial dissociation of the spongy middle zone of the cortex. Few lipid storing nerve cells are present (X); intense proliferative astroglial reaction.

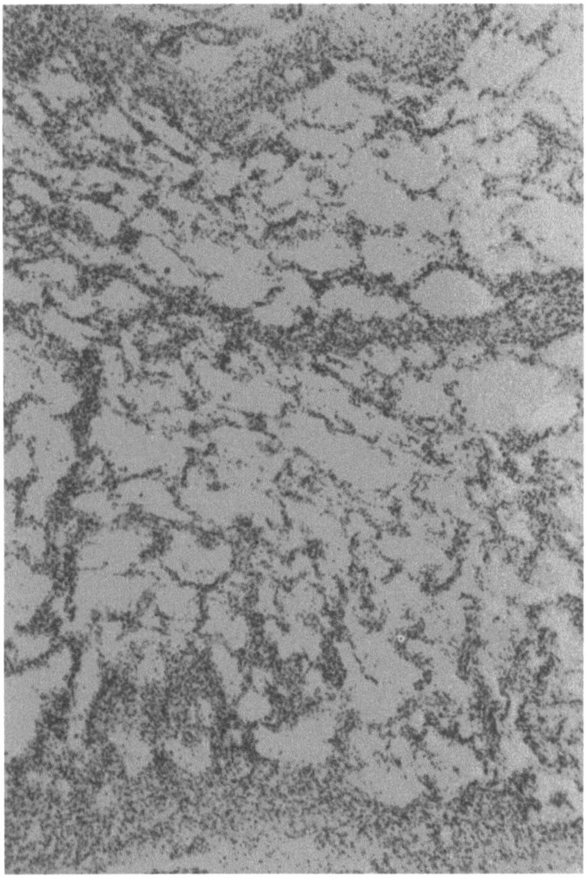

Fig. 3. Spongy lesion of gray and white matter; Subacute leucoencephalitis van Bogaert (Fall Schubert); Cortex frontalis and neuraxis; Formalin, paraffin, Cresyl violet, X44; Coarse, spongy cavities are interspersed in cortex and subcortical zone.

a wider sense "dystrophies of transport structures" (Seitelberger). The morphological changes of this dystrophy develop in a regular sequence.

The following stages can be distinguished: Hypertrophic-proliferative phase, in which the cytoplasmic volume of the astrocyte increases in the pericaryon as well as in the processes (footplates around the capillaries, endings at the nerve cells). At the same time one can observe proliferation and expansion of the cellular processes. Histologically they appear as so-called "plasmatic astrocytes," (Fig. 4, left), the cytoplasm of which gives a positive PAS-reaction.

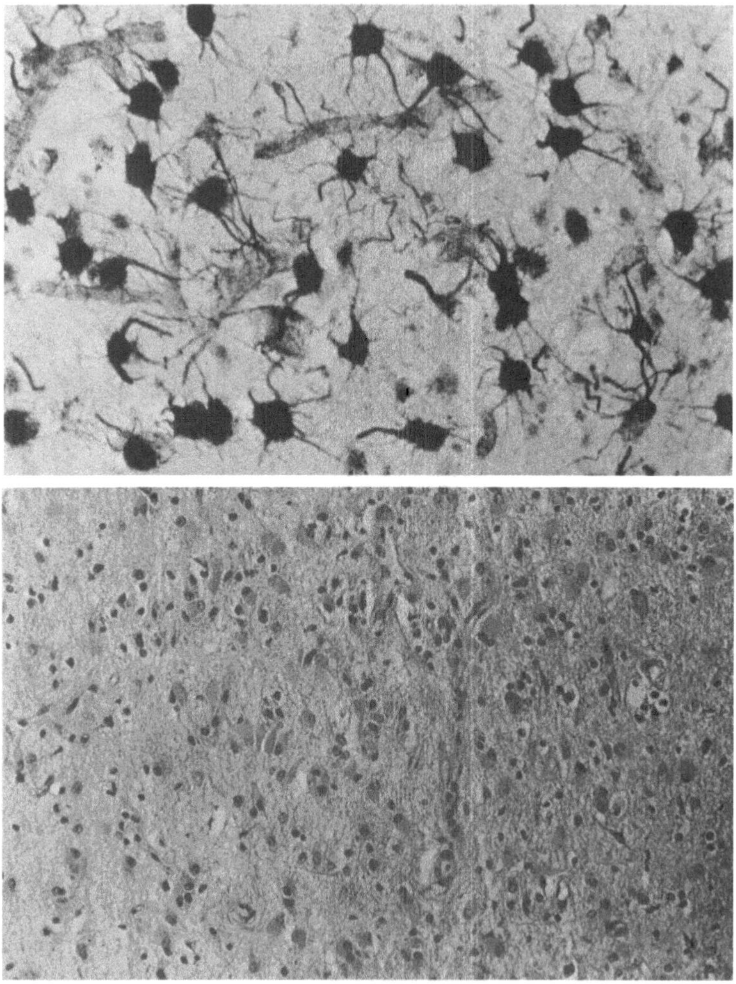

Fig. 4. Gliogenic STSP; Infantile spongy dystrophy; Formalin, paraffin; Left: H & E, X280 (reduced); In the early stage the astrocytes of the inferior cortical layers show swelling with clearly visible hypertrophic eosinophilic cytoplasm; Right: Cajal, X500; (reduced); Impregnation with gold sublimate demonstrates plasmatic swelling and luxuriant processes of the astrocytes

The course of astroglial alteration can be well studied in Cajal preparations (Fig. 4, right). Histochemically the astrocytes in the hypertrophic proliferation phase show a high activity of oxidative (lactic acid dehydrogenase) (Fig. 5) and also of hydrolytic enzymes (acid phosphatase) in the cytoplasm. A local

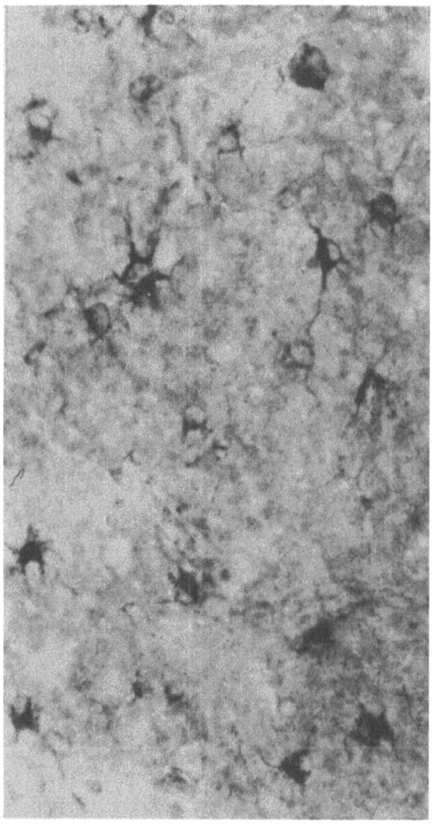

Fig. 5. Gliogenic STSP; Presenile spongy dystrophy; Cortical biopsy (F); Cryostat section, lactic acid dehydrogenase (MTT-method), X350; hypertrophic astrocytes show high activity of lactic acid dehydrogenase in the perikaryon.

aggregation of ballooned astrocytic processes is called by some authors "status precribrousus;" we would rather call it "status prespongiosus" (Fig. 6). Regressive phase, in which with a further increase in volume, the luxuriant processes disintegrate (so-called "Clasmatodendrosis" seen in Cajal preparation) and the ballooned perikaryon dissolves (Fig. 7). These changes are caused by damage to the cellular membrane. The nucleus remains intact for a long period and is found apparently free in the hydropic cytoplasm or in the terminal lacunae. These lacunae caused by disintegration of the ballooned cells vi:

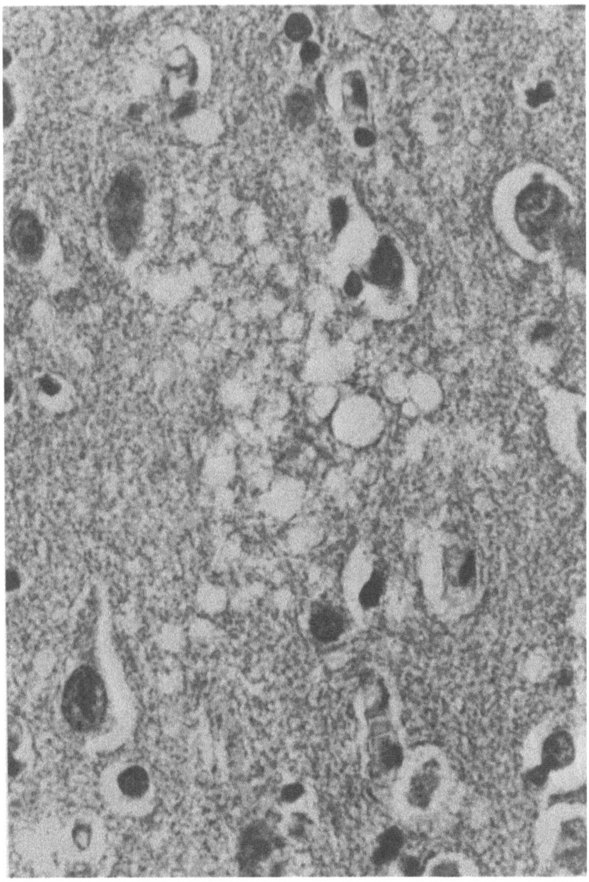

Fig. 6. Gliogenic STSP; Status prae-spongiosus; Presenile spongy dystrophy; Cortex temporalis; Formalin, paraffin, H & E, X560; In the initial stage, in a small area, distended astrocytic processes form a delicate porosity of the neuropil.

humoral decomposition can form small "nest-like" vesiculations. By secondary disintegration of the cellular membranes among the lacunae and their confluence, larger cyst-like systems develop. Ballooning of the perivascular foot-plates leads to a perivascular loosening of tissue (dilatation of Held's perivascular glial chambers); the dilatation and disintegration of the perineuronal processes of astrocytes leads to dilatation of Obersteiner's pericellular interstices which, therefore, do not represent technical artifacts. The defective phase is characterized by the fact that the small number of remainin

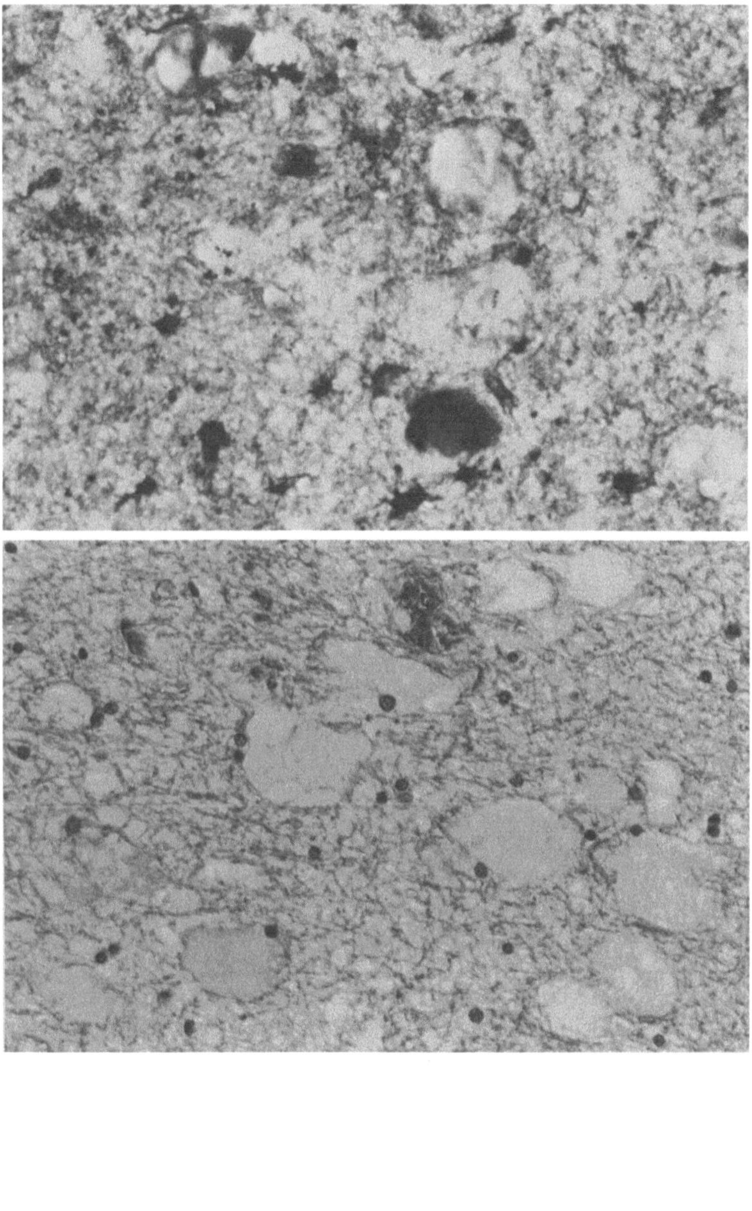

Fig. 7. Gliogenic STSP; Malignant edema accompanying brain tumor; Formalin, paraffin; Left: H & E, X350 (reduced); Tremendous swelling of white matter astrocytes by homogeneous or floccular plasmatic substances; Right: Cajal, X220 (reduced); The content of swollen white matter astrocytes is impregnated in variable intensity by gold sublimate.

astrocytes transformed into "fibrillary astrocytes" cannot sufficientl substitute the tissue defect. Around the lacunae a fibrous meshwork is formed, in which the remaining parenchymal elements (nerve cells and processes, oligodendroglia) are embedded (Fig. 8). The nerve

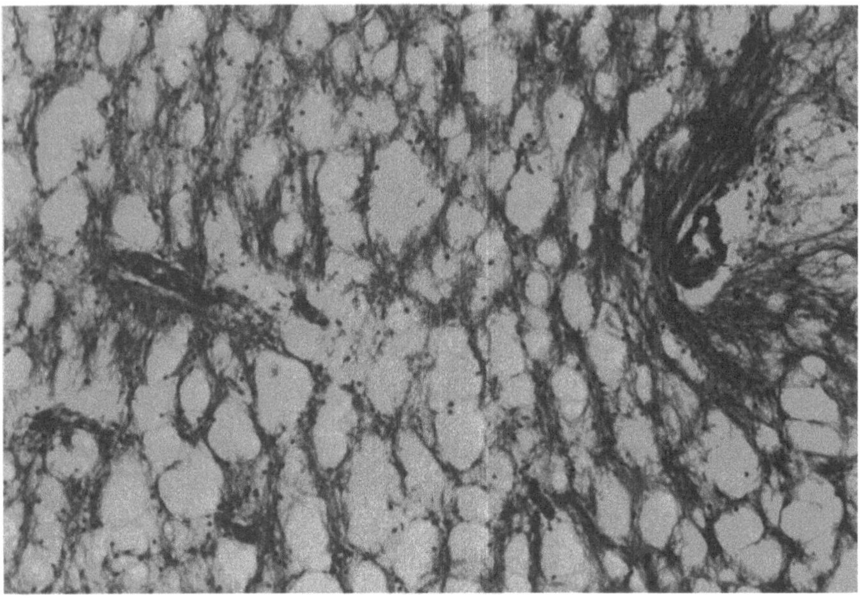

Fig. 8. Gliogenic STSP; Cerebellar white matter; Formalin, paraffin, H & E, X112; In the final stage there is a sieve-like spongiosity of the tissue. In the cavities "free" nuclei of the ballooned astrocytes can be seen. A small number of intact nerve fibers is left between the holes and around blood vessels.

cells which do not primarily participate in these changes at first remain intact but later on, due to the loss of nutritive astroglial element, suffer secondary damage and gradually disintegrate. The facts mentioned above prove that in advanced stages, types of STSP cannot easily be distinguished. The cytologic appearance of remaining nerve cells, the astroglia (astroglia proliferation present in the neurogenic type, lacking in gliogenic type a), and especially the distribution of lesions permit a differential diagnosis. Unlike type 1, the distribution is unsystematic in type 2, it is usually disseminated and patchy or diffusely confluent.

b) In the white matter gliogenic STSP is also pathologically induced by the alteration of the astroglia mentioned before. But it seems that generally interfascicular oligodendroglia are also primarily involved, because, in the absence of neuronal lesions, an intense secondary loss of myelin sheaths and neurites cannot be entirely explained by an alteration of the comparatively sparse astroglial elements of the white matter. This assumption is supported by recent electron microscopical studies which will be discussed later in this symposium by Sluga. In the final stage of the already established STSP of the white matter, however, it is not possible to decide whether it is of astroglial or of oligodendroglial origin.

Representatives of the gliogenic STSP are familial spongy idiocy (van Bogaert & Bertrand), presenile spongy dystrophy and Jakob-Creutzfeldt's disease, which, according to the combination with a neuronal lesion of a type corresponding to Nissl's acute cell disease, can be characterized as glio-neuronal dystrophy. In Morbus-Wilson hepato-cerebral degeneration glial dystrophy is connected with a proliferative vascular dystrophy. Exogenous syndromes of a similar type can be found in a form of "diffuse pontine dystrophy" in chronic alcoholism (Seitelberger & Gross), in other hepatogenic syndromes, and in various toxic-metabolic disturbances. This type of lesions seems to indicate disturbances in protein metabolism.

A special nosologic condition or a syndrome belonging to the oligodendroglial type of STSP is not known, except if one assumes that the spongy lesion of Jacob's "Ödemnekrose" (necrosis due to edema) as well as a pathogenetically similar group of leucoencephalopathies are of gliogenic origin. Relations of this gliogenic lesion type to brain edema have been frequently discussed. Edema, especially in the gray substance, is, according to electron microscopical and biochemical findings, assumed to be an increase of the liquid phase in the astrocytic cytoplasm. Relations between STSP and interstitial edema of the white substance cannot be discussed, because its features have not been sufficiently substantiated.

Mesenchymogenic STSP caused by loss of cerebral vascular structures is, as stressed before, impossible. STSP, which always represents a lesion of neuroectodermal tissue elements, could only be called mesenchymogenic in the sense that it is caused by effects via the vascular and hematogeneous mesenchyme. There are a large number of infections and toxic agents which can induce spongy tissue lesions in this way. However, this would not mean "mesenchymogenic" as we use the term in the present study.

The types of STSP discussed which are caused by a more or less selective loss of single nervous tissue components, represent only a small portion of the types of spongy tissue alterations. From this main group discussed a second one may be distinguished, where not a selective, but a basically non-selective type of lesion causes a spongy alteration of tissue which we call "spongio-necrosis of brain tissue." This group comprises the spongio-necroses that occur: 1) in inflammatory syndromes; 2) in vascular circulatory syndromes, i. e., in arteriosclerosis, in hypertension, and especially in Binswanger's syndrome (Jellinger & Neumayer); 3) in the interstitial hemodynamic brain edema caused by microlaceration of the tissue texture mainly in the centrum ovale; and 4) in post-traumatic encephalopathies. Pathogenetically, the latter represent a combinatior types 2 and 3 but also show sequelae of glio-vascular metabolic dystrophies as described under the gliogenic type of the first main group of STSP. The non-selective spongy lesions of this type, however, should not be called status spongiosus; this term should only be applied to the lesions described in the first main group of the selective type. The kind of lesion involved in the second group ought to be des nated "spongio-necrosis of brain tissue." A detailed discussion of th respective conditions would go beyond this presentation and would al be out of place according to the terminology proposed above. It will be the subject of a further special study.

As examples of the second group, however, spongy lesions due to inflammatory changes encountered in encephalitic syndromes sha be described. In the course of certain encephalitides dense, interstitial, hemato-histiocytic infiltrates may appear. These infiltrates irreparably damage the integrity of tissue either by primary mechanical effects combined with a secondary loss of neuroectodermal struc tures, especially of astroglial elements, or sometimes by means of direct parenchymal injury. In later stages of inflammation after disappearance of infiltrating cells, glio-mesenchymal "Abbau" and reparation can be observed. On account of the locally suppressed glial proliferative capacity there remains finally a spongy focus corresponding in shape and density to the infiltrate. This is a secondary partial necrosis of neuroectodermal tissue components with incomplete glial reparation caused by quantitative astroglial reduction. This type of focal spongy lesions, which may also be called "post-infiltrative spongio-necrosis" appears, according to the polio-encep alitic distribution of the encephalitides concerned, mostly in the gra matter. Post-infiltrative spongio-necrosis is met especially in connection with subacute polio-myelitis in the most severely affected parts of the spinal cord, in the anterior horn, and in the tegmentum of brain stem (Scharenberg; Noetzel; Ule; Busch; Seitelberger & Jellinger) (Fig. 9). It also appears in encephalitis lethargica von Economo and seldom in protracted courses of encephalitides of the Arbor Virus group.

As a pathogenetically related special form, the so-called "focal encephalitic spongio-necrosis" must be mentioned. Here circumscribed spongy areas related to vessels occur in gray or white matter. They have no connection with rupturing of the intraadventitial spaces nor to perivascular gliogenic spongiosis; they repre-

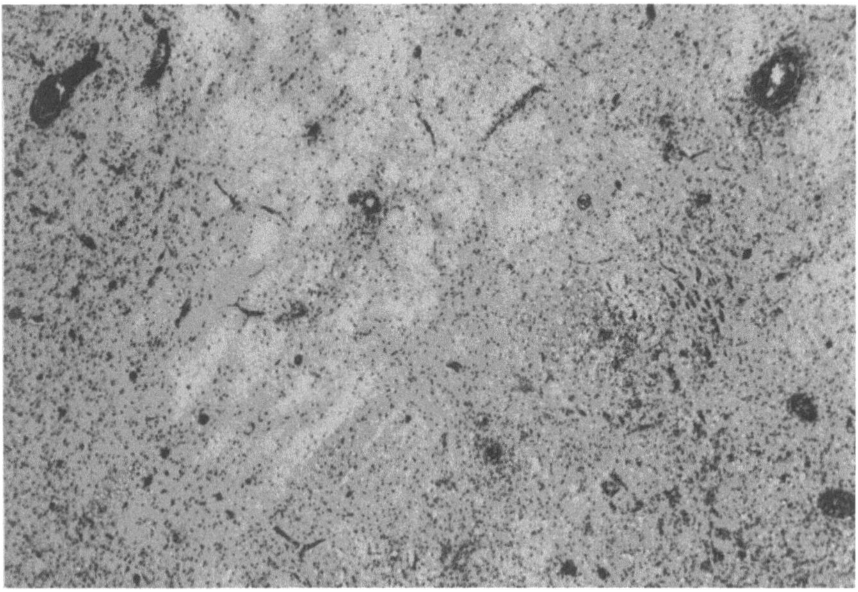

Fig. 9. Focal encephalitic spongio-necrosis; Poliomyelitis; Tegmentum medullae oblongatae, lateral part; Formalin, paraffin, Cresyl violet, X35; diffuse slight spongy alterations following dense interstitial infiltration.

sent the final stage of an interstitial, serous parvicellular infiltration encountered as a symptom of the respective encephalitic syndrome. Histologically, the early infiltrative stage of the process is observed only rarely and with difficulty. It consists of a local permeation of the vascular blood-brain barrier by protein-containing fluid and by a small number of infiltrative cells, among which hypertrophic histiocytes prevail. Soon a delicate loosening of the gray matter, resembling the status pre-spongiosus, and a microglial proliferation in which also compound granular cells appear takes place, while the macroglial element disappears without reaction. Even neuronal structures, especially neurites, deteriorate within these foci. The result is a subtotal cobweb-like rarefication necrosis interwoven by a few glial filaments (Fig. 10). Contrary to type I of STSP, the lesions of this type completely lack astroglial structures except for a small number of glial fibers. Some microglial nuclei and seldom a secondarily damaged nerve cell can be observed. Size and distribution of the foci resemble the nodular foci of interstitial gliomesenchymal infiltration always present in the encephalitides mentioned; intermediate and transitional stages have been confirmed.

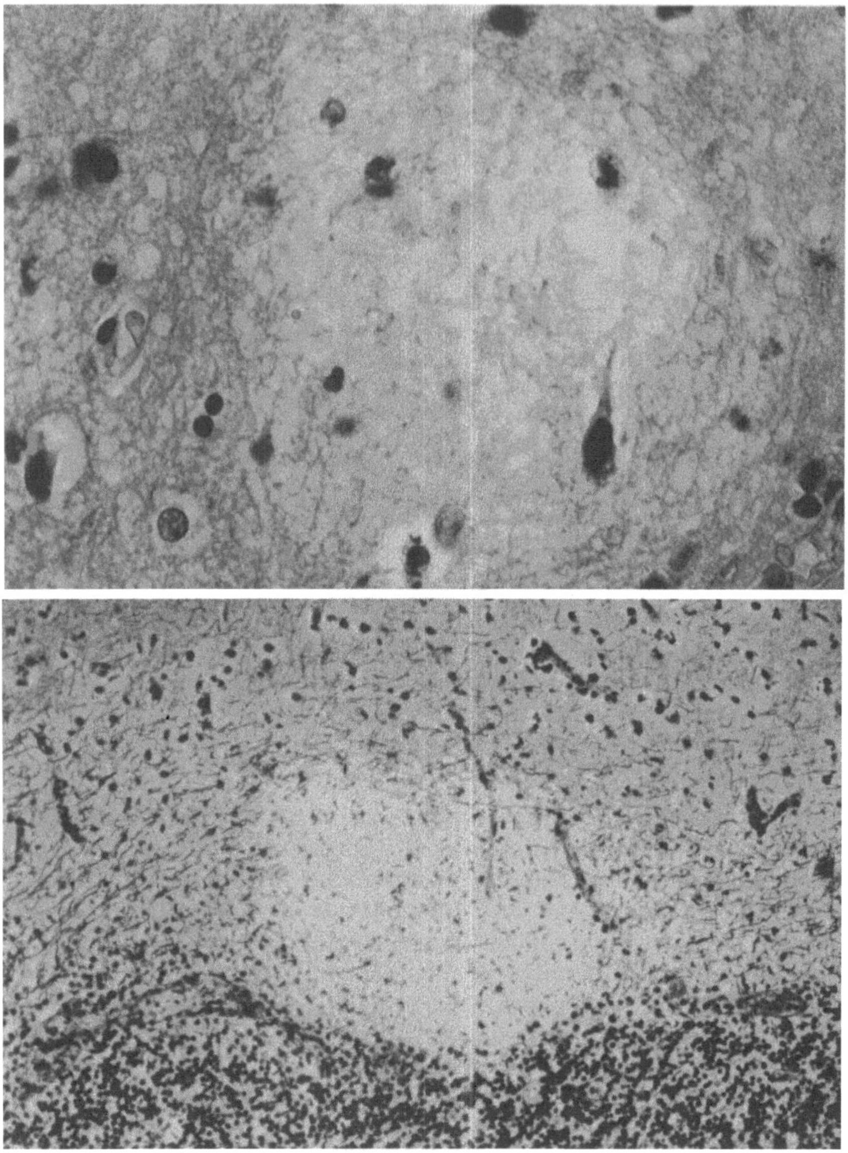

Fig. 10. Focal encephalitic spongio-necrosis; Endemic spring-summer-encephalomyelitis; Top: Cortex occipitalis; Formalin, paraffin, H & E, X560; Circumscribed spongy alteration, in which only one shrunken nerve cell and few macrophages are left. Bottom: Cerebellar cortex; Formalin, paraffin, Bodian, X175; Spongy lesion of the Purkinje cells and the molecular layer. The focal necrosis is devoid of cells and disrupts the passing neurites.

Pathogenetically, a vasogenic infiltrative-toxic lesion of neuroectodermal tissue elements, mainly of macroglia and nerve cell processes (subtotal necrosis) is assumed to be taking place in the course of certain encephalitic syndromes. The noxious effect seems to be caused by the infiltrative histiocytic element, possibly as carrier of immunological factors. Hypothetically we may interpret this as a necrobiotic pendant to the inflammatory nodules of interstitial infiltration. Certainly vaso-circulatory factors such as stasis, capillary spasms or ischemia have no part in the formation of this spongy alteration. Such lesions are especially severe in the viral encephalitis of the Arbor group B: European and Russian spring-summer encephalomyelitis, encephalitis Japonica B, Western equine encephalitis, etc. They are seldom encountered in poliomyelitis.

SUMMARY

The status spongiosus (STSP) is usually defined and histopathologically characterized as a special form of partial necrosis of the central nervous tissue. Theoretically there are three different types of STSP: 1) neurogenic, 2) gliogenic, and 3) mesenchymogenic (non-existent). 1) This form originates in massive selective neuronal loss in the course of atrophies or selective parenchymal necroses, if the neuronal loss, i.e., the loss of nerve cells and of the neuronal component of the neuropil cannot be replaced by glia. Even neuroaxonal dystrophy can cause STSP in the gray matter and sometimes in the white substance, too. 2) This form is caused by selective loss of the astrocytic element of the neuropil ("glial dystrophy"), as it occurs in deficiency syndromes and in disturbances of protein metabolism within the syndromes of "dystrophy of transport structures." The STSP in the white matter is caused by dystrophy of astrocytic glial elements, too. Selective loss of the oligodendroglial element may be involved in the so-called "Ödemnekrose."

There are three phases of the alteration of astroglia: a) proliferative phase: increase of the cell volume with luxuriant production of processes; b) regressive phase: deterioriation of the glial processes ("Clasmatodendrosis") and hydropic ballooning of the cell perikaryon; c) defective phase: desintegration of the cells; formation of holes and secondary confluence to larger cyst-like spaces. Different from this group of STSP due to selective partial necroses are spongy lesions caused by non-selective loss of neuroectodermal structures, for which the term "spongio-necrosis of the brain tissue" is proposed. As an example, spongy alterations found in encephalitic cyndromes are described.

REFERENCES

Bogaert, L. van and I. Bertrand: Sur une idiotie familiale avec dégénérescenece spongieuse du névraxe, Acta Neurol. Belg., 49, 572 (1949).

Busch, W.: Die Poliomyelitis bei Jugendlichen und Erwachsenen, Arch. Psychiat. Z. Neurol., 198, 438-455 (1959).

Crompton, M. R.: A case of subacute spongiform encephalopathy supporting a vascular pathogenesis, Acta Neuropath., 2, 291-296 (1963).

Jellinger, K. and E. Neumayer: Progressive subcorticale vasculäre Encephalopathie Binswanger, Arch. f. Psychiat. u. Zs. f. d. ges. Neurologie, 205, 523-554 (1964).

Noetzel, H.: Über die Rückbildung der Entzündung bei akuter Poliomyelitis, Beitr. path. Anat., 117, 337-342 (1957).

Scharenberg, K.: Pathology of poliomyelitis treated in respirator, J. Neuropath. exp. Neur., 14, 297-304 (1955).

Schubert, P.: Atypischer Fall einer subakuten sklerosierenden Leukoencephalitis (van Bogaert), Acta Neuropath., 6, 93-97 (1966).

Seitelberger, F.: Zur Morphologie und Histochemie der degenerativen Axonveränderungen im Zentralnervensystem. 1er Congrès Internat. des Sciences Neurologiques. Bruxelles 1957: IIIe Congrès Internat. de Neuropath., Rapports, 127-147.

_____: Sonderformen cerebraler Lipoidosen. Histochemische und histologische Befunde, Proc. IVth. Internat. Congr. Neuropath., Sept., 4-8 Munich (1961).

_____: Zur allgemeinen Histopathologie degenerativer Prozesse des Nervensystems, Centenarfeier für Karl Schaffer, Budapest (1964), (In press).

_____, M. Gootz and H. Gross: Beitrag zur spätinfantilen Hallervorden-Spatz'schen Krankheit, Acta Neuropath, 3, 16-18 (1963).

_____ and H. Gross: Über eine spätinfantile Form der Hallervorden-Spatz'schen Krankheit. II. Mitteilung: Histochemische Befunde. Erörterung der Nosologie, Dtsch. Z. Nervenheilk., 176, 104-125 (1957).

_____ and _____: Zur Neuropathologie des Alkoholismus, in: Arbeitstagung über Alkoholismus, Wien, 12-30 (1962).

_____ and _____: Die Läsion der Brücke bei alkoholbedingten Encephalopathien (Zentrale pontine Myelinolyse; diffuse pontine Dystrophie), Sitzung Verein f. Neur. u. Psychiat. in Wien, 25, II. (1963).

_____, H. Jacob and R. Schnabel: The myoclonic variant of cerebral lipidosis, 3rd Internat. Symp. on Sphingolipidoses and allied Diseases, New York (1965), (in press).

_____ and K. Jellinger: Umschriebene Grosshirnatrophie bei Alzheimer'scher Krankheit, Dtsch. Z. Nervenheilk., 178, 365-379 (1958).

_____ and _____: Atypische infantile nekrotisierende Panencephalitis, in: Livre Jubilaire du Dr. van Bogaert, Acta Med. Belg., (Brussels), 713-726 (1962).

_____ and _____: Neuropathologie der Zeckenencephalitis, II. Internat. Symp. on Encephalitides (Warschau) (1965).

Ule, G.: Neuropathologische Aspekte klinischer Verlaufsformen der Heine-Medinschen Krankheit, Internist, 2, 304-307 (1961).

M. KIDD

ULTRASTRUCTURAL ASPECTS OF STATUS SPONGIOSUS

*SOME ELECTRON MICROSCOPICAL OBSERVATIONS**

Cortical biopsies from human cases with spongy changes were examined by electron microscopy. Circular and elliptical spaces containing a watery fluid were found in the gray matter, ranging in size downwards from 10 μ. The smaller pathological spaces were bounded by a single intracellular membrane and therefore corresponded topologically to the normal flattened sacs of the cytoplasm (endoplasmic reticulum, mitochondrial and nuclear membranes). The larger spaces appeared to be similar watery expansions of the cytoplasm itself, sometimes containing irregular membranes.

The smaller spaces could be distinguished from the usual artefacts of fixation by their circular or elliptical profiles in section, which were suggestive of distension under pressure, whereas those of artefactual origin were no more than a moderate separation of the walls of the cytoplasmic sacs.

The cells of origin of the spaces were difficult to identify, but the smaller ones were found sometimes to be in neurons, and the larger ones in astrocytes. Hypotheses of the origin and evolution of these spaces will be presented for discussion.

*This communication was previously given at the European Round Table on the Spongy Degenerations of the Presenium, in Venice, June 1965, and will be published in full in the proceedings of that meeting: Acta neuropath, Supplementum III.

J.-F. FONCIN

ELECTRON MICROSCOPIC OBSERVATIONS IN CREUTZFELDT-JAKOB DISEASE

ULTRASTRUCTURAL STUDY

This discussion of spongiosis in Creutzfeldt-Jakob disease is based on two cases. The first has been published previously (1). The patient was a 59-year-old woman whose previous history remains unknown. She showed a progressive dementia and prominent Korsakov-like amnesic deficiency. Neurological findings were not conclusive; vision appeared grossly normal; muscular wasting was not present and rhythmic clonus appeared only two days before death, which occured approximately four months after onset. An EEG was recorded on six instances but not after the onset of myoclonus and was non-characteristic. Right frontal biopsy was performed for diagnostic purpose after 2 1/2 months. An abnormality was recognized, but no specific diagnosis was made until electron microscopic examination drew attention to the spongiosis which was clearly to be seen on H-E routine preparations in retrospect. Autopsy confirmed the diagnosis with microspongiosis, neuronal rarefaction and heavy gliosis being characteristic. The cerebral cortex was prominently affected, with the occipital regions comparatively spared. An unusual feature was the gross brain atrophy (890 g). The second case is reported here for the first time. A 42-year-old woman without significant previous history developed progressive amnesic deficiency and deteriorated during eleven months. A frontal tumor was suspected, and the patient was referred by Professor Garcin to the neurosurgeon. Ventriculography which was normal and frontal cortical biopsy were performed. Histological features were microspongiosis, neuronal retraction and rarefaction with no significant gliosis. Creutzfeldt-Jakob disease was diagnosed. The subsequent course was not typical for this condition. Mental deterioration has progressed very slowly and the level of

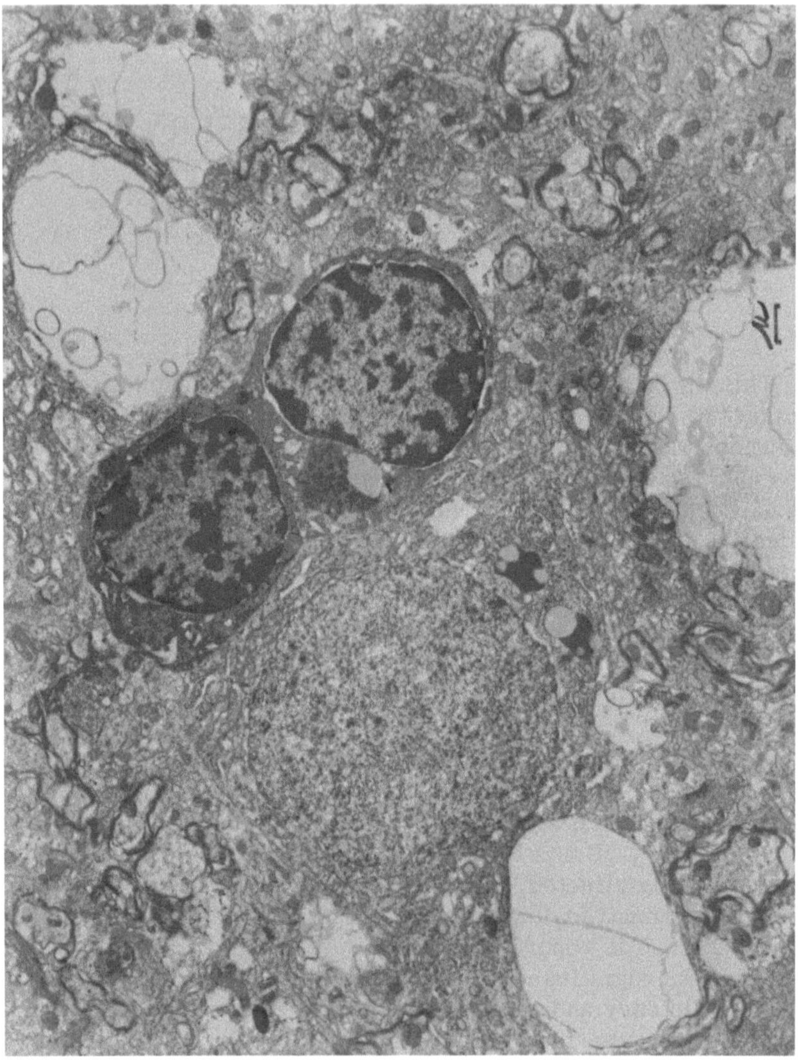

Fig. 1. General field showing nearly normal neuron, two oligodendrocytes, and four large cavities.

consciousness has remained nearly normal. Abnormal movements have appeared, but with complex choreiform-opposition jerks rather than myoclonic movements. A very marked clonic dysarthria is present. Neither visual defect nor peripheral motor neuron defect can be demonstrated. EEG has remained non-specific. The patient is at the present time alive after an illness of one year and a half.

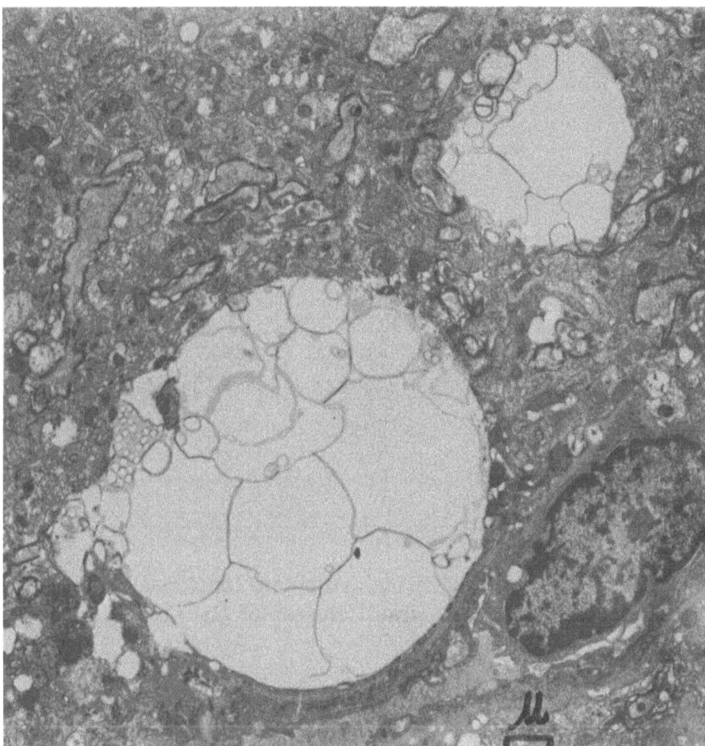

Fig. 2. Low power view with large spherical cavity near a blood vessel. Note normal nerve fiber inside cavity.

The ultrastructural study being restricted in this paper to the aspects of spongiosis, it is felt that the perhaps doubtful diagnosis in the second case is of minor relevance to our purpose, since spongiosis was a prominent feature and quite comparable to that already published with reference to the first case.

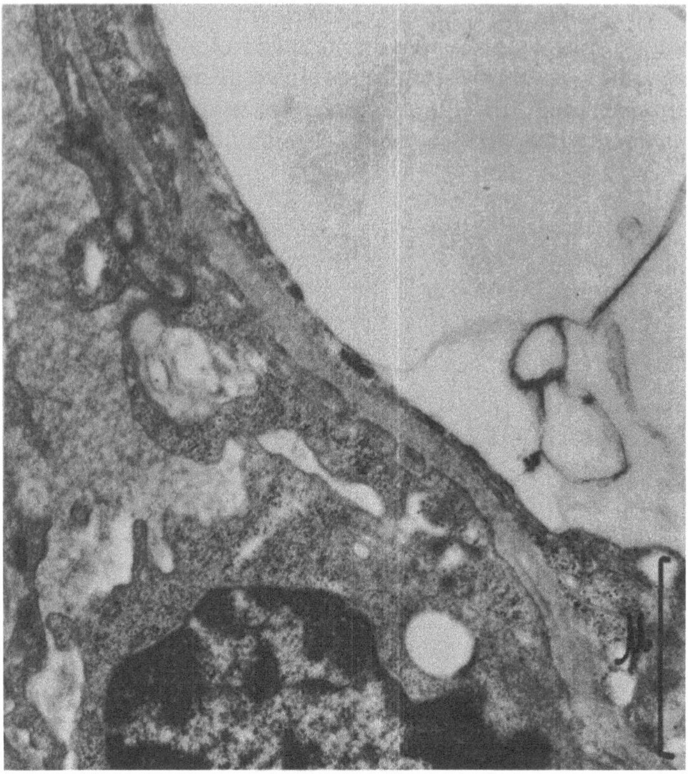

Fig. 3. Part of Figure 2 showing cytoplasm interposed between cavity and basement membrane. Note small cluster of glycogen-like particles between vesicles.

The technique for electron microscopy was as previously described. Embedding was carried in Araldite on a slow schedule according to Barnes. The findings are comparable in both cases and will be described simultaneously.

At low power, the most striking feature is the presence of numerous "holes," looking as if they were punched out of the surround ing tissue. These cavities are mostly nearly circular in section, consistent with a spherical shape, but occasionally they appear deformed by adjacent structure such as nerve cells or myelinated axons. Their diameter is approximately 1 to 10 microns, the larger being found mostly in the second case. Their content is generally electron-optically clear except for the presence of numerous smoot membrane profiles which delimit vesicles, the confluence of which seems to result in a cavity. "Daughter vesicles" are often contained in the larger ones; these are more exactly circular in section, whereas the larger appear deformed, as if squeezed together. It is difficult to ascertain whether the membrane between adjoining vesicles is double, but in certain instances a small amount of cytoplasm is retained between two vesicles containing numerous glycogen-like particles. Very rarely glycogen particles in clusters are found free in the cavity.

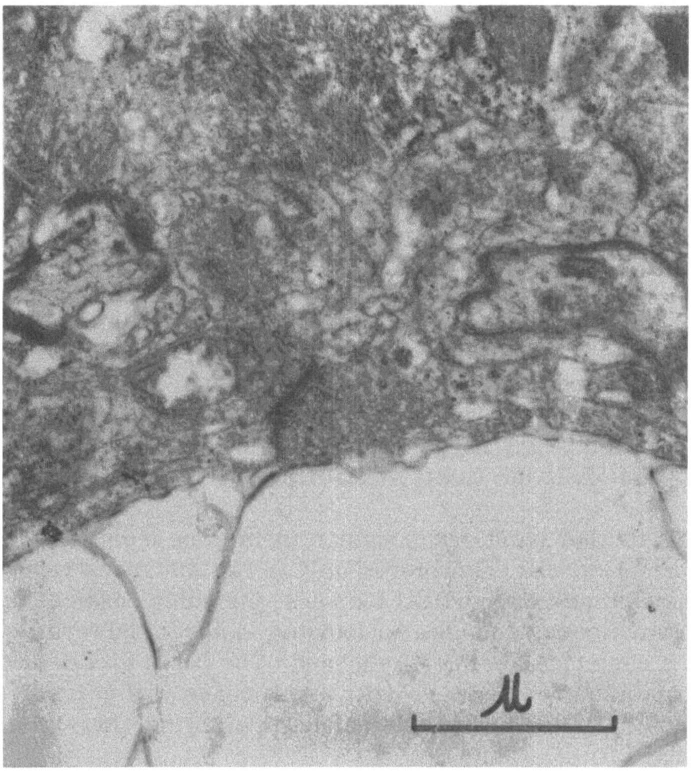

Fig. 4. Border of a cavity, with reflected membrane. Note small layer of clear cytoplasm between cavity and presynaptic element.

The confines of the cavities themselves are often difficult to study. Most spherical cavities are clearly membrane-bound, and the membrane limiting the component vesicles is continuous with the membrane limiting the cavity. In such instances the cavity is separated from other structures, e.g., presynaptic terminal or base ment membrane, not only by the above-mentioned proper membrane but by a cytoplasmic layer containing glycogen granules. This situation (membrane-bound cavity) is readily interpreted as fundamenta inasmuch as the absence of clearly visible limiting membrane can more easily be explained as artefactual rupture of a membrane than the converse.

The origin of the cavities is also a matter of interpretation. The preceding discussion, and especially the occurrence of substructure in the cavities, is deemed a sufficient proof that they are, at least primitively, intracellular. The question then arises concerning the type of cells in which they take origin. They are never seen in a neuronal perikaryon or myelinated axon. They never appear as an appendage of an abnormal myelin sheath. On the contrary, the sheaths usually remain quite normal when running along a cavity. The obvious contiguity between cavities and glial cytoplasm, particularly when glycogen particles are found between adjoining vesicles indicates a probable glial origin of the cavities. The isolated dilatation of the perinuclear cistern discussed in our first paper was not found in the second case. Nevertheless, since the de novo formation of such a membrane system is improbable, we retain the hypothesis that they arise from the smooth endoplasmic reticulum.

As indicated above, the present discussion is limited to the spongiosis. It is nevertheless to be noted that there is no evidence in the specimen of any necrosis or tissue destruction; normal structures coexist along the cavity. Glial fiber accumulation only can be noted.

As a further point of discussion, it is to be mentioned that such cavity formation was encountered only in two instances reported her among more than fifty cortical biopsies, including cases of cerebral edema from various causes. An isolated instance, however, was found in a case of Alzheimer's disease. The basic lesion was identical to that described above, but its significance was certainly different, inasmuch as the cavity was unique in many sections from several blocks.

The implications of these findings and discussion with regard to our topic are now to be considered. Concerning brain edema, we must bear in mind that neither of the two brains were edematous (the first one on anatomical evidence, the second one on clinical, neurosurgical and pneumoencephalographic evidence). Our findings then point out that appreciable amounts of fluid can be accumulated or at least segregated without any edema or swelling; morphological fluid accumulation in the brain and brain edema in the gross sense are not necessarily synonymous.

Concerning cortical spongiosis, it is felt that, in the cases presented here, ultrastructural images show it as a positive intracellular fluid accumulation or segregation process and not as the negative image of a destruction without reaction as often expressed by the classical school of neuropathology.

REFERENCE

Foncin, J.-F., J. Gaches, and J. Le Beau: Encéphalopathie spongiforme (Biopsie étudiée au microscope électronique, confirmation autopsique), Rev. Neurol., 111, 507-515 (1964).

DISCUSSION

JELLINGER: May I add some words to Dr. Feigin's excellent report concerning the course and sequelae of cerebral edema? First I would like to comment on what he called the "intermediate stage" of evolution of brain edema. We may observe this type in cases with prolonged post-traumatic coma following severe closed brain injury that we proposed to call "protracted form of post-traumatic encephalopathy." In a large series of post-mortem cases with survival periods from a few hours to 300 days, we were able to find all stages from acute cerebral edema to severe late effects characterized by various stages of diffuse, or rarely focal, myelin destruction with comparatively good preservation of axons and variable degree of progressive astroglial reaction without marked sclerosis in the deep and subcortical white matter, the arcuate fibers being comparatively well preserved. A high number of these patients didn't suffer from skull fractures, and in about 30% concussional foci were missed, whereas almost all of them clinically showed aspiration asphyxia in the acute post-traumatic stage with acute symptoms of intracranial pressure increase and compression syndromes indicating severe cerebral swelling (Jellinger, et al., 1963; Jellinger, 1965).

In comparatively early stages we found all signs of acute edema of the cerebral white matter with separation of myelin sheaths and axons and with various degrees of initial myelin changes indicated by some birefringent sudanophobic (lipid) globules as well as by myelin pallor and swelling. Later stages revealed progressive diffuse myelin loss from incomplete to subtotal necrosis of the white matter with a special type of predominantly steady degradation: almost no neutral fats, but a high rate of crystallin mostly birefringent degradation products, biochemically characterized by a strong rise of cholesterol esters with decrease of free cholesterol (Holländer and Pilz; Personal communications). The final stages after long survival periods are known as severe post-traumatic hydrocephalus with marked atrophic demyelination of the cerebral white matter with or without focal cystic lesions and secondary tract degenerations.

These myelin lesions of "reactive" post-traumatic type were compared by us with other types of anoxic-vascular leucoencephalopathies, e.g., carbon monoxide leucoencephalopathy, which can be separated from the classical "intervallary" type of Grinker's myelinopathy. Pathogenetically, we suggested a superposition of at least two principal factors, generalized cerebral edema and focal vaso-circulatory disorders causing a critical breakdown of tissue supply. This pathogenic interpretation in some respects could account for myelin lesions in post-traumatic encephalopathy, too, though here a greater complexity of pathological noxae has to be admitted.

The second point of discussion is Binswanger's encephalopathy (ESCP). I cannot quite follow Dr. Feigin's suggestion that its morphological picture is primarily or merely the end result of antecedent cerebral edema, and above all, that the lesions of the cerebral vessel walls are merely secondary to edema. We often may find severe organic lesions of the cerebral vessels belonging to the type of angio- and angiolosclerosis, hyalinofibrosis or subintimal fibrosis, and typical hyalinosis of hypertensive angiopathy. These lesions are to be found in the basal ganglia, followed by typical status lacunaris or small focal necroses. Similar vascular lesions are seen in the deep and subcortical white matter as well as in the small extracerebral vessels with comparatively good preservation of the cortical vessels. With the exception of these localizing characteristics, they don't demonstrate any significant differences from vascular lesions in hypertensive disease and arteriosclerosis without severe affection of the cerebral white matter. Therefore, we cannot believe the vascular changes to be secondary to the tissue process. These data, however, indicate that the diffuse and focal lesions of cerebral white matter in ESCP are sequelae of organic and functional cerebrovascular disturbances, which we assume to be a special type of cerebral hypertensive arteriosclerosis (Jellinger and Neumayer, 1964).

As to the pathogenesis of myelin lesions in ESCP, the vascular dependence of which has been accepted since the time of Alzheimer, we would like to state that they comprize (a) diffuse myelin pallor with or without glial sclerosis as consequence of chronic edema and (b) focally accentuated myelin lesions from partial to subtotal myelin necrosis with comparatively good preservation of axons and slight amounts of degradation, whereas focal total necrosis are exceptionally rare. We considered these focal lesions, comparable to those in Fahr's disease and other anoxic-vasal leucoencephalopathies, to be process-dependent lesions secondary to chronic and/or recurrent edema in combination with various intermittent vaso-circulatory disturbances in the course of general hypertensive disease and the resulting organic and functional cerebrovascular disorders. The morphological picture of ESCP, therefore, seems to us the end result of a combination of chronic or relapsing cerebral edema based upon protracted disturbances of cerebral circulation and barrier function in hypertensive arteriosclerosis, modified and complicated by intermittent local and general vaso-circulatory lesions causing focal subtotal and rarely even total necroses. ESCP could be considered as a kind of "dystrophy of vascular genesis."

REFERENCES

Holländer, H.: Histochemische Untersuchungen von Markabbauprodukten

bei der protrahierten Form der posttraumatischen Encephalopathie. Arch. Psychiat. Z. Neurol. 206, 161-164 (1964).
Jellinger, K.: Komatöse Form der "CO-Leukoencephalopathie." Acta neuropath. (Berl.) 1, 411-415 (1962).
____: Protrahierte Formen der posttraumatischen Encephalopathie. Beitr. gerichtl. Med. 23, 65-118 (1965); Proc. 8th Int. Congr. Neurol., Tom I, 405-408 (1965).
____: Zur Morphologie komatöser und postkomatöser Encephalopathien. Abstr. 5th Int. Congr. Neuropath. Zürich (1965).
____ and E. Neumayer: Progressive subcortical vasculäre Encephalopathie Binswanger. Arch. Psychiat. Z. Neur. 205, 523-554 (1964).
Seitelberger, F. and K. Jellinger: Zur Frage der "CO-Leukoencephalopathie." Wiener klin. Wschr. 72, 422-429 (1960).

BRIGHTMAN: Professor Zülch spoke of the splitting of the myelin sheaths. From the micrographs, however, the sheaths appeared normal. At sites where splitting did occur, was this separation random and artifactual or was there a cleavage of the intermediate lamina? Such a cleavage, as Robertson showed, can occur in the myelin of peripheral nerve soaked in hypotonic media and would represent an opened diffusion channel communicating with the periaxonal fluid. The question, then, is whether the separation occurred at the interperiod lamina.

FEIGIN: I am very happy to hear that Dr. Jellinger has seen many instances of what we called the intermediate stage of degeneration due to edema, the stage of active myelin degeneration which must intervene between the intact myelin of the acute stage and the myelin loss of the obsolete cases. We have seen only a few such cases, probably because we do not have an opportunity to study many acute traumatic cases in New York for medico-legal reasons. Such cases are autopsied by the Medical Examiner. Dr. Jellinger's observations are an essential link in our understanding of the course of cerebral edema.

We believe that the hyaline vascular change in Binswanger's encephalopathy is the primary lesion which causes the white matter degeneration. This type of vascular change is relatively common, being observed in the brains of some hypertensive individuals without tissue damage, and being observed in some normotensive individuals in association with lesions of greatly varying and non-specific character, of which edema is only one example.

Cases of obsolete edema may be seen in which this vascular change is present or absent. We have seen cases of hypertensive individuals with bilateral, diffuse zones of white matter degeneration like that of Binswanger's encephalopathy, except that the vascular change is not evident. For these reasons, we prefer to focus our attention on edema as the pathogenetic mechanism, with the vascular change as a secondary phenomenon due to the edema, the hypertension or both.

ZÜLCH: What we saw in light microscopy was twofold. There was a ballooning of the myelin sheath and a fine vacuolar swelling like a bunch of grapes. Now we wanted to try to correlate these findings in the light microscope with the electron microscope. I think the ballooning has been convincingly shown in one of the pictures. With regard to the splitting-up of the sheath which would correspond to the fine vacuolar swelling, I rely upon my co-worker in this field of electron-microscopy, who is very critical. May I ask Dr. Wechsler to answer the question?

WECHSLER: We have seen the splitting of the intermediate or intraperiod lines of the myelin complex. But there are also more severe forms of destruction of the lamellas of the myelin sheath; e. g., it is interesting to see that there are some relationships between these alterations of the myelin sheath and the alterations found in the supporting oligodendroglia.

TERRY: Dr. Gonatas, Mr. Weiss and I have studied electron microscopically two biopsies of patients with autopsy-proven Jakob-Creutzfeldt's disease and our findings were somewhat different from those demonstrated by Drs. Kidd and Foncin. Most important, we were not impressed by the presence of a membrane surrounding the clear areas within the cytoplasm. These clear zones were found frequently within reactive or fibrous astrocytes and rarely in neurons, and they surely correspond to the spongy state as seen by the light microscopists. The clear zone in the cytoplasm was not separated from the normal cytoplasm by any sort of membrane or other visible structure. It is, I think, something of a presumption to say that the membrane-bounded space is an earlier phenomenon than the clear zone without a membrane. There is no evidence for its being earlier or later. The clear zone might be the result of a change in the permeability of the plasma membrane, or perhaps a sac of endoplasmic reticulum or Golgi apparatus might imbibe fluid through the rest of the cytoplasm.

KIDD: First of all, I would like to say that I found the discussions I had with Dr. Terry in New York and Dr. Sarah Donahue in Indianapolis useful on this subject, though we come to different conclusions. I agree that this is a presumption that these vacuoles that Foncin and I showed ruptured to produce these spaces. I haven't said what makes them rupture or why they rupture; after all, these changes in histology occur over a period of a year, presumably.

I agree that the vacuoles could have formed by pinocytosis. I simply took the simplest hypothesis, fitting the pictures together into a sequence, and I agree that other deductions are possible, but, as you notice, I do also see spaces not surrounded by a membrane inside the cytoplasm. It is simply that the other spaces seem to be significant as well.

FONCIN: These pictures are strikingly different from mine. Perhaps, by coincidence, my two cases could have been from another type of condition,

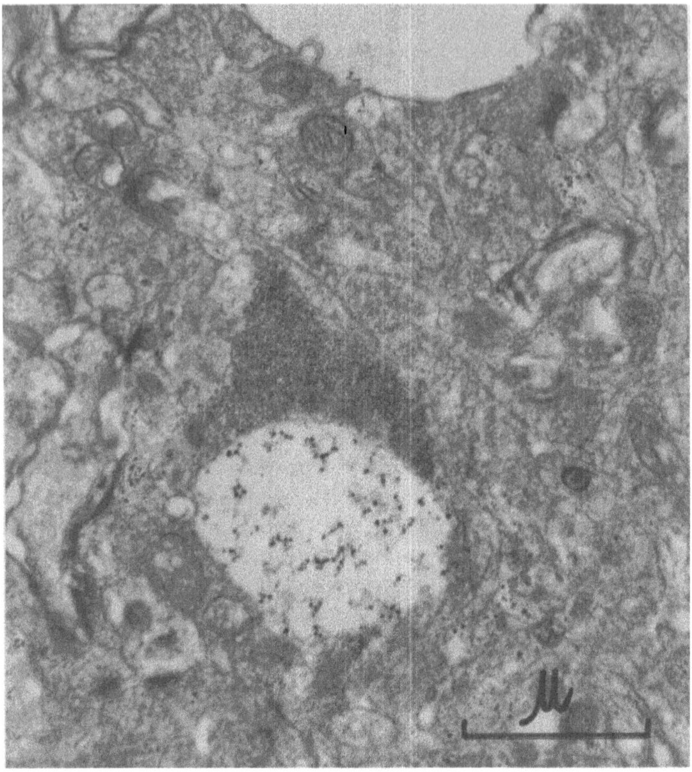

Fig. 3. Electron micrograph referred to by Dr. Foncin.

since the unity of Jakob-Creutzfeldt disease is by no means established. Occasionally, however, I found images comparable to Dr. Terry's. In the upper part of the picture you can see part of a cyst like those I demonstrated, and at the bottom, a cavity without bordering membrane and containing numerous glycogen granules. Such appearances were rare.

Concerning the possible mechanism of the phenomenon, I want to stress that the glia is remarkably normal except for the cyst formation. As a consequence, this formation must be primary and not due to a regional cause, as could be partial necrosis or the like.

McMENEMEY: Would the biochemists like to contribute to this particular discussion?

LOWENTHAL: I think Dr. Terry has some chemical results on Jakob-Creutzfeldt's disease. I would like to know if they are comparable to the results obtained in brain edema.

KATZMAN: We do not have any electrolyte analyses to report on Jakob-Creutzfeldt's disease, but we do have results that have been published by

Drs. Suzuki, Korey and Terry (Journal of Neurochemistry, 11:403, 1964) in reference to the protein metabolism in which they were unable to demonstrate any abnormality of the incorporation of labelled amino acids into proteins by the ribosomal fraction of tissue obtained at cerebral biopsy.

II. Brain Edema in Human Pathology (Continued)

Chairman: ***J. E. Gruner***

J. N. CUMINGS

CHEMICAL ASPECTS OF EDEMATOUS BRAIN

Some biochemical aspects of human cerebral edema associated with tumor, abscess and vascular disorders have already been described (Cumings, 1961, 1962). These examinations demonstrated that the soluble cerebral proteins, extracted from the brain tissue by 0.3 M sucrose, contained numerous proteins but only included albumin from the area of the edema, which was most frequently in the white matter. The proteins present were at that time visualized following starch gel electrophoresis, while the patterns of a number of different enzymes associated with the various protein fractions were also studied. There were some slight changes in enzyme pattern between the normal and the edematous areas, more especially in the white matter and it was then concluded that when cerebral edema occurred in the white matter in association with either a tumor or an abscess, much of the fluid could be extracellular. Nevertheless, when the edema was associated with a cerebrovascular lesion the findings were equally compatible with some or possibly most of the edema fluid being within the myelin sheath and the myelin cell.

Edema in the rat and cat brain was produced experimentally by organic tin compounds (Kalsbeck & Cumings, 1963), and the results obtained were interpreted as being very similar to those found in human vascular lesions. Both from biochemical and histological studies it was concluded that much of the edema fluid was within the myelin sheath or cell and only a small amount in the extracellular space. Edema in the cerebral cortex only rarely occurs in man or in organic tin induced edema in animals in our experience, so that studies on the white matter of brain only are of real significance.

A further study in experimentally produced edema has recently been made (Herschkowitz, et al., 1965). Cerebral edema was produced in monkeys by the administration of intravenous distilled water and various enzyme systems, electrolytes, lipids, protein and water were estimated. The conclusions of these workers from the biochemical results were that while some of the fluid was extracellular, much was within the myelin sheath or cell. Dr. W. G. P. Mair was given some of the material from these monkeys, and mention will be made later concerning his views from an electron microscopic study of the material. Confirmatory evidence was obtained from measurements of impedance and the electroencephalogram recordings of the white matter of the brain.

Further biochemical studies on human cerebral edema have been made; these will be described in a comparison with the observations already made.

Portions of normal and edematous brain from the same patients were obtained at autopsy from cases of cerebral tumor and cerebrovascular lesions. The white matter only was examined and suitable pieces of known weight were sectioned at 20 μ in the cryostat (cold microtome) at −18°C and the sections extracted with 0.3 M sucrose. One piece of edematous tissue exuded edema fluid and this fluid was analyzed. Polyacrylamide disc electrophoresis as used previously (Monseu & Cumings, 1965) as well as starch gel electrophoresis were carried out in every case and all demonstrated the presence of albumin as well as many other proteins. This is illustrated in Figure 1, and the results are identical with those obtained previously.

Total nitrogen, potassium, sodium, alkaline phosphatase, lactate dehydrogenase, aldolase, phosphohexose isomerase, glucose-6-phosphate, phosphocreatine kinase and water were estimated. Swelling per cent (SP) was calculated using the formula of Elliott and Jasper (1949). The results in the various conditions are seen in Figures 2-6 where SP is given followed by a comparison of the protein content, electrolyte and enzyme levels. In each case the normal, as calculated for fresh tissue, has been regarded as 100 per cent and the changes in the edematous side recorded.

Figure 2 shows the white matter changes seen in cases of edema associated with tumor, examples being given in descending order of SP. Protein, sodium and water are invariably increased; potassium shows little change except in one case, and phosphocreatine kinase and aldolase are lower. The levels of lactate dehydrogenase are variable. The edema fluid which separated out from the case with a SP of 89.4 was examined directly and showed on analysis a composition almost identical with that of the sucrose extracted fluid from the edematous brain.

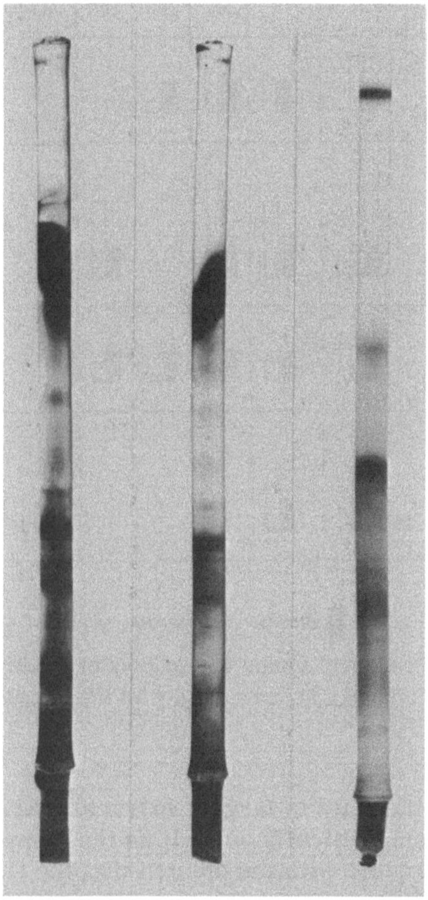

Fig. 1. Polyacrylamide disc electrophoresis of edema fluid, sucrose extracted edematous white matter from a case of cerebral tumor and sucrose extracted normal white matter (from left to right).

These findings can be compared with some of the originally published results (Cumings, 1962) when calculated in the same manner and are seen in Figure 3. There is a raised protein content, but the enzymes then studied were all lower in amount despite a SP of 58.0. There is thus a close similarity between the original findings and the present ones.

The absence of any increase in glutamic oxalacetic transaminase and more especially of creatine kinase, taken in conjunction with no increase in potassium, apart from one case, strongly sup-

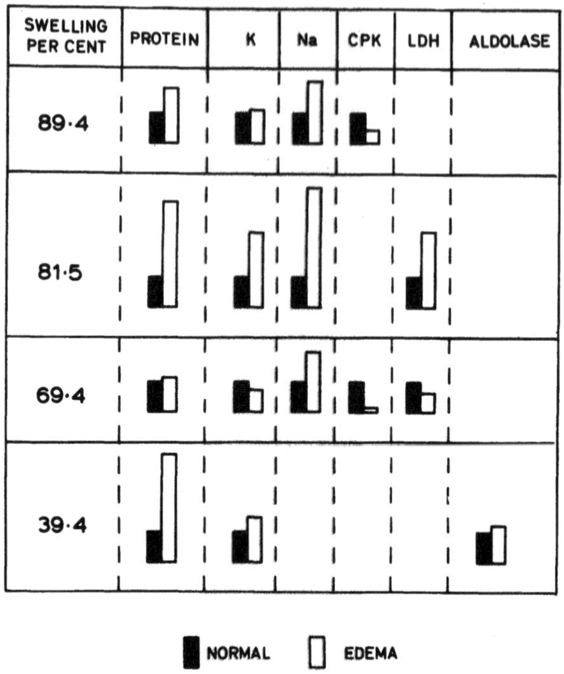

Fig. 2. Case of cerebral tumor with edema of the white matter. Changes in various substances as compared with the normal white matter.

ports the view that the fluid is largely extracellular. The protein pattern seen electrophoretically as well as the composition of the fluid would be compatible with the opinion that the fluid was derived from blood plasma.

Figure 4 illustrates the results found in two cases of cerebrovascular lesion, where it is seen that when there is a high SP, potassium and some enzyme levels are elevated. When SP is negligible, few significant changes are present.

Similar methods of calculation have been applied to the results of the experiments on cats given organic tin, and on monkeys infused with distilled water. The results are not exactly comparable. Figure 5 illustrates the findings in the cat, in which most enzymes apart from acid phosphatase were lower in the edematous region. Similarly in the monkey, as seen in Figure 6, SP was 17.9 but here the results were more like those in human cases of vascular disease. There was a lowered potassium and creatine kinase but a raised sodium and lactate dehydrogenase, and an increased anaerobic glycolysis.

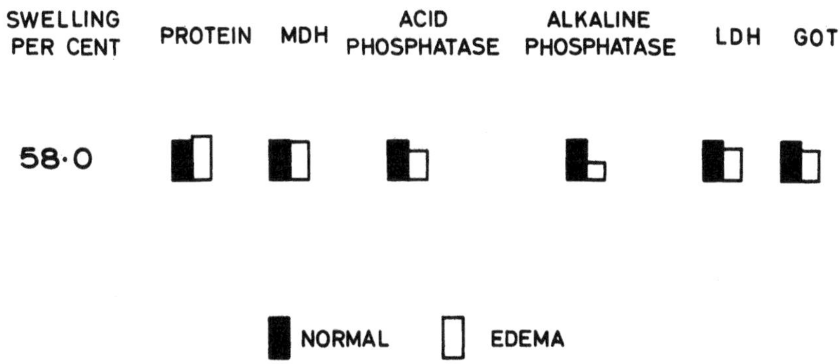

Fig. 3. A similar comparison as in the previous figure obtained from earlier results (Cumings, 1962).

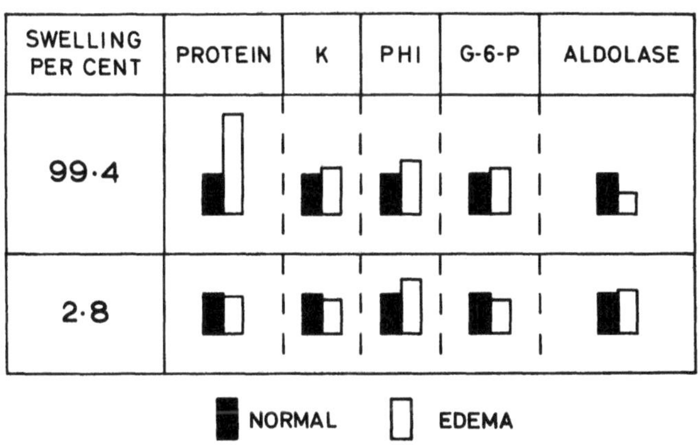

Fig. 4. A similar comparison as in Figure 2 but in patients with cerebrovascular disease with associated edema.

While the findings in human cerebral edema associated with a tumor or abscess are strongly suggestive of the presence of an increased extracellular fluid of proteinous nature, the changes in cases of vascular occlusion or small hemorrhage are more closely paralled by the findings in the animal experiments. Some of the edema fluid may well be extracellular as judged by both the biochemical and the electrophysiological experiments, but much of the fluid is undoubtedly within the myelin sheath or myelin cell in the white

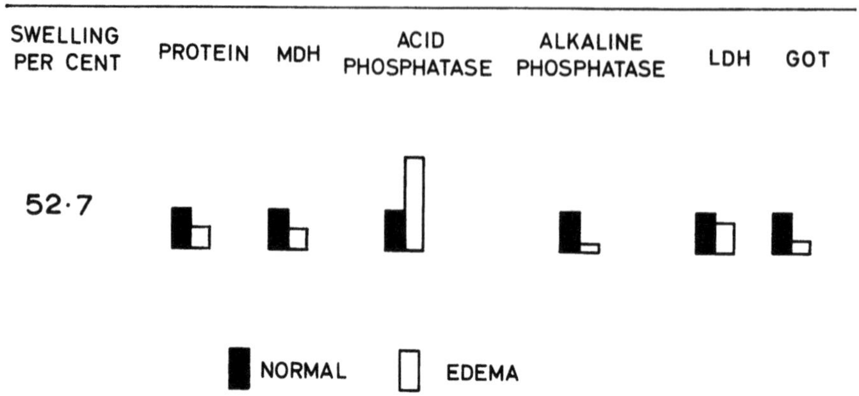

Fig. 5. Similar to Figure 2 but in cats given organic tin with resulting edema (see Kalsbeck & Cumings, 1963).

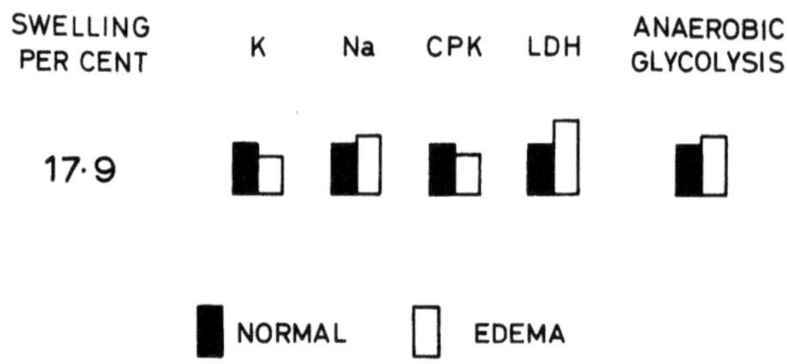

Fig. 6. Results in the monkey's white matter given distilled water (see Herschkowitz, MacGillivray & Cumings, 1965).

matter. This latter view has been partly confirmed by the electron microscopic studies of Dr. W. G. P. Mair on our material, for he has demonstrated some most interesting changes. Figure 7 shows the cortex of the brain in a control animal given a glucose infusion. This animal showed no edema biochemically and no raised SP yet the astrocytic processes (AP) around the capillary are greatly distended.

Figure 8 is of the white matter in a monkey which received distilled water. There is again a marked distension of the astrocytic processes (AP). The oligodendrocyte cytoplasm contains numerous dilated vesicles. There is also some separation of the lamellae in some of the myelinated fibres. These findings are those of Dr. Mair, but I believe it can be seen that the extracellular spaces are also somewhat enlarged and that these findings are compatible with the biochemical and electrophysiological results already mentioned.

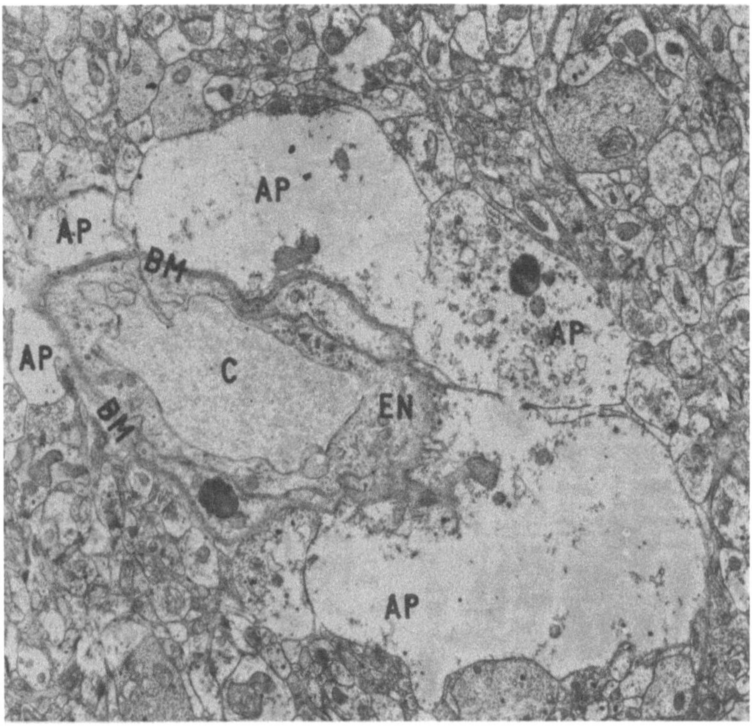

Fig. 7. Electron microscopy of a monkey's cerebral cortex following intravenous glucose but no edema biochemically. AP, astrocyte processes; C, capillary; EN, endothelium; BM, basement membrane. X15000 (reduced).

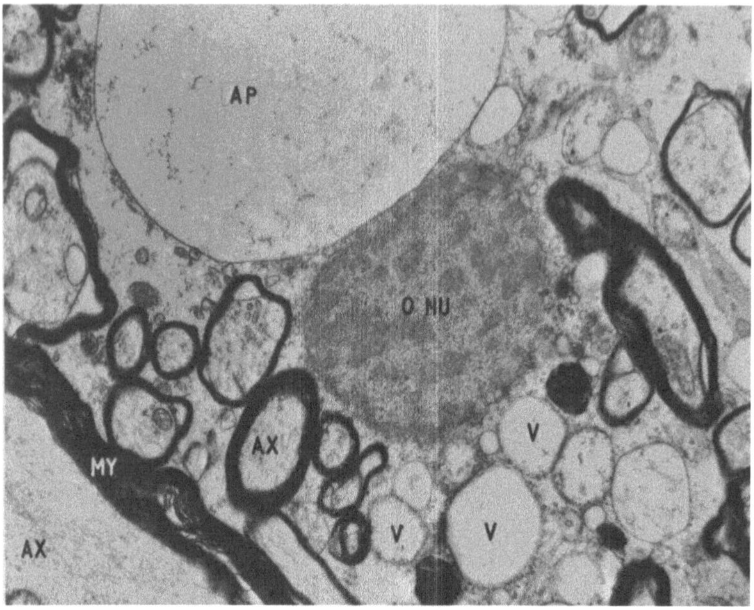

Fig. 8. Electron microscopy of a monkey's cerebral white matter following intravenous distilled water with edema. AP, astrocyte processes; AX, axis cylinder; V, vesicles; MY, myelin; O NU, oligodendroglia nucleus. X18000 (reduced).

REFERENCES

Cumings, J. N.: Soluble cerebral proteins in normal and oedematous brain, J. Clin. Path., 14, 289-294 (1961).

_____: Water soluble proteins and enzymes in normal and in oedematous brain tissue, Proceedings of IV. International Congress of Neuropathology, München, Thema I, Vol. I, (1961), (ed. by H. Jacob), Stuttgart: Georg Thieme Verlag, 157-161 (1962).

Elliott, K. A. C. and H. Jasper: Measurement of experimentally induced brain swelling and shrinkage, Amer. J. Physiol., 157, 122-129 (1949).

Herschkowitz, N., B. B. MacGillivray and J. N. Cumings: Biochemical and electrophysiological studies in experimental cerebral oedema, Brain, 88, 557-584 (1965).

Kalsbeck, J. E. and J. N. Cumings: Experimental edema in the rat and cat brain, J. Neuropath. exp. Neurol., 22, 237-247 (1963).

Monseu, G. and J. N. Cumings: Polyacrylamide disc electrophoresis of the proteins of cerebrospinal fluid and brain, J. Neurol. Neurosurg. Psychiat., 28, 56-60 (1965).

D. KARCHER
A. LOWENTHAL

HYDROSOLUBLE PROTEINS OF EDEMATOUS HUMAN NERVOUS TISSUE*

In edematous brain tissue, water content and sodium concentration, expressed in wet or in dry weight, are increased. Potassium content is practically unchanged. At autopsy, alterations are at a maximum in periventricular white matter (Lowenthal, 1959). After having defined edematous tissue, we wanted to study with the method described previously in our laboratory (Van Sande, 1962) the hydrosoluble proteins. We used only edematous tissue taken during neurosurgical procedure. Brain edema was diagnosed by macroscopic examinations and confirmed by optical microscope. Until now, only very few studies have been made on edematous human brain (Kyota, 1959; Cumings, 1961; Van Sande, 1962).

The agar gel pherogram of human hydrosoluble proteins extracted from edematous human brain is characterized by the increase of fast-moving fractions. In the same region of the pherogram we described also increases of protein fraction in some neurological diseases in the cerebrospinal fluid (CSF). Similar increases are characteristic for the hydrosoluble proteins in some other locations of the central nervous system. Indeed, in the CSF fast-moving alpha globulins predominate in fresh lesions of nervous parenchyma (Fig. 1). In spinal cord extracts and in brain stem and chiasm extracts (Van Sande, 1962, 1964) the fast-moving fraction also reaches a high level (Fig. 2). The mobility rate of that fraction is not always the same. Isolated, after preparative agar gel electrophoresis, this fraction precipitates with serum anti-albumin (Van Sande, 1964).

*Work accomplished with grants from Fonds de la Recherche Medicale, The National Multiple Sclerosis Society of the U.S.A., and the Van Hinderdael Foundation.

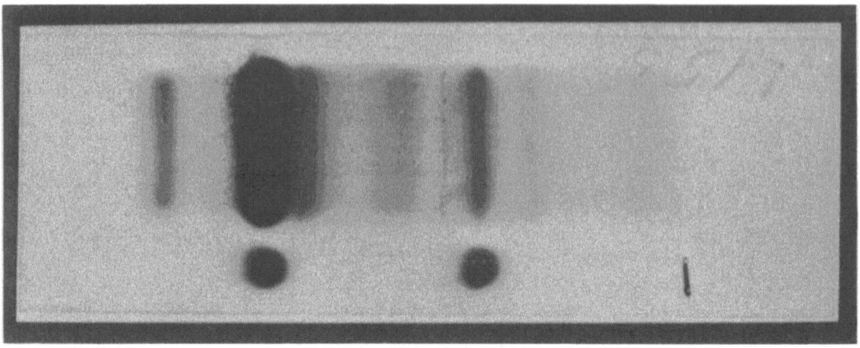

Fig. 1. Agar gel pherogram of cerebrospinal fluid proteins with an increase of fast-moving alpha globulin.

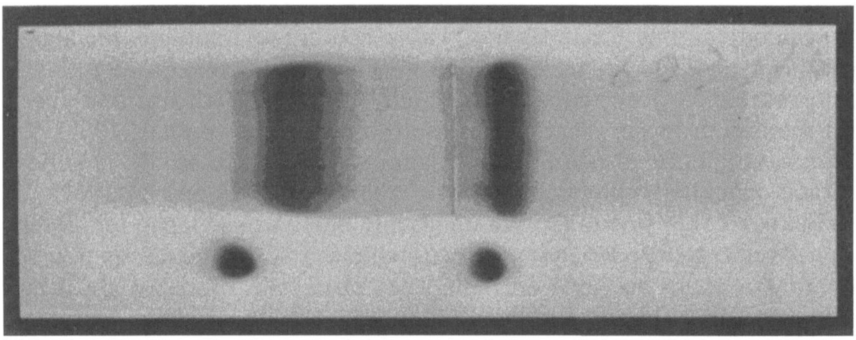

Fig. 2. Agar gel pherogram of hydrosoluble protein of spinal cord.

Keeping in mind those results we attempted a better definition of hydrosoluble proteins extracted from edematous tissue.

METHODS

Thirty-nine brain pieces were studied. They were taken from 22 patients operated for meningioma (6 cases: 6 fragments of gray matter, 6 of white matter and 1 of cerebellum); for neurinoma (3 cases: 3 fragments of gray matter, 2 of white matter, 2 of cerebellum); for glioblastoma (13 cases: 2 fragments of gray matter, 14 of white matter, 2 of cerebellum and 1 of basal ganglia). All extractions were done as previously described (Van Sande, 1962). Every extract was submitted to agar gel electrophoresis and to LDH enzymo-electrophoresis. Fractions were isolated on Sephadex G200 column, phosphate buffer 0.045 M, pH 7.5, ionic strength 0.1. The fraction under study is pointed out with the aid of a Uvicord recording instrument at 253 mμ. After dialysis and concentration by ultrafiltration, the protein is further purified on the Sephadex DEAE (diethylaminoethyl) cellulose buffered with 0.050 M triethanolamine and 0.005 M (disodium ethylenediamine tetra-acetate dehydrate), complexon III, pH 7.5 with NaCl gradient maximum of 0.6 M. Purity of the fraction is confirmed by agar gel and acrylamide electrophoresis.

Molecular weight is estimated after passage on Sephadex columns by measuring the elution volume necessary to reach a peak of the eluted protein. Human albumin, serum alpha-two globulin, fast-moving fraction of the spinal cord, and anodic fraction of edematous brain were compared. The total protein concentration of the extracts was determined. The different protein fractions were precipitated after diffusion in agar gel according to Feinberg.

The extracts were finally added to trypsin in a proportion of fifty to one. The mixture was then placed into an incubator at 37°C for five hours, a similar enzyme quantity was added, and incubation was prolonged for two hours.

This means that we were able to determine for the isolated fractions: 1) molecular weight by comparison; 2) immunologic characteristics by using the Feinberg method; and 3) sensitivity to trypsin action by comparison with action on serum albumin.

RESULTS

Our results were as follows: the agar gel pherograms of human edematous brain hydrosoluble proteins obtained by biopsy show a predominance of two fast fractions (Fig. 3); one has a mobility rate identical to that of human serum albumin and the other is a slower one but is always seen in the region of the fast alpha globulins. The second one has no sharp limits as does the first. After isolation of the fractions (Fig. 4) by passage on Sephadex G200 columns, we could show that the edematous alpha globulin has the highest molecular weight and that this weight is the same as that of the human serum alpha-two globulin. Brain tissue albumin molecular weight is lower than that of serum albumin. The fraction with alpha mobility isolated from spinal cord extracts has a molecular weight similar to that of serum alpha-two globulin.

By incorporating anti-serum to agar gel, we precipitated different fractions in extracts from total proteins or from isolated fractions. By using suitable proportions of protein solutions and anti-serum, comparable precipitation lines were obtained for serum,

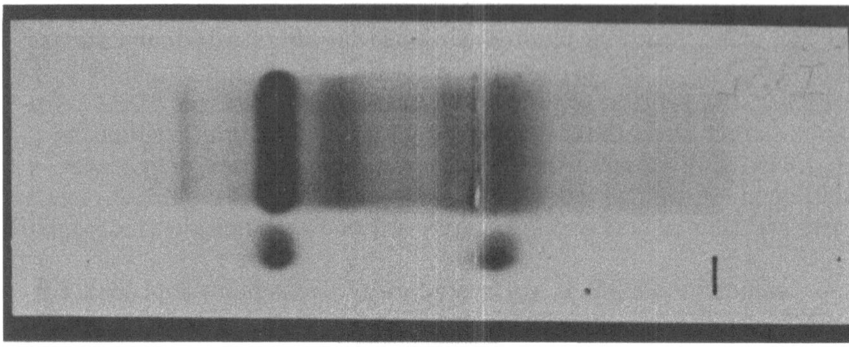

Fig. 3. Agar gel pherogram of hydrosoluble protein of human brain edema with two increased fast-moving fractions.

spinal cord extract and edematous brain extract. Isolated fast fraction of spinal cord and edematous extracts give precipitating lines that cross (Fig. 5) with serum albumin lines and are confluent. They reveal between these different fractions an antigenic parenty but show that they are not identical.

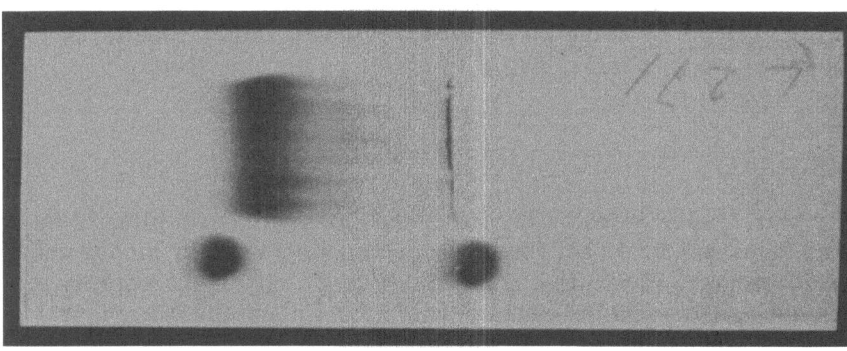

Fig. 4. Agar gel pherogram of isolated and purified fast-moving fractions of brain edema.

By trypsin, human albumin was split into two fractions which have molecular weights after passage on Sephadex that are similar. One, however, migrates with the same mobility as the albumin and the other as an alpha-one serum globulin. Trypsin action in the same proportion on edematous albumin is less important. A slow fraction is also obtained but represents only a small proportion of the total albumin. Trypsin action on edematous albumin and on serum is quite different (Fig. 6). One could think that in edematous

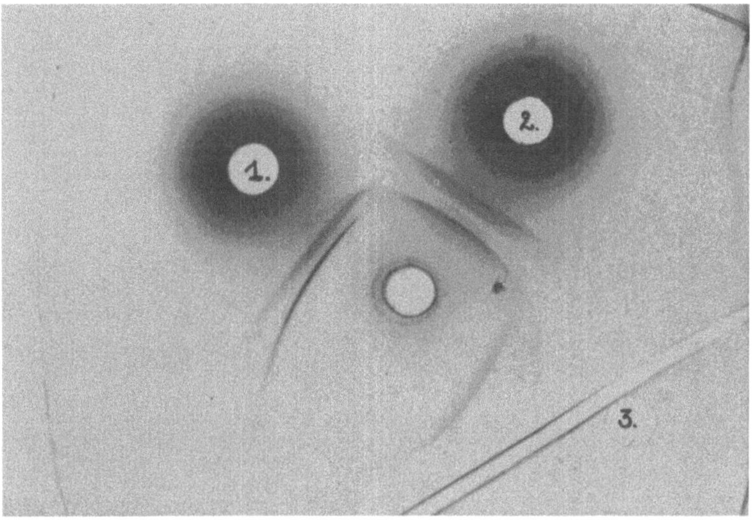

Fig. 5. Spinal cord extract (1), edematous tissue extract (2), and isolated fast moving protein of the spinal cord (3). Interrupted precipitation line crosses between 3 and 2 and 2 and 1.

tissue an enzymatic reaction takes place acting on the albumin and causing a slower migrating fraction. This could explain that edematous albumin does not react with trypsin. The suspected enzymatic reaction in edema could be compared to trypsin action and could be eventually a proteolysis.

DISCUSSION

The above mentioned results prove that in brain edema fast moving protein fractions can be isolated. Their mobilities are comparable to that of human serum albumin or to alpha-two globulin. Molecular weights and sensitivity to trypsin action are different from those of serum albumin. Those fractions are antigenically related to human albumin but are not identical. One can say that we found protein fractions related to modified serum albumin. In two uremic brains taken at autopsy and in one diabetic brain from a patient who died in a diabetic coma with encephalopathy, we did not find those fractions.

Two hypotheses could explain the properties of this fraction. It could be an abnormal protein synthesized in cells undergoing abnormal physiological conditions during brain edema, or it could also

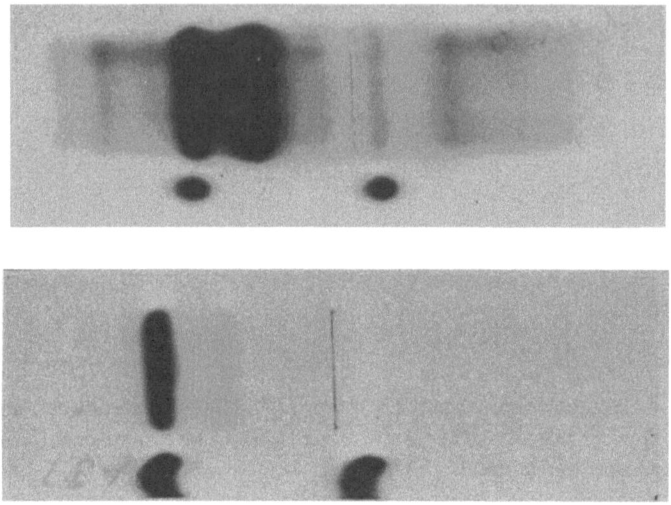

Fig. 6. Trypsin action on serum albumin (Top) and fast-moving protein of human edematous nerve tissue (Bottom).

be, and this seems more probable, that an albumin of extra-cerebral origin, contained in the edema liquid is modified in edematous cells by an abnormal metabolic process. Further investigations taking into account this last hypothesis could allow to bring further information on metabolism of edematous nervous tissue cellular components.

CONCLUSION AND SUMMARY

Human edematous nerve tissue, due to development of brain tumor, is characterized by increase of water and sodium content as well as by fast-moving hydrosoluble proteins. These proteins migrate as the albumin or the serum alpha globulins. They are related to human serum albumin but have different mobility rates, molecular weight, sensitivity to trypsin action, and also immunological properties. We suppose that these proteins come from the serum or from the extra-cellular fluid and are modified by the edematous cellular tissue components. We believe that the study of these proteins could show the biochemical modifications of nervous tissue cellular constituents during brain edema.

REFERENCES

Cumings, J. N.: Soluble cerebral proteins in normal and oedematous brains, J. Clin. Pathol., 14, 289 (1961).
Feinberg, J. G.: Immunology, 2, 346 (1959).
Kiyota, K.: Electrophoretic protein fractions and hydrophylic property of brain tissue. The proteins of brains with oedema, J. Neurochem., 4, 209 (1959).
Lowenthal, A.: Composition du cerveau en certains éléments minéraux et essai sur leur signification en pathologie, Les Editions Acta Medica Belgica, Bruxelles (1958).
Van Sande, M.: Contribution à l'étude des protéines cérébrales et de deux enzymes (la déhydrogénase de l'acide lactique et la déhydrogénase de l'acide malique) du système nerveux central, Annales de la Société Royale des Sciences Médicales et Naturelles de Bruxelles, 15, 1-2, 1-120 (1962).
_____, D. Karcher and A. Lowenthal: Caractérisation électrophorétique des protéines spinales. Protides of the Biological Fluids (ed. by H. Peeters), 253-254. Amsterdam: Elsevier Publishing Company (1964).

J. E. GRUNER

ELECTRON MICROSCOPIC OBSERVATIONS ON HUMAN BRAIN EDEMA STUDIED IN BIOPSY MATERIAL

Some years ago, I studied biopsies of human brain edema. Samples were obtained during surgical operations for tumors, abscesses or hematomas, after putting some drops of cold osmic acid in situ on the adjacent white matter. This process is not dangerous since the periventricular gray matter is at quite a large distance and the osmic acid is hardly penetrating. Samples were then taken of perifocal edema in the later stages. They were taken far from the edematous focus and we may have missed the most typical lesions of the blood-brain barrier. Samples were said to have been taken from the centrum ovale; it is possible that some of them were taken either deeper than I thought or from the arcuate fibers by perforation of a convolution. As in cortical edema samples, the most typical lesion was the swelling of astroglia as well as of oligodendroglia (Fig. 1).

Perivascular glial processes were clustered without any enlargement of the spaces between or outside them (Fig. 2). They were pallid and had many vesicles in cases of abscess. Tumoral glial cells in the marginal zone of the glioblastomas were swollen the same way. Glia appeared swollen near the outer margin of the myelin sheaths. The spirals of myelin lamellae were not distended. The fact that there were mitochondria in the periaxonal clear zone and that there was a double membrane around proved that it was a cytoplasmic swelling. Now and then, spaces between the thick myelin fibers were too wide (Figs. 3, 4). I did not think this was a sign of edema because I had observed the same in demyelinating processes where I thought it was rather the result of a rupture of

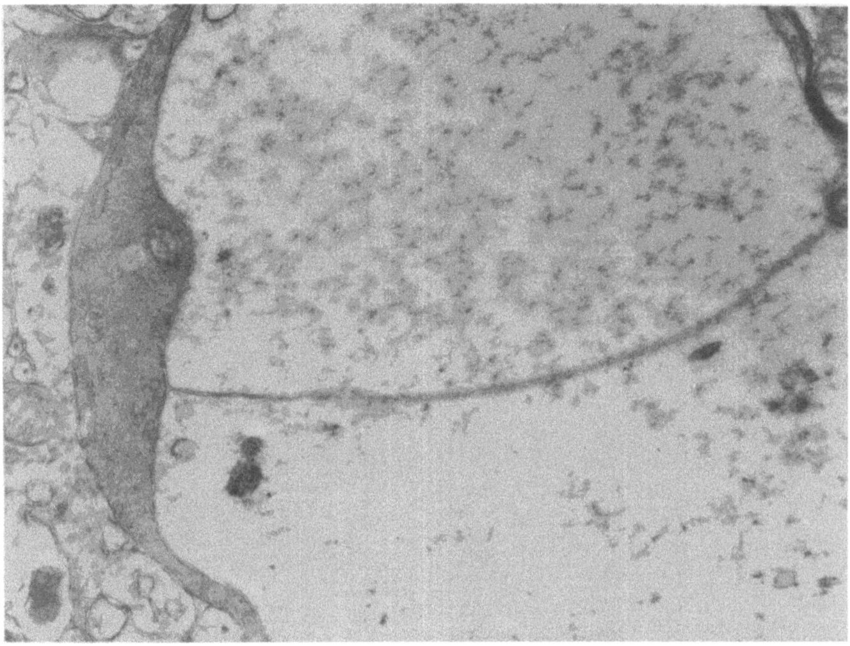

Fig. 1. Edema; swelling of astroglia in contact with a dark cell.

the membranes of glial cells. Some cytoplasmic ruptures seemed to be the result of an artificial shrinkage in biopsies prepared with metracrylate; however, the spaces did not disappear in samples taken half an hour after urea had been injected and had reduced the swelling of the brain.

My conclusion was that edema, wherever it was located, was a glial swelling. This notion was in accordance with what other researchers had found in cortex and in white matter. But it fitted neither the optical observations of experimental edemas nor the fluorescent microscopic pictures of Klatzo and his colleagues. It was not adapted to the electron-microscopic pictures of experimental edema, such as the ones shown by Zimmermann and his colleagues, with abnormal intercellular fluid. And finally it was not in agreement with the macroscopic and microscopic contrast between the cortex and the white matter swelling, especially in the Jaburek areas, where there is little astroglia reaction even in the kind of edema I studied; that is, perifocal edema.

I had then to obtain new biopsies closer to the focus (tumors, hematomas, etc.), in more recent cases of edema. I used glutaraldehyde fixation and araldite embedding. Then I had to admit that my concept was wrong or, at least, an oversimplification. In the

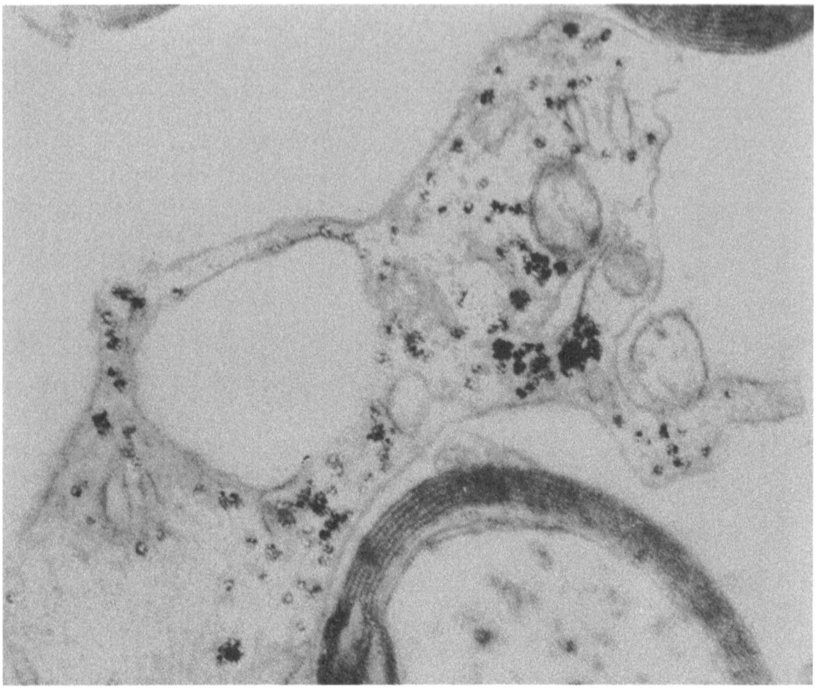

Fig. 2. Edema adjacent to a glioblastoma; enlargement of spaces between the glial cells.

new pictures the presence of dilated spaces is evident in certain cases. This is particularly clear in the areas with thick parallel myelin fibers and even clearer in some particular cases as an abscess around which the brain "weeps" as an Emmenthaler cheese and in hematoma and tuberculoma cases (Figs. 4, 5). Clearly visible after overcoloration, the fluid spreads between the sheaths and the astroglia; in the subcortical area it may penetrate between the glial membranes and reach a synaptic connection. Brain swelling seems then a result of three associated phenomena: accumulation of fluid between cells, bubbles in the myelin sheaths, and swelling of the astrocytic processes. The importance of each differs from one biopsy to the other. The dilation of the spaces is considerably less in volume than the two others. Astrocytic swelling is the most important process, either close to the intercellular edema or as the only noticeable sign, more often appearing as a swelling of the clear glial cells than of granular (that is, vesicular) glia. Perivascular glia are always swollen; the clear glia between the thick myelin fibers are differently swollen from one case to the other, and, in each case, from one sample to the other. The bubbles in the myelin

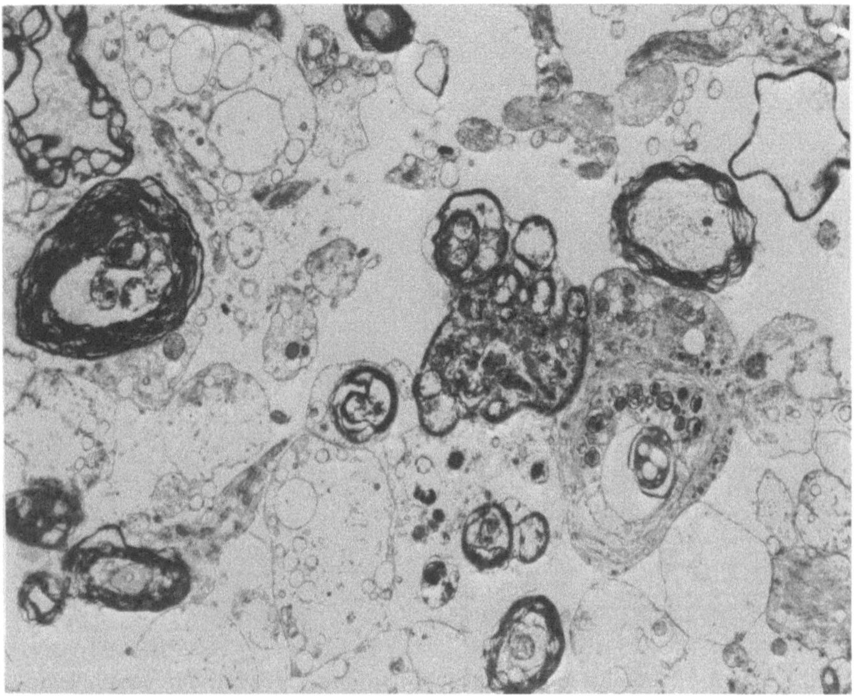

Fig. 3. Wall of a cyst in the neighborhood of glioblastoma; irregular and dilated spaces with more or less osmiophilic contents.

sheaths are very irregularly distributed (Figs. 4, 5). Some sheaths look quite normal, even where they are not normally spaced, neighboring others which are partly disrupted. The swelling of the juxta-axonal area is less frequent.

I never saw fluid between vessels and glial cells or between vascular glial processes, similar to what was shown by Hirano and Zimmermann. This does not mean it does not exist; one can never be sure of having reached the most typical point of the lesion since samples are so small. The characteristics of brain edema certainly vary from one type of edema to another and according to its age. As for the type of perifocal inflammatory edema I studied, I think that the increase of fluid and enlargement of spaces are mainly visible after destruction of tissues or after extravasation of red blood corpuscles. It seems to me that glial swelling, whether primary or secondary, soon becomes the dominant lesion in the histological pattern of edema, but I would not like to conclude once more too promptly.

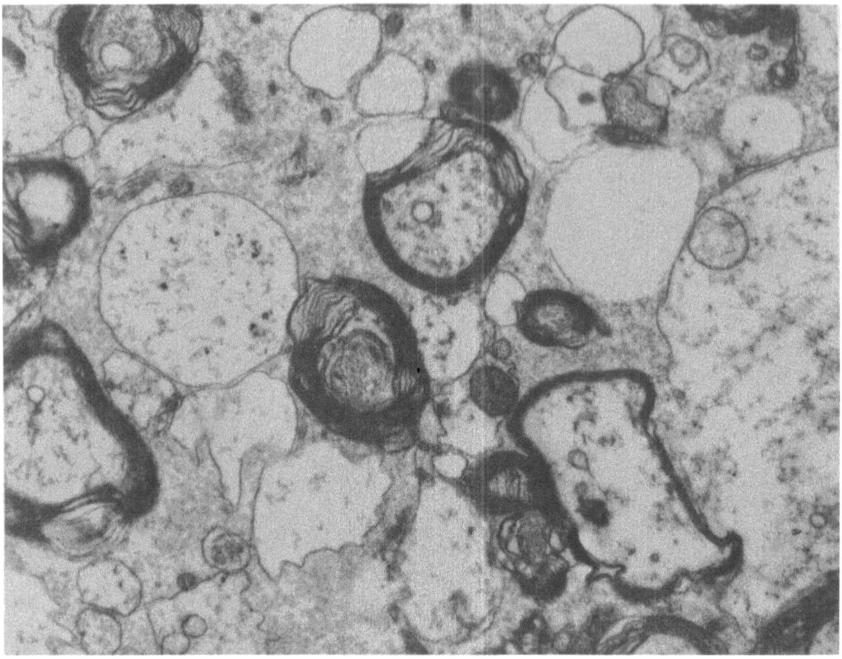

Fig. 4. Edema with parietal tuberculoma; intercellular osmiophilic edema; astroglial swelling; ballooning of myelin sheaths.

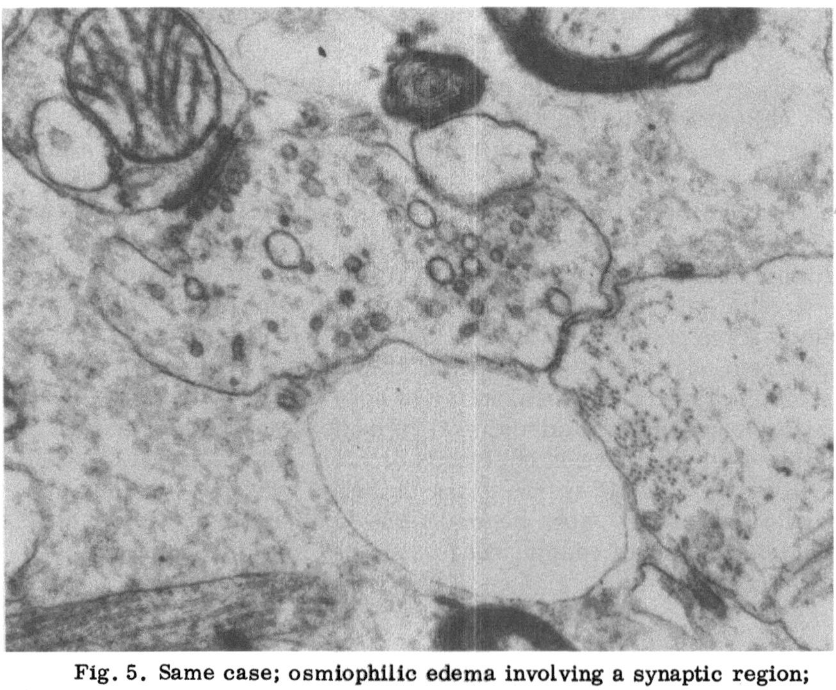

Fig. 5. Same case; osmiophilic edema involving a synaptic region; ballooning of myelin sheaths.

P. LAMPERT
F. GARRO
A. PENTSCHEW

LEAD ENCEPHALOPATHY IN SUCKLING RATS*

AN ELECTRON MICROSCOPIC STUDY

The morphology of lead encephalopathy in infants and children is well documented by light microscopy (Blackman, 1937; Pentschew, 1958; Smith, et al., 1960; Popoff, et al., 1963; Pentschew, 1965). Vascular damage and serous exudation followed by endothelial, microglial and astrocytic prolifereation are prominent features. The cerebellum is most frequently affected. Similar morphological alterations develop in the brains of suckling rats when their mothers are fed a diet containing lead carbonate (Pentschew, et al., 1966). The purpose of this paper is to present some electron microscopic observations on this lead encephalopathy in suckling rats together with an account on the vascular permeability to Trypan Blue and Thorotrast, an electron dense tracer.

MATERIAL AND METHODS

The principles of laboratory animal care as promulgated by the National Society for Medical Research were observed during this study. Long-Evans rats were mated and the dams were kept in individual cages. At delivery the dams were put on a diet of Purina laboratory chow containing four percent lead carbonate (Fisher Scientific Company). They remained in good health but their offspring, getting lead through lactation, grew less well than normal control

*This investigation was supported in part by Research Grant NB-02275 from the National Institute of Neurological Diseases and Blindness, National Institutes of Health, Bethesda, Maryland, and the Veterans Administration Central Laboratory for Anatomic Pathology and Research, AFIP, Washington, D.C.

litters. About 20 to 30 days after birth the suckling rats, regardless of sex, developed a sudden onset of paraplegia of their hind legs. Most of them died two or three days thereafter. A few recovered even while on a lead diet. If put on a normal diet at the onset of the paraplegia, all animals recovered.

For light microscopic studies, groups of suckling rats were sacrificed by formalin perfusion before and at the onset of the paraplegia. At either one or 24 hours before sacrifice, some of these animals were given intravenous or intraperitoneal injection of 0.5 ml. of a 1:100 dilution of Trypan Blue. Control rats of the same age but of greater weight were given 1 ml. of the diluted Trypan Blue.

For electron microscopy, eight suckling rats from different litters were sacrificed by osmium perfusion at the onset of the paraplegia, i.e., 19 to 31 days after birth. Five of these rats were given an intravenous injection of 0.25 or 0.5 cc. of Thorotrast (colloidal thorium dioxide, Fellows Testagar, Detroit) one hour before sacrifice. One paraplegic rat received 0.5 cc. of Thorotrast 20 hours before osmium perfusion. One normal control rat, 25 days old, received 0.5 ml. of Thorotrast one hour before sacrifice and two normal controls, 26 and 30 days old, were killed 24 hours after the intravenous injection of Thorotrast.

The animals were anesthetized with Nembutal. Their chest was opened, the right atrium incised, the left ventricle cut, and a cannula inserted into the aorta. The blood was first flushed for 30 seconds with Palay's balanced salt solution which was followed for about 30 minutes by Dalton's osmium fixative. A flow of about three drops per second, as observed in a drip chamber three feet above the animal, was maintained throughout the perfusion. The black, firm brain were removed and dissected with the aid of a dissecting microscope. Small blocks were cut from the striatum and cerebellum, dehydrated and embedded in epon according to Luft. Thin sections were stained with uranyl acetate or lead tartrate and examined with an RCA EMU 3G electron microscope operating at 50 kv.

RESULTS

The cerebellum of paraplegic animals presented a reddish brown discoloration due to the presence of abundant petechial haemorrhages (Fig. 1b, c) One hour after the intravenous injection of Trypan Blue, staining of the brain was visible in certain areas, most strikingly in the striatum, the occipital lobes, the cerebellum, and the lower spinal cord (Fig. 1b). Twenty-four hours after the intraperitoneal injection of Trypan Blue staining of the brain was more widespread, but was still most intense in the above mentioned sites

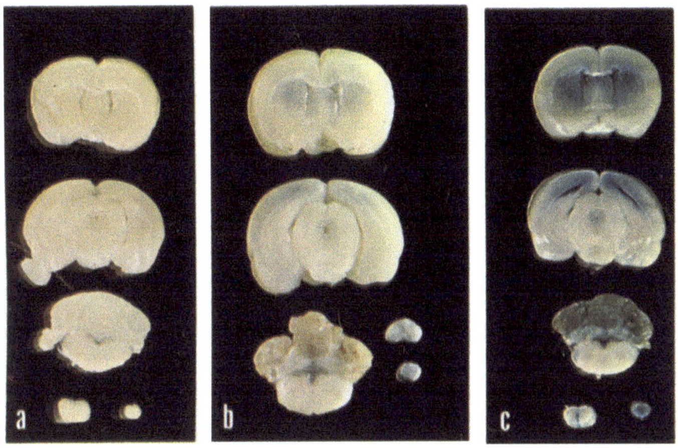

Fig. 1. a) Normal brain of 25-day-old rat 24 hours after intraperitoneal injection of Trypan Blue. No staining of the brain occurred. b) Brain of lead poisoned, 25-day-old rat one hour after the intraperitoneal injection of Trypan Blue. Some staining is visible in the striatum, occipital lobes, cerebellum, and spinal cord. c) Brain of lead poisoned, 26-day-old rat 24 hours after intraperitoneal injection of Trypan Blue. Staining of the brain is more intense and widespread.

(Fig. 1c). Animals sacrificed at 15 days after birth, i.e., before they became paraplegic, presented no hemorrhages in the cerebellum but permeability to Trypan Blue was already noted at this stage. Control animals of the same age showed no staining of the brain, except in areas known to be permeable, i.e., the area postrema, pineal gland, neurohypophysis and choroid plexus (Fig. 1a).

Light microscopy of the severely affected cerebellum demonstrated perivascular hemorrhages which were sprinkled throughout the molecular and granular layers as well as in the white matter. Subpial hemorrhages were particularly numerous. There were large cyst in the white matter. The margin of these cysts presented widely separated but intact myelinated fibers and glial cells. The neurons of the granular layer and the Purkinje cells were generally well preserved. Macrophages and a few reactive astrocytes were present. Proliferated capillaries with prominent endothelial cells were striking in the molecular layer. In the striatum smaller and less frequent perivascular hemorrhages occurred. A separation of individual myelinated axons within fiber bundles was noted. There were also a few proliferated microglial cells and astrocytes. The oligodendroglial cells were normal. Further light microscopic observations on lead encephalopathy in suckling rats are reported in greater detail elsewhere (Pentschew, et al., 1966).

Electron microscopy of the striatum and cerebellum of paraplegic rats revealed the following observations. The extracellular space was enlarged in the gray and white matter (Figs. 2, 4, 5). While this was widespread in the white matter it occurred only in foci around vessels or hemorrhages in the gray matter. In the latter, the presence of red cells squeezed within a compact neuropil suggested that normal, narrow intercellular spaces were restored (Fig. 3). Fine granular material, possibly precipitated plasma proteins, was found in widened extracellular spaces.

Nerve cells were well preserved. Axons occasionally presented spheroid enlargements filled with mitochondria, dense bodies and vesicular elements. Some axons presented a clumped, amorphous axoplasm and a myelin sheath with loosened myelin lamellae. The latter, degenerating axons were often engulfed by microglial cells. Myelin sheaths around normal axons were remarkably well preserved even in white matter exhibiting enormously widened extracellular spaces (Figs. 4, 5). Occasionally, however, wide splits within compact sheaths occurred. Large spaces between axons and surrounding myelin sheaths or "empty" loops of myelin were also noted.

Oligodendrocytes were well preserved (Fig. 4). They were identified by their location, i.e., arranged in rows in the white mat-

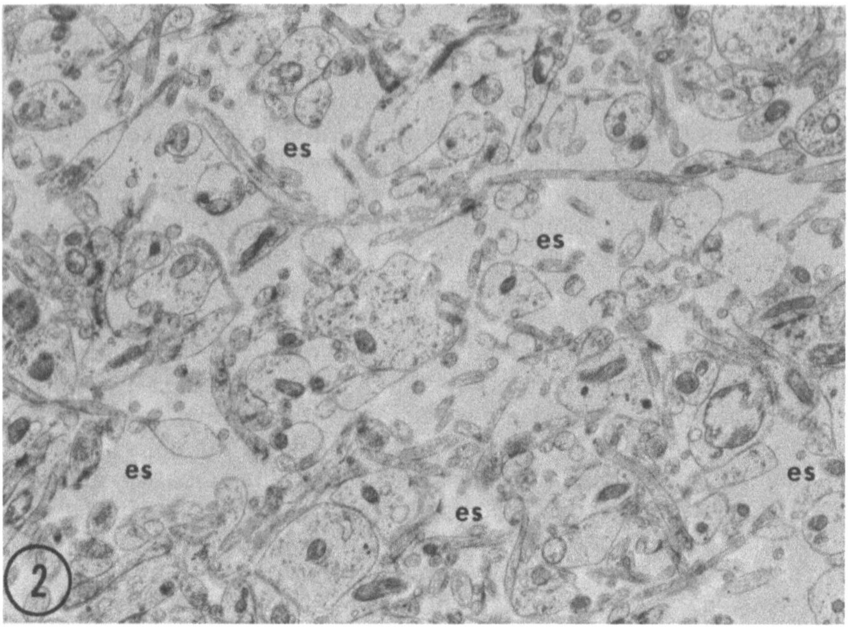

Fig. 2. Striatum of lead poisoned, 19-day-old rat. Note widened extracellular spaces (es). X10,000 (reduced).

ter and as satellites around nerve cells. They had a "dark" cytoplasm rich in ribosomes and devoid of filaments. They did not exhibit phagocytic properties.

Astrocytes were identified by their "clear" cytoplasm and by the attachment of their processes to vessels and to neurons. A few glycogen granules and bundles of filaments were characteristic components of the astrocytic cytoplasm. Filaments were scanty in astrocytes of normal gray matter. In the paraplegic rats some astrocytes, particularly in the white matter, contained an increased number of filaments, mitochondria and ribosomes in their cytoplasm (Fig. 5). Cytoplasmic swelling was not observed. Foot processes alongside abnormal vessels sometimes contained vacuoles filled with amorphous material. An increase of glycogen granules, some lipid droplets and occasional myelin figures were observed in a few astrocytic processes.

Microglial cells were numerous. They had a "dark" cytoplasm rich in ribosomes. They usually contained abundant phagocytosed de-

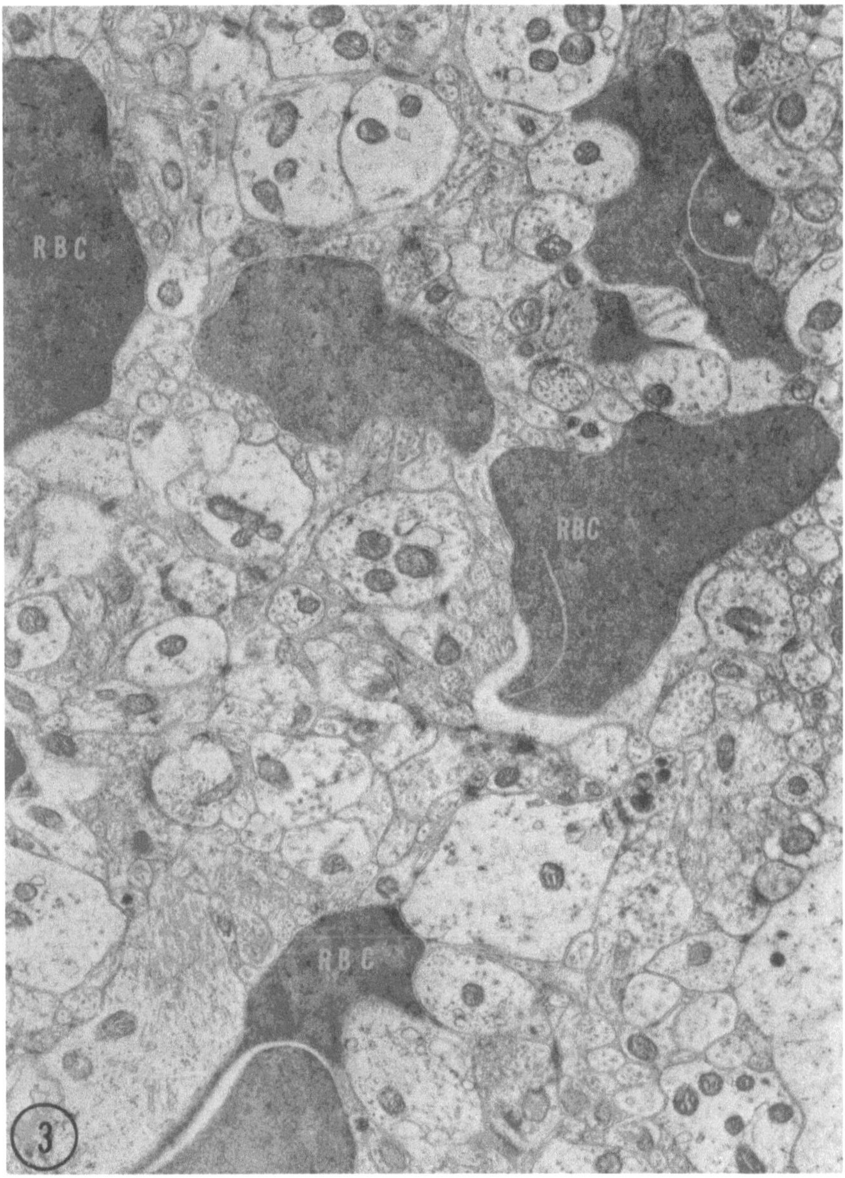

Fig. 3. Striatum of lead poisoned, 28-day-old rat. Red blood cells (RBC) are squeezed within compact neuropil. There are normal, narrow intercellular spaces between neuronal and glial processes. X11,500 (reduced).

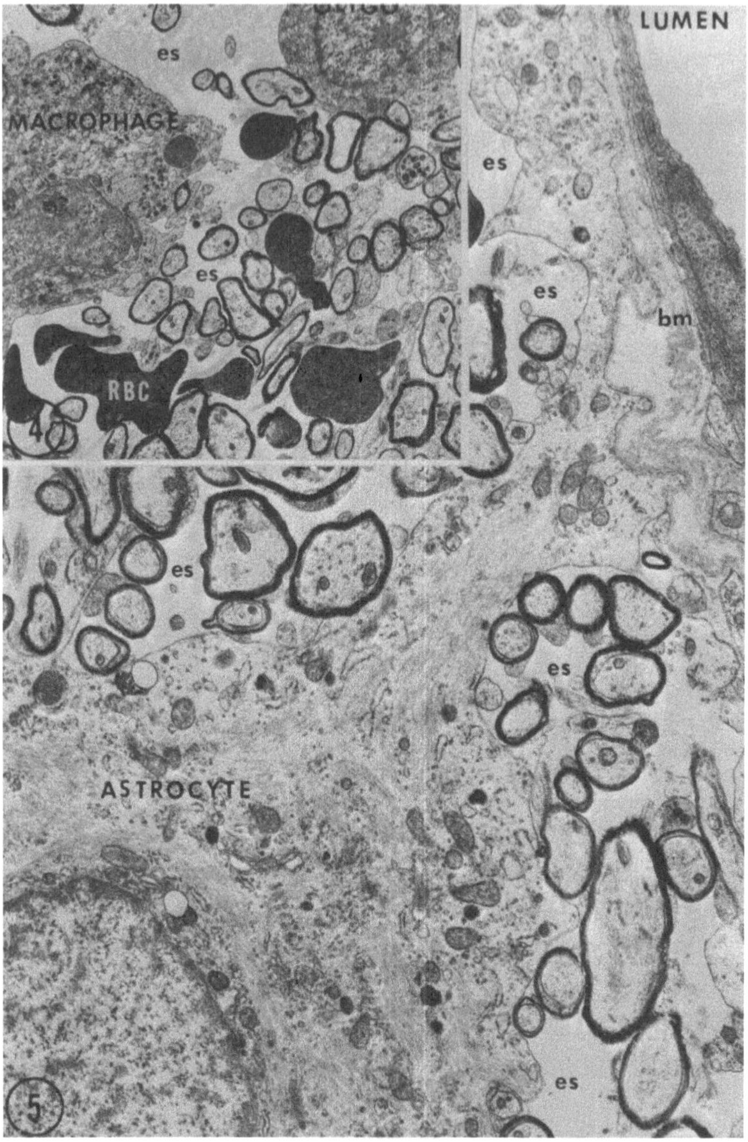

Fig. 4 (Top). Large extracellular spaces (es) are present in the white matter. Note well-preserved oligodendrocyte, myelin sheaths, red blood cells (RBC), and a macrophage filled with debris. Cerebellar white matter, lead poisoned, 19-day-old rat. X3,000 (reduced).

Fig. 5 (Bottom). Fibrous astrocyte filled with glial filaments in white matter with abundant extracellular spaces (es). Note the attachment of the astrocytic foot process to a vessel with loosened basement membrane (bm). Myelin sheaths are well preserved. Cerebellar white matter, lead poisoned, 19-day-old rat. X7,000 (reduced).

bris including breakdown products of red blood cells. Their shape varied. In regions showing abundant extracellular space these stuffed microglial cells or macrophages were round with a peripheral nucleus. In other areas where narrow intercellular spaces prevailed, e.g., the gray matter, these cells were slender with elongated nuclei. Dense bodies or lysosomes were scanty in these cells prior to phagocytosis but numerous thereafter.

The appearance of vessels varied considerably. The majority showed no visible changes at all. Some, particularly those located in tissue with abundant extracellular space, presented numerous, large vacuoles in their endothelial cells (Fig. 6). Overlapping endothelial processes were sometimes noted beneath or above the vacuolated endothelium. The basement membrane of vessels altered in this fashion appeared loosened and astrocytic foot processes were sometimes missing (Fig. 6). There were also capillaries which, on cross section, presented several big endothelial cells and a prominent pericyte (Fig. 7). Such proliferating vessels were generally found in compact neuropil, particularly in the molecular and granular layer of the cerebellum.

In normal control rats, no permeability to Thorotrast was demonstrated one or 24 hours after its intravenous injection. There was no uptake of Thorotrast particles by endothelial cells. In paraplegic rats Thorotrast traversed the wall of small vessels by passing through gaps between adjacent endothelial cells (Fig. 8). The electron dense particles then spread throughout the basement membrane and penetrated into the surrounding neuropil by migrating between and through glial cells. While passing through glial cells the particles were generally found within membrane bound compartments (Fig. 8). Amorphous material, possibly plasma proteins, escaped from the vessel in a similar fashion. The Thorotrast particles diffused readily throughout intercellular spaces and often collected in areas where intercellular clefts converge (Fig. 9). In the animal sacrificed 20 hours after the intravenous injection of Thorotrast, most of the particles were found within microglial cells (macrophages) (Fig. 10) but some particles were still encountered in intercellular spaces. It is of interest to note that so far we have not been able to demonstrate a permeability to Thorotrast in vessels with vacuolated endothelial cells.

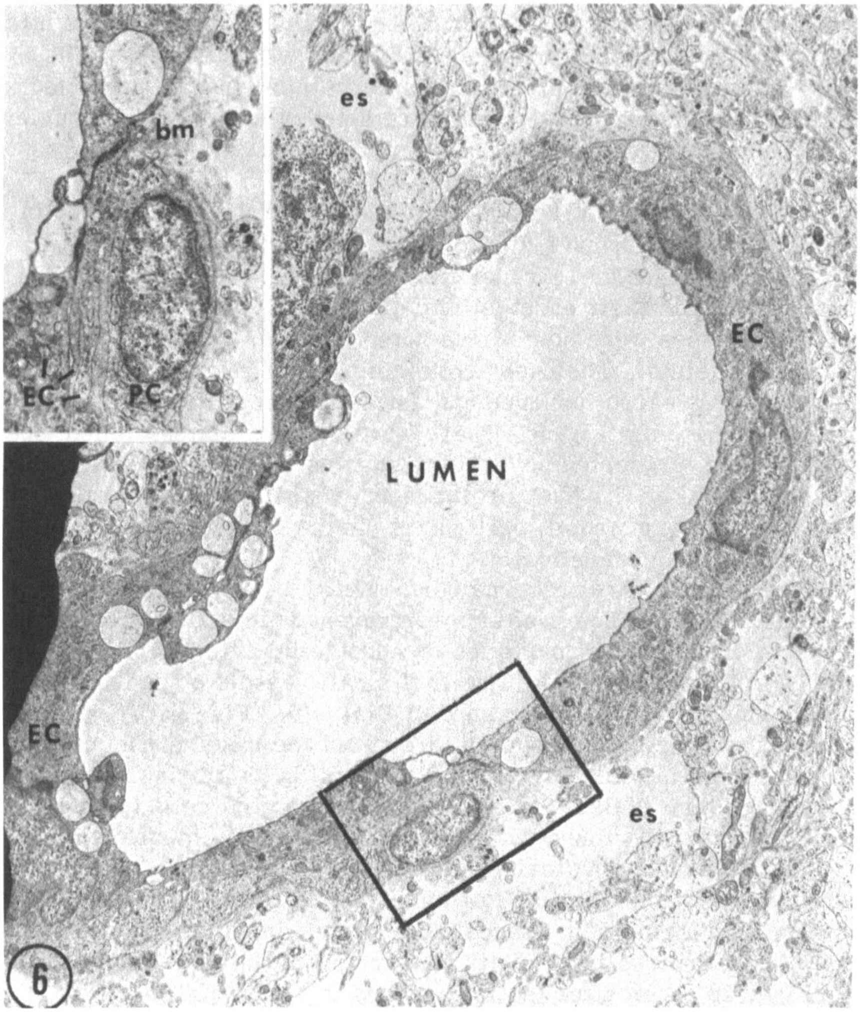

Fig. 6. Vessel with vacuolated endothelial cells within tissue showing abundant extracellular spaces (es). X3,000. Insert shows overlapping endothelial cells (EC), a well-preserved pericyte (PC), and a loosened basement membrane (bm). Astrocytic foot processes are missing. Striatum, lead poisoned, 19-day-old rat. X6,000 (reduced).

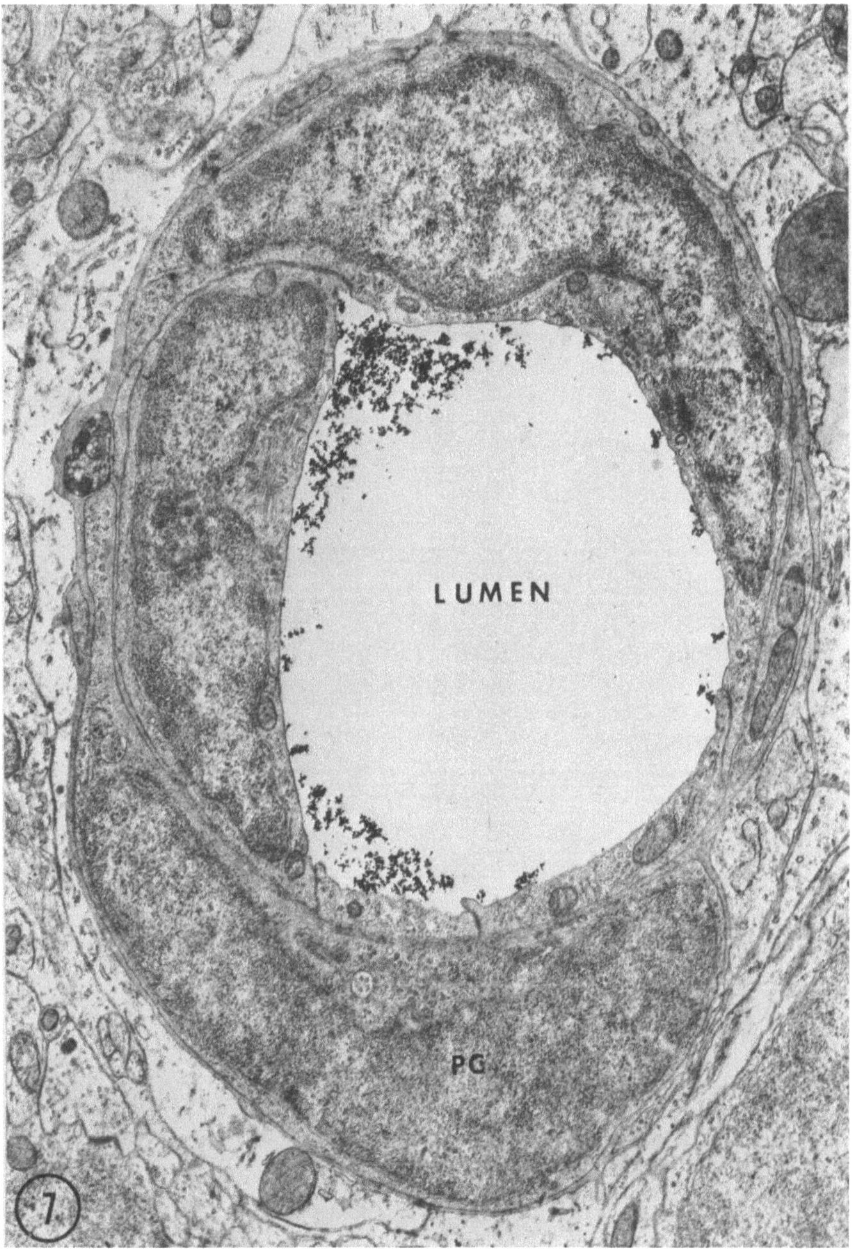

Fig. 7. Proliferated capillary in compact granular layer of the cerebellum. Several endothelial cells and a prominent pericyte (PC) are seen. Thorotrast particles are present within the lumen of the vessel but not between or within cells. Lead poisoned, 28-day-old rat. X10,000 (reduced).

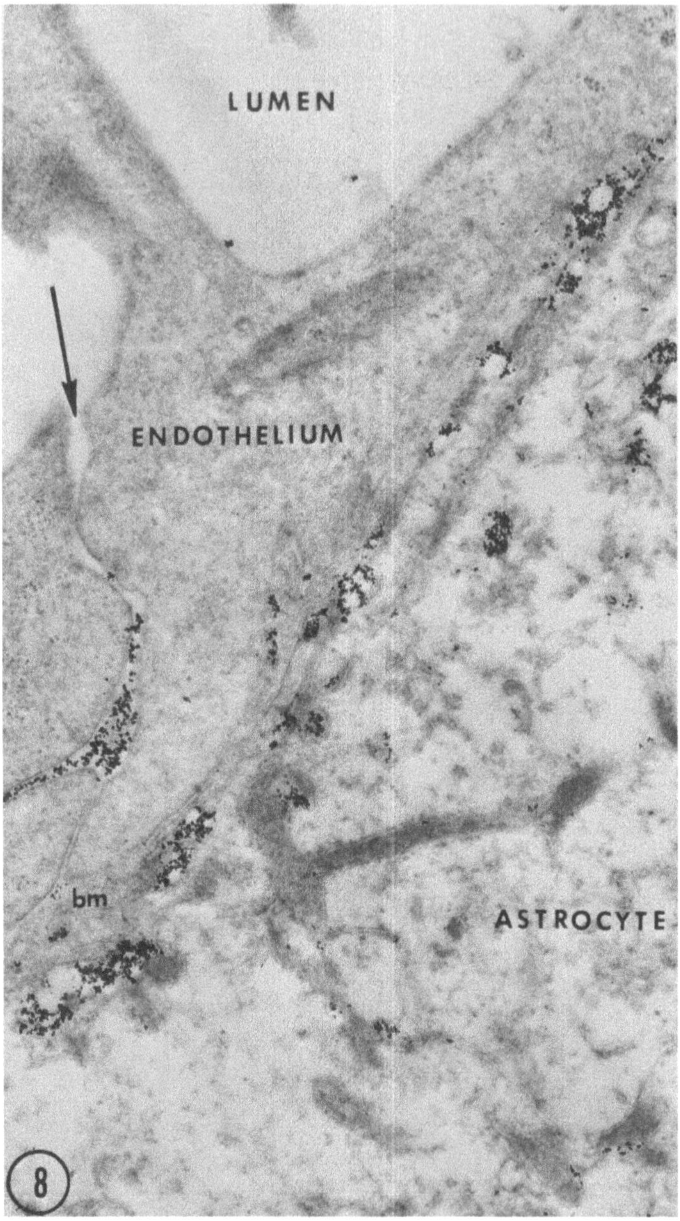

Fig. 8. One hour after intravenous injection of Thorotrast. The electron dense particles are found between endothelial cells (arrow), within the basement membrane (bm), and within vesicular structures inside an astrocytic process. Amorphous material, possibly plasma proteins, are also seen within membrane lined structures in the cytoplasm of the astrocyte. Cerebellar cortex, lead poisoned, 25-day-old rat. X28,000 (reduced).

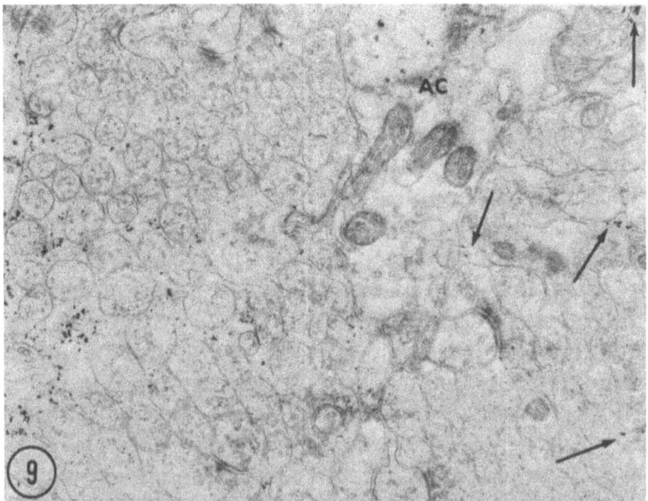

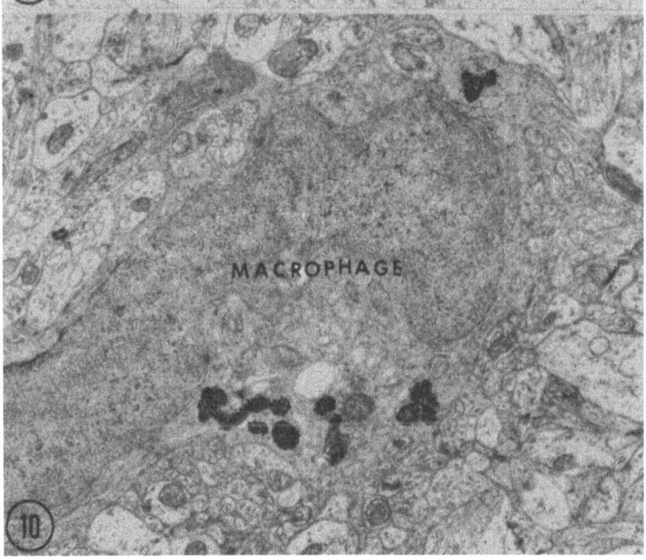

Fig. 9 (Top). One hour after intravenous injection of Thorotrast. The electron dense particles are noted within enlarged extracellular spaces. At right, farther away from the leaking vessel, a few particles in intercellular spaces are indicated by arrows. Molecular layer of cerebellum, lead poisoned, 25-day-old rat. X22,000 (reduced).

Fig. 10 (Bottom). Twenty hours after intravenous injection of Thorotrast. The particles are collected within membrane bound compartments inside a macrophage. The neuropil presents normal intercellular spaces. Striatum, lead poisoned, 28-day-old rat. X10,000 (reduced).

DISCUSSION

Lead encephalopathy of suckling rats belongs to the so-called "dysoric encephalopathies," a group of diseases with similar histopathological features (Pentschew, et al., 1966). They are characterized by an abnormal vascular permeability, i.e., a dysfunction of the blood-brain barrier or "dysoria." This disturbance develops in selective areas of the brain which are not necessarily the same in each disease. The neurons remain relatively well preserved in spite of severe tissue changes. Astrocytes and microglial cells proliferate. The classical example of such a disease is Wernicke's encephalopathy where these alterations are observed in the mammillary bodies and certain nuclei of the brain stem.

The electron microscopic study reported here contributed direct morphological evidence of a vascular dysfunction in lead encephalopathy. Thorotrast (colloidal thorium dioxide), which does not penetrate through normal vessels, did so in the striatum and cerebellum of lead poisoned rats. The electron dense particles traversed the vessel wall by passing between endothelial cells and through the basement membrane (Fig. 8). The same separation of normally tightly joined endothelial cells and the escape of plasma and Thorotrast from vessels has also been described in early lesions of allergic encephalomyelitis (Lampert & Carpenter, 1965). Most likely this endothelial separation represents an unspecific reaction to injury similar to observations on increased vascular permeability in other organs after a variety of injuries (Majno & Palade, 1961; Movat & Fernando, 1963a, b; Casley-Smith, 1965). The significance of vacuolated endothelial cells is not clear at present. Vessels with vacuolated endothelium have been described in cerebral edema (Struck & Umbach, 1964; Herzog, et al., 1965). In the study reported here, vessels altered in this fashion, as well as capillaries with endothelial proliferation, did not show a permeability to Thorotrast.

The use of Thorotrast consisting of colloidal thorium dioxide suspended in dextrin as supplied by Fellows Testagar, Detroit, has been criticized as a means for testing vascular permeability. Rowley (1963) demonstrated that dextrin will induce a degranulation of mast cells with the subsequent release of histamine, an agent capable of producing a permeability change. According to Ashton and Cunha-Vaz (1965), histamine does not produce an increased permeability of cerebral and retinal vessels, however, in contrast to vessels in other organs. This would confirm our experience since we have not seen Thorotrast pass through vessels in normal young or adult rats.

Once past the endothelial and basement membrane, Thorotrast spreads between glial and neuronal processes. This finding suggested that narrow intercellular spaces represent no barrier for the diffusion of colloidal substances. In allergic encephalomyelitis, a similar spread of plasma proteins and Thorotrast throughout intercellular spaces has been described (Lampert & Carpenter, 1965). There is evidence that the migration of particles is facilitated in areas where normally wider extracellular spaces exist, i.e., in the white matter (Levine, et al., 1963; Hirano, et al., 1964). For the same reason, a rapid spread of particles is anticipated in regions with abnormally widened extracellular spaces as observed in lead encephalopathy in the white and gray matter (Figs. 2, 4, 5). The fact that red cells are found squeezed within compact gray matter (Fig. 3) whereas they float freely within widened extracellular spaces in the white matter (Fig. 4), may be interpreted that in the gray matter narrow intercellular spaces are either more quickly restored or less easily created. We favor the former more dynamic interpretation.

Thorotrast particles and possibly also plasma proteins were not only observed in intercellular spaces in the affected regions of the brain but also within vesicles in astrocytic processes (Fig. 8). This finding is consistent with the observations by Klatzo and Miquel (1960) who showed that astrocytes incorporate proteins by pinocytosis. Similar observations have been described by Tani and Evans (1965) who observed the uptake of Ferritin by astrocytic processes in the edematous cat brain. Some astrocytes, particularly in the white matter, were further characterized by features known to be present in reactive, proliferating cells, i.e., they showed an increase of glial filaments, ribosomes and mitochondria.

Our study has not yet revealed any clues in regard to the origin of the numerous microglial cells or macrophages. The axonal changes, consisting of axoplasmic enlargements filled with mitochondria, dense bodies and vesicular elements, are interpreted as non-specific axonal reactions to injury. Such axonal enlargements have been described in a variety of conditions including trauma to axons (Lampert & Cressman, 1964). Since we also found degenerating axons, it must be assumed that axons were severed. This undoubtedly occurred in advanced cerebellar lesions in which the white matter was replaced by large cystic spaces. In this respect, it is even more remarkable that myelin sheaths around intact or altered axons at the margin of cysts remained well preserved.

SUMMARY

1. Lead poisoning of suckling rats produces an abnormal vascular permeability in the brain particularly in the cerebellum, striatum, occipital lobes, and lower spinal cord.

2. The striatum and cerebellum were examined with the electron microscope. A considerable widening of the extracellular space was observed in both gray and white matter, but this was a transitory phenomenon in the gray matter.

3. Microglial, astrocytic, and endothelial proliferation occurred. Neurons, oligodendrocytes and myelin sheaths remained well preserved.

4. Intravenously injected Thorotrast (colloidal thorium dioxide), an electron dense tracer, traversed vessel walls by passing between but not through endothelial cells. After penetration of the basement membrane, the particles spread throughout intercellular spaces between glial and neuronal processes. Thorotrast was also noted within membrane-bound compartments of astrocytic processes. Twenty hours after intravenous injection of Thorotrast, most of the particles were found within macrophages but some were still in intercellular spaces.

5. These morphological features are characteristic of "dysoric encephalopathies."

REFERENCES

Ashton, N. and J. G. Cunha-Vaz: Effect of histamine on the permeability of the ocular vessels, Arch. Ophthal., 73, 211-223 (1965).

Blackman, S. S.: The lesions of lead encephalitis in children, Bull. Johns Hopkins Hosp., 61, 1-62 (1937).

Casley-Smith, J. R.: Endothelial permeability, II, The passage of particles through the lymphatic endothelium of normal and injured ears, British J. Exp. Path., 46, 35-49 (1965).

Dalton, A. J.: A chrome-osmium fixative for electron microscopy, Anat. Rec., 121, 281 (1955).

Herzog, I., W. A. Levy and L. C. Scheinberg: Biochemical and morphologic studies of cerebral edema associated with intracerebral tumors in rabbits, J. Neuropath. & Exp. Neurol., 24, 224-255 (1965).

Hirano, A., H. M. Zimmerman and S. Levine: The fine structure of cerebral fluid accumulation, III: Extracellular spread of cryptococcal polysaccharides in the acute stage, Am. J. Path., 45, 1-19 (1964).

Klatzo, I. and J. Miquel: Observations on pinocytosis in nervous tissue, J. Neuropath. & Exp. Neurol., 19, 475-487 (1960).

Lampert, P. and S. Carpenter: Electron microscopic studies on the vascular permeability and the mechanism of demyelination in

experimental allergic encephalomyelitis, J. Neuropath. & Exp. Neurol., 24, 11-24 (1965).
_____ and M. Cressman: Axonal regeneration in the dorsal columns of the spinal cord of adult rats: an electron microscopic study, Lab. Invest., 13, 825-839 (1964).
Levine, S., H. M. Zimmerman, E. J. Wenk and N. K. Gonatas: Experimental leukoencephalopathies due to implantation of foreign substances, Am. J. Path., 42, 97-117 (1963).
Luft, J. M.: Improvement in epoxy resin embedding methods, J. Biophys. Biochem. Cytol., 9, 409-414 (1961).
Majno, G. and G. E. Palade: Studies on inflammation, I, The effect of histamine and serotonin on vascular permeability. An electron microscopic study, J. Biophys. Biochem. Cytol., 11, 571-605 (1961).
Movat, H. Z. and N. V. Fernando: Acute inflammation. The earliest fine structural changes at the blood-tissue barrier, Lab. Invest., 12, 895-910 (1963a).
_____ and _____: Allergic inflammation, I: The earliest fine structural changes at the blood-tissue barrier during antigen- antibody interaction, Am. J. Path., 42, 41-50 (1963b).
Palay, S. L., S. M. McGee Russell, S. Gordon and M. A. Grillo: Fixation of neural tissue for electron microscopy by perfusion with solutions of osmium tetroxide, J. Cell Biol., 12, 385-419 (1962).
Pentschew, A.: Intoxikationen; in Handbuch der speziellen pathologischen Anatomie und Histologie (ed. by W. Scholz), Vol. XIII, 2, 1929-1971 (1958).
_____: Morphology and morphogenesis of lead encephalopathy. Acta Neuropathologica, 5, 133-160 (1965).
_____, F. Garro and P. Schweda: Systemized dysoric encephalopathy in the suckling rat produced by lead, Proceedings Vth Intern. Congress Neuropath., Excerpta Medica, 730-733 (1966).
Popoff, N., S. Weinberg and I. Feigin: Pathologic observations in lead encephalopathy with special reference to the vascular changes, Neurology, 13, 101-102 (1963).
Rowley, D. S.: Mast cell damage and vascular injury in the rat. An electron microscopic study of a reaction produced by Thorotrast, British J. Exp. Path., 44, 284-290 (1963).
Smith, J. F., R. L. Laurin, J. B. Nichols and A. Ashbury: Studies in cerebral edema and cerebral swelling. The changes in lead encephalopathy in children compared with those in alkyl tin poisoning in animals, Brain, 83, 411-429 (1960).
Struck, G. and W. Umbach: Vergleichende elektronenoptische Untersuchungen an der menschlichen Hirnrinde vor und nach Odemtherapie, Virch. Arch. Path. Anat., 337, 317-327 (1964).

Tani, E. and J. P. Evans: Electron microscopic studies of cerebral swelling. I. Studies on the permeability of brain capillaries, using Ferritin molecules as tracers, Acta Neuropath., 4, 507-526 (1965)

E. SLUGA

OBSERVATIONS ON THE WHITE MATTER IN HUMAN BRAIN EDEMA

The ultrastructural pathological changes in brain edema demonstrate not only a dichotomy between gray and white matter but vary also according to the cause of edema. In the gray matter, the type of affected morphological structures and the development of the pathological changes are observed to be consistently of the same kind. Between the different forms of gray matter edema there are only differences in the results of the biochemical examinations (Aleu, et al.). In the white matter there are also differences in the pathomorphological changes: swelling of the astroglial cells, increase in extracellular space (PPD edema: Gonatas, et al.; extradural compression: Raimondi, et al.; Evans & Tani), or the primary occurrence of vacuoles and large clefts between the lamellae of myelin sheaths (triethyl tin poisoning: Terry, et al.). Tani and Evans also have observed changes in the oligodendroglial cells.

It seems that in white matter edema the primarily affected morphological structures may be different and different morphological structures may be altered as the condition develops. The common effect in all kinds of white matter edema is the development of myelin sheath changes. The pathogenesis of the myelin alteration and the actively participating structures are an unanswered problem of white matter edema.

Electron microscopic observations on human brain material of the white matter edema form the basis of this report. The excised material was taken from three cases of different primary neurological diseases. There was one case of spongiform encephalopathy; the two other cases showed edema concomitant with encephalitis (one was a subacute sclerosing leukoencephalitis). The white matter affected by a slight edema showed swelling of the astroglial cells and processes as well as alterations of oligodendroglial cells which will be described in detail in this paper. The observed alterations of the myelin sheaths have been analyzed in relation to the changed oligodendroglial cells. This paper does not deal with the problem of extracellular space.

The remarkable alterations of the oligodendroglia varied in intensity in the individual cells. All examined specimens showed some cells of normal structure; others revealed all kinds of pathological changes up to the disintegration of cells. The initial alteration of the oligodendroglial cells consists of the formation of perinuclear cleft (Fig. 1). It becomes enlarged and can distend to vesicle-like formations (Figs. 2, 3). The next step in the development of the patho logical alterations can be seen in other oligodendroglial cells. In their cytoplasm, vesicle-like formations are established (Fig. 4), which are bounded by membranes and sometimes bordered by ribosomes (Fig. 5). Their origin could be deduced as cysternae of the endoplasmic reticulum. In consequence, a progressive augmentation and confluence of these vesicles takes place and cells can be observed in which most of their cytoplasm is transformed into large lacunae (Figs. 6, 7). The last state of these progressive pathological alterations seems to be manifested by cells of structural disintegration. Sometimes a nucleus surrounded only by multilocular large lacunae is seen (Fig. 8).

The sensitivity of oligodendroglial cells in the course of white matter edema is well documented by light microscopy. Penfield and Cone described the "acute swelling" and Bailey and Schaltenbrand the so-called "mucous degeneration" of the oligodendroglial cells in edematous white matter. Zülch described the swelling of oligodendroglia in brain edema as "simple swelling" and he suggested that the different forms of oligodendroglial cell swelling represent merely different stages of the pathological change in these cells occurring in the course of white matter edema. It was Jakob who considered the "acute swelling" of oligodendroglia as a sensitive indicator of initial changes in white matter edema. His observations dealt mostly with the changes of the nuclear structure. The frequently discussed problem was the nature of the change in these cells since unaltered oligodendroglial cells were also described by many authors observing white matter edema (Scheinker, Greenfield).

Ultrastructural observations cannot so far resolve the problem of oligodendroglial participation in the pathological changes of white matter edema. In the course of the studies of Terry, et al., Gonatas, et al., Raimondi, et al., and Schröder and Wechsler, there was no description of altered oligodendroglia. Tani and Evans, however, observed in the oligodendroglia evaginations of the outer membrane of the nucleus, with appearance of lacunae, distension of the endo-

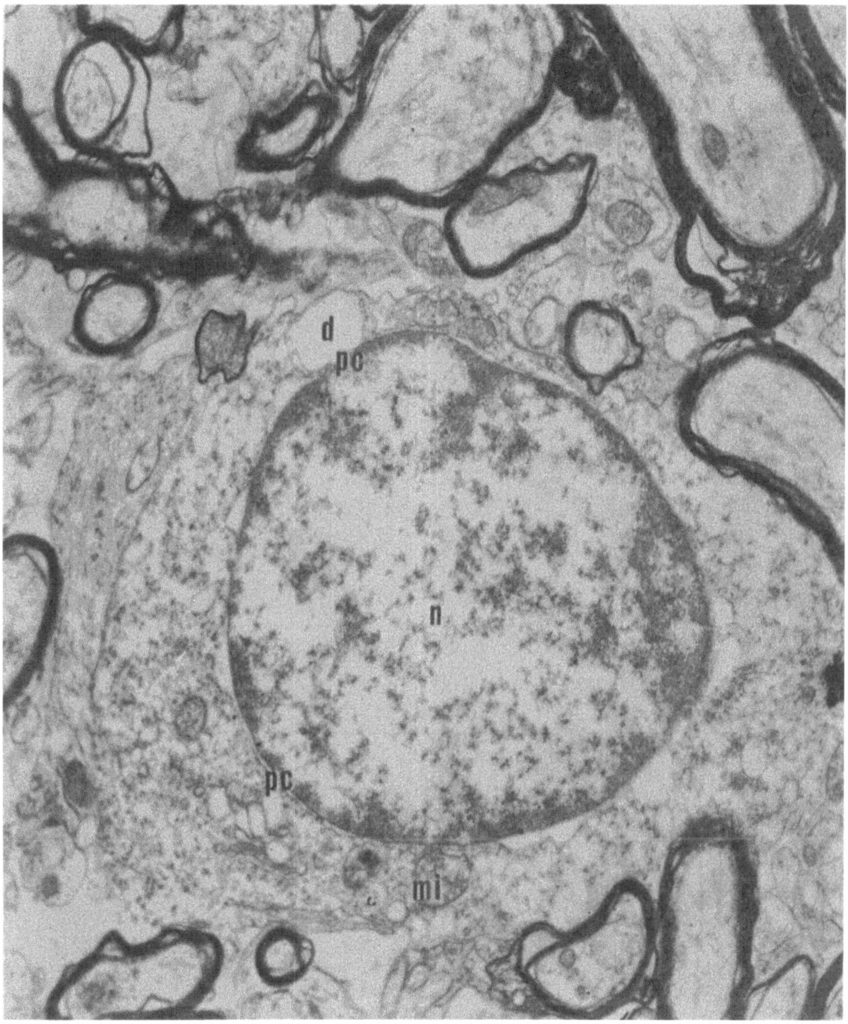

Fig. 1. Interfascicular oligodendroglial cell; nucleus — n; perinuclear cleft — pc with a localized distension — d; mitochondria — mi; X12,000.

plasmatic reticulum and display of vesicles. They suggest that these pathological alterations correspond to the "hydropic swelling" of light microscopy. According to the author's own observations, the

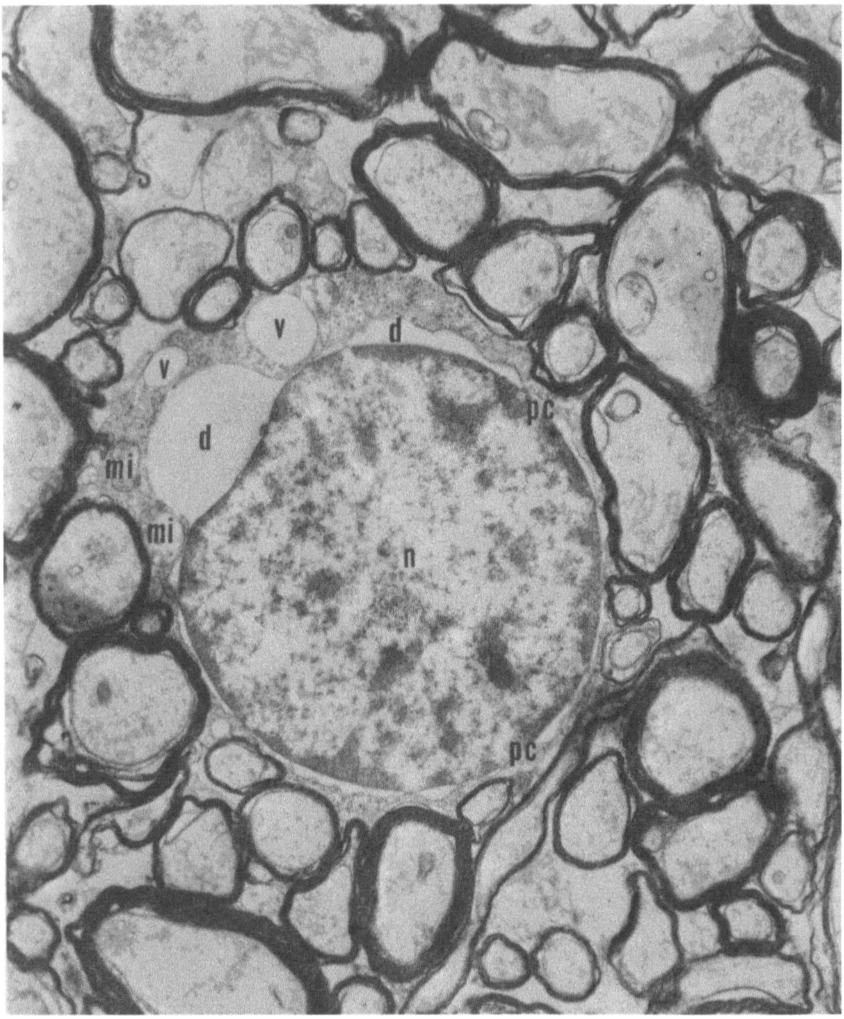

Fig. 2. Interfascicular oligodendroglial cell,nucleus — n; perinuclear cleft — pc with plurilocal distensions — d; and beginning formation of vesicle-like formations; some vesicles — v in the cytoplasm — c; mitochondria — mi; X10,000.

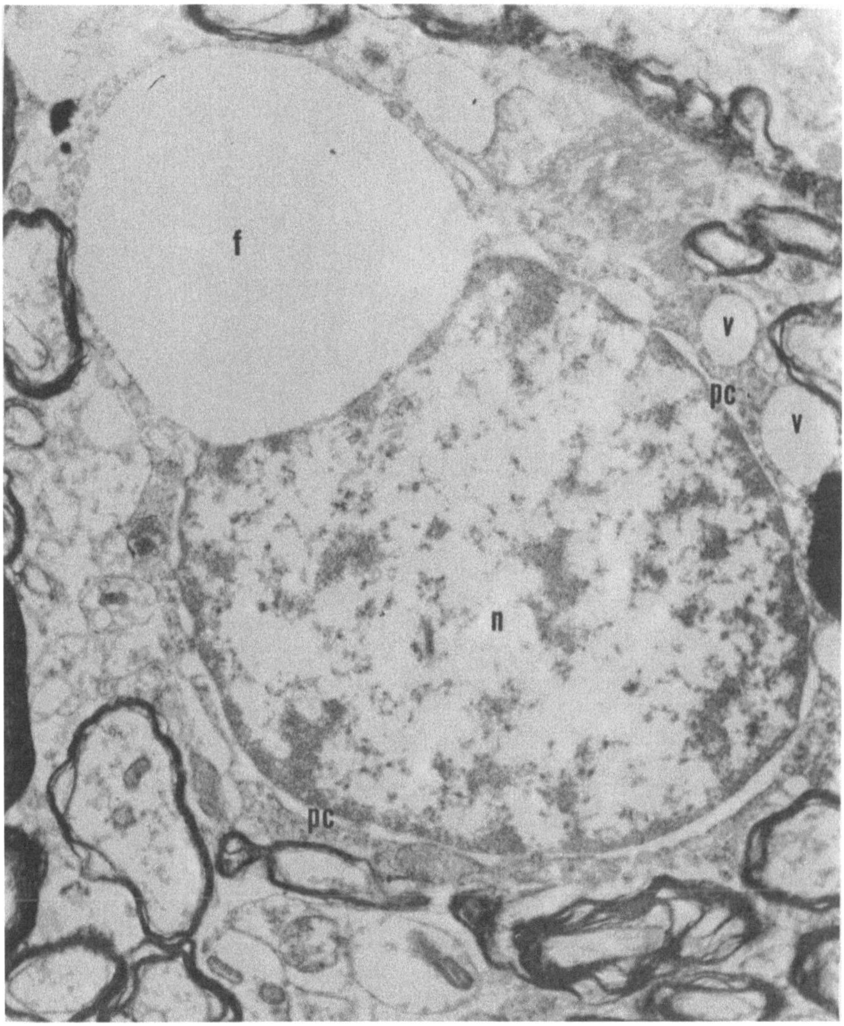

Fig. 3. Interfascicular oligodendroglial cell; nucleus — n; perinuclear cleft — pc with a large vesicle-like formation — f; some vesicles — v in the cytoplasm — c; X12,000.

alteration of oligodendroglial cells, from the occurrence of distension of the perinuclear cleft up to the formation of large lacunae with terminal cell destruction, are suggested as different develop-

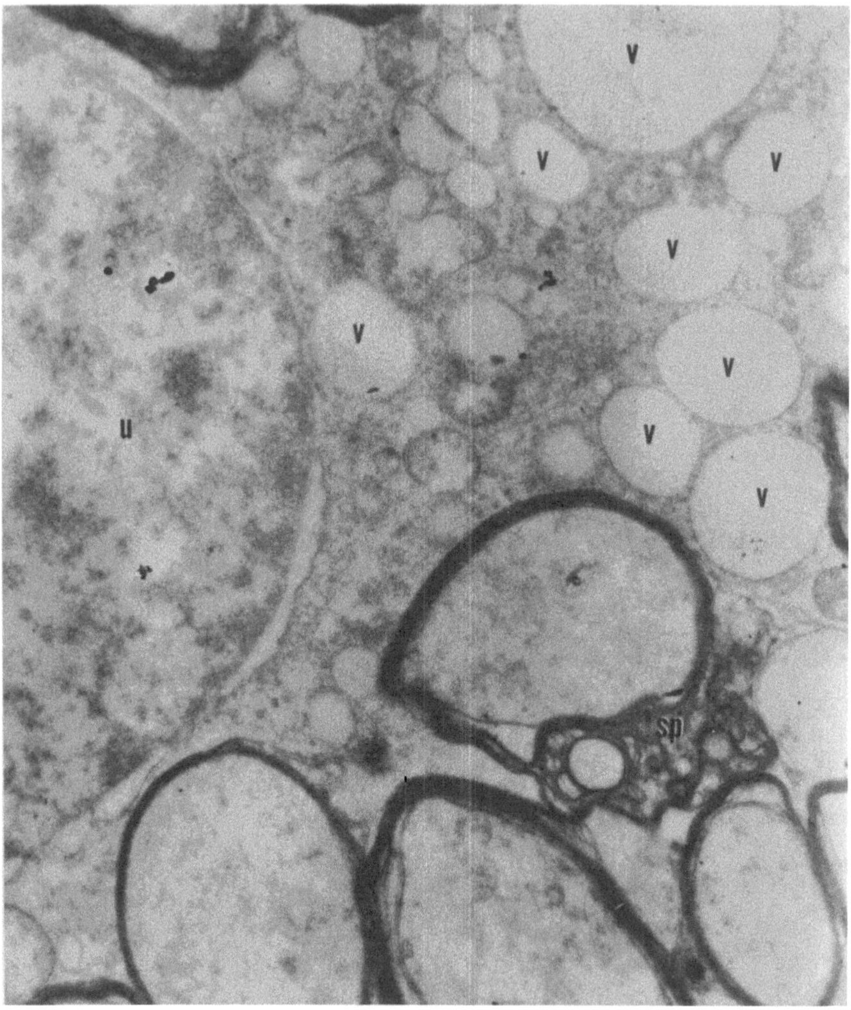

Fig. 4. Interfascicular oligodendroglial cell; nucleus – n; appearance of vesicles – v in the cytoplasm – c; splitting – sp of myelin of one neuron in connection with the changed cell; X20,000.

mental stages of cell alteration in the sense of cell swelling. The swelling spreads in the intracysternal compartment and has to be

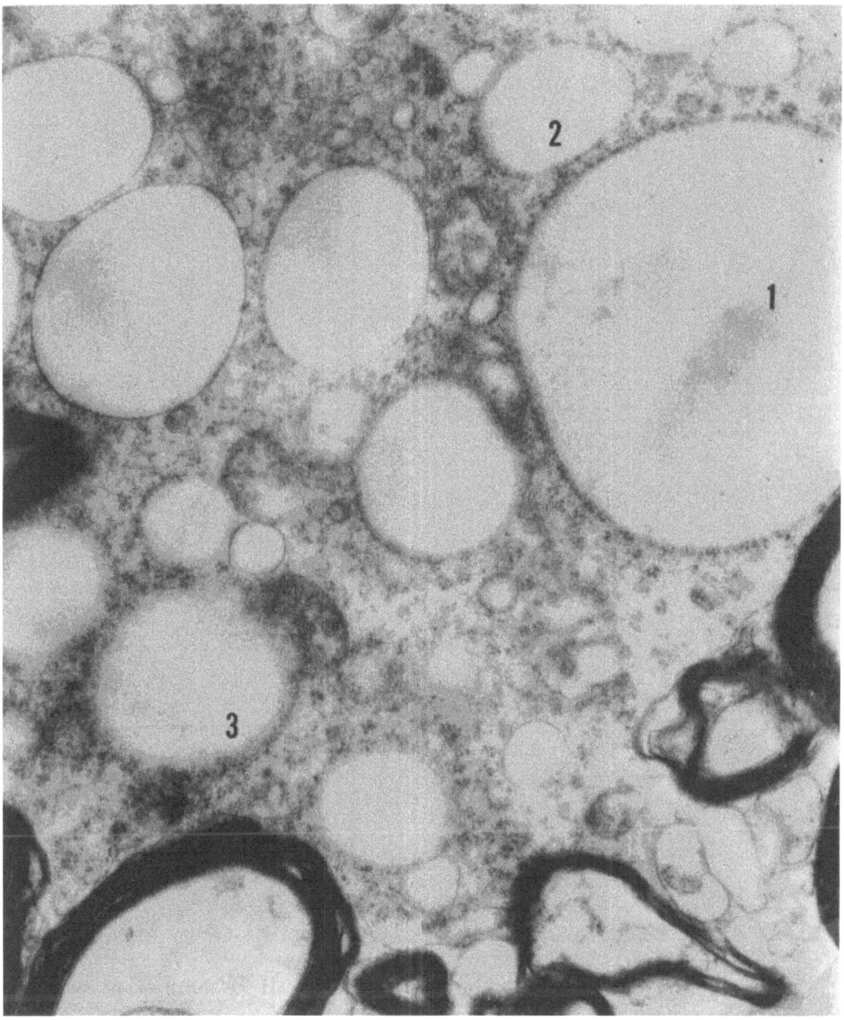

Fig. 5. Cytoplasm of an oligodendroglial cell; membrane-bounded large vesicles 1, 2, 3, are bordered by ribosomes; X30,000.

considered as related intravitally to the pathogenetic processes of white matter edema.

The relationship and the temporal course of the alteration in astroglial cells and the extra-cellular space to the oligodendroglia

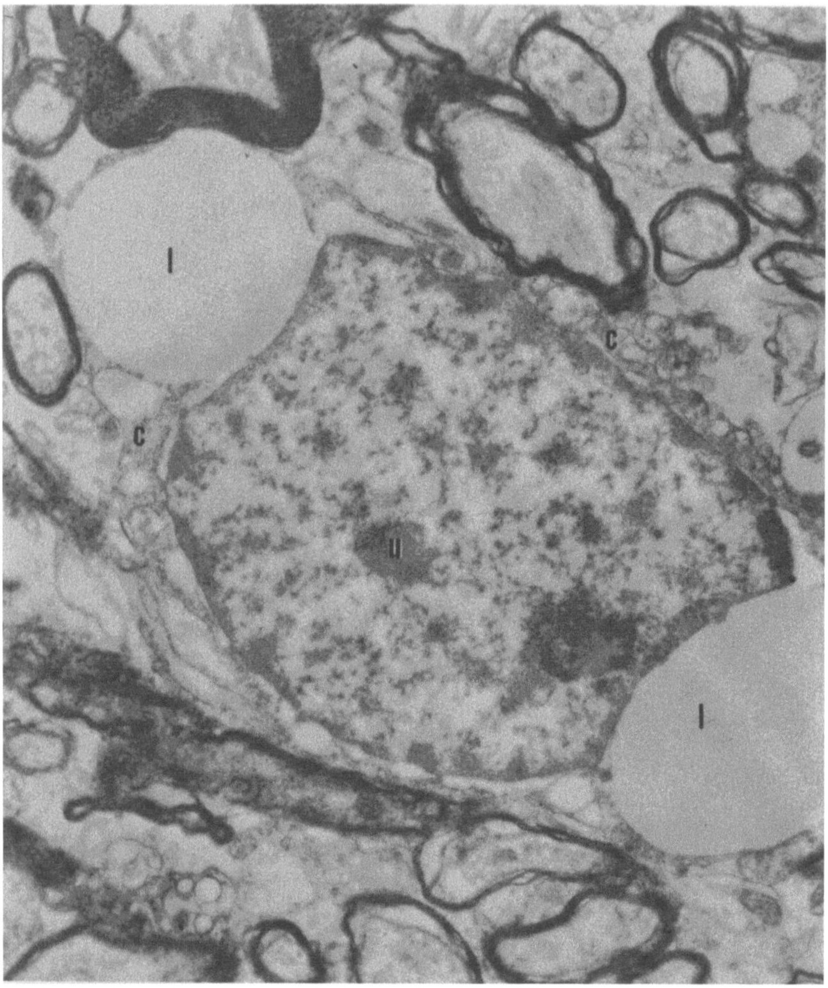

Fig. 6. Interfascicular oligodendroglial cell; nucleus — n; two lacunae — 1 replace the majority of the cytoplasm — c; X12,000.

cannot be absolutely stated from these observations. In the material of all three cases there was no region in which the oligodendroglial cell changes alone could be observed, so it is likely that the oligodendroglial changes appear as the result of the other abnormalities.

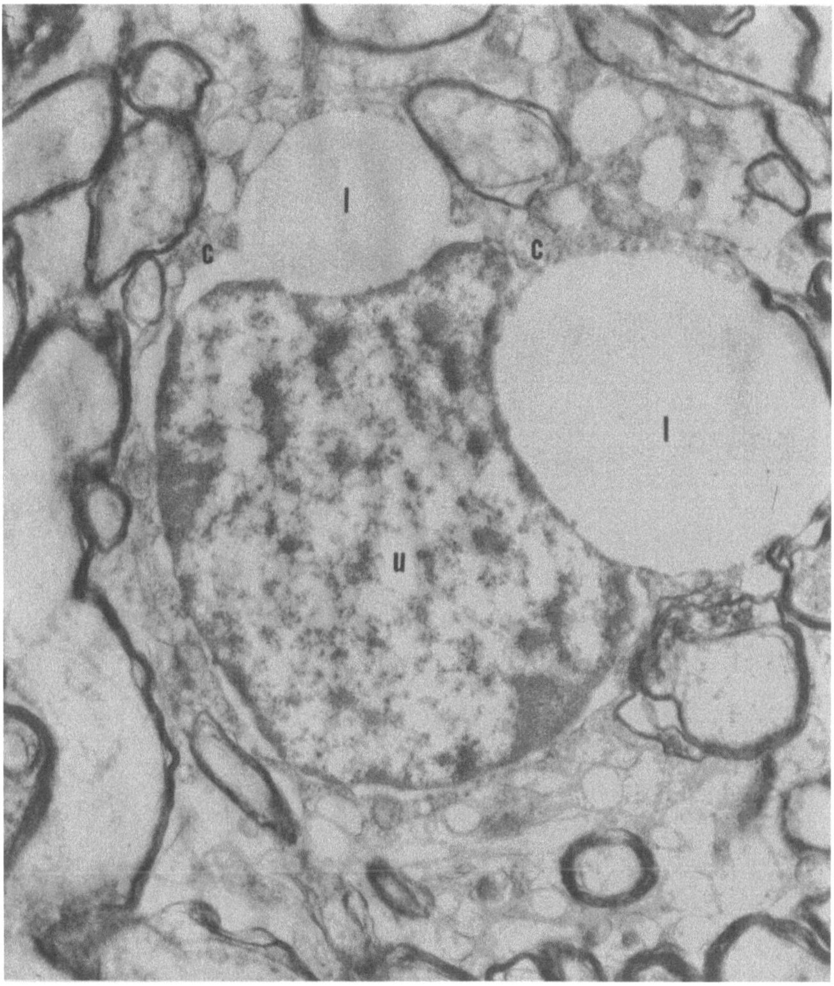

Fig. 7. Interfascicular oligodendroglial cell; nucleus — n; two lacunae — l replace the majority of the cytoplasm — c; X12,000.

A relationship between altered oligodendroglial cells and alteration of myelin sheaths was constantly evident in our material. Light-microscopic studies, especially by Zülch, gave evidence of such a connection. Ultrastructural examinations of the different

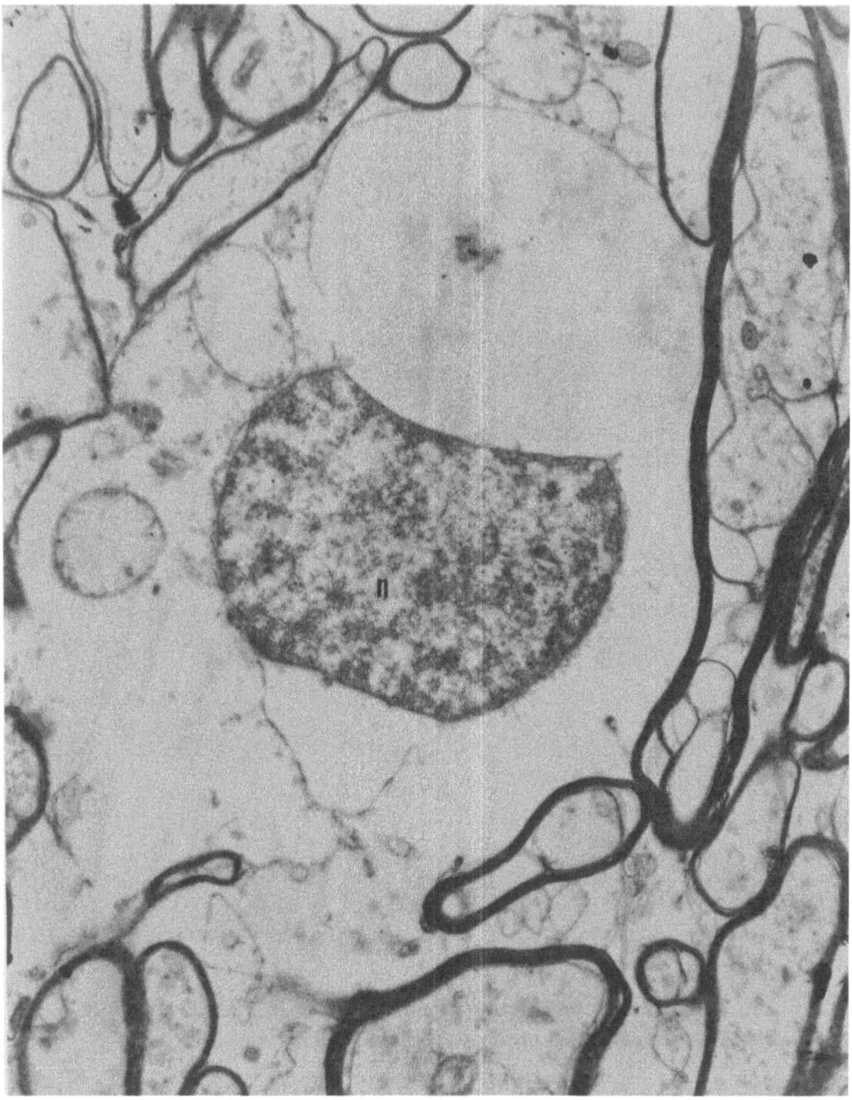

Fig. 8. Interfascicular oligodendroglial cell in structural disintegration; nucleus – n; multilocular lacunae replace the whole cytoplasm; X12,000.

types of white matter edema have not so far given sufficient information concerning the modality of myelin alteration. One fact that is uniformly described is that the splitting of myelin lamellae occurs in the intraperiod line. The question of the re-opening of the extracellular space between the myelin lamellae is an unresolved problem in triethyl tin edema (Aleu, et al.). Tani and Evans produced edema by extradural compression and described myelin splitting associated with the appearance of small cytoplasmic profiles derived from myelin-forming glial cells. They suggest that this process is the reverse of myelinogenesis and that the myelin-forming glial cells may have an important role in myelin splitting or myelin disintegration. Our studies support a similar explanation of the damage of the myelin structures.

As known, in the central nervous system it is difficult to relate the individual myelinated axons to their original oligodendroglial cell; but as far as it is possible, our material demonstrates that either altered myelin sheaths were situated in the vicinity of severely damaged oligodendroglial cells (Figs. 4, 9, 10) or that the alteration takes place in those areas of the myelin sheath which were covered by the oligodendroglial cell process (Figs. 11, 12). The observed alterations of the myelin sheaths consisted mainly of splitting of the lamellae of the compact myelin. Between the split myelin lamellae, vesicles of different size were observed (Figs. 10, 11, 12). These vesicles were sometimes surrounded by small cytoplasmic strips (Fig. 13). Because of these observations a relation is assumed between altered cells and the damage of the myelin.

Concerning the mechanism of those alterations, only a working hypothesis can be suggested. Under certain pathological conditions in the compact adult myelin elements of cytoplasm can appear in those areas where they were located in the developing loose myelin. It seems possible that the degeneration of the oligodendroglial cell in the course of edema is one of these pathological conditions and the spreading of pathologically changed cytoplasm might be one of the factors causing myelin splitting. The progressive destruction of the oligodendroglial cell could cause further and, probably, irreversible, damage of the myelin sheaths. These constant findings in the white matter altered by edema may be important in understanding the problem of myelin sheath destruction, a well-known sequel of brain edema. An experimental study on cold-induced edema in rabbits is under way and should give some clarification to the mechanism of myelin alteration in cerebral edema.

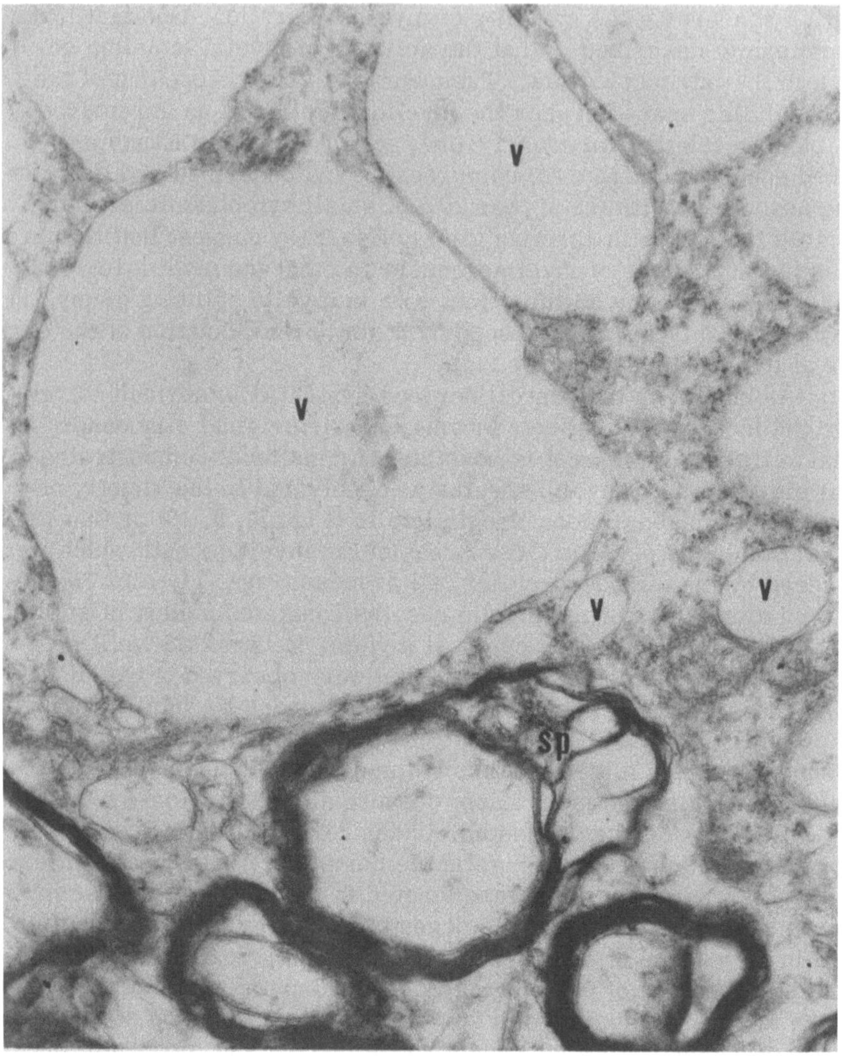

Fig. 9. Altered myelin sheath at the border of an associated swollen oligodendroglial cell; large vesicles — v of a swollen oligodendroglia; splitting — sp of myelin lamellae; X25,000.

REFERENCES

Aleu, F. P., F. L. Edelman, R. Katzman and L. C. Scheinberg: Ultrastructural and Biochemical Analysis in Cerebral Edema Associated with Experimental Mouse Gliomas, J. Neuropath. Exp. Neurol., 23, 235-263 (1964).

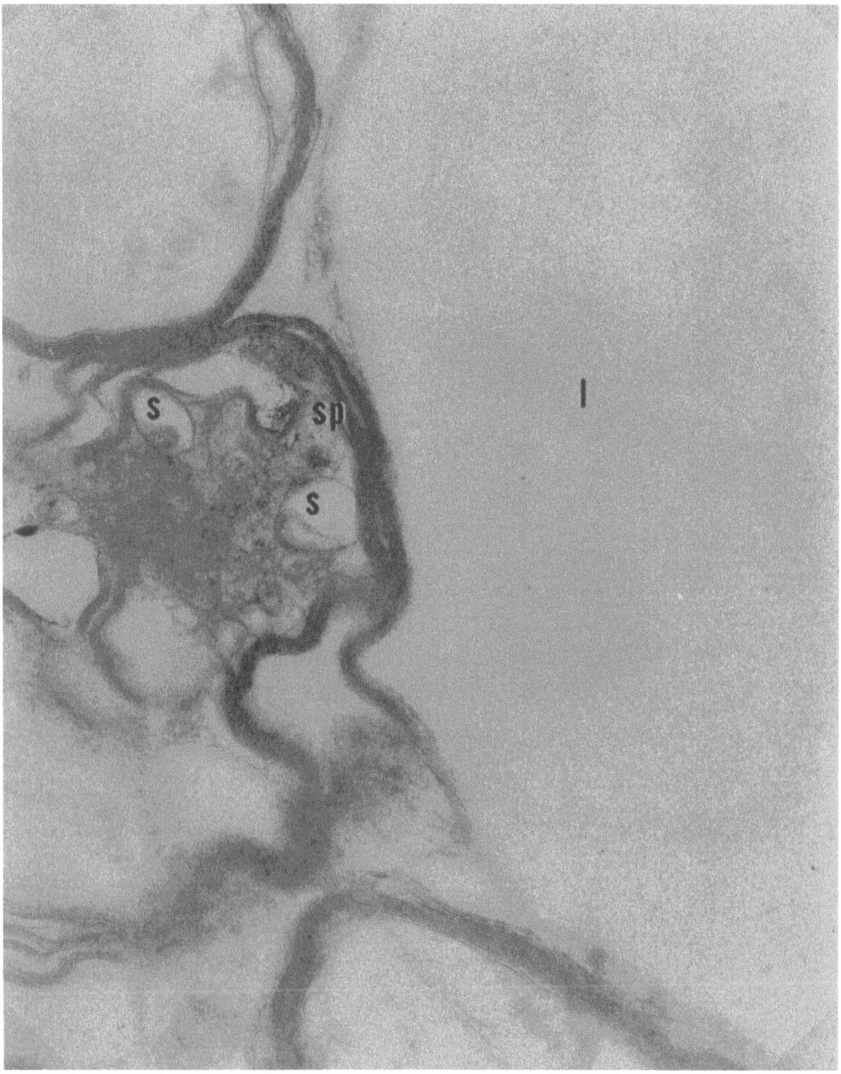

Fig. 10. Altered myelin sheath at the border of an associated swollen oligodendroglial cell; lacunae — l of the oligodendroglia; splitting — sp of myelin lamellae with appearance of vesicles — s; X40,000.

______, R. Katzman and R. D. Terry: Fine Structure and Electrolyte Analysis of Cerebral Edema Induced by Alkyltin Intoxication, Ibid., 22, 403-413 (1963).

Bailey, P. and G. Schaltenbrand: Die mukôse Degeneration der Oligodendroglia, Dtsch. Z. Nervenheilk., 97, 231-237 (1927).

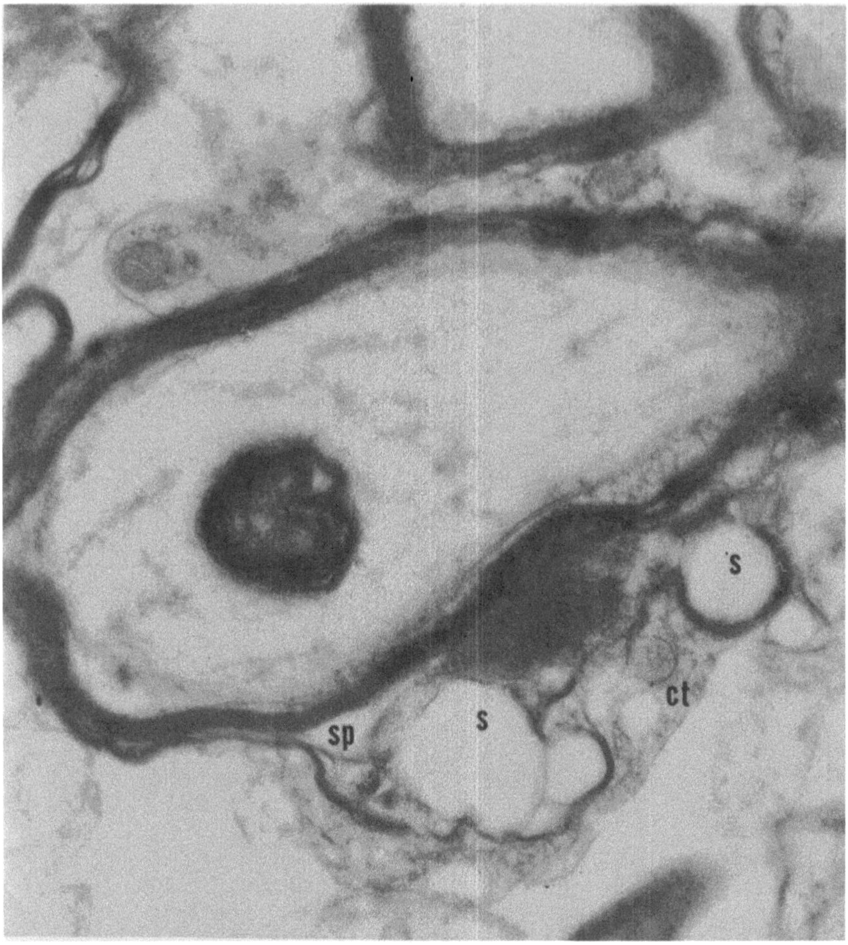

Fig. 11. Altered myelin sheath in the area of oligodendroglial cell-tongue; cell tongue — ct; splitting — sp of myelin lamellae with appearance of vesicles — s; X32,000.

Greenfield, J. G.: The Histology of Cerebral Edema Associated with Intracranial Brain Tumours, Brain, 62, 129-152 (1939).
Gonatas, N., H. M. Zimmermann and S. Levin: Ultrastructure of Inflammation with Edema in the Rat Brain, Am. J. Path., 42, 455-469 (1963).

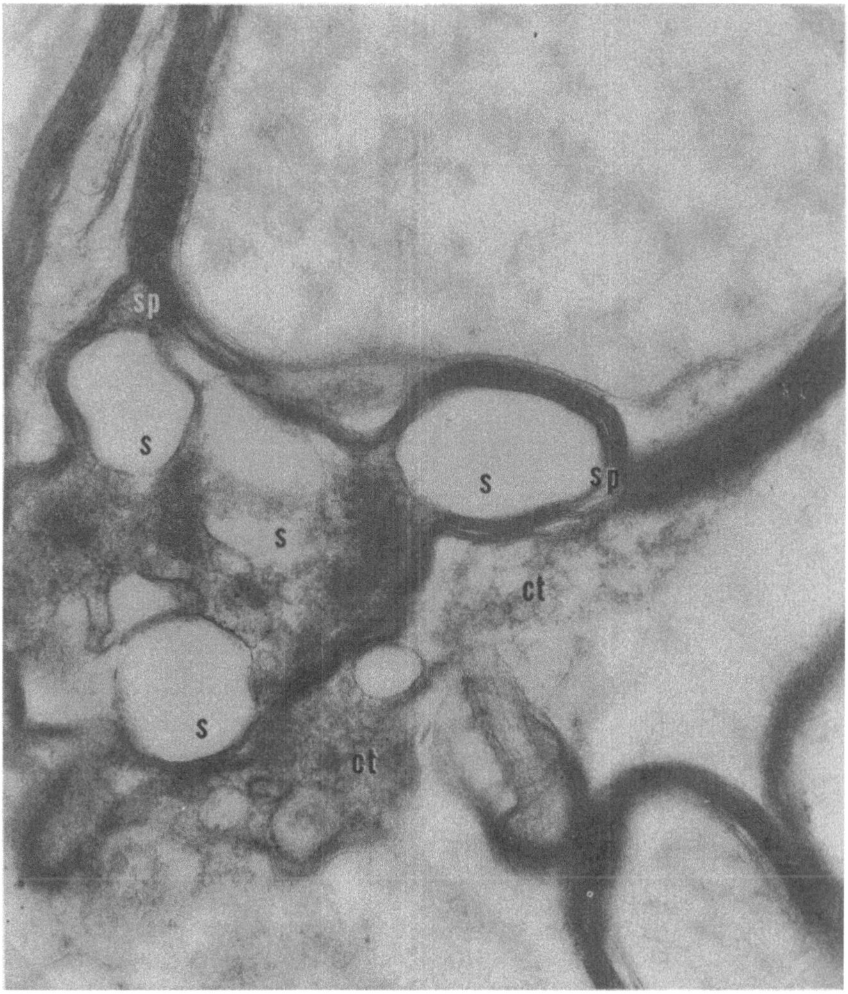

Fig. 12. Altered myelin sheath in the area of oligodendroglial cell-tongue; cell tongue — ct; splitting — sp of myelin lamellae with appearance of vesicles — s; X40,000.

Jakob, H.: Die Kernhomogenisierung der akut geschwollenen Oligodendroglia und der prae-amöboiden Glia beim Hirnödem, Arch. f. Psych. und Z. ges. Neurol., 206, 690-704 (1965).

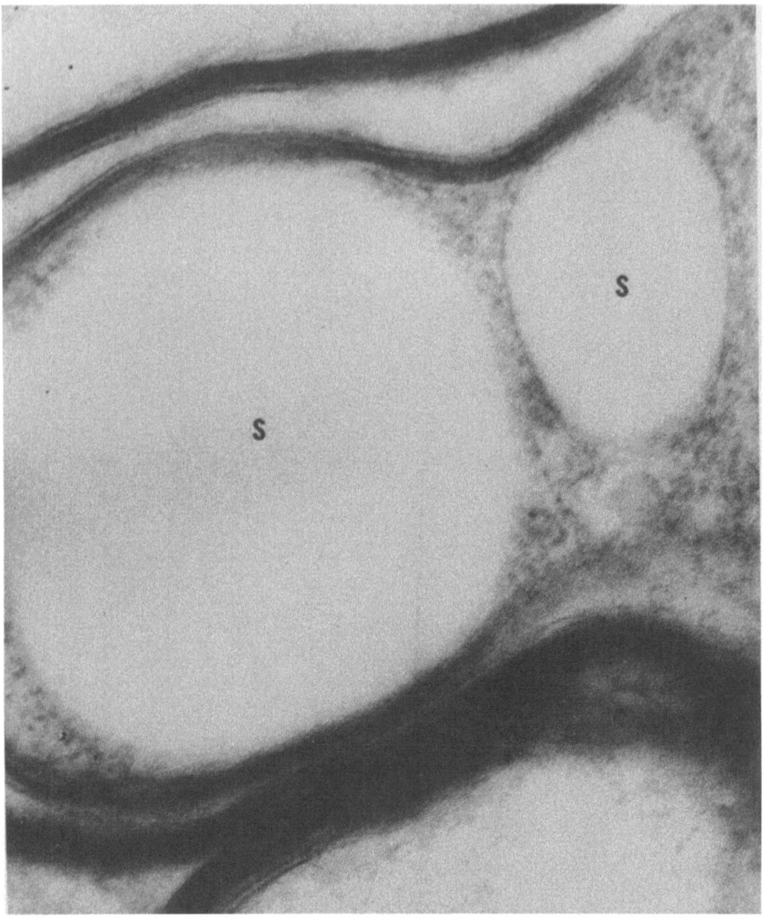

Fig. 13. Split myelin lamellae with vesicles — s, surrounded by small strips of cytoplasmic appearance; X92,000.

Penfield, W. and W. Cone: Acute swelling of Oligodendroglia, a Specific Type of Neuroglial Change, A. M. A. Arch. Neurol., 16, 131-153 (1926).

Raimondi, A. J., J. P. Evans and S. Mullan: Studies of Cerebral Edema, III, Alteration in the White Matter. An Electron Microscopic Study Using Ferritin as Labelling Compound, Acta Neuropath., 2, 177-197 (1963).

Scheinker, I.: Zur Histopathologie des Hirnödems und der Hirnschwellung bei Tumoren des Gehirns, Dtsch. Z. Nervenheilk., 147, 137-162 (1938).

Schröder, J. M. and W. Wechsler: Ödem und Nekrose in der grauen und weissen Substanz beim experimentellen Hirntrauma, Acta Neuropath., 5, 82-111 (1965).

Tani, E. and J. P. Evans: Electron Microscope Studies of Cerebral Swelling. II. Alterations of Myelinated Fibers. Ibid., 4, 604-623 (1965).

_____ and _____: Electron Microscope Studies of Cerebral Swelling. III. Alterations in the Neuroglia and the Blood Vessels of the White Matter, Ibid., 624-639 (1965).

Zülch, K. J.: Morphologische Befunde bei Hirnschwellung. Zbl. Neurochirurgie, 5, 166-175 (1940).

_____: Hirnödem und Hirnschwellung, Virch. Archiv., 310, 1-58 (1943).

J. ESCOLÁ *
W. KRÜCKE
E. THOMAS

EDEMA IN PERIPHERAL NERVES

In 1922 Bielschowsky and Valentin, and later Denny-Brown, et al., (1945), described in detail the morphological changes in locally frozen nerves. Edema and "Seröse Entzündung" was considered by Krücke (1941) to be an essential first step towards "Mukoide Degeneration" and "Bindegewebige Sklerosierung" of the nerve. Decrease of birefringence of the myelin sheath due to low temperature was observed by Tomity and Csillik (1964).

In order to get further information on the non-Wallerian type of nerve degeneration after application of low temperature, we chille the nervus ischiadicus of rats with dry ice for half a minute or longe The animals were killed after 4, 24, or 48 hours respectively. The procedure of damage leaves the nerve macroscopically fully intact, but when the animals were killed a local swelling of the nerve due to edema could be observed in situ.

Cutting fresh frozen cryotome sections avoids embedding artifacts and gives the true topographical picture in the severed nerve as compared with the intact portion proximal to the lesion. For elec tron microscopic investigation the material was fixed in situ with buffered osmium textroxide and embedded in Vestopal or Epon.

Four hours after freezing it is possible to observe with light microscopy local swelling and a pale staining of myelin layers in the damaged area as revealed by the OTAN method for the demonstration of myelin. A separation of nerve fiber bundles as well as of single fibers is evident. Also, poorly stained homogenous exudative material often with a network-like appearance and with only a very few scattered cells can be seen (Fig. 1).

Oxidative enzymes and hydrolytic enzyme activities are much diminished in the chilled area, but accumulations of enzymes are noted proximal and distal to the lesion (Fig. 2).

*Deceased.

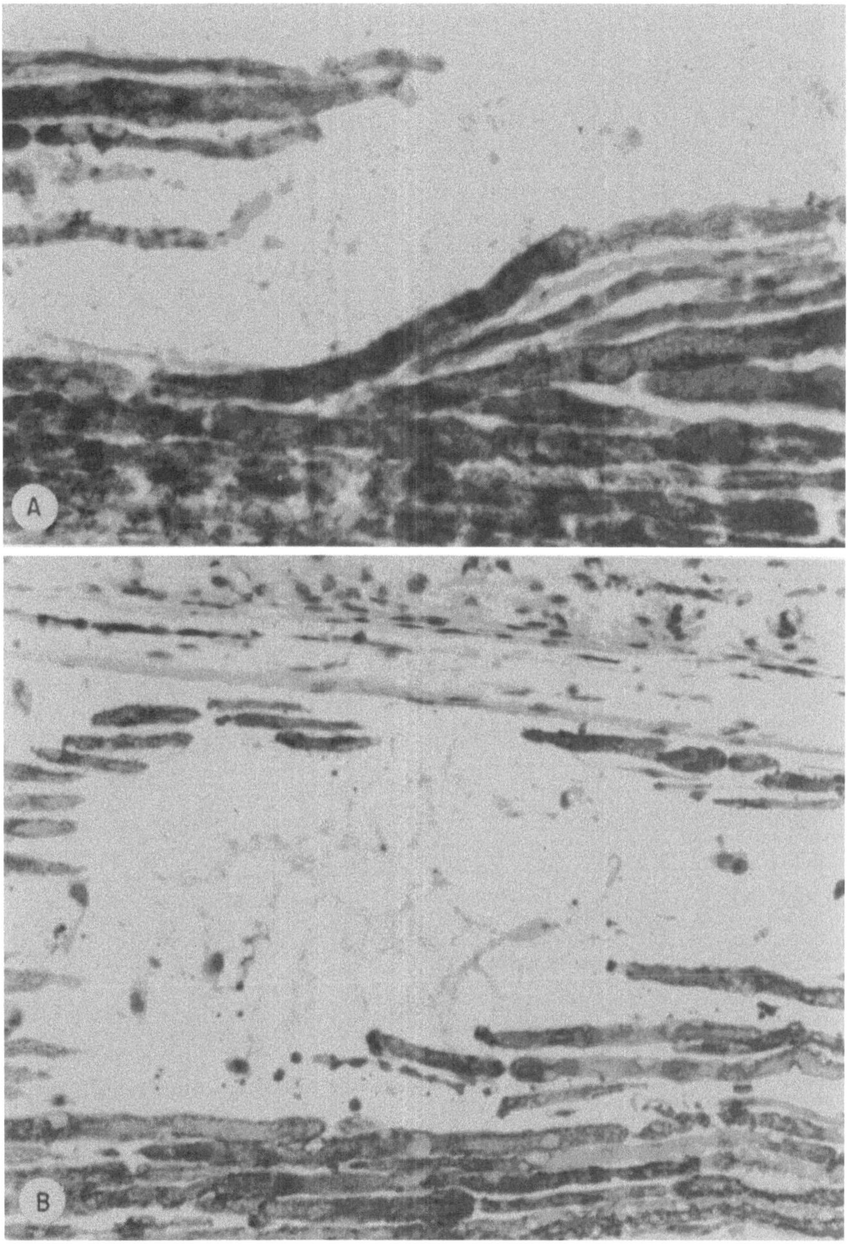

Fig. 1. Nervus ischiadicus of rat, frozen 4 hours before sacrifice; a) plasmal reaction; exudative non-stainable material between seperated nerve fibers; X400; b) Fettrot 7B-Meyer's haemalum stain. A network-like exudation between disconnected fibers is poorly stained. Only a few cells are visible. X250.

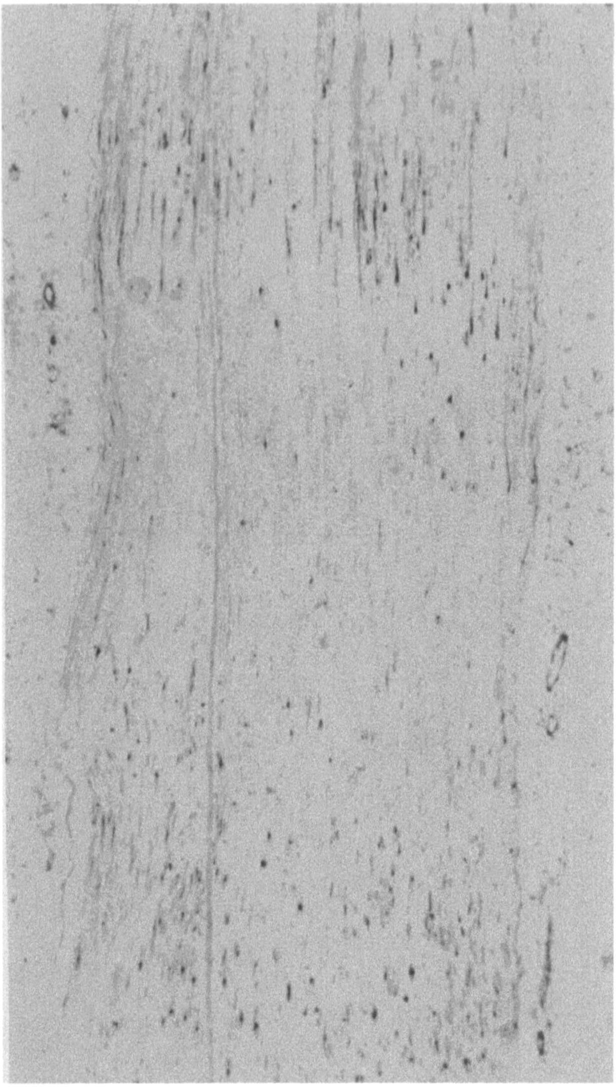

Fig. 2. As Fig. 1; reaction for lactate dehydrogenase with TNBT, counterstained with carmalum; accumulation of enzymes proximal and distal to the lesion; in the chilled part enzyme activity is highly reduced. X38.

The myelin sheaths of the large fibers show signs of disintegration as seen in various stains, particularly the copper phthalocyanine method and the plasmal reaction. The latter method is especially suitable for the demonstration of alterations in the peripheral myelin sheath. In the course of time larger parts of the sheath will become plasmal-negative and often a swelling of the fiber in diameter is observed (Fig. 3). Occasionally the plasmal re-

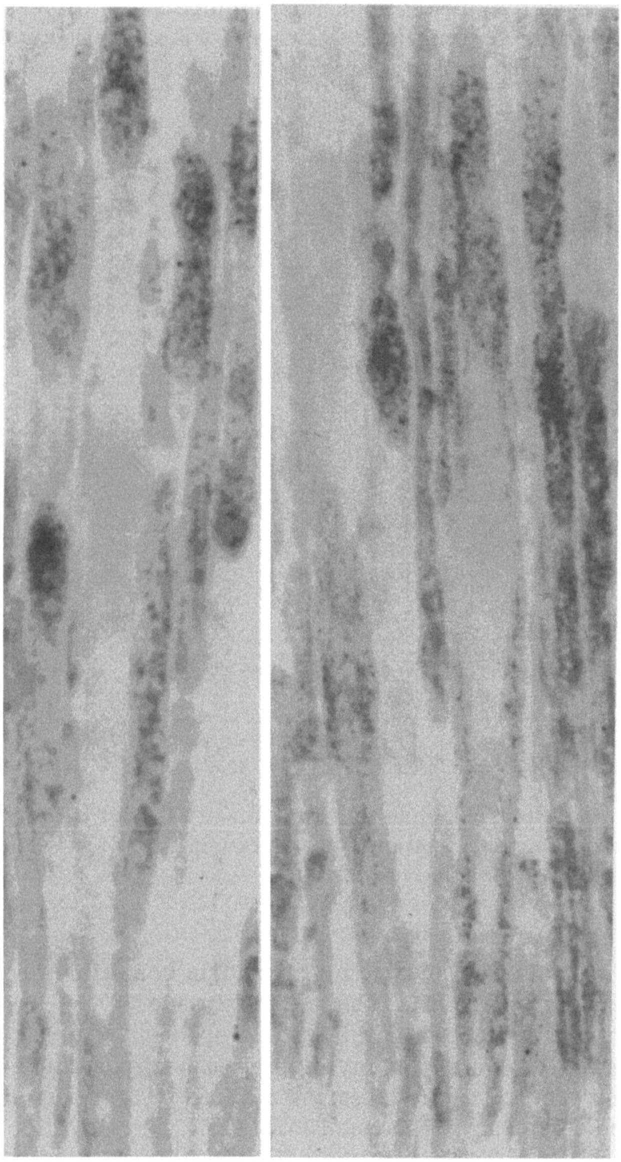

Fig. 3. Nervus ischiadicus of a rat, frozen 24 hours before sacrifice; plasmal reaction. Swelling and partial negativity of fibers can be seen. Fine plasmal-positive granules are also observed. X400.

action appears unevenly in the sheath. At times we observed numerous small plasmal-positive granules distributed in the remaining parts of the myelin sheath.

Fine structural observations with the electron microscope detected highly separated myelin lamellae 24 hours after operation. A striking and repeated observation was numerous small vesicles of different size lying accumulated between a widely split myelin (Figs. 4-7). In contrast, the axis cylinders seemed relatively unaffected.

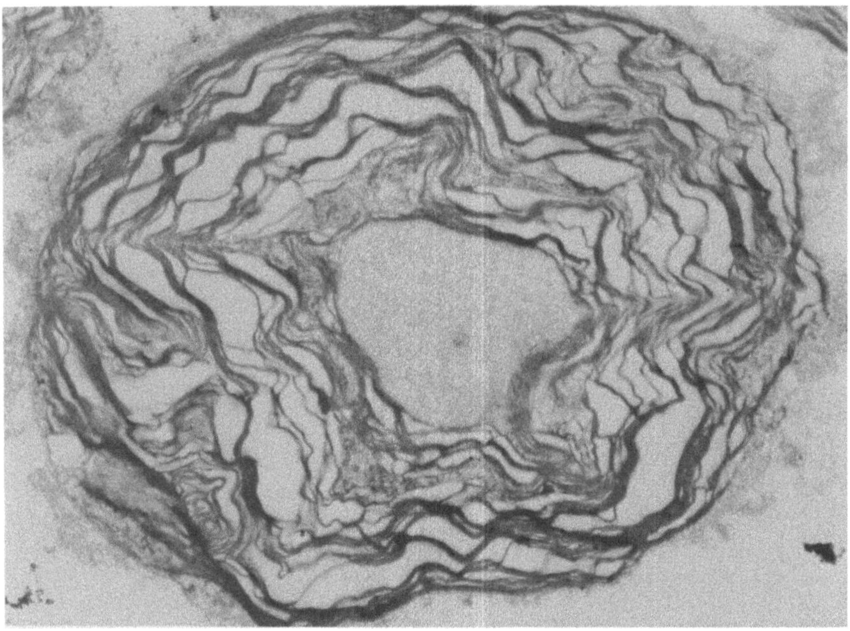

Fig. 4. Nervus ischiadicus of a rat, frozen 24 hours before sacrifice. Electron microscopic examination reveals accumulations of vesicles between seperated myelin lamellae. X5,000.

They were not enlarged and the mitochondria sometimes seemed of normal appearance, while others were swollen.

Ice crystal formation resulting in a splitting of dense lines and intermediate bands of the myelin sheath was considered to be the cause for structural modification induced by freezing and thawing (Fernandez-Moran & Finean, 1957).

Our results not obtained immediately after chilling but after various survival intervals indicate that injury of a nerve by low temperatures is followed by an early edema between the single nerve

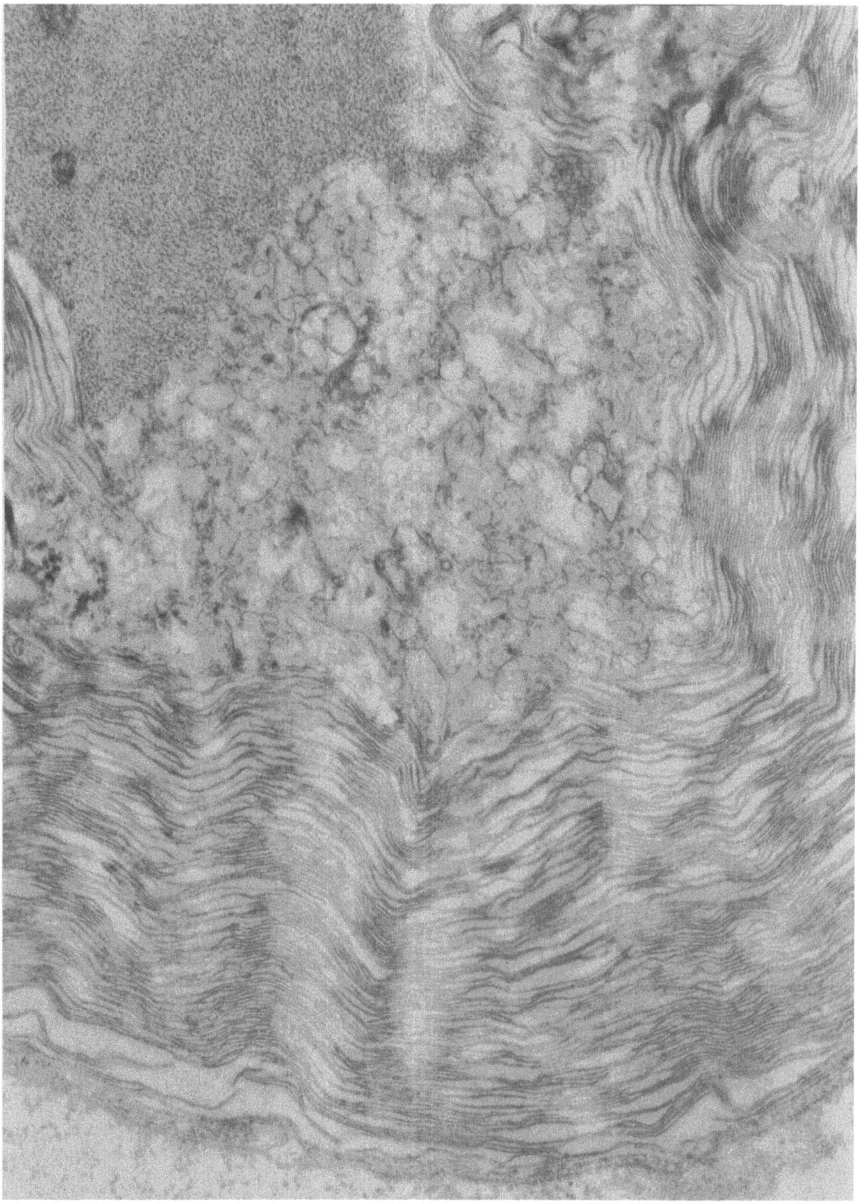

Fig. 5. Accumulation of numerous vesicles neighboring the axis cylinder. X20,000.

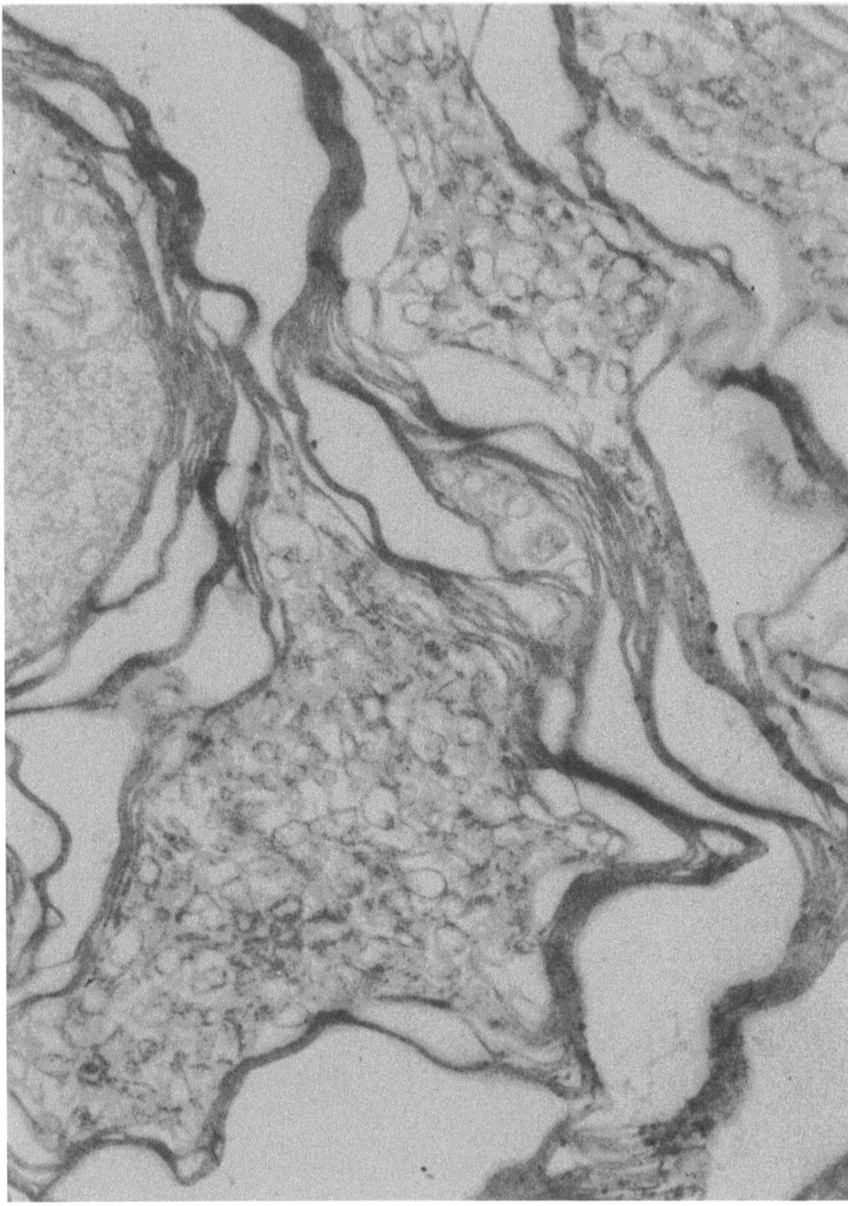

Fig. 6. Highly split myelin lamellae around areas of small vesicles and other unidentifiable formations. X24,000.

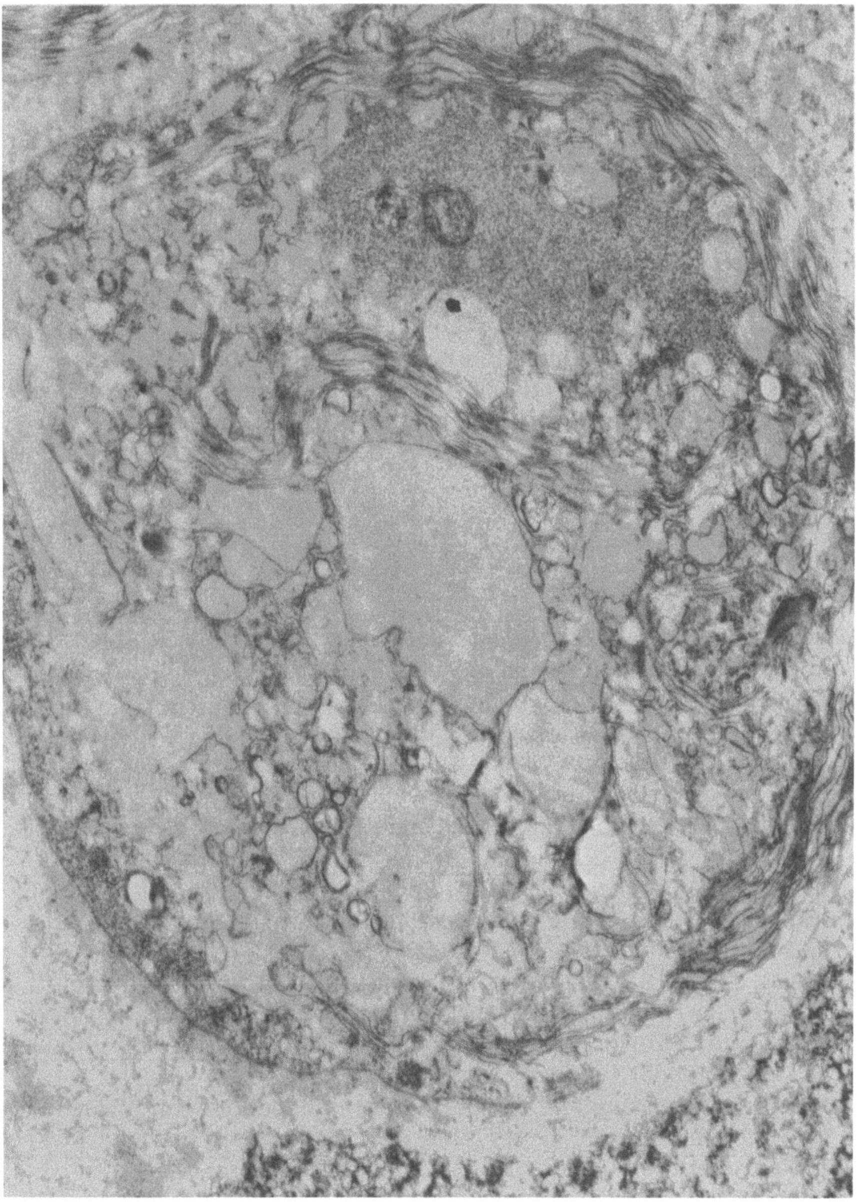

Fig. 7. Large vacuoles between myelin lamellae and vesicles of different size and shape. Note an unaffected inner portion of the axis cylinder and a well-preserved mitochondrion. X18,000.

fibers and the fiber bundles. Furthermore, the myelin sheaths themselves are affected as seen by a separation of the myelin lamellae. It can be assumed that this is due to the crystallization of water during the process of freezing. Another sequel of damage seems to be the appearance of accumulated vesicles lying between the separated myelin lamellae.

In addition to the edema, a highly reduced enzymatic activity in the chilled area (Thomas, 1965) seems to be another factor involved in a slow type of degeneration without early "Fettabbau" and without cellular infiltration. The process observed in the nerve fiber may be compared with the "Mukoide Degeneration" of the nerve (Krücke, 1941) and is as such to be separated from the Wallerian type of degeneration and other observations made on the mechanism of demyelination (Lampert & Carpenter, 1965; Lampert, 1965; Thoma & Sheldon, 1964).

REFERENCES

Bielschowsky, M. and B. Valentin: Die histologischen Veränderungen in durchfrorenen Nervenstrecken., J. Psychol. u. Neurol., 29, 133-152 (1922).

Denny-Brown, D., R. D. Adams, Ch. Brenner, and M. M. Doherty: The pathology of injury to nerve induced by cold, J. Neuropath. Exp. Neurol., 4, 305-323 (1945).

Fernandez-Moran, H. and J. B. Finean: Electron microscope and low-angle X-ray diffraction studies of the nerve myelin sheath, J. Biophys. Biochem. Cytol. 3, 725-748 (1957).

Krücke, W.: Ödem und seröse Entzündung im peripheren Nerven, Virchow's Arch., 308, 1-13 (1941).

Lampert, P. and S. Carpenter: Electron microscopic studies on the vascular permeability and the mechanism of demyelination in experimental allergic encephalomyelitis, J. Neuropath. exp. Neurol., 24, 11-24 (1965).

_____: Demyelination and remyelination in experimental allergic encephalomyelitis. Further electron microscopic observations, J. Neuropath. exp. Neurol., 24, 371-385 (1965).

Thomas, E.: Histochemistry of the peripheral nervous system, Report on the Vth Int. Congress of Neuropathol., Zürich, Aug. 30-Sept. 3, 1965, Proc. by Excerpta Medica, Amsterdam S. 396 (1966).

Thomas, P. K. and H. Sheldon: Tubular arrays derived from myelin breakdown during Wallerian degeneration of peripheral nerve, J. Cell. Biol., 22, 715-718 (1964).

Tomity, I. and B. Csillik: Submicroscopic alterations of myelin sheath ultrastructure due to low temperature, Acta Morphol. Acad. Sci. Hung., 12, 387-394 (1964).

K. A. HOSSMANN

MORPHOLOGICAL SUBSTRATE OF THE BLOOD-BRAIN BARRIER IN HUMAN BRAIN TUMORS

It is a well-established fact that in human brain tumors the so-called blood-brain barrier system is severely affected. This has been proved by the use of indicator substances such as dyes (3, 6) or radioactive isotopes (2, 19, 25). Gamma-encephalography, a current diagnostic method, is based on this principle (25).

Considering the interrelationship between edema and disturbances of the blood-brain barrier, it would be advisable, while investigating the peritumoral edema, not to ignore the changes within the tumor itself. We have carried out such an investigation with the object of determining whether the breakdown of the blood-brain barrier in tumors is connected with morphological pecularities of the actual tumor vessel system.

The previously postulated morphological substrate of the blood-brain barrier in normal brain tissue involved the capillary endothelial cells (2, 23, 28), the interstitial ground substance (16), the pia-glial membrane (13, 27), the basement membrane (4, 8) and the perivascular glial cells (14, 18, 31). Comparative morphology of the brain capillaries and other capillaries of the body by means of electron microscopy has shown, however, that there is no basic difference in the structure of the vessel walls (1, 5, 10, 11, 15). The minute intercellular space of brain tissue does not offer an explanation for the barrier phenomenon, since substances which enter the brain by way of the cerebrospinal fluid do not necessarily do so from the blood vessels. The most significant morphological feature seems to be the lack of a perivascular space around the small vessels of the brain, where the basement membranes of the capillaries and small veins are fused with the glial membranes so that the processes of the perivascular glial cells are in direct contact with the vessel walls. This phenomenon, which we would like to refer to as the "histotopographical precondition for a blood-brain-barrier system" (17), is considered now by most authors as the essential morphological substrate of the blood-brain barrier (1, 10, 12, 15 a. o.).

The present communication is based on a series of human brain tumors which Dr. Wechsler and I examined in the last three years. Some of our results could be correlated with earlier observations (7, 20, 24, 26, 29, 30, 32). Our investigations deal with the capillaries and small vessels; we did not examine the morphological properties of the vessel wall only but also tried to find out whether there were morphological signs of disturbances of fluid transport mechanisms. For this purpose we analyzed the perivascular spaces and the perivascular tissue within the tumor. Marked differences occurred between glial and non-glial tumors.

Isomorphic gliomas. In isomorphic gliomas (spongioblastoma, astrocytoma, oligodendroglioma, ependymoma) the electron microscopic findings in the vessels of regions without regressive changes do not differ essentially from those in normal brain vessels (Fig. 1a-b). The lumen of the vessel is surrounded by a poreless endothelium and the endothelial cells are of variable size but do not exceed the normal range of variability. The basement membrane around the endothelial cells does not show any fenestration; occasionally it encloses a normal pericyte. The width of the basement membrane ranges from 0.1 to 1.0 μ. A marked variation as compared to normal blood vessels is not only found in different tumors but also in different regions of the same tumor. The vascular basement membranes of the capillaries are fused with the basement membranes of the perivascular tumor cells and as in normal brain tissue, a free perivascular space does not occur. The tumor cells form a complete glial sheath around the vessels, the intercellular spaces between the perivascular cells and processes being generally in the range of only 200 Å. We call this fact the "replacement of the astrocytic glial sheath by a tumor sheath" (17). The fine structure of the perivascular cells is identical to that of the rest of the tumor. Thus in tumors such as fibrillary astrocytomas or spongioblastomas, the perivascular cells show a fibrillary differentiation in contrast to normal astrocytic sucker feet. The size of the pericapillary cell processes differs greatly. In protoplasmatic astrocytomas some processes enclose more than three quarters of the vessel's circumference.

Pinocytotic vesicles are found in abundance. They are concentrated directly under the outer cell membranes of the endothelial cells or pericytes but never under the cell membranes of the peri-

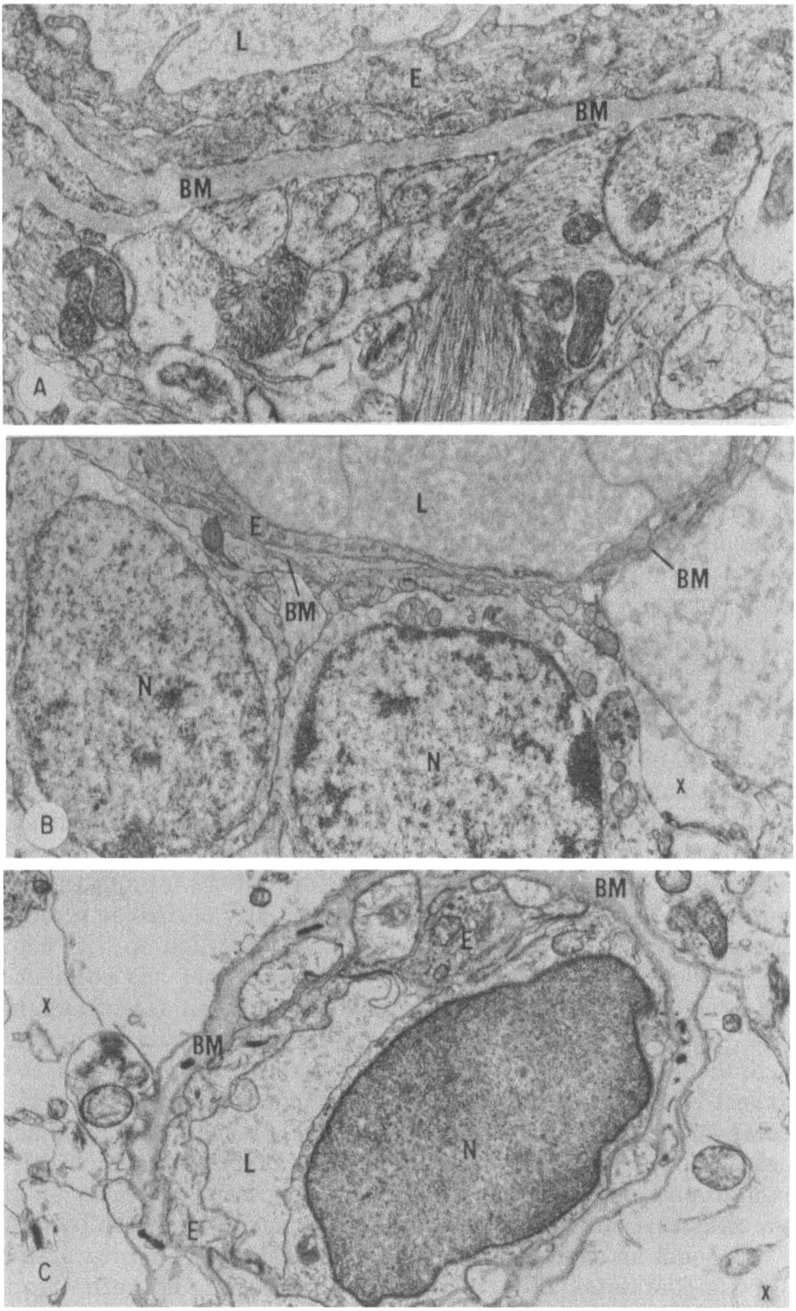

Fig. 1. Capillaries of isomorphic gliomas: a) fibrillary astrocytoma, X15,000; b) oligodendroglioma, X10,000; c) protoplasmic astrocytoma (regressive area) X10,000; L — lumen of the capillary; E — endothelial cell; N — nucleus; BM — basement membrane; x — enlarged extracellular space.

vascular glial cells. The number of vesicles seems to be independant of the dimensions of the endothelial cells or the basement membranes and of the fine structure of the respective tumor cells (protoplasmic or fibrillary differentiation). Furthermore, the correlation was not found between the number of the vesicles and edema which was observed by Cervos-Navarro in the course of x-irradiation (7).

In regressive tumor areas, alterations of the tumor cells (swelling of the endoplasmic tubuli and mitochondria, general swelling of the cytoplasm, disruption of cell membranes) are always accompanied by an enlargment of the extracellular space. This process starts farther away from the vessels. Only at an advanced stage does the enlargement of the extracellular space affect the perivascular tumor sheath. Even then the cell membranes of the tumor cells are not detached from the vessel walls until extensive cell damage and necrosis occur (Fig. 1c). The glial sheath thus seems to have the greatest resistance to regressive changes.

Although there is a break-down of the blood-brain barrier in isomorphic gliomas, the histotopographical relationship between vessels and surrounding tissue in areas without regressive changes remains the same as in normal brain tissue. The only marked difference as opposed to brain areas with an effective blood-brain barrier system is the replacement of the astrocytic glial sheath by a tumor sheath. The efficiency of the barrier is consequently related to the functional efficiency of the glial sheath. It is not astonishing that in astrocytomas the water content is the highest of all gliomas.

Malignant gliomas. In malignant gliomas (glioblastoma, malignant astrocytoma, polymorphic oligodendroglioma) the described histotopographical relationship between the capillaries and the surrounding tissue occurs only in non-proliferated vessels. If there is a proliferation of the small vessels, as typically occurs in glioblastomas, a perivascular space is visible which is filled up with numerous cell processes, branching basement membranes and collagen fibrils (Fig. 2 a-b). The glial basement membranes are often fenestrated. Processes of the cells lying in the perivascular space pass through these gaps into the tumor tissue around the vessel. In these regions it is difficult to detect a clear boundary between the perivascular space and the surrounding tumoral tissue. The cytoplasm of these cells is polymorphic, occasionally anaplastic, which indicates a tumoral growth, though whether they are of vascular or glial origin cannot be determinated exactly. Torack is of the opinion that they represent an adventitial response to destructive tumor activity (30). Luse postulates an infiltration of neoplastic glial cells into the perivascular space (20).

The enlarged perivascular space is, however, not a free diffusional space. As in areas far from the vessels the intercellular

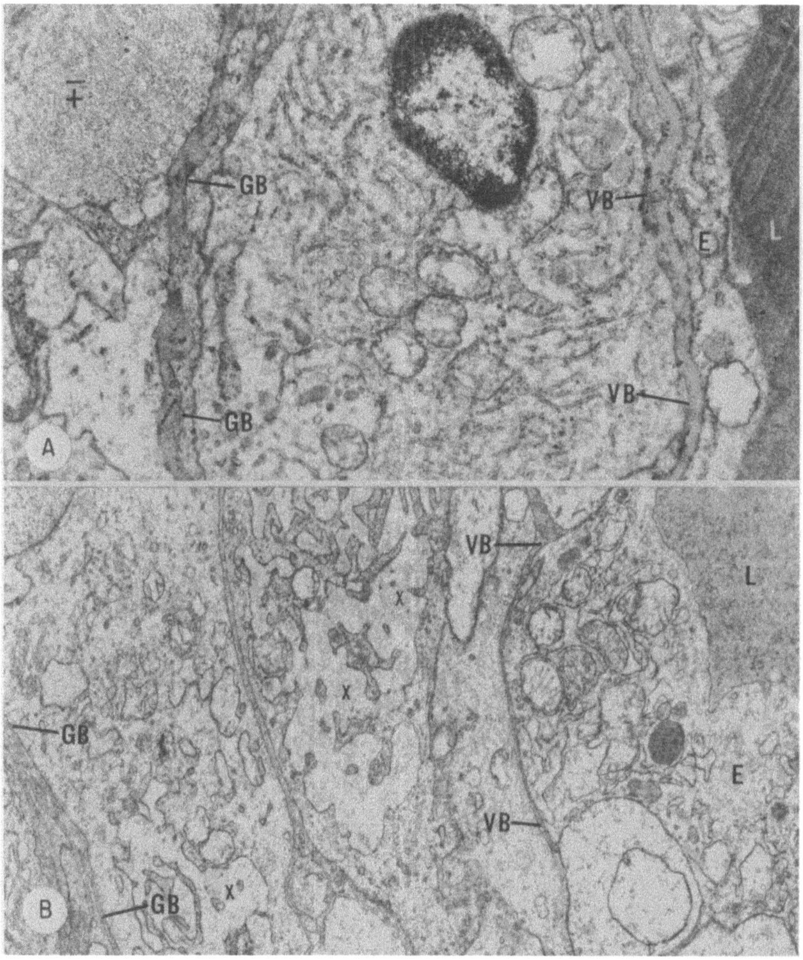

Fig. 2. Capillaries of glioblastomas; a) X20,000; b) X15,000; L — lumen of the capillary; E — endothelial cells; VB — vascular basement membrane; GB — glial basement membrane; F — fibrillary cell process; x — enlarged endoplasmic tubuli.

space between the above mentioned cells generally does not exceed 200 Å. The perivascular glial sheath is formed by a continuous cell layer, as in isomorphic gliomas. In malignant gliomas the sheath consists of fibrillary and protoplasmic as well as anaplastic cells. In regressive areas the endothelial cells and the adventitial cells may be swollen.

Non-glial tumors. The described histotopographical relationship between the vessels and the surrounding tissue is dependant on the existence of a glial matrix. In non-glial tumors (Fig. 3 a-b) the

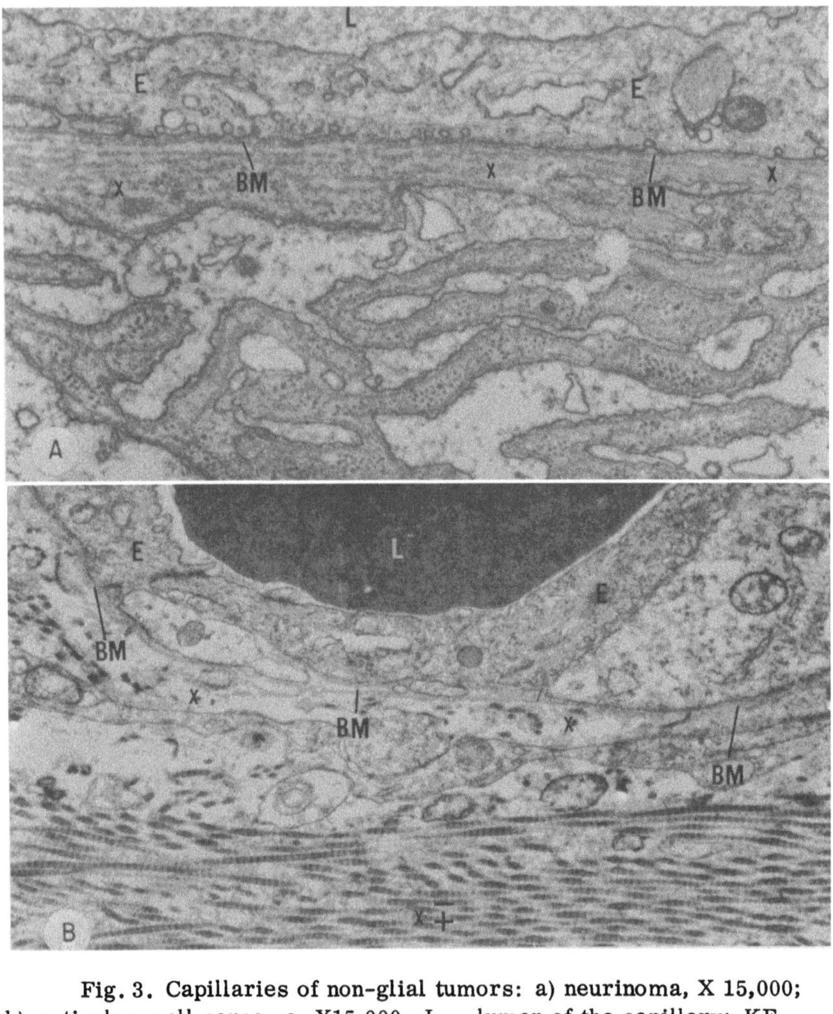

Fig. 3. Capillaries of non-glial tumors: a) neurinoma, X 15,000; b) reticulum cell sarcoma, X15,000. L — lumen of the capillary; KF — collagen fibrils; x — perivascular space.

histotopographical properties resemble more or less those of extracerebral organs. The capillaries of all these tumors are surrounded by a true perivascular diffusional space which has a free connection with the corresponding ground substance. In neurinomas, for instance, this intercellular ground substance is formed by basement membrane-like material and collagen fibrils. In reticulum cell sarcomas the perivascular space is especially large and filled up with thick bundles of collagen fibrils. In meningiomas we found, in accordance with Yoshida, et al. (32), a very thin endothelium, which occasionally exhibits fenestration. A continuous cell layer ressembling the perivascular neoplastic glial sheath does not occur in any of these tumors. Thus the morphological basis for a barrier similar to that of the brain cannot and does not exist.

CONCLUSION

Our results can be summarized as follows (Fig. 4). In normal brain tissue with an effective blood-brain barrier system the lumen of the capillaries is surrounded by a poreless endothelium and a continuous cell membrane. The vascular and the glial basement

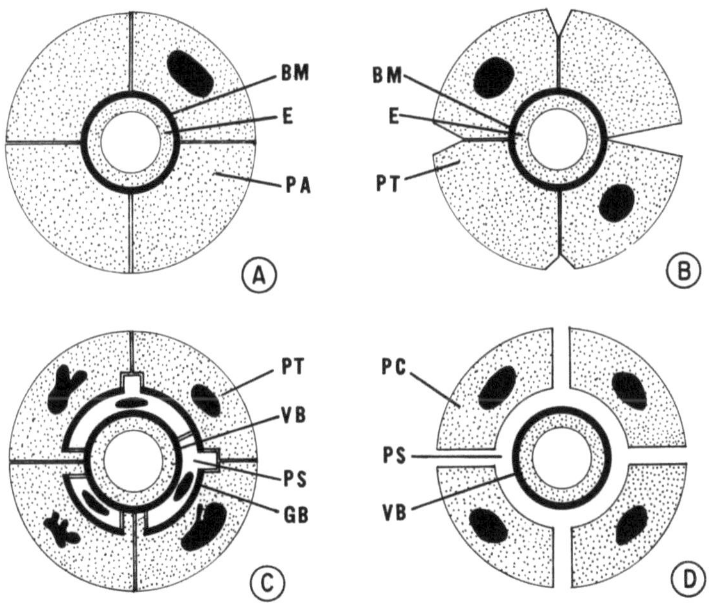

Fig. 4. Schematic representation of the histotopographical relationships between vessels and surrounding tissue: a) normal brain; b) isomorphic gliomas; c) malignant gliomas; d) non-glial tumors; E: endothelial cell; BM: basement membrane; PA: perivascular astrocytic glial sheath; PT: perivascular tumor glial sheath; PC: perivascular tumor cells; PS: perivascular space; GB: glial basement membrane; VB: vascular basement membrane.

membranes are fused; a perivascular space does not occur. The vessels are enclosed by an astroglial sheath; the intercellular space does not exceed 200 Å. The isomorphic gliomas possess a poreless endothelium and a continuous basement membrane, too. There is no perivascular space. The crucial difference is the replacement of the astrocytic glial sheath by a tumor sheath. The extracellular space may be expanded in a region far from the vessels, but only in highly regressive areas does the enlargement affect the perivascular tumoral sheath. In malignant gliomas the proliferated vessels are also surrounded by a neoplastic glial sheath, but here the perivascular space is enlarged and filled up with different kinds of cells. Since a free diffusional space does not exist, the breakdown of the blood-brain barrier in gliomas must be referred to a functional insufficiency of the perivascular blastomatous glial sheath. In non-glial tumors the free perivascular space does not allow the establishment of a barrier phenomenon.

It would be interesting to analyze the relationship between the disturbances in fluid transport mechanisms in the tumor and the peritumoral edema. As has been pointed out by several authors, in the gray matter there is a domination of the swelling of the astroglia and in the white matter the enlargment of the perivascular space. This pattern seems to be typical for edema of varying pathogenesis, as Dr. Wechsler will show you in experimental edema models. We suppose that there is no fundamental morphological difference whether the increased fluid influx that leads to edema comes by way of the extracellular spaces or astroglial cells. It is remarkable, however, that peritumoral edema is concentrated around the vessels, although there are no morphological signs of vessel damage in the edematous brain tissue. The solution to this fundamental problem is probably not a morphological one.

REFERENCES

1. Bairati, A.: Perivascular relationship of the neuroglia cells, in: Biology of Neuroglia, (ed. by W. F. Windle). Springfield, Ill.: Charles C. Thomas, XIV, 340 pp (1958).
2. Bakay, L.: The blood-brain barrier with special regard to the use of radioactive isotopes, Springfield, Ill: Charles C. Thomas, XII, 154 pp. (1958).
3. Bates, J. I. and J. Kershman: Selective staining of experimental brain tumors during life, J. Neuropath., 8, 411-418 (1949).
4. Breemen, V. L. van and C. D. Clemente: Silver deposition in the central nervous system and the hematoencephalic barrier studied with the electron microscope, J. Biophys. Biochem. Cytol., 1, 161-165 (1955).

5. Broman, T.: On basic aspect of the blood-brain barrier, Acta Psychiat. Kbh., 30, 115-124 (1955).
6. Brunschwig, A., R. L. Schmitz and Th. H. Clarke: Intravital staining of malignant neoplasms in man by Evans blue, Arch. Path. 30, 902 (1940).
7. Cervos – Navarro, J. C.: Die Bedeutung der Elektronenmikroskopie für die Lehre vom Stoffaustasch zwischen dem Zentralnervensystem und dem übrigen Körper, Dtsch. Z. Nervenheilk., 186, 209-237 (1964).
8. Dempsey, E. W. and G. B. Wislocki: An electron microscopic study of the blood-brain barrier in the rat, employing silver nitrate as a vital stain, J. Biophys. Biochem. Cytol., 1, 245-256 (1955).
9. Dobbing, J.: The blood-brain barrier, Guy's Hosp. Rep., 105, 27-38 (1956).
10. Edström, R.: An explanation of the blood-brain barrier phenomenon, Acta Psychiat. Kbh., 33, 403-416 (1958).
11. Farquhar, M. G. and J. F. Hartmann: Electron microscopy of cerebral capillaries, Anat. Rec. 124, 288-289 (1956).
12. Gardner, W. J.: The blood-brain barrier: an expression of the absence of interstitial spaces in ectodermal tissue?, Perspect. Biol. Med., 6, 169-176 (1961).
13. Gärtner, W.: Die Blut-Liquorschanke, Z. Biol., 86, 115-139 (1927).
14. Gerschenfeld, H. M., F. Wald, J. A. Zadunaisky and E. D. P. De Robertis: Function of astroglia in the water-ion metabolism of the central nervous system. An electron microscope study, Neurology, 9, 412-425 (1959).
15. Hager, H.: Die feinere Cytologie und Cytopathologie des Nervensystems, Stuttgart (1964).
16. Hess, A.: The ground substance of the central nervous system and its relation to the blood-brain barrier, World Neurol., 3, 118-124 (1962).
17. Hossmann, K. A., M. Schröder and W. Wechsler: Elektronenmikroskopische Untersuchungen zum morphologischen Substrat der Bluthirnschranke, Verh. Dtsch. Ges. Pathol., 49, 350-356 (1965).
18. Ishii, S. and E. Tani: Electron microscopic study of the blood-brain barrier in brain swelling, Acta Neuropath., 1, 474-488 (1962).
19. Kramer, S., L. K. Burton and N. G. Trott: Radioactive isotopes in the localisation of brain tumors. Acta Radiol. Stockh., 46, 415-424 (1956).
20. Luse, S. A. and B. Harris: Electron microscopy of the brain in experimental edema, J. Neurosurg., 17, 439-446 (1960).
21. Maynard, E. A., R. L. Schultz and D. C. Pease: Electron micros-

copy of the vascular bed of rat cerebral cortex, Amer. J. Anat., 100, 409-433 (1957).
22. Nyström, S. H.: Electron microscopical structure of the wall of small blood vessels in human multiforme glioblastoma, Nature (London), 184, 65 (1960).
23. Peters, A.: Plasma membrane contacts in the central nervous system, J. Anat. (London) 96, 237-248 (1962).
24. Pineda, A.: Submicroscopic structure of acoustic tumours, Neurology, 14, 171-184 (1964).
25. Planiol, T.: Diagnostic use of gamma encephalography in neurosurgery, IInd Int. Congr. Neurol. Surg. (Washington, D. C., 1961); Excerpta Med., N. 36, E4-E5 (1961).
26. Raimondi, A. J., S. Mullan and J. P. Evans: Human brain tumors: an electron-microscopic study, J. Neurosurg., 19, 731-752 (1962).
27. Schaltenbrand, G. and P. Bailey: Die perivasculäre Piagliamembran des Gehirns, J. Psychol. Neurol. Lpz. 35, 199-278 (1928).
28. Spatz, H.: Die Bedeutung der vitalen Färbung für die Iehre vom Stoffaustausch zwischen dem Zentralnervensystem und dem übrigen Körper. Arch. Psychiat. Nervenkr. 101, 267-358 (1933).
29. Tani, E. and S. Ishii: Ontogenic Studies on the Rat Brain Capillaries in Relation to the Human Brain Tumor Vessels, Acta Neuropath., 2, 253-270 (1963).
30. Torak, R. M.: Ultrastructure of capillary reaction to brain tumors, Arch. Neurol., 5, 416 (1961).
31. Tschirgi, R. D.: The blood-brain barrier, in: Biology of Neuroglia (ed. by W. F. Windle, ed.(Springfield, Ill: Charles C. Thomas, XIV, 340 pp. (1958).
32. Yoshida, N., I. Ohmaru and T. Sato: Electron microscopic studies on human brain tumor, V. Intern. Congr. Electron microscopy: Philadelphia, 2 (1962).

DISCUSSION

FLEISCHHAUER (to Dr. Lampert): What is the reason for the difference in staining with trypan blue of the upper and lower parts of the spinal cord? In your pictures the upper pars are much less densely stained than the lower parts. Is there any explanation?

LAMPERT: We were impressed with the deeper Trypan blue staining of the lower spinal cord just as we were struck by the selective staining of the occipital lobes, striatum and cerebellum. We have no answer at present why the endothelial cells should be more vulnerable in these areas.

ZÜLCH: Is this observation limited to young animals still suckling, or is it the same with adult animals?

LAMPERT: These observations were done on suckling rats. Adult animals showed no changes after lead poisoning. We noted with interest that a few suckling rats recovered even on a continuous lead diet.

EVANS (to Dr. Brightman): Professor Zülch has anticipated my question in part. These are very beautiful and convincing demonstrations. They are, however, so at variance with the observations of Raimondi on the passage of ferritin that I should like to ask about the influence upon the results of the age of the animals, of species difference and of possible difference in the micromaterial used.

ZÜLCH: May I add one question: does myelination play a role? Do you have myelin preparations of this particular age? Does myelination progress from above downwards as in man in the spinal cord? I have published such observations.

LAMPERT: In regard to Dr. Evans' comment about the Ferritin studies of his team on the vascular permeability in cerebral edema, I wish to state that we must be very careful in interpreting the dissemination of Ferritin. I have also tried this tracer, but I became discouraged because the slightest artefactual disruption of cellular membranes apparently permits the penetration of this material into cells. Dr. Brightman has just published some interesting findings in this regard (J. Cell Biol., 26, 99, 1965) and I am sure he will comment on this topic in his paper. Of course, Ferritin may behave differently from Thorotrast.

Dr. Zülch asked about the relation of myelination to the permeability changes. In the examined tissues, i.e., the striatum and cerebellum, myelination was complete. I have no electron microscopic observations on the lower spinal cord nor on animals at earlier stages before they became paralyzed when they already demonstrated a permeability change to Trypan blue. However, since the vascular alterations manifested themselves predominantly in grey matter regions, I doubt that myelination plays a role.

WOLMAN (to Dr. Gruner): I was very pleased to notice that you mention that there were differences in findings in your first series of biopsies as compared to the later series because of fixation. If it is permitted to air some unorthodox opinions, I would like to suggest the following. We all know that cell membranes are made of lipoproteins. We also know that they are not the stable structures as we see them with an electron microscope. They change, they may undergo phase reversals and form vesicles. We have evidence indicating that a suspension consisting mainly of cell walls (homogenate of white matter) can be transformed into emulsions having the hydrophilic layer once on the inside of droplets and once on the outside. We may produce such changes by using different fixation procedures, and I imagine that something similar may happen in vivo. I wonder whether the finding of the edema fluid in some instances outside cells, and on other occasions, inside cells, may not be correlated with observations which have been reported by a number of electron microscopists who saw the same structures, once in a vesicular form and once in a lamellar form. It is possible that what we are really showing are just so many Equivalent-bilder which are, however, not quite equivalent, since some are fixed in one way with more hydrophilic substances, and some are fixed in another.

GRUNER: I thank you for a comment to which I have nothing specific to answer.

BRIGHTMAN: Dr. Lampert, you have shown very elegantly the intracellular passage of your marker. Do I understand correctly from your description that although some of these cells, the ones which you identify as microglial cells, are able to phagocytose the marker, whereas the neurons are not? Is that correct?

LAMPERT: One hour after intravenous injection I found Thorotrast within vesicles inside astrocytes. After 24 hours the particles were predominently within microglial cells or macrophages. I did not see Thorotrast within neurons.

BRIGHTMAN: One short subquestion: I would very much like to know how you can distinguish a microglial cell from a macroglial cell.

LAMPERT: My identification of microglial cells or macrophages is done by exclusion, i.e., I believe being able to recognize neurons and astrocytes. I find it difficult to distinguish oligodendrocytes from resting microglial cells. Since I have as yet not found a satisfactory clue in my studies which would suggest that oligodendrocytes might become phagocytes, I still like to call the cell illustrated in Figure 10, a microglial cell or macrophage.

BRIGHTMAN: As we will see, Ferritin in our experiments had the unhappy tendency to spread across membranes which looked quite intact. However, the cell membranes can have discrete ruptures and one can be fooled by the widespread artifactual deposition of freely dispersed micelles within the cytoplasm. Your marker was convincingly restricted to membrane-bounded inclusions.

KATZMAN: I have just two questions at this time, one for Dr. Cumings and one for Dr. Lowenthal. I wanted to ask Dr. Cumings what was the reference unit in his figures and in the graphs that he showed. Did you refer the content of sodium, potassium, and enzyme activity to the wet weight or the dry weight? It was not clear to me. Dr. Lowenthal, your finding that the protein from the edematous brain electrophoretically resembles serum albumin but is not identical to serum albumin is of very great importance. I wonder, however, if you could tell us about the preparative methods for your serum albumin as well as brain proteins. Were these identical? Could there be any possibility that the difference in preparing the proteins from these two sources might have contributed to the small change in apparent molecular weight that you found?

CUMINGS: The reference is, as I mentioned, to wet weight in every case. I did actually calculate them all for dry weight as well. It made no difference to the ratios, really, which were used, for you get the same relative ratio in each case.

KATZMAN: If you referred this to dry weight, wouldn't your enzyme activity be normal?

CUMINGS: The transaminase and creatine kinase, for instance, are reduced in the edematous side, whether wet weight or dry weight was used for reference.

ZEMAN: I would like to address a question to Dr. Cumings in respect to triethyl tin poisoned animals. If I read his slide correctly, he found high acid phosphatase and low alkaline phosphatase values, and I just wonder at what state of the process these estimates were obtained. We have done similar studies and also found high acid phosphatase values, but only in the very early stage of the edema, when the animal is not really sick. But if we follow the animal two or three days, then the acid phosphatase values drop about 30%, and similar findings were obtained for alkaline phosphatase.

CUMINGS: On the whole, most of the animals we used were definitely showing evidence of poisoning by organic tin. Most of these findings were, in fact, reported in Kalsbeck's and Cumings's paper; all the data are actually there. The animals were in what I think you would regard as a relatively late stage rather than a relatively early stage.

CLASEN: I believe you stated in the paper which you published with Dr. Kalsbeck (J. Neuropath. Exp. Neurol., 22: 237-247) that there was not an increase in total water-soluble protein in triethyl tin edema. Is this correct?

CUMINGS: No this is not correct. No statements about the total water-soluble protein in this condition were made in that paper.

CLASEN: In view of the above, this question should be eliminated.

CUMINGS: There was no increase in the white matter, although the distribution of the proteins varied a little from the normal.

LOWENTHAL: Dr. Katzman, we not only isolated the albumin of the brain edema, but also the albumin of the serum, the albumin of the spinal cord, and the serum albumin after the action of trypsin on the Sephadex column, and then we compared them.

HUSZÁK: The sodium as well as the water pump depend on the oxidative activity of the cells. I would like to ask Professor Cumings whether he has some experience concerning the activity of oxidative enzymes. In general, the glycolytic enzymes are not so sensitive to the anoxic state and to the water content of the cells as the oxidative enzymes present in the mitochondrial particles. The same experience can be obtained by experimental isolation of the mitochondrial system, chiefly in the white matter.

CUMINGS: This is a difficult question to answer, because the best experiments are those relating to the monkey. It is much more difficult to judge in the human material, where all the material was obtained post-mortem, but in the monkey anaerobic glycolytic enzymes and some of the others were done at biopsy. Now this paper from which I am quoting and the results will be published in about a month's time. So it will be all available for you and will be quoted in the actual reference (Brain. 88, 557-584, 1965).

LOWENTHAL: I would like to put a question related to what I said and would like to direct it to Dr. Seitelberger, because we once had a biopsy of a Creutzfeldt-Jakob case and we did not find any abnormal protein in that biopsy. Dr. Seitelberger said this morning that in Jakob-Creutzfeldt's disease there is an abnormal protein metabolism. I would like to have some comment on this.

SEITELBERGER: The table I showed about the general characters of glial dystrophies concerned degenerative types which occur in inborn metabolic errors such as hepato-cerebral degeneration or maple syrup disease. From the results of the studies on these diseases and the glial reactions in chronic alcoholics correlated to certain clinical findings, we brought up the hypothesis that changes in protein metabolism, which may be connected in several instances with hepatic lesions, can produce glial dystrophies. A special kind of glial dystrophy is also the anatomical basis of Jakob-Creutzfeldt's disease.

BROWNSON:* I would like to mention briefly some studies undertaken jointly with Dr. Larry W. McDonald,** related to early brain response to insult, with special reference to Dr. Jacob's referral to acute swelling of oligodendroglia. Our study utilized white male rats, 30 days of age. The experimental animals received total-head radiation (3/4 inch diameter beam defining aperture) of high energy (900 MeV) alpha particle radiation administered from the 184-inch cyclotron, using the plateau of the Bragg curve. The radiated animals received 10 k rads and were sacrificed during intervals of 50 minutes, 1.5, 2, 3, and 8 hours following exposure to the beam. All animals were anesthetized with pentobarbital-sodium and received intracardiac injection of sodium nitrite and heparin, followed by glutaraldhyde perfusion fixation. Tissue samples were removed from the corpus callosum, minced in buffered 1% osmium tetroxide, processed in araldite, sectioned on the Porter-Blum MT-2, double stained with uranyl acetate-lead citrate, and examined with the Hitachi (HU-11) electron microscope.

Preliminary results indicate that the fine structure of cells identified in earlier reports by light microscopy as degenerating oligodendrocytes undergoing acute swelling may be observed. The nucleus was round and eccentrically located, usually showing dense granules near the nuclear membrane. Lesser amounts of irregularly arranged aggregates of light and dark nuclear material were observed in the center of the nucleus. The inner nuclear membrane was intact and noticeably separated from the outer nuclear membrane, which consisted primarily of dense granules. Early cytoplasmic changes showed swollen mitochondria, enlarged Golgi apparatus and abundant vesicles. Although the nuclear membranes of degenerating cells were intact, their plasma membrane consistently showed interruptions suggesting that they had ruptured. A second plasma membrane, also showing interruptions, and apparently belonging to a cell surrounding the oligodendrocyte was encountered. The frequent breaks in opposing plasma membranes often co-existed over the same circumference between which fragments of debris appeared to be in passage. The cytoplasm of the surrounding cell was comparatively clear with scattered rough-surfaced endoplasmic reticulum, multi-sized vesicles and occasional mitochondria. A variety of

*Work supported by U. S. A. E. C. and N. I. H.

**N. I. H. Special Post-doctoral Fellow and Visiting Professor.

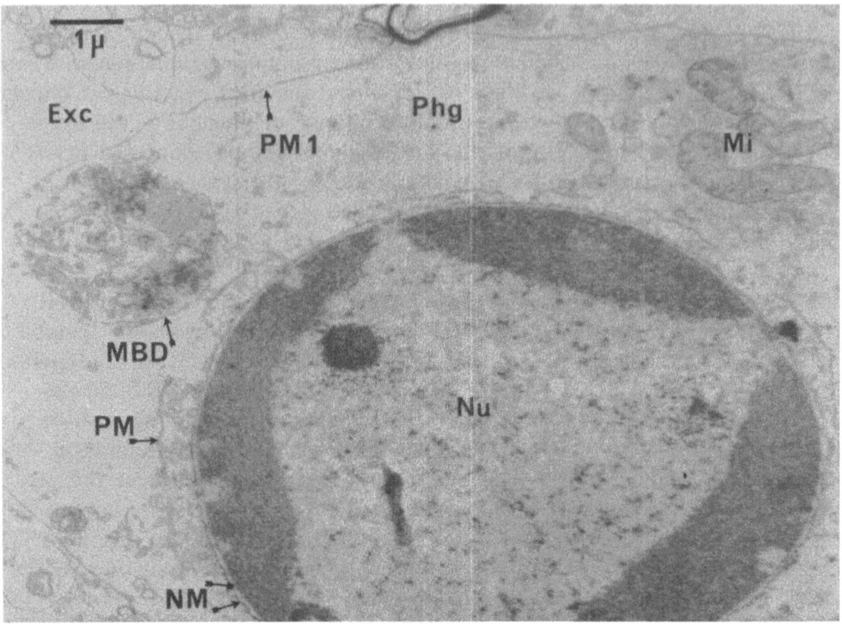

Interfascicular cell necrosis and phagocytosis, 6—hours. Clumping and margination of nuclear material (Nu). Nuclear membrane (NM) and adjacent plasma membrane of interfascicular cell (PM) and phagocyte cell (PM1). Watery phagocyte cytoplasm (Phg) containing swollen mitochondria (Mi) and membrane bound debris (MBD). Enlarged extracellular space is noted (Exc). X15,000.

different forms of necrotic cells were encountered, nearly all of which appeared to be damaged interfascicular glial cells, presumably oligodendroglia. The morphologic differences varied from early increased nuclear density accompanied by swelling of organelles to nearly total nuclear density and complete aggregation of cytoplasmic structures into dense irregular masses with interspersed membranes and dark granules. A condition common to all degenerating cells was the complete surrounding of the cell or cell remnant by a watery cytoplasm and isolation of fragments by limiting membranes suggesting a process of engulfment. The extremely early appearance of this phenomenon in 6 hours, the absence of an associated nucleus in the field and occasional appearance of fibrils within the engulfing cytoplasm suggests astrocyte involvement. Radiosensitive cells such as monuclear cells, phagocytic cells, or some hematogenous elements that may have been in the brain when radiated would seemingly suffer suppression or inactivation. Astrocytes on the other hand are not acutely inactivated by this dose level, but on the contrary appear to become more active with time. It has been my purpose here to call attention to the subject of acute swelling of oligodendroglia and the possible astrocyte role in phagocytosis.

KLIMKOVA-DEUTSCHOVA: Dr. Lampert, this fact of selectivity is very interesting. There is a local, developmental, and ontogenetic selectivity. As I have experience with human pathologic states of intoxication with workers in lead factories, I want to ask you whether you made any experiments with adult rats, because it is a well known fact that in adults we often see polyneuropathies, whereas in young people we more often see encephalopathies.

LAMPERT: Adult rats, even when poisoned with a large amount of lead carbonate, did not get sick. Only suckling rats developed this encephalopathy.

TORACK: (1) In these leaking vessels, were the junctions between endothelial cells normal or abnormal? (2) Did you think that these large vessels were venules or capillaries? (3) Were any thorotrast particles found in spaces not larger than 200 A° ?

LAMPERT: (1) Leaking vessels presented endothelial cells which were separated from each other, i.e., the junctions between endothelial cells were open. (2) Leaking vessels were interpreted as venules. (3) Thorotrast generally collected in extracellular spaces which were larger than 200 Å in width but individual particles were also found in "normally sized" intercellular clefts. I believe that the relative lack of an extracellular space in the gray matter as compared to the white matter limits but does not prevent the in vivo spread of colloidal substances. In this respect the following study is releveant (J. Neuropath. Exp. Neurol, 25: 531-541, 1966). We focused a LASER beam on the exposed skull of rats that were given an intravenous injection of Thorotrast just prior to LASER radiation. Underneath the impact area of the LASER beam we found a focal necrosis of the cerebral cortex which was surrounded by a zone of edema. Thorotrast particles which had escaped from disrupted vessels in the necrotic cortex were found for a short distance between swollen astrocytic processes in intercellular spaces of the edematous cortex (Fig. 1). In the subcortical edematous white matter very large extracellular spaces were encountered which apparently allowed for a more massive and widespread dissemination of Thorotrast (Fig. 2).

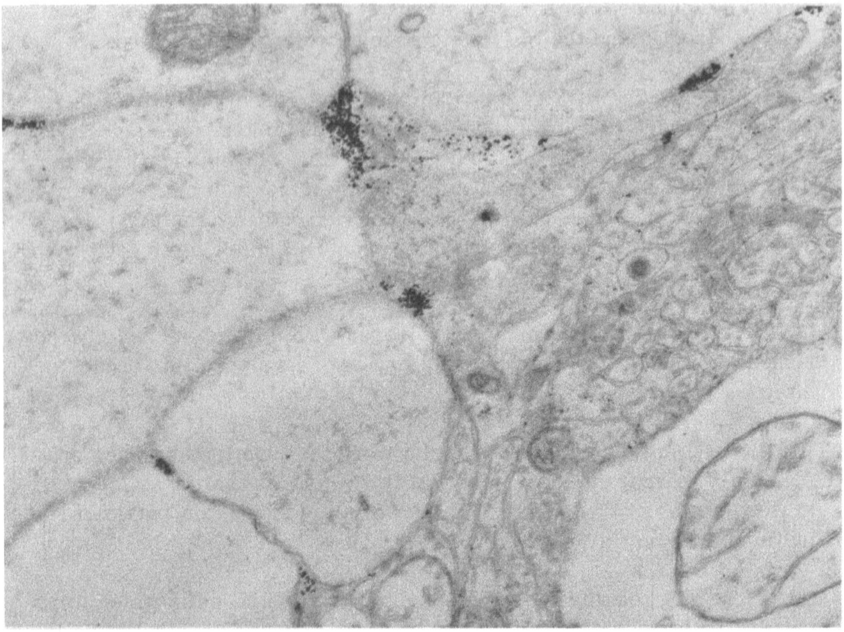

Fig. 1. Edematous cerebral cortex of rat one hour after LASER radiation. Thorotrast which was injected intravenously just prior to LASER radiation is seen in intercellular spaces between swollen astrocytic processes. X28,000.

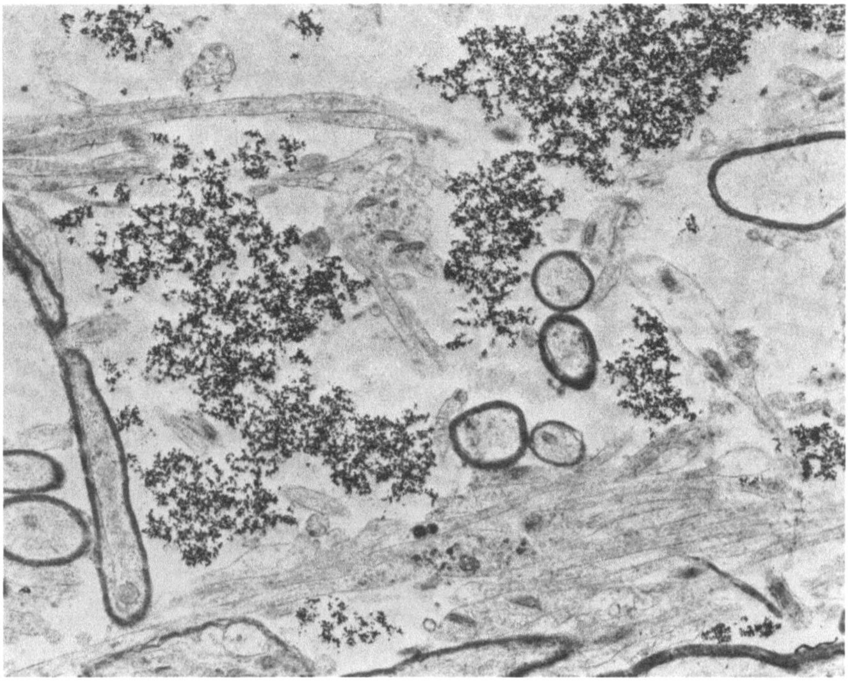

Fig. 2. Edematous subcortical white matter of rat 24 hours after LASER radiation. There are very wide extracellular spaces with massive deposits of Thorotrast which was injected intravenously just prior to LASER radiation. X10,000.

III. Fluid Compartments, Electrolytes and Transport Mechanisms

Chairmen: ***T. Broman and D. B. Tower***

MILTON W. BRIGHTMAN

MOVEMENT WITHIN THE BRAIN OF FERRITIN INJECTED INTO THE CEREBROSPINAL FLUID COMPARTMENTS

INTRODUCTION

It is appropriate at the outset of a symposium concerned with cerebral fluid compartments to examine the morphological evidence for and against the very occurrence of such compartments. Though preparative procedures are responsible for the large pericellular spaces within cerebral tissue visualized by light microscopy (Patek, 1944; Woolam & Millen, (1955), much smaller "gaps" of about 200 Å between all cells have been demonstrated electronmicroscopically. These intervals have been interpreted not as artifact but as representing the apposed lipid leaflets of adjacent cell membranes (Sjöstrand, 1958), or as the middle leaflets together with the fused outer leaflets of contiguous unit membranes (Schultz & Karlsson, 1965). According to either interpretation, there is no appreciable intercellular space except that of the synaptic cleft and other specialized junctions (Schultz & Karlsson, 1965). This view was supported by the observation that, following hydration of the brain, the 200 Å-wide interval remains constant while the glial cells become greatly distended. The excess water is envisioned as having moved from one cell directly into a neighboring cell across their contiguous plasmalemmas; the water so remains within the intracellular compartment (Gerschenfeld, Wald & Zadunaisky, 1959). However, the penetration of ferrocyanide into the 200 Å-wide gaps of the toad's retina (Lasansky & Wald, 1964) and of ferritin into the Schwann cell channels in the toad's spinal ganglion (Rosenbluth & Wissig, 1964) support Robertson's conclusion (1957) that these gaps are open, hydrated channels.

The observations reported here demonstrate that the intercellular clefts of the mammalian brain are also true spaces along which the protein molecule, ferritin, can freely move (Brightman, 1965b).

MATERIALS AND METHODS

Ferritin was selected as the tracer because it is a protein, each molecule of which is discernible, and because it occurs endogenously within the brain (Diezel, 1955). Ferritin solutions, from which the cadmium had been removed, were injected into the lateral cerebral ventricles of 12 male rats and into the cisterna magna of four male rats in amounts ranging from 15 mg (0.15ml) to 100 mg (1.0 ml) of ferritin. After periods of 12 minutes to 3 1/2 hours, the brains were fixed by perfusion of buffered osmium solutions through the cerebral ventricles or the aorta. Glutaraldehyde was perfused through the aorta of one animal. In order to ascertain the significance of ferritin that was freely dispersed within the cytoplasm, the ependyma and subependymal neuropil of two additional rats were fixed with osmium solution for two hours prior to the injection of the protein. The ependyma and subependymal neuropil of the ventricular system, the anterior medullary velum, and the adjacent medulla oblongata and cerebellum were examined electronmicroscopically. Details of the experiments are given elsewhere (Brightman, 1965a).

RESULTS

The ferritin molecule, about 100 Å in diameter, appears in the ensuing micrographs as a dense black sphere about 60 Å in diameter. This sphere represents the ferric core of the molecule, the surrounding apoferritin, protein shell being invisible. The molecules entered the interstices of the parenchyma by crossing its inner (ependymal) or outer (pia-glial) borders.

The epithelium lining the cerebral ventricles is exceptional in that at the ventricular lumen, the junction between adjacent cells is usually open (Fig. 1) rather than closed (cf. Farquhar & Palade, 1963). Closures of the interspace usually occur at variable distances from the ventricle in the form of discrete "fasteners" rather than encompassing girdles. As a consequence, ferritin can enter the interspace of the luminal junctions and thence along the entire intercellular space by circumventing these short, intermembranous fusions (Brightman, 1965a). The basal plasmalemma of the ependyma was not subtended by a continuous basement membrane (Tennyson & Pappas, 1962; Brightman & Palay, 1963). Instead, the extracellular

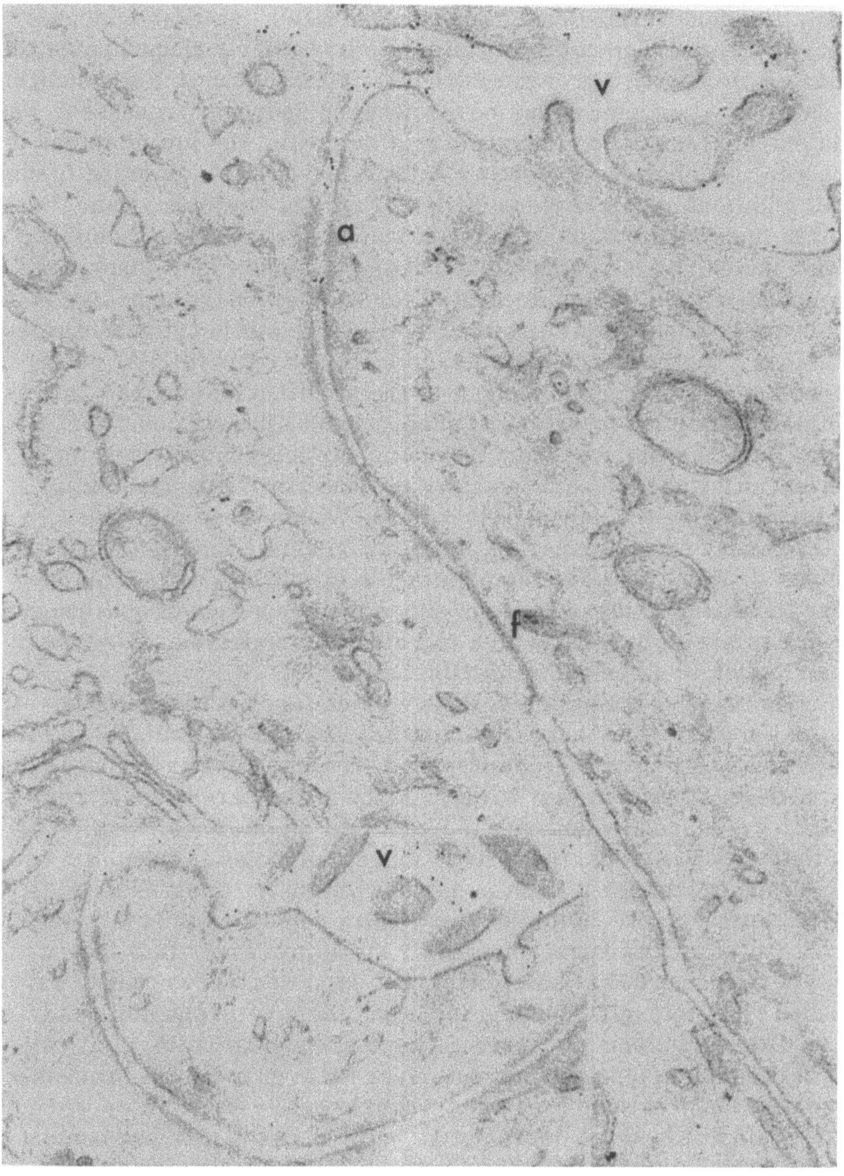

Fig. 1. Ferritin molecules have moved from the ventricle (v) into the interspace of an adhering zonule (a) between two ependymal cells. A few micelles occur on either side of an obliquely sectioned intercellular fusion (f). X75,000.(reduced). Ferritin lies within two uncoated pinocytotic pits formed by the luminal plasmalemma and within the open, arcuate junction communicating with the ventricle (v). X75,000 (reduced). Ventricle IV; glutaraldehyde-fixed; stained with lead salts.

space between the bases of adjacent cells was focally distended to contain a moderately dense, amorphous "filler" similar in appearance to basement membrane material. Irregularly shaped pools of dense material also occured infrequently throughout the parenchyma between glial processes but never between neuronal processes. Near the pia-glial border at the surface of the brain, the invaginations of the glial plasmalemma together with its basement membrane formed still additional pools of dense filler. Ferritin micelles accumulated within the ubiquitous though discontinuous system of extracellular filler including the perivascular basement membrane. Pinocytosis by ependymal cells also accounted for an additional accumulation of molecules which were stored intracellularly within cytoplasmic inclusions. The result of this intracellular and extracellular entrapment was a filtering out of most of the micelles leaving only a few colloidal particles to enter the subependymal interstices.

However, in most animals, many particles moved well into the parenchymal interspaces after pouring across damaged glial cells bordering the subarachnoid fluid. Within these processes, micelles lay freely dispersed in the cytoplasmic matrix (Fig. 3). Such a distribution was also obtained in ependymal cells fixed before the introduction of protein. Since the deposition of non-bounded micelles was coincident with a ruptured plasmalemma, this type of distribution was considered artifactual.

In many of the animals, though much ferritin had initially entered the interstices across a damaged glial border, numerous micelles had penetrated the interspaces, including synaptic clefts (Fig. 5), at least 30 μ from this border. Much of the parenchymal interspace was mured by apparently intact cell membranes (Figs. 4, 5). In the deeper regions, there were more molecules in the clefts between the processes than in inclusions within the processes (Figs. 4, 5). Furthermore, micelles were more numerous in focally distended confluences between three or more processes than they were within the usual 200 Å-wide clefts, but particles were entirely excluded from interglial fusions including the myelin sheaths. Intermembranous fusions occurred between ependymal cells, glial cells, or between both types of cell but never between neuronal processes. The proximity of such fusions to a focal confluence (with or without filler) emphasized the degree of variability in the size and content of the extracellular space. The plasmalemmas lining the deeper reaches of the interspace were not only intact, but capable of pinocytosing micelles (Figs. 3, 6).

Apparently, a cell process must be at least 300 Å-wide before it can form pinocytotic indentations (Brightman, 1965b). For example, where the perivascular attenuations of glial end-feet were thinner than approximately 300 Å, pinocytotic pits were not evident while, in

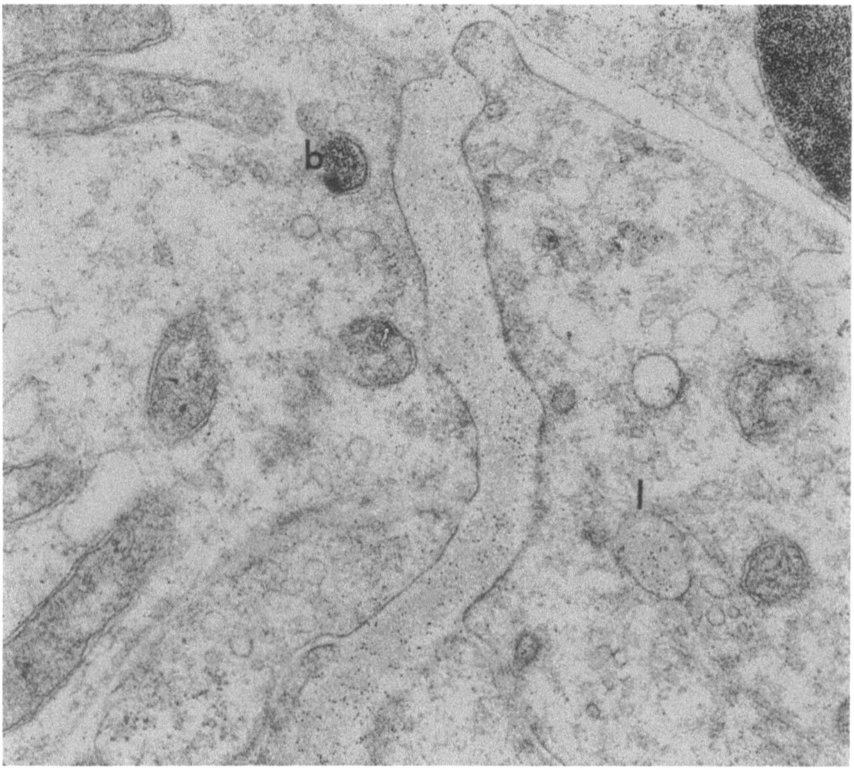

Fig. 2. The distended interspace between two adjacent ependymal cells contains a dense "filler" within which ferritin accumulates. A small dense body (b) packed with ferritin may be compared with a transversely sectioned invagination of the filler (i). A portion of a large dense body in an adjoining glial cell is packed with ferritin molecules (upper right corner); the cytoplasm of this cell contains freely dispersed micelles. X50,000 (reduced).

an adjacent thicker portion of the same process, ferritin-laden vesicles were present in the cytoplasm (Fig. 3). Ferritin-containing vesicles were encountered far more frequently in astrocytic and ependymal processes than they were in neuronal processes. In all processes, some particles were enclosed within large vesicles bearing a granular or filamentous coat. Most often, however, the wall of the pinocytotic vesicle was not densely rimmed, the wall being identical to the remainder of the adjacent plasmalemma. The micelles were often segregated within multivesicular bodies and sometimes in crystalloid array within dense bodies of ependymal and glial cells. Occasionally, ferritin-containing vacuoles occured within pericytes and within a few endothelial cells.

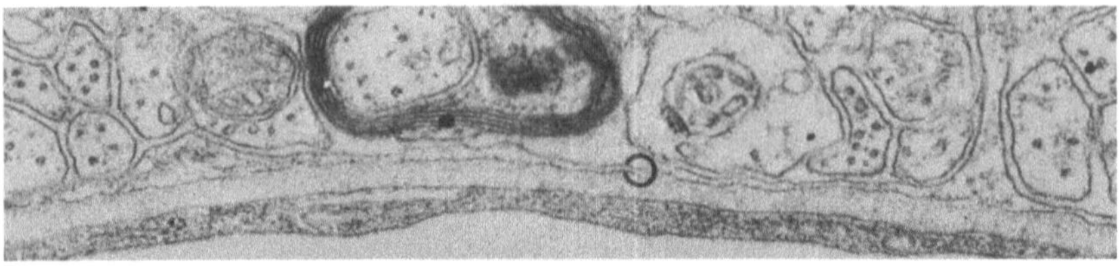

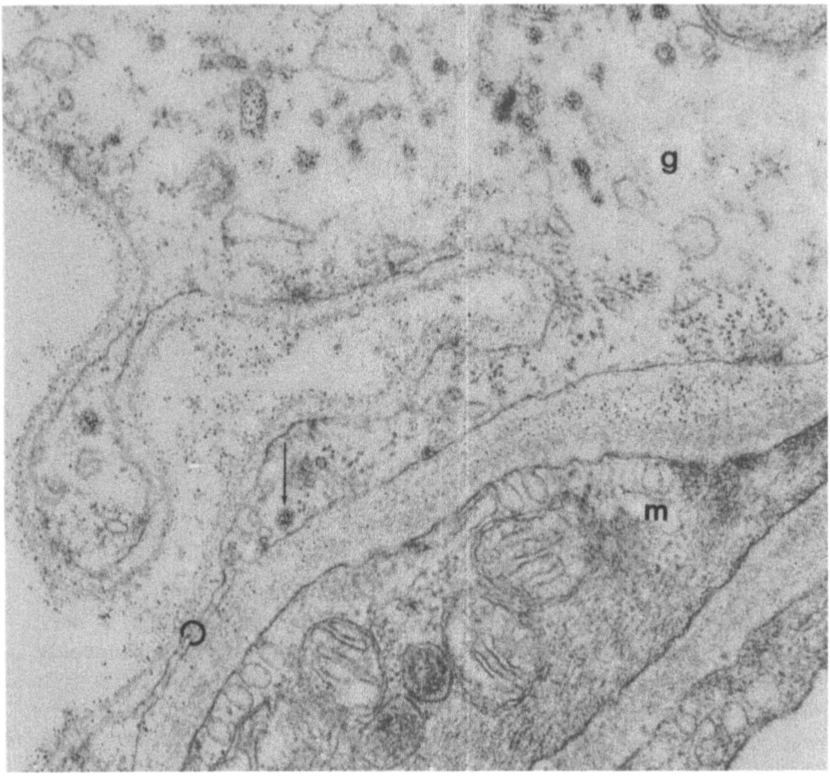

Fig. 3. The broad portions of a glial cell (g) fronting a large parenchymal vessel contains many ferritin-laden vesicles (arrow, e.g.). The attenuated portion (encircled) contains no vesicles. Ferritin has accumulated in the basement membranes shared by the glial and smooth muscle cell (m), but none has reached the vesicles of this cell or of the endothelial cell (lower right). The glial cytoplasm also contains freely dispersed micelles. Medulla oblongata. X65,000 (reduced). Portions of the perivascular sheath are T-shaped, the cross-bar being an attenuated sheet (encircled) that does not contain vesicles. Subependyma of ventricle III; hamster; lead-stained. X55,000 (reduced).

Within neuronal somata and processes, especially the dendritic ones, ferritin was sequestered predominantly within multivesicular bodies. Coated pinocytotic indentations occurred at any point along

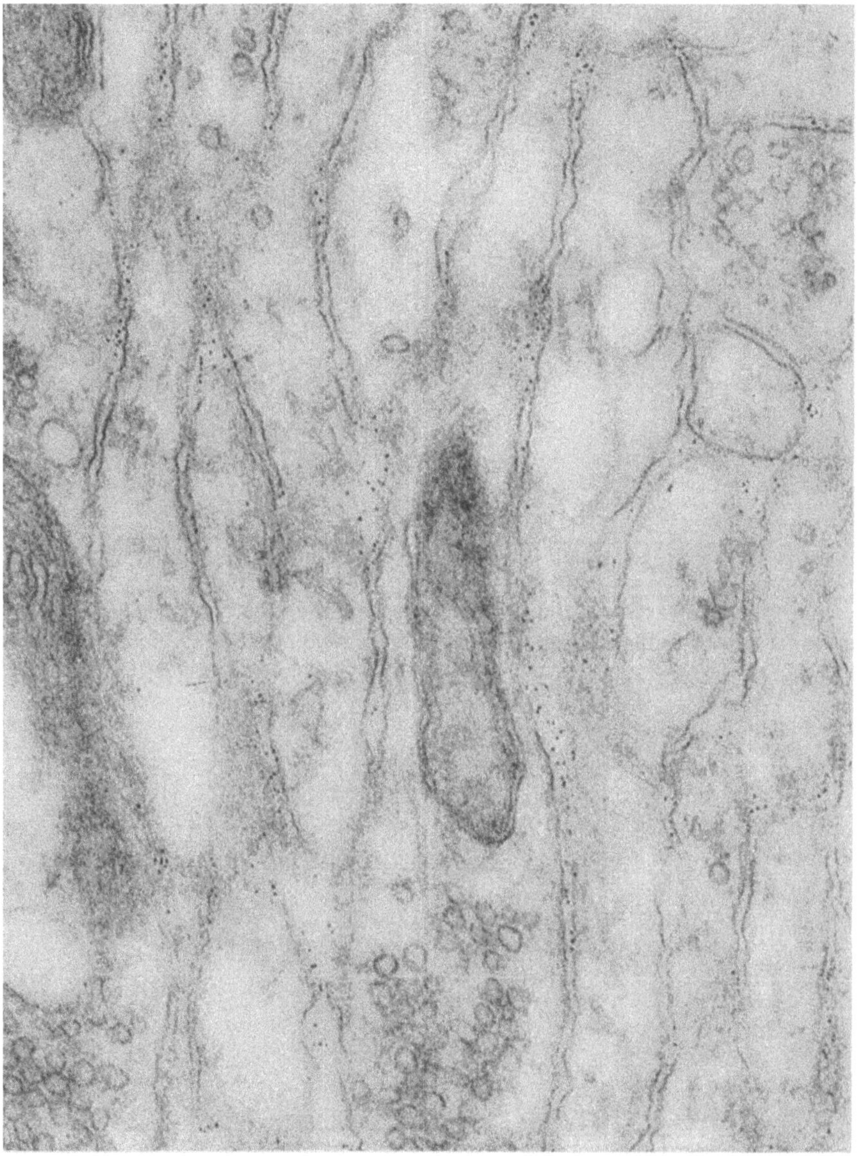

Fig. 4. The electron lucent clefts between neuronal and glial processes of the cerebellar parenchyma contain many ferritin molecules. There are no pinocytosed micelles in this field. Molecular layer of the cerebellum. X90,000 (reduced).

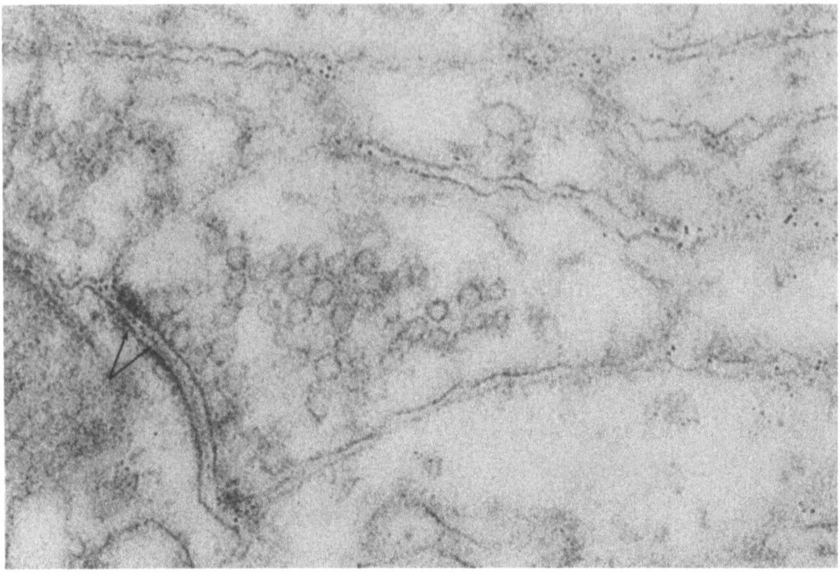

Fig. 5. Ferritin molecules occur within the electron lucent channels and the synaptic cleft (arrows) of the periaqueductal neuropil. X90,000 (reduced).

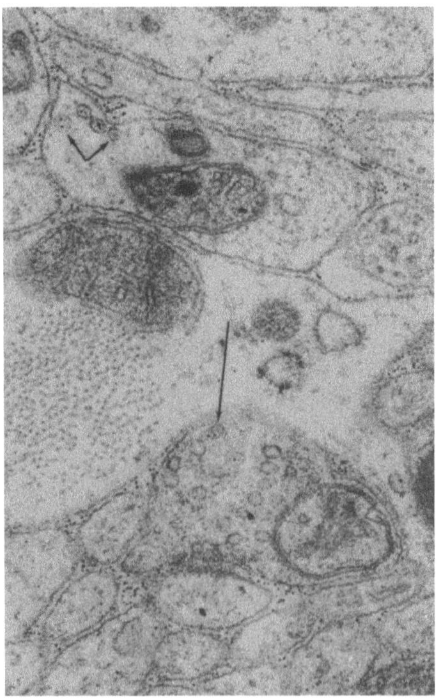

Fig. 6. Ferritin lies within the intercellular channels of the cerebral parenchyma and within vesicles inside one process that is probably glial (short arrows) and within a single vesicle near the plasmalemma of a presynaptic ending (long arrow). Iter. X58,000 (reduced).

the neuronal plasmalemma, and were easily distinguished from synaptic vesicles by virtue of their extraneous coat and their larger diameter. However, an occasional uncoated vesicle, indistinguishable from the neighboring synaptic vesicles, also contained micelles (Figs. 6, 7, 8). Such vesicles usually occurred singly, directly beneath the plasmalemma.

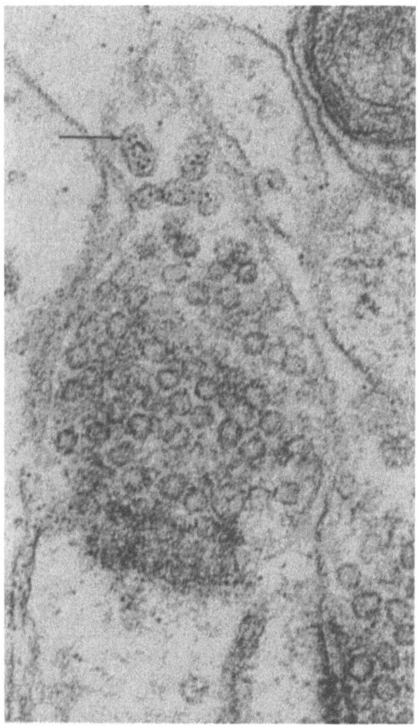

Fig. 7. One end of a pre-synaptic terminal contains five vesicles enclosing ferritin. The upper two vesicles (arrow) are large and irregular in shape. The lower three vesicles are more similar in size and shape to the synaptic vesicles filling the rest of the terminal. Iter. X100,000 (reduced).

DISCUSSION

It is concluded that the 150 to 200 Å-wide electron lucent clefts between cell processes of the rat brain represent true, patent spaces along which the large protein molecule, ferritin can move. The space between neuronal processes is often narrowed at the synaptic cleft by a short constriction about 40 Å-wide (Van Der Loos, 1963), which is too narrow to allow passage of the ferritin molecule. However, as the stricture is usually confined to one end of the cleft, micelles would be able to penetrate via the opposite, wider end as far as the dense lamina within the cleft (Brightman, 1965b).

Whereas the focal distentions of the interspace containing dense filler and the perivascular basement membranes "trap" ferritin some micelles may still be accessible to the bordering plasmalemmas. However, the occluded portions of the interspace that are formed by interglial fusions entirely exclude the molecules. These five-layered fusions occur invariably between ependymal cells near the ventricular lumen and between perivascular glial processes. Their occurrence between glial cells elsewhere in the parenchyma appears random in position and variable in extent. It is likely that these fusions are usually not very extensive but short and circumventable. Intermembranous fusions do not occur between neuronal processes in the portions of the rat brain examined, nor are they as extensive as those recently described in swollen cerebral tissue fixed in glutaraldehyde (Schultz & Karlsson, 1965). The formation of these apparently artifactual five-layered junctions in swollen tissue, however, indicates caution in interpreting the disposition of micelles in the interspace on either side of, but never within, an intermembranous fusion. Thus, if intracellular swelling, be it artifactual or real, developes <u>after</u> the penetration of ferritin, micelles would be squeezed from an obliterating interspace; if intracellular swelling occurs <u>before</u> the introduction of ferritin, the protein would be prevented from entering the already occluded interstices. But, if fixation with osmium solutions is adequate, then what intracellular swelling that may occur is insufficient to obliterate the interspaces. The ubiquitous occurrence of the large ferritin molecule within the 200 Å-wide clefts and within the distended confluences of osmium-fixed brains is hardly consistent with the speculation that, following such fixation, there is a "virtual disappearance" of the extracellular space (Rall, Oppelt & Patlack, 1962).

The attenuated portions of the perivascular glial end-feet which usually cap part of the endothelium would be expected to offer a relatively slight barrier to the diffusion of gases, water and solutes. But such thin processes would act as formidable though localized barrier to the passage of colloids insofar as these processes have not been

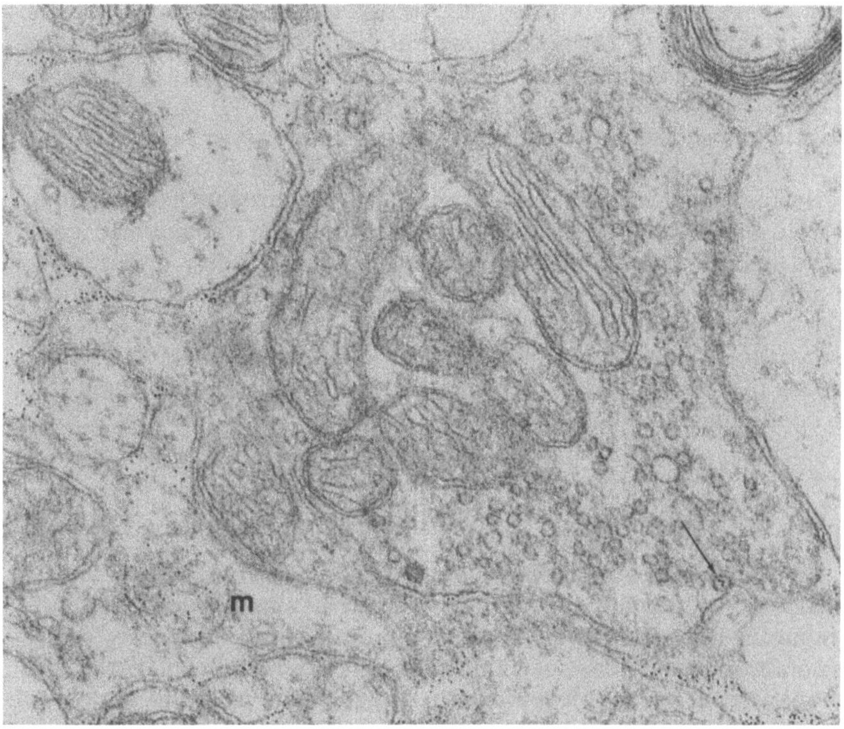

Fig. 8. This pre-synaptic ending contains many vesicles of different dimensions. The smaller vesicles are regarded as synaptic. One vesicle (arrow), uncoated and about as big as the synaptic vesicles, lies next to the plasmalemma and contains three ferritin molecules. Micelles also lie within the multivesicular body (m) of an unidentified process and within the intercellular clefts. Ventricle IV. X65,000 (reduced).

observed to form pinocytotic invaginations. The absence of pinocytotic vesicles may be due to such factors as increased viscosity of the narrowed cytoplasm, and a heightened mutual electrostatic repulsion of the approximated membranes (Brightman, 1965b). Furthermore, Curtis has suggested (1965) that the drainage of aqueous medium from the attenuated process would probably be so slow, that any further approximation of the plasmalemmas, i.e., pitting, could not occur within a reasonable time.

The limiting plasmalemma of glia and neuronal processes that are sufficiently broad can form pinocytotic vesicles that are usually uncoated and about as big as synaptic vesicles. Within pre-synaptic endings, the occasional incorporation of ferritin within vesicles that are indistinguishable from synaptic vesicles (Figs. 6, 7, 8) suggests several interpretations: (1) though the great majority of vesicles are synaptic, a few are pinocytotic; (2) synaptic vesicles arise from the plasmalemma only infrequently and, in so doing, pinocytose whatever is present in the immediate interspace; (3) a preformed synaptic vesicle situated near the plasmalemma may fuse with it, becoming pinocytotic in response to the presence of protein in the interspace (an unlikely series of events). The present results demonstrate that, although localized variations in the dimensions, configuration, and content of true pericellular spaces may either slow the movement of colloid or entirely exclude it, large protein molecules are, nevertheless, able to permeate the interstices of the brain. A substance placed in a cerebral ventricle can penetrate the far reaches of the interspace to become directly available not only to glial cells and neuronal somata, but to synaptic endings as well.

SUMMARY

Within the brain of the rat, the 200 Å-wide pericellular spaces, visualized electronmicroscopically, are true spaces along which ferritin molecules can move. This movement is stopped locally by intermembranous fusions, of variable extent, between contiguous glial and ependymal cells. Movement is also impeded by pools of dense, amorphous "filler" between ependymal cells, glial cells, and about the smooth muscle cells and endothelial cells of parenchymal and subarachnoid vessels. This filler accumulates large numbers of particles. Nevertheless, many of these protein molecules penetrate the parenchymal interstices at least 30 μ from the subarachnoid border by moving pinocytotically and, in places, intercellularly across the glial border primarily and the ependymal border to a lesser extent.

Once inside the interspaces, some of the micelles are pinocytosed and segregated predominantly by glial processes which must, however, have a minimal width of approximately 300 Å before pinocytotic indentations can be formed. Endothelial cells and neuronal processes incorporate less of the protein. Occasionally, ferritin-laden vesicles occur among synaptic vesicles from which they are indistinguishable. Thus, substances placed in the ventricle can move intercellularly as well as intracellularly to eventually be incorporated directly from the interspace into all cell processes, including synaptic terminals.

REFERENCES

Brightman, M. W. and S. L. Palay: The fine structure of ependyma in the brain of the rat, J. Cell Biol., 19, 415-439 (1963).

_____: The distribution within the brain of ferritin injected into cerebrospinal fluid compartments. I. Ependymal Distribution, J. Cell Biol., 26, 99-123 (1965a).

_____: The distribution within the brain of ferritin injected into cerebrospinal fluid compartments. II; Parenchymal distribution, Am. J. Anat., 117, 193-200 (1965b).

Curtis, A. S. G.: Personal communication (1965).

Diezel, P. B.: Iron in the brain: A chemical and histochemical examination, in: Biochemistry of the developing nervous system (ed. by H. Waelsch), New York: Academic Press, pp. 145-152 (1955).

Farquar, M. G. and G. E. Palade: Junctional complexes in various epithelia, J. Cell Biol., 17, 375-412 (1963).

Gerschenfeld, H. M., F. Wald, J. A. Zadunaisky and E. D. P. De Robertis: Function of astroglia in the water-ion metabolism of the central nervous system, Neurology, 9, 412-425 (1959).

Lasansky, A. and F. J. Wald: The extracellular space in the toad retina as defined by the distribution of ferrocyanide, A light and electron microscope study, 15: 3, 463-480 (1963).

Patek, P.: The perivascular spaces of the mammalian brain, Anat. Rec., 88, 1-24 (1944).

Rall, D. P., W. Oppelt and C. S. Patlak: Extracellular space of brain as determined by diffusion of inulin from the ventricular system, Life Sciences, 2, 43-48 (1962).

Robertson, J. D.: New observations on the ultrastructure of the membranes of frog peripheral nerve fibers, J. Biophys. Biochem. Cytol., 3, 1043-1048 (1957).

Rosenbluth, J. and S. L. Wissig: The distribution of exogenous ferritin in toad spinal ganglia and the mechanism of its uptake by neurons, J. Cell Biol., 23, 307-326 (1964).

Schultz, R. L. and U. Karlsson: Fixation of the central nervous system for electron microscopy by aldehyde perfusion, II, J. Ultrastr. Res., 12, 187-206 (1965).

Sjöstrand, F. S.: Ultrastructure of retinal rod synapses of the guinea pig eye as revealed by three-dimensional reconstructions from serial sections, Ibid., 2, 122-170 (1958).

Tennyson, V. M. and G. D. Pappas: An electron microscope study of ependymal cells of the fetal, early postnatal and adult rabbit, Zeit. f. Zellforsch., 56, 595-618 (1962).

Van Der Loos, H.: Fine structure of synapses in the cerebral cortex, Ibid., 60, 815-825 (1963).

Woolam, D. H. M. and J. W. Millen: The perivascular spaces of the mammalian central nervous system and their relation to the perineuronal and subarachnoid spaces, J. Anat., 89, 193-200 (1955).

HERMANN HAGER

MORPHOLOGICAL COMPARTMENTS IN THE CENTRAL NERVOUS SYSTEM

During the physiological studies on the functional compartments (extracellular space, glial space, neuronal space) of the central nervous system, the need for a comparison of these measurements with the morphological characteristics of the nervous tissue, and for the correlation of these two approaches, became apparent. In addition to the functional compartmentation, the structural delineation of the cerebral spaces would be of paramount importance for the interpretation of the pathological changes which are characteristic of cerebral edema. Various investigations were undertaken to determine the functional extracellular space in the brain. Determinations of the chloride space (Tower, 1958) and measurements of cortical impedance (van Harreveld & Ochs, 1956) tend to substantiate a space of 25-30%. However, the functional extracellular compartment, as measured with radioactive sulfate (Woodbury, 1958), thiocyanate (Streicher, 1961), and C -sucrose (Reed & Woodbury, 1960), was significantly smaller (4-15%) than the chloride space. Light microscopic investigations of the morphological spaces using any or all of the histological methods at our command demonstrated nerve cell bodies, myelinated and unmyelinated nerve fibers, coarser ramifications of dendrites and neuroglia cells with their processes. However, there remained a space between the ramifications of all these elements, the nature of which could not be resolved. Nissl (1903) called these spaces "nervöses Grau." Campbell (1905) referred to the "terra incognita" which remained when cells, fibers and neuroglia were substracted. The presence of a ground substance of a protein-carbohydrate nature occupying these spaces was suggested by Hess (1953) using histochemical staining. Electron microscopy has revealed a complete filling of these spaces with cell processes (Fig. 1). These

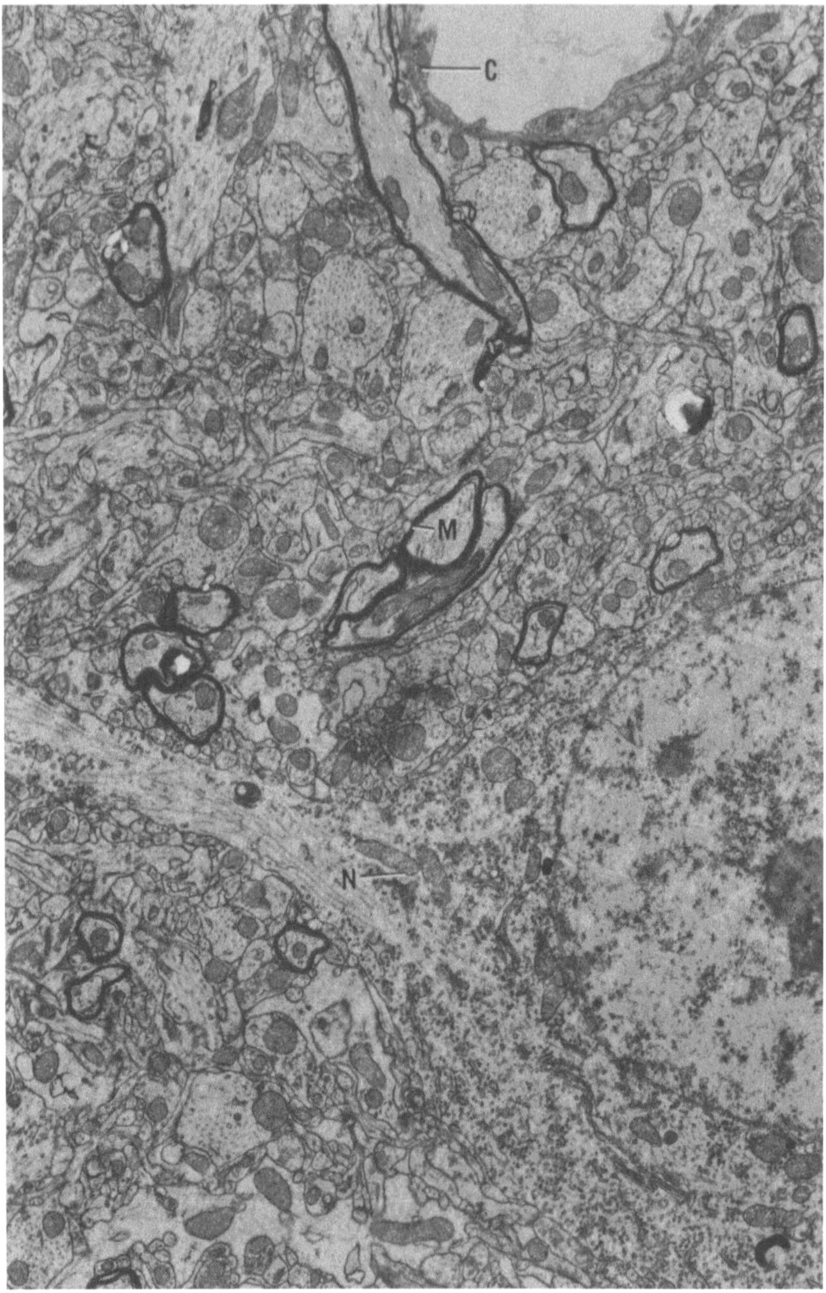

Fig. 1. Survey micrograph of the parietal cortex of the rabbit brain. Part of a nerve cell (N) and a capillary (C) are included in the field. At this magnification all cellular processes of the neuropil are closely apposed. Note the close contact of the cell processes with the capillary wall. M = Myelinated nerve fibers. Fixation by glutaraldehyde perfusion. X9,000 (reduced).

processes, which form the neuropil in the submicroscopical range, are closely packed together. The surface membranes of neighboring elements are separated by a constant distance of 150-200 Å. Consequently, this results in a continuous system of extracellular gaps. The extracellular space is limited to these gaps (Niessing & Vogell, 1957; Horstmann, 1957; Hager, 1959; Horstmann & Meves, 1959). The measurements in electron micrographs of osmium tetroxide fixed tissue show that in the central nervous system the mean percentage of extracellular space does not exceed 5% of the total volume (Horstmann & Meves, 1959). Some speculations have been made about the nature of the intercellular gap substance. Robertson (1958) has proposed that the gap substance is composed of a highly hydrated gel which is probably a mucopolysaccharide. Sjöstrand had originally suggested that the light zone between paired membrane structures was composed of compact lipid layers. However, according to his newer theory (Sjöstrand, 1960), a single surface membrane has an over-all thickness of approximately 125 Å, and a true extracellular space does not exist between the apposed membranes.

Recently, Karlsson and Schultz (1964, 1965) and Schultz and Karlsson (1965) used buffered glutaraldehyde of low concentration (2.5%, pH 7.4) for perfusion fixation of the central nervous system. With this method they often found a much closer cell to cell membrane relationship than after osmic acid fixation, and at times a complete occlusion of the intercellular gap.

Another important finding was a difference in the appearance of the plasma membrane (Fig. 2). After glutaraldehyde fixation the membranes appeared triple layered as first shown by Robertson (1957) and interpreted by him in terms of a general pattern of molecular organization (Robertson 1959, 1960, 1962). A five-layered membrane complex is also often formed by the fusion of the outer membrane lamellae. This was interpreted as favouring Sjöstrand's concept mentioned above. Nevertheless, the structure of the fused or separated paired membranes can be readily understood in terms of the unit membrane concept of Robertson.

In our laboratory we use a considerably higher concentration of buffered glutaraldehyde solution (6.5%, pH 7.4) for perfusion fixation of the central nervous system (Rewcastle, 1965). Excellent tissue preservation was obtained by this method. We occasionally found variations in the distance between surface membranes of the cell processes forming the neuropil, at times including fusion of the apposed membranes (Fig. 2). For the most part, however, there was an extracellular gap greater than 100 Å.

Van Harreveld, on the other hand, disagrees with the concepts referred to in the preceding discussion. He suggests that the han-

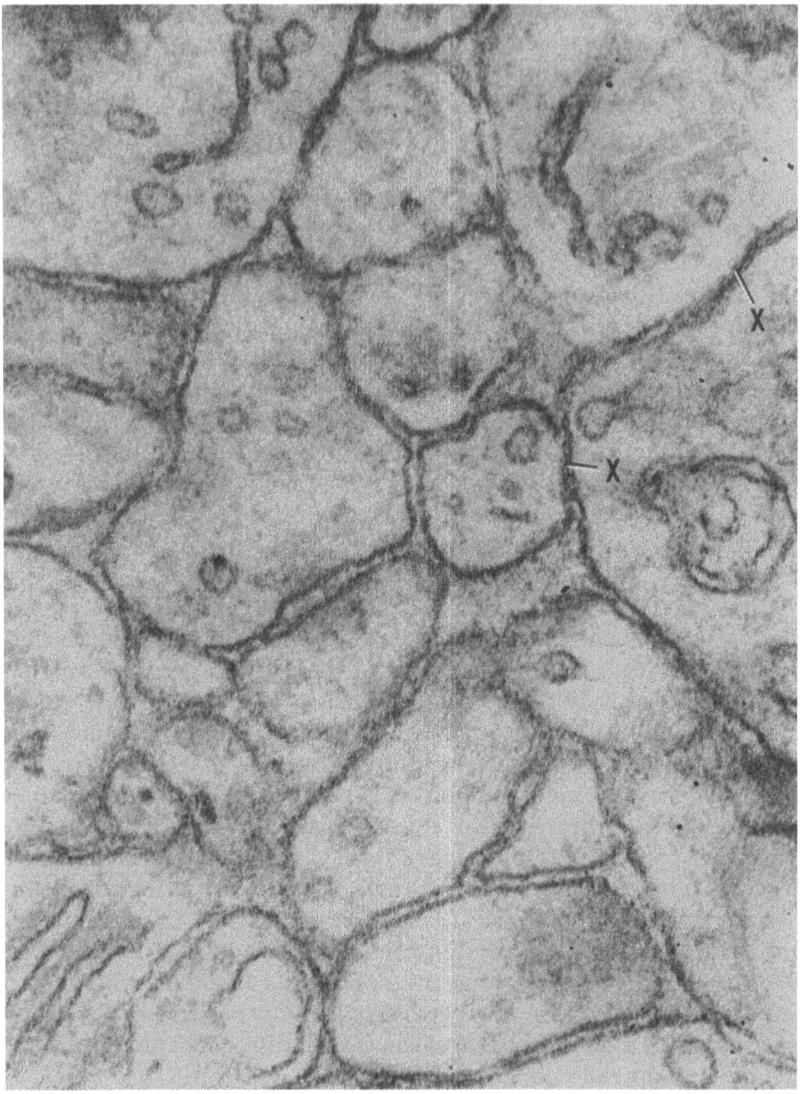

Fig. 2. Part of the neuropil of the parietal cortex of the rabbit brain. The cell processes are surrounded by a thin extracellular space. Occasionally (X) a close apposition of the triple layered membranes, forming a five-layered complex can be seen. Fixation by glutaraldehyde perfusion. X120,000.

dling of the tissue during fixation results in hypoxia and a rapid intracellular movement of chloride and water from the extracellular compartment. As he points out, the high concentration of extracellular electrolytes in the central nervous system and the low specific impedance represent indirect evidence for a large extracellular space (van Harreveld, 1957; Van Harreveld & Ochs, 1956). Additional suggestive evidence includes the large impedance rise observed following arrest of the blood supply to the brain (van Harreveld & Ochs, 1956) and after asphyxiation (Schadé, 1963). On the basis of impedance measurements, the volume of free extracellular fluid would have to be approximately 30% of the total volume of the cortex. To support their contention van Harreveld and Crowell (1964) subjected the cerebellar cortex to substitution fixation. In tissue frozen immediately after circulatory arrest, an extracellular space of approximately 24% was observed. In tissue frozen after 8 minutes, asphyxiation, the extracellular spaces had disappeared. If the observations of van Harreveld and his co-workers are correctly interpreted and swelling of the intracellular compartment causes a diminution of the extracellular space, then the results of osmic acid and glutaraldehyde fixation must be erroneous.

In considering the changes which occur in cerebral edema, it is also of importance to establish the volume of extracellular space normally present in the white matter. As in the cerebral cortex we have observed that the myelinated fibers and other cell processes of the white matter are closely packed together. Other investigators have described extracellular spaces consisting mostly of triangular wedges with an average diameter of 500-1000 Å between the surface membranes of these processes (Gonatas, Zimmerman & Levine, 1963; Brambring, 1965). The measured volume of the extracellular space, using electron micrographs, was 10% of the total volume of the white matter. We are convinced that shrinkage of the compact myelin sheath during fixation and embedding can produce such an enlargement of the extracellular compartment. That a considerable shrinkage of the layer spacings occurs as a result of the preparative procedures has been established by electron microscopy and analysis of X-ray diffraction patterns (Fernandez-Moran & Finean, 1958).

The evidence obtained from electron microscopic examination of the extracellular space may be summarized as follows: The volume of extracellular space in comparison to that in other organs is very small. This volume corresponds well to the functional space as measured with radioactive sulfate and thiocyanate. Numerous investigators have demonstrated that fixation and other preparative procedures do affect the extent of this space demonstrable in the electron microscope. Therefore, these observations are not entirely conclusive with respect to the extent of the extracellular space *in vivo*.

In the central nervous system, perivascular spaces can be observed around arteries and larger veins (Figs. 3, 4). Basement membranes have a special significance as limiting structures of these spaces. The inner lining of the perivascular space in the brain is

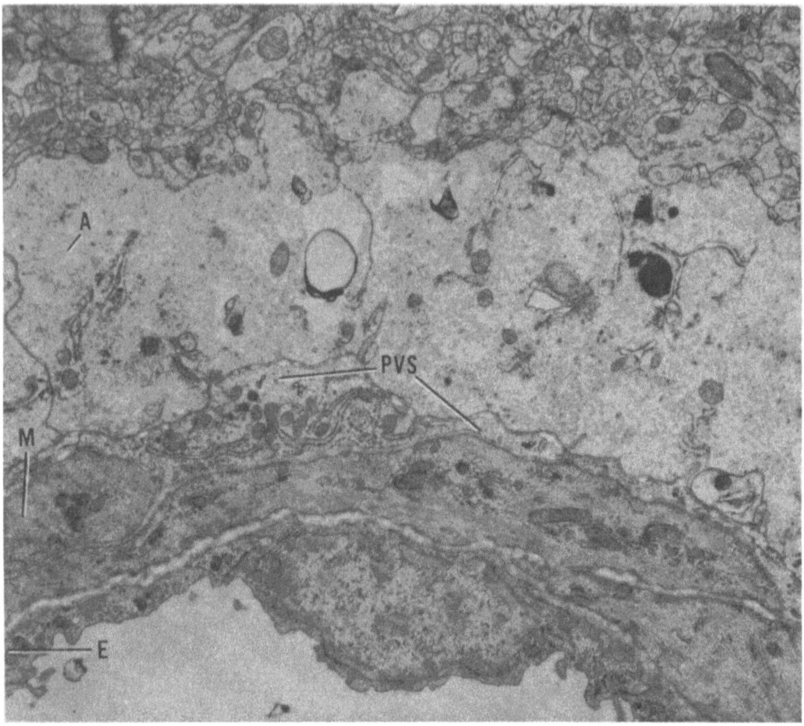

Fig. 3. Perivascular space around a transversely sectioned small artery in the cerebral cortex. The outer border of this space (PVS) is formed by a layer of astrocytic processes (A) and their overlying basement membrane. Adventitial cell processes can be seen. Several smooth muscle cells (M) are completely enclosed by vascular basement membrane which is continuous with that of the endothelium (E). X9,000 (reduced).

the basement membrane of the vessel wall. The outer lining is the basement membrane which covers the perivascular astrocytic processes (Nelson, Blinzinger & Hager, 1961; Hager, 1961). Adventitial elements are always found within this space. As the vascular channels proceed to the capillary level the outer and inner lining basement membranes fuse resulting in an obliteration of the perivascular space. Here the surface membranes of the astrocytic processes which form a complete sheet around the capillary are in

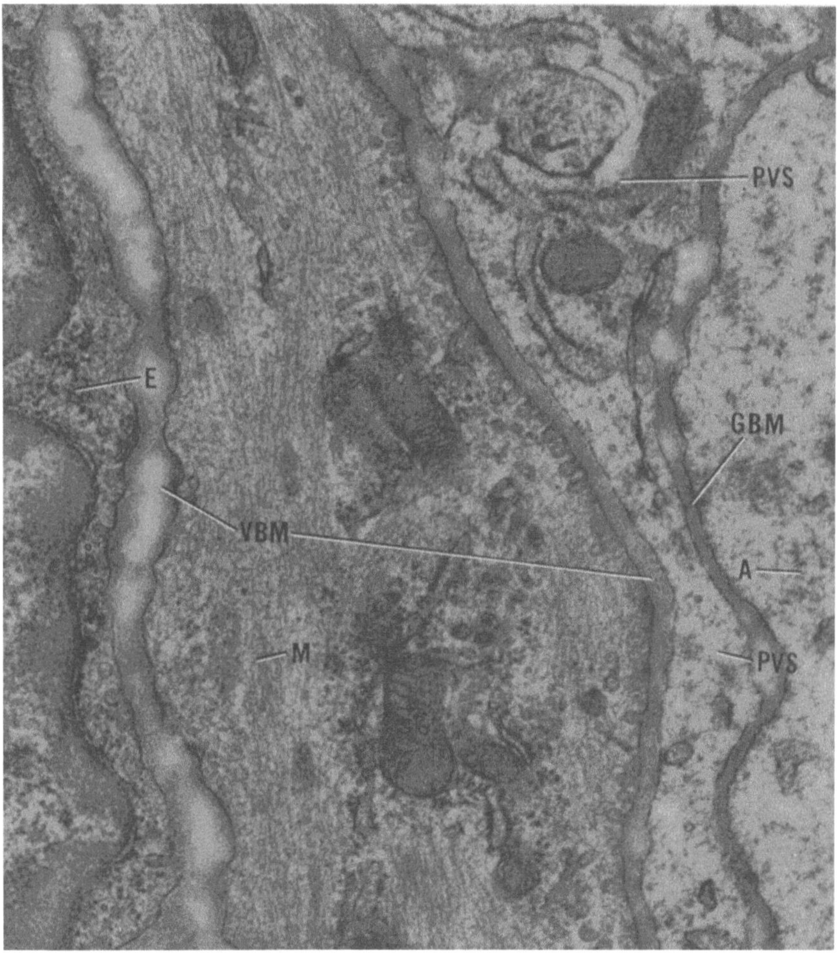

Fig. 4. Borders of the perivascular space around a small artery in the cerebral cortex. A continuous vascular basement membrane complex (VBM) lines the endothelium (E) and encloses the smooth muscle cells (M), and together with the glial basement (GBM) covering the perivascular astrocytic processes (A), forms the boundaries of the perivascular space (PVS) which contains an adventitial process. X45,000 (reduced).

close contact with the vessel wall (Fig 5). The lack of an extended pericapillary space, which is generally found in other organs, is thought to be the essential morphological substrate of the so-called blood-brain barrier (Hager, 1961). The direct contact of the surface membrane of the astrocytic end-feet on the capillary basement membrane complex apparently has an inhibitory function on the transport

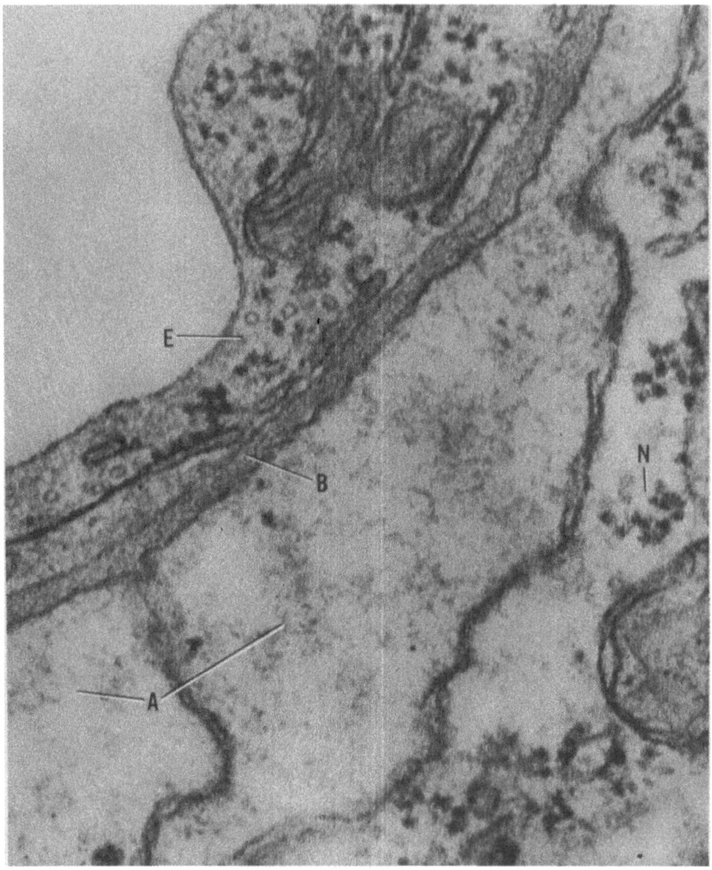

Fig. 5. Portion of a capillary in the cerebral cortex. The surface membranes of the pericapillary astrocytic foot process (A) are in close contact with the single basement membrane (B). E = endothelium, N = part of neuronal cytoplasm. Fixation by glutaraldehyde perfusion. X120,000 (reduced).

of materials. The absence of a perivascular space around capillaries prevents free diffusion which can occur around the capillaries of other organs. The pathway for the transfer of fluid, electrolytes and metabolites from blood vessels to neurons is represented by a cellular compartment, the astrocytic space.

Koch, Ranck and Newman (1962) brought further confirmation to the view that the large chloride space of the nervous system may represent the fluid of both the extracellular and the astroglial compartments as first suggested by Woodbury (1958). This astroglial compartment of the tissue may account for the cortical impedance findings interpreted by van Harreveld as favoring a large extracellular space.

In the electron microscope the astrocyte exhibits a "watery" clear cytoplasm (Fig. 6). The low density of the cytoplasmic matrix may reflect a relatively high intravital hydration. The poorly developed endoplasmic reticulum consists of small tubules and cisternae. A small amount of ribosomes is present. The Golgi zone is well developed. The mitochondria vary considerably in size and shape. A special form of mitochondria can be observed in subpial and perivascular astrocytes (Blinzinger, Rewcastle and Hager 1964, 1965). The interior structural pattern of these unusual mitochondria is characterized by the presence of numerous equilateral prismatic tubules having a highly regular arrangement. This structural pattern may be of special functional significance.

Further suggestions of the metabolic importance of the astroglial compartment comes from the histochemical and electron microscopic demonstration of glycogen accumulations in reactive and edematous, swollen astrocytes (Figs. 7-11), (Hager, 1964a,b). With histochemical methods (PAS-Bauer reaction, Best-stain, combined with enzymatic controls) one can demonstrate such accumulations of glycogen in reactive astrocytes in traumatic lesions of mammalian cerebral cortex. The distribution and quantity of the glycogen are similar to that described by others (Klatzo, Miquell, Haymaker, Tobias & Wolfe, 1962; Wolfe, Klatzo, Miquell, Tobias & Haymaker, 1962) under comparable conditions. In the electron microscope one can find in the cytoplasmic matrix of reactive astrocytes round granules of uniform size which are sometimes arranged in small groups (Fig. 11). These particles were evident following lead hydroxide staining of sections from experimental perifocal edema as early as 16 hours after injury. In the processes of swollen protoplasmic astrocytes accumulations of these granules are also demonstrable. Of special interest is their presence in the pericapillary cytoplasmic feet (Figs. 7-10) and in the perineuronal processes of glia cells (Fig. 8).

The glycogen nature of this particulate component in the astrocytic cytoplasm is evident from the results of Fawcett (1958), Revel, Napolitano and Fawcett (1960) and Themann (1963) who examined particulate glycogen from different tissues and organs. Fawcett also established the morphological criteria for the identification of this particulate polysaccharide. These criteria were derived from ob-

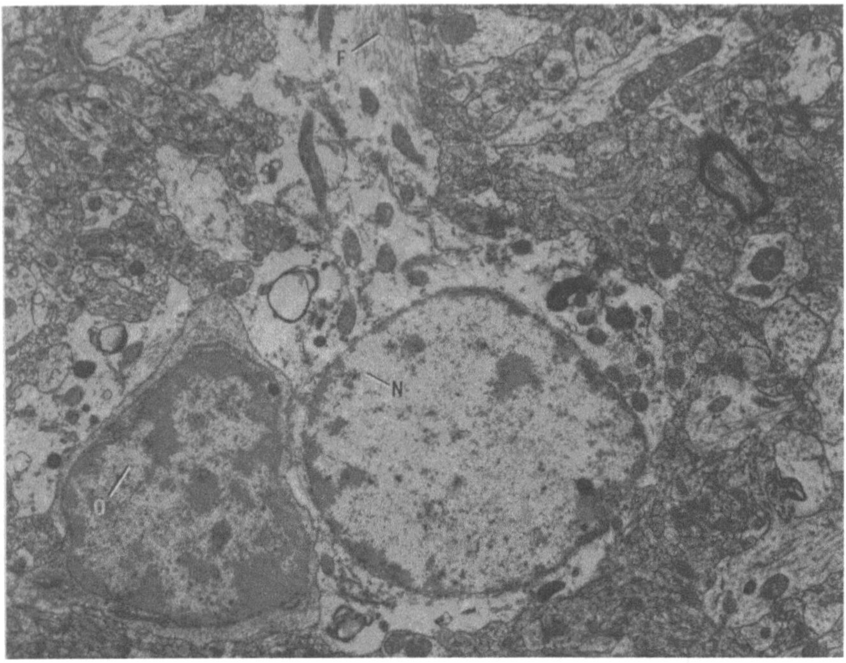

Fig. 6. Astrocyte in the parietal cortex of the rabbit brain. The cytoplasm is relatively clear and contains cisternae of the endoplasmic reticulum, mitochondria and a few free ribosomes. A bundle of glia filaments (F) is present in the cytoplasm. Note the appearance of an adjacent oligodendrocyte (O). Both the cytoplasm and the nucleus of this cell show a considerably greater density. N = nucleus of the astrocyte. Fixation by glutaraldehyde perfusion. X9,000 (reduced).

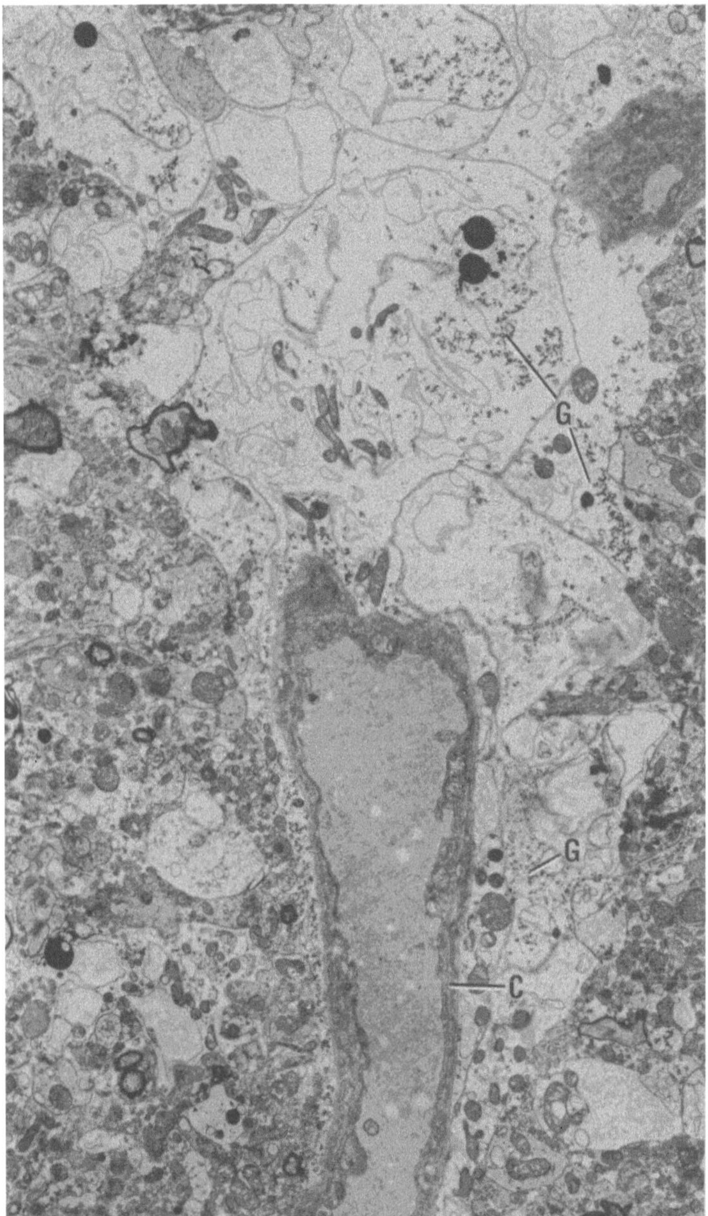

Fig. 7. Perifocal edema of the cerebral cortex 16 hours after experimental injury. The pericapillary astrocytic feet are swollen. Cytoplasmic accumulations of glycogen particles (G) are evident. C = capillary. Glutaraldehyde fixation, stained with lead hydroxide. X5,700.

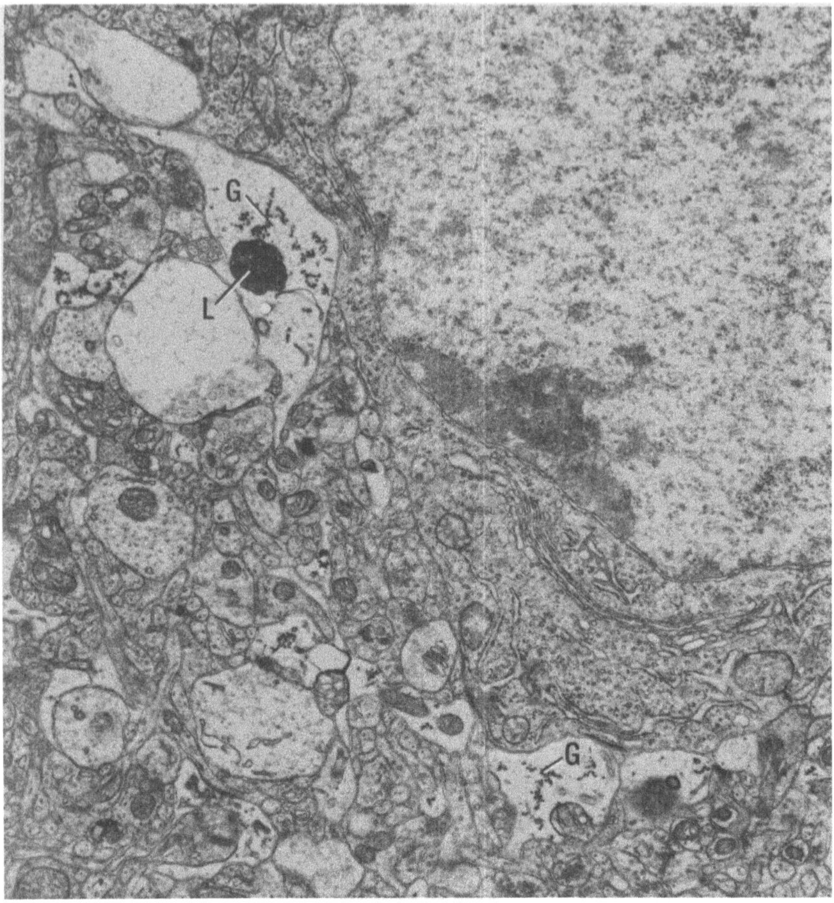

Fig. 8. Accumulation of glycogen particles (G) in the cytoplasm of astrocytic processes which are in close contact with the surface membrane of a neuron. L = lipid droplets. Section of a 16-hour-old experimental traumatic lesion of the cerebral cortex. Glutaraldehyde fixation, stained with lead hydroxide. X9,000.

servations of unstained and stained ultrathin sections and of the glycogen pellets which were isolated from representative tissues by centrifugation. The pathologic accumulation of particulate glycogen in astrocytes may be attributable to the inhibition of aerobic glycolysis associated with the lowered metabolic rate as a result of tissue alteration. The glycogen accumulation suggests that the astrocytic compartment plays an important role in the carbohydrate metabolism of the brain. Furthermore, these findings stress the functional importance of this cellular compartment as a metabolic pool which links the blood stream with the metabolic activities of the neuron.

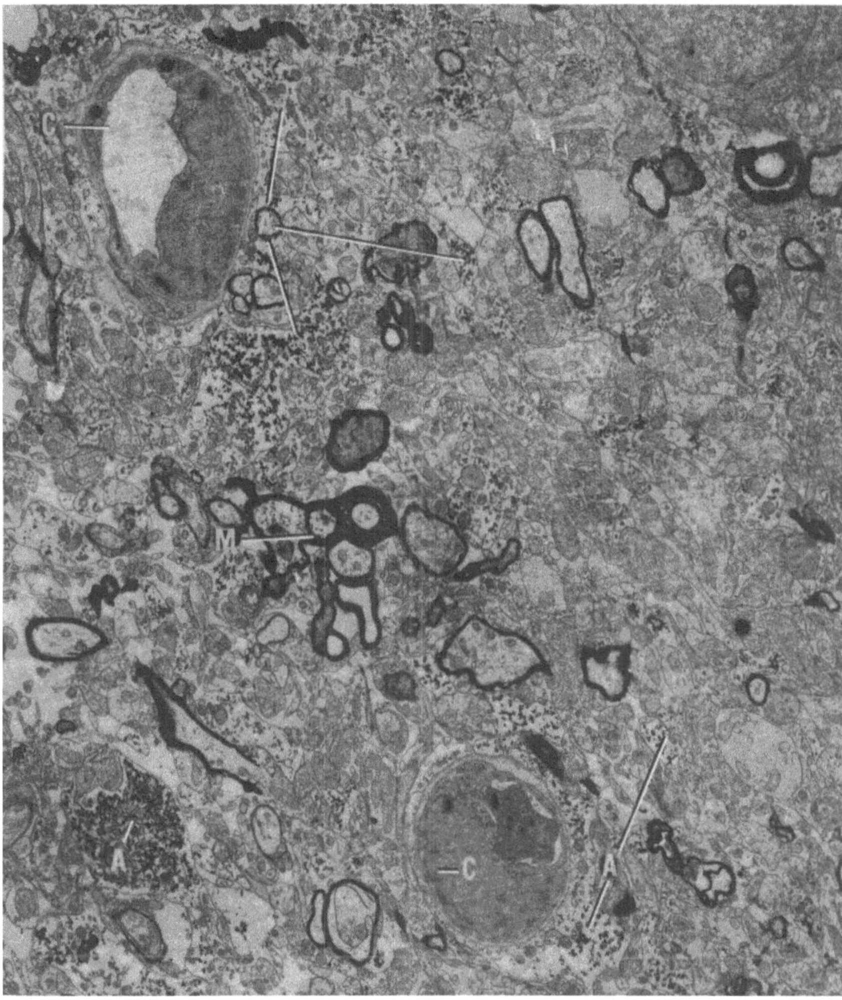

Fig. 9. Distribution of glycogen particles in the altered cortex in a 7-day-old experimental traumatic lesion. The cytoplasm of astrocytic processes (A) contains many glycogen particles. C = capillary. M = myelinated nerve fibers. Glutaraldehyde fixation, stained with lead hydroxide. X5,700.

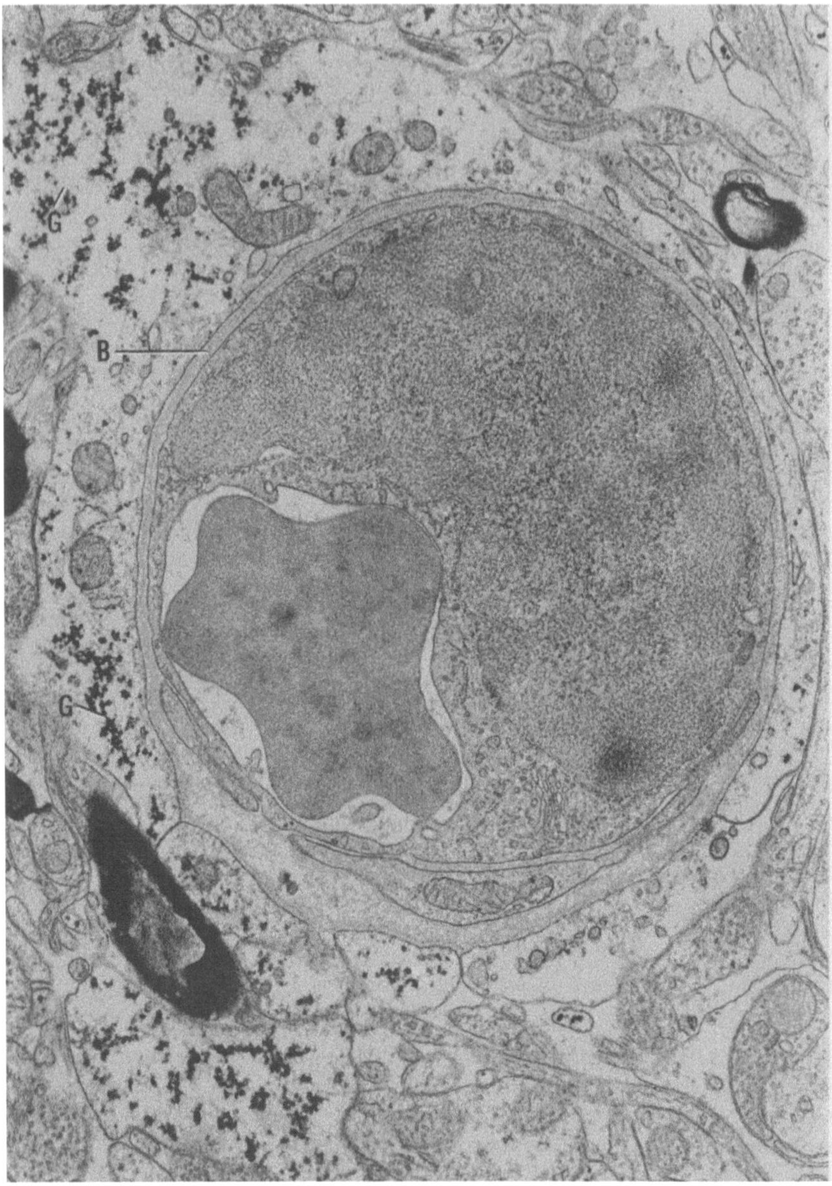

Fig. 10. Accumulation of glycogen particles (G) in an astrocytic foot process which ensheathes a capillary. B = basement membrane. A 7-day-old traumatic lesion of the cerebral cortex. Osmium fixation stained with lead hydroxide. X24,000 (reduced).

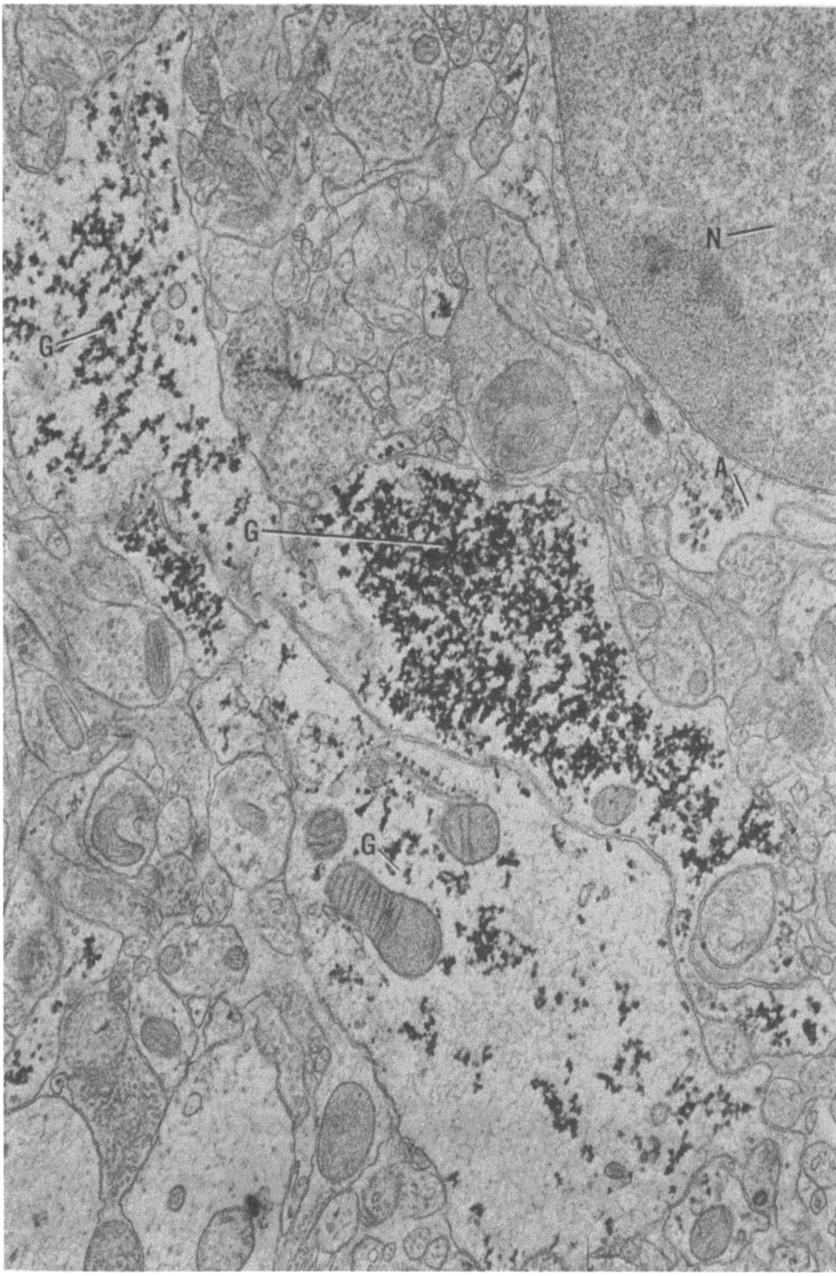

Fig. 11. Large numbers of glycogen particles (G), stained with lead, are present in the cytoplasmic processes of astrocytes in a 7-day-old traumatic lesion in the cerebral cortex. The cell body of an astrocyte (A) contains only a few particles, other cell processes forming the neuropil are free of these deposits. (N = nucleus of astrocyte). X24,000 (reduced).

REFERENCES

Blinzinger, K. H., N. B. Rewcastle and H. Hager: Beobachtungen über Mitochondrien mit eigenartiger Innenstruktur (Prisma-Typ) in Astrozyten des Goldhamster gehirns, Zschr. Naturforsch., 19 b (1964).

_____, _____ and _____: Observations on prismatic-type mitochondria within astrocytes of the Syrian hamster brain, J. Cell Biol., 25, 293-303 (1965).

Brambring, P.: Elektronenmikroskopische Untersuchungen über die Weite des Extrazellularraumes im Grosshirnmark, Acta Neuropath., 4, 317-325 (1965).

Campbell, A. W.: Histological Studies on the Localization of Cerebral Function, Cambridge University Press, p. 360 (1905).

Fawcett, D. W.: Identification of particulate glycogen and ribonucleoprotein in electron micrographs, J. Histochem. Cytochem., 6, 95 (1958).

Fernandez – Moran, H. and J. B. Finean: Electron microscope and low-angle X-ray diffraction studies of the nerve myelin sheath, J. Biophys. Biochem. Cytol., 3, 725-748 (1957).

Gonatas, N. K., H. M. Zimmerman and S. Levine: Ultrastructure of inflammation with edema in the rat brain, Amer. J. Path., 42, 455-469 (1963).

Hager, H.: Elektronenmikroskopische Untersuchungen über die Feinstruktur der sogenannten Grundsubstanz der Gross- und Kleinhirnrinde des Säugetiers, Arch. Psychiatr., 198, 574-600 (1959).

_____: Elektronenmikroskopische Untersuchungen über die Feinstruktur der Blutgefässe und perivasculären Räume im Säugetiergehirn. Ein Beitrag zur Kenntnis der morphologischen Grundlagen der sogenannten Bluthirnschranke, Acta Neuropath., 1, 9-33 (1961).

_____: Die feinere Cytologie und Cytopathologie des Nervensystems, dargestellt auf Grund elektronenmikroskopischer Befunde. Veröffentlichungen aus der morphologischen Pathologie, No. 67, Stuttgart: Gustav Fischer Verlag (1964).

van Harreveld, A.: Changes in volume of cortical neuronal elements during asphyxiation, Amer. J. Path., 191, 233-242 (1957).

_____ and J. Crowell: Extracellular space in central nervous tissue, Fed. Proc., 23, 304 (1964).

_____ and S. Ochs: Cerebral impedance changes after circulatory arrest, Amer. J. Physiol., 187, 180-192 (1956).

Hess, A.: The ground substance of the central nervous system revealed by histochemical staining, J. Comp. Neurol., 98, 69-92 (1953).

Horstmann, E.: Die Struktur der molekularen Schichten im Gehirn der Wirbeltiere, Naturwiss., 44, 448 (1957).

_____ and H. Meves: Die Feinstruktur des molekularen Rindengraues und ihre physiologische Bedeutung, Zschr. Zellforsch., 49, 569-604 (1959).

Karlsson, U. and R. L. Schulz: Plasma membrane apposition in the central nervous system after aldehyde perfusion, Nature, 201, 1230-1231 (1964).

_____ and _____: Fixation of the central nervous system for electron microscopy by aldehyde perfusion I. Preservation with aldehyde perfusates versus direct perfusion with osmium tetroxide with special reference to membranes and the extracellular space, J. Ultrastruct. Res., 12, 160-186 (1965).

Klatzo, J., J. Miquell, W. Haymaker, C. Tobias and L. S. Wolfe: Observations on appearance of histochemically demonstrable glycogen in the rat brain as an effect of alpha particle radiation, in: Effect of ionizing radiation on the nervous system, Internat. Atomic Energy Agency, Vienna, 285-296 (1962).

Koch, A., J. B. Ranke and B. L. Newman: Ionic Content of Neuroglia, Exper. Neurol., 6, 186-200 (1962).

Nelson, E., K. Blinzinger and H. Hager: Electron microscopic observations on the subarachnoid and perivascular spaces of the Syrian hamster brain, Neurology, 11, 285-295 (1961).

Niessing, K. and W. Vogell: Das elektronenoptische Bild der sogenannten Grundsubstanz der Hirnrinde, Zschr. Naturforsch., 12b, 641-646 (1957).

Nissl, F.: Die Neuronenlehre und ihre Anhänger, Jena: Gustav Fischer Verlag (1903).

Reed, D. J. and D. M. Woodbury: Kinetics of C -sucrose distribution in cerebral cortex, Cerebrospinal fluid and plasma of rats, Fed. Proc., 19, 80 (1960).

Revel, J. P., L. Napolitano and D. W. Fawcett: Identifications of glycogen in electron micrographs of thin tissue section, J. Biophys. Biochem. Cytol., 8, 575 (1960).

Rewcastle, N. B.: Glutaric acid dialdehyde; a routine fixative for central nervous system electron microscopy, Nature, 205, 207-208 (1965).

Robertson, J. D.: The cell membrane concept, J. Physiol., 140, 58 (1957).

_____: Structural alterations in nerve fibers produced by hypotonic solutions, J. Biophys. Biochem. Cytol., 4, 349-364 (1958).

_____: The ultrastructure of cell membranes and their derivatives, Biochem. Soc. Symposia, 16, 3-43 (1959).

_____: A molecular theory of cell membrane structure, Vierter Internationaler Kongress für Elektronenmikroskopie, Berlin, 1958, Verh., Vol. II, 159-171. Berlin-Göttingen-Heidelberg: Springer-Verlag (1960).

_____: The unit membrane of cells and mechanisms of myelin formation, in: Ultrastructure and metabolism of the nervous system, Research Publications, Association for Research in Nervous and Mental Disease, Vol. 40, 94-158. Baltimore: Williams & Wilkins (1962).

Schadé, J. P.: Functional correlates of ionic movements in the cerebral cortex, in: Selective Vulnerability of the Brain in Hypoxaemia (ed. by J. P. Schadé and W. H. McMenemey), Oxford: Blackwell Scientific Publications, 89-99 (1963).
Schultz, R. L. and U. Karlsson: Fixation of the central nervous system for electron microscopy by aldehyde perfusion; II: Effect of osmolarity, pH of perfusate, and fixative concentration, J. Ultrastruct. Res., 12, 187-206 (1965).
Sjöstrand, F. S.: Electron microscopy of myelin and of nerve cells and tissue. in: Modern Scientific Aspects of Neurology (ed. by J. N. Cummings), London: Edward Arnold Ltd., 188-231 (1960).
Streicher, E.: The thiocyanate space of rat brain, Amer. J. Physiol., 201, 334 (1961).
Themann, H.: Elektronenoptische Untersuchungen über das Glykogen im Zellstoffwechsel, Veröffentlichungen aus der morphologischen Pathologie, 66. Stuttgart: Gustav Fischer Verlag (1963).
Tower, D. B.: The neurochemical substrates of cerebral function and activity, in: Biological and Biochemical Bases of Behavior (ed. by H. F. Harlow and C. M. Woolsey), Madison: University of Wisconsin Press (1958).
Wolfe, L. S., J. Klatzo, J. Miquell, C. Tobias and W. Haymaker: Effect of alpha-particle irradiation on brain glycogen in the rat, J. Neurochem., 9, 213 (1962).
Woodbury, D. M.: Discussion remarks, in: Biology of Neuroglia, (ed. by W. F. Windle), Springfield: Charles C. Thomas, 120-127 (1958).

DONALD B. TOWER

DISTRIBUTION OF CEREBRAL FLUIDS AND ELECTROLYTES *IN VIVO* AND *IN VITRO*

Older concepts of brain edema based on gross changes of brain volume and fluid content (Elliott & Jasper; Schaltenbrand & Bailey; Weed, et al.), have been modified by recognition that some forms of edema affect cerebral cortex primarily while others involve subcortical white matter rather selectively. Recognition of swelling of cerebral cortex may be credited to Elliott, and the phenomenon has been subsequently investigated in detail by Leaf; by Pappius, et al. (1956, 1958, 1962); and by Varon and McIlwain among others. Selective edema of white matter was demonstrated in the classic study by Stewart-Wallace and has more recently been studied experimentally by Aleu, et al., and by Pappius and Gulati, among others. Much of the current morphological and biochemical work in these fields is represented by contributions to this conference and need not be reviewed here.

Despite the importance of these advances for our understanding of brain edema, the basic problem of interpreting changes of fluid content and electrolyte distribution in terms of tissue and cellular morphology remains. There is little unanimity of opinion on how to define by suitable quantitative means the fluid compartments of cerebral tissues and the distribution of electrolytes between and within these compartments. Current controversy and confusion over extracellular *versus* intracellular fluid spaces in brain is sufficiently familiar to require no elaboration here (for discussion, see Bourke, et al.). To a considerable extent the problem seems to stem from a general reluctance to modify the preconceived concept of a simple, two-compartment model in order to take account of the highly complex and heterogeneous nature of cerebral tissues. Based on current morphological observations, we should anticipate a number of membrane-bound and membrane-enclosed fluid compartments each with potential or actual differences in accessibility to solutes and electrolytes. Hence, detailed studies with various indicator solutes, such as chloride, thiocyanate, sucrose and inulin, can be expected to provide a complex and not easily interpretable picture.

Some investigations of this type form the subject of this presentation. For obvious technical reasons the majority of the studies has been limited to cerebral cortex slices in vitro. The previous contributions to this field from the laboratories of Professor McIlwain in London and Professor Elliott in Montreal deserve acknowledgement because of their value for the design and interpretation of the present studies. Appropriate references to these contributions appear in the subsequent text. It is to be emphasized that the investigations summarized here and reported elsewhere in greater detail (Bourke, et al.; Bourke & Tower; Tower & Bourke), are in no sense definitive with respect to the problems already alluded to. At best these data may serve to exemplify some of the complexities of interpretation which confront us, both under relatively physiological conditions and in the presence of obviously pathological situations of swelling and edema in cerebral tissues.

METHODS

Details of methods employed have been reported elsewhere for both in vivo studies (Bourke, et al.), and in vitro studies (Bourke & Tower; Tower, 1958; Tower & Bourke). Special aspects relating to specific experiments are indicated subsequently in the text or illustrative data. Accordingly only some basic information on methods is included here for general orientation.

With the exception of chloride, all indicator solutes were added in trace amounts (0.4 to 1.0 μc), using inulin-carboxyl-C^{14} (S.A. 1.14 μc/μM), uniformly-labelled sucrose-C^{14} (S.A. 3.02 μc/μM), and K-thiocyanate-C^{14} (S.A. 2.63 μc/μM). Chloride normally present in fluids and tissue samples was determined by amperometric titration. Analytical and counting procedures and the method of calculating indicator solute spaces are detailed in the paper by Bourke, et al. All data presented here are expressed per unit fresh tissue weight (see discussion by Bourke and Tower).

Studies in vivo were carried out on various mammalian species under anesthesia and with special attention to procedural, temporal and analytical details, as specified in the original report (Bourke, et al.). Isotopically-labelled indicator solutes were administered by injection into cisternal cerebrospinal fluid (CSF) and were allowed to equilibrate with the cerebrospinal systems for appropriate intervals (as determined experimentally) before samplings and space determinations were carried out. For calculations of indicator solute spaces in cerebral cortex samples, reference was invariably made to the solute concentration in subarachnoid CSF immediately overlying the tissue sample at the time of biopsy.

Studies in vitro, with the exception of those on corpus callosum, utilized incubated slices of cat cerebral cortex prepared and handled essentially as specified by Tower (1958). Only "first" or pial slices of cortex (100-150 mg., 0.5 mm. thick) were employed in order to facilitate handling and to minimize cut surfaces. The friability and "stickiness" of white matter precluded slicing, so that cat corpus callosum was exposed in situ by blunt dissection and cut longitudinally in two portions for incubation directly. (By area and weight measurements it was calculated that such sections of corpus callosum were approximately 0.5 mm. thick and never exceeded 0.6 mm.). For all samples special attention was paid to the time between sacrifice and start of incubation, the time being held rigidly to 10-15 minutes with no more than 5 minutes of the period devoted to gassing of incubation vessels (i.e., contact of slices with incubation medium at room temperature before complete oxygenation) (Varon & McIlwain). Unless specified otherwise, incubations were at 37° in media of the following basic composition (in mM/liter): $NaHCO_3$ 25, $CaCl_2$ 1.3, $MgSO_4$ 1.2, KH_2PO_4 0.4, glucose 20, and NaCl 120 and KCl 5 (5 K medium) or NaCl 98 and KCl 27 (27 K medium), with the gas phase 95% O_2-5% CO_2. Additions and/or substitutions to these basic media are indicated for specific situations in the subsequent text. All slices were weighed initially (fresh weight) and after incubation (final weight) on a torsion balance. For final weights, slices were carefully separated from media by the gentlest possible suction filtration and minimal drainage on No. 54 Whatman filter discs (cerebral cortex) or Millipore 0.45 μ (HA) filter discs (corpus callosum) and rapidly weighed (Bourke & Tower). Further handling of tissue and media samples for analysis and counting were as specified by Bourke, et al.

RESULTS

The data considered here have been drawn from three groups of studies. The first comprises observations on fluid spaces in adult mammalian cerebral cortex accessible in vivo to various indicator solutes. These observations provide indications of interspecies relationships and serve as reference points for the second group of data concerned with similar studies on incubated slices of adult cat cerebral cortex in vitro. Additional data relevant to the interpretation and significance of these in vitro studies are provided by the third group of observations involving comparable studies in vitro on cerebral cortex of neonatal and maturing kittens and on corpus callosum of adult cats. Subsequent discussion considers the relevance of these various findings to morphological parameters and to changes in cerebral cortex associated with circulatory arrest in vivo.

1. Cortical Fluid Spaces IN VIVO

Results of a rather extensive investigation of the accessibility in vivo to cerebral cortex fluids of chloride, thiocyanate, sucrose and inulin are summarized in Tables 1 and 2 and Figure 1, taken from the original report by Bourke, et al. For a given species (Table 1), the cortical sucrose and inulin spaces are identical, the

TABLE 1

CORTICAL FLUID SPACES IN VIVO

	Cat	Monkey (M. mulatta)	Cat vs. Monkey P value
Total Brain Weight (g.):	31.0	88.5	–
Cerebral Cortex Spaces (%):			
Sucrose [4/5]*	27.1 (±0.9)	33.6 (±2.95)	{ < 0.001
Inulin [2/3]	27.9 (±0.15)	33.8 (±1.05)	
Chloride [5/4]	34.5 (±0.95)	38.4 (±1.5)	{ < 0.001
Thiocyanate [2/2]	35.5 (±1.6)	40.4 (±2.7)	
Sucrose-Inulin vs. Chloride-Thiocyanate: P value	< 0.001	< 0.001	

Values tabulated represent means (± S.D.) and are taken from Bourke, et al.
*Figures in brackets denote the number of experiments on cats and monkeys respectively.

cortical chloride and thiocyanate spaces are identical, and the latter are only slightly, albeit significantly larger than the former. This finding obtains for all mammalian species examined (Table 2), but between any two species there is clearly a significant difference in the sizes of both sets of spaces (Tables 1 and 2). Thus, from smaller to larger species there is a progressive increase in the size of

TABLE 2

CORTICAL FLUID SPACES IN VIVO:
CALCULATED AND EXTRAPOLATED VALUES

Species	Species Brain Weight (g)	Sucrose - Inulin Spaces (%)	Chloride - Thiocyanate Spaces (%)
Mouse	0.4	[8.5]*	[17.0] *
Rat	1.6	[14.5]	[23.0]
Guinea Pig	4.75	19.4	27.5
Rabbit	9.3	22.5	30.1
Cat	31.0	28.0	34.9
Monkey (M. mulatta)	88.5	32.8	39.1
Sheep	109	33.8	[39.9]
Chimpanzee	380	39.5	[44.8]
Beef	380	[39.5]	[44.8]
Man	1320	[45.2]	[49.8]
Whale (B. physalus)	6785	[52.7]	[56.3]

*Values in brackets denote extrapolated values; all others were calculated from observed values as detailed by Bourke, et al. See Figure 1 for correlation of spaces with brain weight.

these spaces, and, as summarized in Figure 1, when these data are plotted as a function of the logarithm of the average species brain weights, a straight line plot is obtained with a highly significant correlation ($P < 0.001$), slopes for each set of space data all being of the same order of magnitude. A similar correlation for cortical chloride content, covering additional species, has also been demonstrated (Bourke, et al.).

There are a number of implications of these in vivo observations. The close similarity and parallelism of the sucrose-inulin and chloride-thiocyanate spaces are especially noteworthy and suggest that the bulk of the fluid accessible to these solutes is functionally, if not actually, extracellular. This suggestion is based primarily on the inulin data, since the inulin molecule is not normally considered capable of penetrating cell membranes. The small excess of chloride-thiocyanate spaces over sucrose-inulin spaces most probably reflects an intracellular locus for a portion (15-20%) of the total tissue content of chloride or thiocyanate (Davson & Spaziani; Thomas & McIlwain; Van Harreveld & Schadé). Also noteworthy is the fact that the spaces for solutes examined are not identical for all species. Hence one cannot generalize in this respect, and clearly this factor may explain some of the current confusion

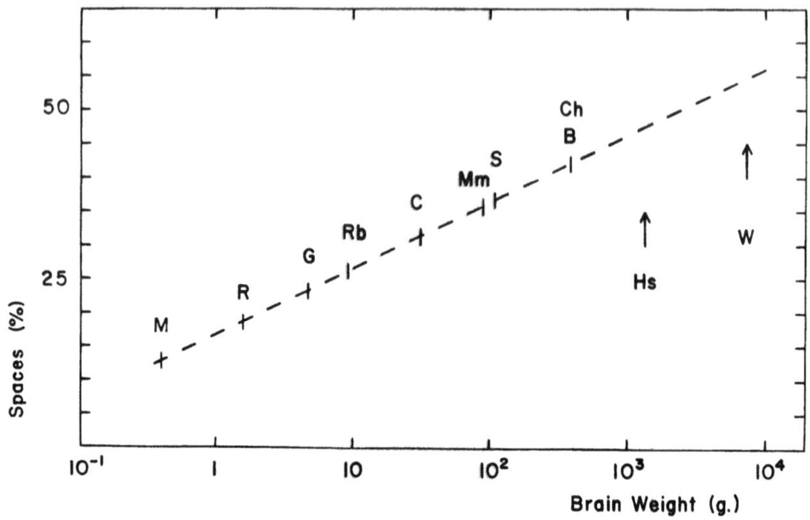

Fig. 1. Depiction in summary form of the correlation between cortical fluid spaces (ordinate) and species brain size (abscissa, log scale). The plotted curve represents an approximation of the individual curves for in vivo cortical fluid spaces accessible to sucrose, inulin, chloride and thiocyanate as reported by Bourke, et al. Actual slopes of the curves (calculated by the method of least squares) vary between +9.153 and +10.530, and the correlation coefficients are statistically highly significant ($P < 0.001$). Species for which one or more sets of data were obtained are indicated by small vertical lines intersecting the curve. (Key to species: M, mouse; R, rat; G, guinea pig; Rb, rabbit; C, cat; Mm, monkey; S, sheep; Ch, chimpanzee; B, beef. The predicted positions for man (Hs) and whale (W) on the curve are indicated.)

over sizes of fluid spaces in the central nervous system. Whether the suggested extrapolations (Table 2) for human and whale cerebral cortex are valid remain to be tested experimentally. However, it is obvious that attempts to compare extracellular space estimates based on electron micrographs of sub-mammalian brains (Horstmann & Meves) or rat cerebral cortex (Farquhar & Hartmann; Gerschenfeld, et al.), with estimates based on impedance studies of rabbit and cat cerebral cortex (Freygang & Landau; Van Harreveld & Schadé) are hardly permissible (Table 2), regardless of any other aspects involved in such comparisons. For technical reasons, previous reports on sizes of indicator solute spaces in mammalian cerebral cortex are not directly comparable with those reported here (see discussion by Bourke, et al.). However, observations on dog and rat cortex indicate appreciable spaces accessible to inulin and sucrose (Rall, et al.; Reed & Woodbury), and numerous studies on chloride spaces in cerebral cortex of various species report values of the same order of magnitude as predicted by our data.

2. Swelling and Fluid Spaces of Adult Cortex IN VITRO

(a) Swelling: Some characteristics of the swelling of cat cerebral cortex slices incubated in vitro are summarized in Figure 2 (Bourke & Tower). Regardless of conditions or attention to technique, cortical slices invariably swell in vitro, and the uptake of extra fluid begins immediately upon introduction of the slices into suspending or incubation media (Elliot; Varon & McIlwain). This phenomenon is illustrated for the 5-minute period devoted to gassing samples in media at room temperature (22°) immediately prior to incubation (37°) (Fig. 2, left-hand two points plotted). Immersion of

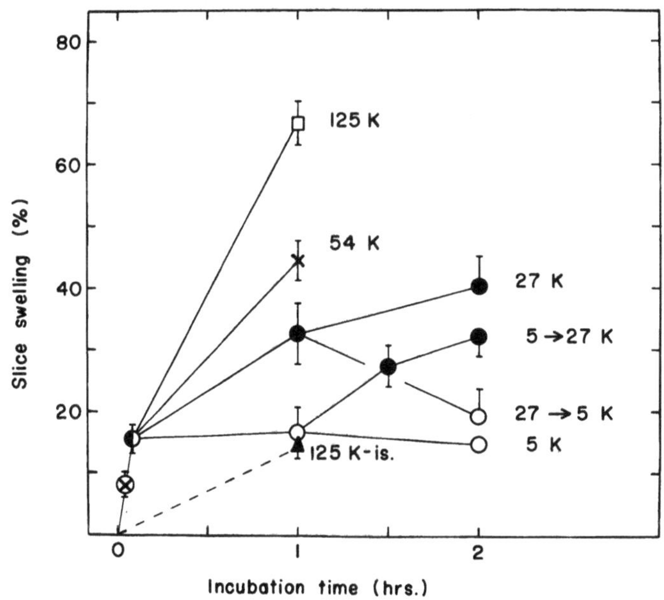

Fig. 2. Effects of external (medium) K^+ and Cl^- on swelling of cortical slices incubated in vitro. Slices of cat cerebral cortex were incubated aerobically in bicarbonate-saline-glucose media containing the K^+ concentrations (mM) indicated. Chloride (125 mM) was present in all media except those denoted K-is (solid triangle) where isethionate$^-$ (125mM) was substituted for Cl^-. Incubations were for the time intervals indicated (abscissa) and were all carried out at 37°, except for the 2.5 and 5 min. samples which were immersed for these periods in 5 K medium at 22° while being gassed with 95% O_2 -5% CO_2. Each plotted point represents the mean of four or more experiments and S. D. of means are indicated by the vertical bars. See text for discussion.

slices in incubation medium (5 K) for 2.5 minutes results in swelling averaging 8.1% and for five minutes averaging 15.5% of the initial fresh weight of slices. These values compare well with those obtained under similar conditions for guinea pig cortical slices by Varon and McIlwain and Keesey, et al.

These investigators attribute this initial swelling to two processes: (1) adherent incubation medium, accessible to inulin and amounting to swelling of some 6-8% and probably attributable primarily to the cut surface of the slices (Keesey, et al.); and (2) swelling during the period slices are in contact with incubation medium and air (not oxygen) at room temperature, amounting to additional swelling of some 7-12% for the 5-minute gassing period. Varon and McIlwain found this type of swelling to be inaccessible to inulin, irreversible on subsequent incubation under optimal conditions, and progressive with time of preparation. Our experience conforms to their view, since slices left in medium for prolonged periods under such sub-optimal conditions swell markedly (up to 50% or more of the initial fresh weight). This factor may account for the relatively higher values of swelling reported for rat cerebral cortex slices by Pappius and Elliott and Pappius, et al. (1958, 1962).

Additional swelling during incubation in 5 K medium is minimal (Fig. 2). After one-hour incubation, cat cortex slices exhibited total swelling of 16.8%, a value which compares well with the one-hour average of 13.5% for guinea pig cortex slices (Keesey, et al.). However, if the K^+ concentration of the incubation medium is significantly increased, additional swelling during slice incubation occurs (Fig. 2), as originally noted by Pappius and Elliott and Pappius, et al (1958). With cat cortex slices in 27 K medium, this extra swelling is largely complete by 30-minute incubation time (cf. 5 → 27 K, Fig. 2) and results in total swelling after one hour averaging 32.7% of the initial fresh weight or about twice the swelling in 5 K medium. Additional swelling occurs as medium K^+ concentrations are raised still further, reaching as much as 70% in 125 K medium.

This K^+-induced swelling is largely reversible or preventable. As shown in Figure 2, slices incubated for one hour in 5 K medium and for a second hour in 27 K medium (5 → 27 K) exhibit a final total swelling identical with controls incubated thus for two hours, Conversely, slices incubated for one hour in 27 K medium and for a second hour in 5 K medium (27 → 5 K) exhibit a final total swelling only slightly greater than controls incubated for 1-2 hours in 5 K medium. To our knowledge this is the first demonstration of extrusion of a substantial portion of slice fluid during incubation in the absence of a hypertonic medium. The extrusion of fluid on changing from 27 to 5 K media averages 13.3 µl./100 mg of slice or over 40 per cent of the total extra fluid of swelling originally present.

All K^+-induced swelling can be prevented by omitting chloride from the incubation medium and substituting the non-diffusible anion, isethionate (2-hydroxyethane sulfonate), as indicated for 125 K-isethionate medium (125 K-is) in Figure 2. Compared to 125 K-Cl controls in which swelling averaged 67%, the 125 K-isethionate slices exhibited a swelling of only 14%. Isethionate is a major intracellular anion in squid axoplasm (Koechlin) and normal constituent of mammalian cardiac muscle (Welty, et al.). As might be expected from studies with other chloride-free media (Thomas & McIlwain), the use of isethionate, chloride-free media was found to be without effect on the usual parameters of cortical slice oxidative metabolism.

The studies summarized in Figure 2 demonstrate two important factors contributing to swelling of incubated cortical slices: the external K^+ concentration and the presence or absence of a diffusible anion (chloride). At least two effects of excess external K^+ may contribute to K^+-induced swelling: hydration of cellular membranes (Tobias) and partial depolarization of cell membranes (Gibson & McIlwain) with consequent influx of extracellular ions (Na^+, Cl^-) and water. No ready explanation for the effects of substituting isethionate for chloride can be offered at this time.

(b) Fluid Spaces IN VITRO: The foregoing data on swelling of incubated cortical slices become more intelligible upon consideration of results of measuring accessibility to slice fluids of the solute indicators, chloride, thiocyanate, sucrose and inulin. Some of these studies are summarized in Tables 3 and 4 (Bourke & Tower). From data in Table 3 it is clear that despite the two-fold difference of slice swelling between samples incubated in 5 K and 27 K media, there is no difference in the size of the spaces accessible to chloride or thiocyanate in the two sets of samples. Thus, the K^+-induced swelling associated with 27 K medium seems to occur in a non-chloride, presumably intracellular compartment(s). This conclusion is supported by experiments in which medium K^+ was changed during incubation (5 → 27 K or 27 → 5 K, Fig. 2) with attendant fluid shifts but with no change in chloride content or size of chloride space of the slices. However, if the external K^+ concentration is increased to 125 mM, the slice chloride space essentially doubles. We can speculate that the K^+-induced, chloride-inaccessible swelling may relate to the membrane-hydration phenomenon proposed by Tobias, whereas the K^+-induced, chloride-accessible swelling may reflect depolarization with attendant major ion and water shifts (Gibson & McIlwain).

It should be pointed out that the data for chloride and thiocyanate spaces given in Table 3 represent studies under ideal conditions where slice swelling was minimized in terms of the component attri-

TABLE 3

FLUID SPACES IN INCUBATED CORTICAL SLICES

Incubation for 60 min. Medium	Time indicator added (min.)	[n]	Slice Swelling (%)	[n]	Chloride or SCN Space (%)	[n]	Sucrose or Inulin Space (%)
5 mM K^+	0	[34]	16.8 (±4.0)	[13]	62.2 (±3.5)	[7]	46.7 (±2.5)
	40					[6]	40.4 (±3.3)
27 mM K^+	0	[102]	32.7 (±4.9)	[19]	64.1 (±3.9)	[33]	42.3 (±2.5)
	40			[4]	63.7 (±4.4)*	[32]	29.4 (±2.5)†

Slices were incubated aerobically at 37° for 1 hr. in bicarbonate-saline-glucose media containing the K^+ concentrations indicated. Values tabulated represent means (±S.D.) for the number [n] of experiments shown.

*Data obtained with thiocyanate (SCN) only.

No significant change up to 40 min. after addition of sucrose or inulin. Identical results obtained with raffinose and isethionate.

butable to the preparative phase preceding incubation (Varon & McIlwain), as discussed above. When this component of slice swelling is not well controlled, the slice chloride and thiocyanate spaces vary directly as a function of slice swelling (Bourke & Tower). By extrapolating to zero swelling, a slice chloride space (in 5 K media) of approximately 43% is obtained, a value of a similar order of magnitude to the in vivo space value (Table 1). Nevertheless, it seems evident that in vitro, chloride and thiocyanate gain access to a compartment(s) which is not accessible to sucrose or inulin (Table 3) and which presumably represents the compartment(s) characterized by Varon and McIlwain as associated with sub-optimal conditions of slice preparation.

The possibility that this chloride-accessible compartment(s) represents glial (astrocyte) cytoplasm seems reasonable, as has been inferred by a number of previous investigators (Farquhar & Hartmann; Gerschenfeld, et al.; Katzman; Koch, et al.; Reed, et al.; Schultz, et al.; Streicher). When considered with respect to the normal in vivo situation, this concept may not be valid (Bourke, et al.). There is little difference in vivo between cortical fluid spaces accessible to sucrose-inulin and to chloride-thiocyanate (Table 1), whereas in vitro there can be a very large difference (Table 3). Furthermore, mammalian brain chloride content during growth and maturation of the brain decreases by almost 50% from high fetal and neonatal levels to much lower adult levels (Flexner & Flexner; Lajtha; Vernadakis & Woodbury) more or less coincident with a considerable absolute increase of cortical glial cell density (Brizee and Jacobs; Vernadakis & Woodbury). Finally in a well-documented, invertebrate situation, glial cells do not function as the extracelluar compartment for the neurons they invest (Kuffler & Potter; Nichols & Kuffler). We have suggested, therefore, that glial cells (astrocytes) in vivo may have the capacity normally to exclude chloride and that this capacity is lost or impaired under in vitro conditions (Bourke, et al.).

The situation in incubated cortical slices with respect to sucrose and inulin spaces (Table 3) is more complex. When these indicator solutes are present in the incubation medium from the time of slice immersion or start of incubation, spaces of the order of 42-47% are observed, always slightly but significantly higher in 5 K than in 27 K media. However, if the indicator solutes are added after incubation under optimal conditions is in progress (after 30-40 minutes incubation time), significantly smaller spaces are found especially in 27 K medium. These differences associated with time of solute addition are not attributable to a diffusion factor (Bourke & Tower), and the smaller spaces persist unchanged up to 40 minutes after addition before gradually expanding to values close to the larger-sized spaces. Furthermore, neither set of spaces bears any relationship to variations in slices swelling (in contradistinction to chloride spaces), and the differences between 5 K and 27 K spaces (0 addition time) are demonstrable in experiments where shifts from 5 → 27 K or 27 → 5 K during incubation are effected. Closely comparable findings have been obtained with raffinose and with S^{35}-labelled isethionate (Bourke & Tower).

It seems reasonable to infer that at least two fluid compartments of incubated slices are involved, one of which seems to be more permeable to sucrose and inulin during early stages of incubation than later when energy-yielding systems of the slices are operating optimally. The coincidence of space values for sucrose-inulin in vivo (Table 1) with those observed for slices incubated in 27 K medium with solute addition at 40 minutes (Table 3) must be considered fortuitous without additional evidence to the contrary. Similar studies have not been reported by others and the inter-species differences (Table 2) make comparisons with previously published data rather difficult. Keesey, et al., using guinea pig cortex slices incubated in 5 K medium with inulin present from the beginning, observed a relationship between the inulin and chloride spaces comparable to that observed for cat cortex slices here (Table 3). Thus, there appears to be substantial qualitative agreement between the data and interpretations already reported by McIlwain and co-workers (Varon & McIlwain; Keesey, et al.), and our own, but much less so for data and interpretations reported by Pappius and Elliott and Pappius, et al. (1962), on incubated slices of rat cerebral cortex. In view of the markedly greater swelling, close correspondence of sucrose and thiocyanate spaces, and the significantly smaller inulin spaces observed in the rat cortex studies, it seems possible that various technical factors (Varon & McIlwain) may have unfavorably influenced the results obtained. Consequently the conclusions drawn by Pappius, et al. (1962), that the inulin space represents a "damage space" and that there is normally a virtual absence of extracellular space in brain tissue require serious reservations at this time.

As suggested by the difference in size of the sucrose-inulin spaces depending on time of addition of the solutes to incubating cortical slices (Table 3), the possibility of metabolic and environmental factors influencing permeability of membranes within the slices requires consideration. The dynamic nature of fluid compartments and accessibility thereto by various indicator solutes is further illustrated by effects of varying incubation conditions, summarized qualitatively in Table 4. These studies are not considered here in any detail since they are only partially relevant and since complete data and discussions are provided elsewhere (Bourke & Tower). Table 4 is included primarily to illustrate that when various substi-

TABLE 4

EFFECTS OF VARYING INCUBATION CONDITIONS ON INCUBATED SLICE SWELLING AND SPACES

Medium or Conditions	Changes from Control†		
	Swelling	Chloride Space	Sucrose Space*
98 mM Li^+/25 mM Na^+	+	+	+
98 mM $choline^+$/25 mM Na^+	-	o	+
No Ca^{++}	-	o	+
27 mM Rb^+/no K^+	o	o	+
125 mM $isethionate^-$/no Cl^-	-	o	o
+ ouabain 10^{-5} M	+	+	o
+ L-glutamate 10^{-3} M	+	o	o
+ 2-deoxy-D-glucose 10^{-3} M	o	+	o
Incubation at 10°	-	+	+
5 mM K^+ (aerobic)	-	o	+
5 mM K^+ (anaerobic)	+	+	o

Key: +, significant increase; −, significant decrease; o, no change from values for control slices incubated aerobically at 37° for 1 hour in a medium containing (in mM/l): K^+ 27, Na^+ 123, Cl^- 125, HCO_3^- 25, Ca^{++} 1.3, Mg^{++} 1.2, SO_4^{--} 1.2, PO_4^{---} 0.4, and glucose 20. See Table 3 for values obtained therewith.

*As determined by addition of indicator at 40 min. incubation time.

tutions, omissions, or additions to the incubation medium are made, the slice parameters of swelling, chloride spaces, and sucrose spaces generally vary quite independently of each other. These observations should dispel any lingering illusions that fluid compartmentation in cerebral cortex is a simple or static situation. Some of the effects listed in Table 4 for Na^+-substituted media, low Ca^{++} media, added glutamate, and anaerobiosis have been reported previously (Leaf; Keesey, et al.; Pappius, et al., 1956, 1958; Stern, et al.), but no one study has hitherto examined the full set of parameters under idential experimental conditions.

3. Swelling and Fluid Spaces in Neonatal Cortex and Adult Corpus Callosum IN VITRO

Some of the questions and difficulties of interpretation posed by the foregoing studies on adult cat cerebral cortex *in vitro* can be clarified by consideration of data obtained under the same *in vitro* conditions on neonatal and maturing kitten cortex and on adult cat corpus callosum. Such studies are summarized in Table 5 (Tower & Bourke).

(a) Neonatal and Maturing Kitten Cortex: Incubated slices of cerebral cortex from kittens within four days after birth exhibit none of the characteristics of adult cortex slices. The slices do not swell, regardless of the K^+ concentration of the incubation medium. The chloride space is significantly smaller than that of adult slices and close to the size of the sucrose-inulin spaces. The sucrose-inulin spaces, although apparently equivalent in size to spaces in adult slices (for solute addition at 0 minutes), are uninfluenced by time of solute addition or K^+ concentration of the medium. [At this age, the brain is one-fifth of the adult size, and the cerebral cortex is only about one-third of its thickness at maturity, contains less solids (dry weight) and does not yet exhibit myelination of pyramidal axons (Noback, et al.; Tower & Bourke).]

At four weeks post-natal age, incubated slices of kitten cortex exhibit no change from the neonatal slices in chloride or sucrose spaces but the slices now exhibit swelling, averaging 12.3% of the slice initial fresh weight, in 27 K medium but no swelling in 5 K medium. Thus, at this stage the K^+-induced swelling has made its appearance. [At this time the brain weight is triple the neonatal value or about two-thirds the adult size, and the cerebral cortex is double the width at birth and exhibits morphological and physiological maturity of neurons and axonal myelination in progress (Noback, et al.; Tower & Bourke; Voeller, et al.).] Accordingly, it seems reasonable to suggest that the K^+-induced swelling observed for cortical slices at this age is probably associated with cortical neurons.

Over the next 4-6 weeks or up through two months post-natal age (the age of weaning), incubated slices of kitten cortex show little change from the situation at four weeks with the exception of a significant decrease in the size of the sucrose space (from 42-43% to 35%). [During this period cortical neurons undergo some final proliferation of dendrities, and axonal myelination is over 50% complete (Noback, et al.). Both total and supratentorial brain weights are close to the adult range by this time, and the cerebral cortex contains essentially the adult complement of solids (dry weight) and exhibits the adult levels of free amino acids including compartmentation of glutamate metabolism (Berl; Berl & Purpura; Tower & Bourke).] It is possible that the reduction in size of the sucrose space may reflect encroachment on interstitial spaces by enlarging neurons, additional cell processes and laying down of myelin along axons. If this be so, the persistence of a larger chloride space would suggest beginning acess of chloride to an additional (? glial) compartment(s). Alternatively, the disparity between sucrose and

TABLE 5

SLICE SWELLING AND FLUID SPACES: COMPARISON OF ADULT CEREBRAL CORTEX WITH NEONATAL CORTEX AND ADULT CORPUS CALLOSUM

	Aerobic Incubation 1 hr. at 37° in 27 mM K^+ medium						
						Sucrose Space (%)	
Type of Sample	[n]	Slice Swelling (%)	[n]	Chloride Space (%)	[n]	Added at 0 min.	Added at 40 min.
Neonatal:							
1.5 - 4 day cortex	[15]	− 1.5 (±3.3)	[13]	52.0 (±1.6)	[13]	43.4 (±3.1)*	
26 - 28 day cortex	[7]	+ 12.3 (±4.4)†	[6]	52.6 (±2.7)	[6]	41.7 (±3.0)	
45 to 64 day cortex	[10]	12.75 (±5.4)	[8]	50.9 (±4.1)	[8]	35.8 (±1.5)	
83 - 90 day cortex	[13]	23.7 (±3.7)‡	[10]	59.9 (±4.9)	[6]	40.9 (±2.1)	35.2 (±2.7)
120 day cortex	[4]	24.3 (±2.7)	[4]	61.8 (±4.3)	[2]	43.4 (±1.4)	32.0 (±0.7)
Adult:							
Cortex	[102]	32.7 (±4.9)	[19]	64.1 (±3.9)	[33]	42.3 (±2.5)	29.4 (±2.5)
Corpus Callosum	[20]	6.7 (±3.3)††	[15]	47.3 (±4.8)	[9]	45.6 (±4.1)#	—§
Liver	[19]	8.0 (±4.3)	[4]	63.7 (±4.0)	[3]	53.8 (±1.0)**	—

*Inulin space [3] 42.2 (±2.0). †With 5 mM K^+ medium, swelling [3] + 0.2 (±1.5).
‡With 5 mM K^+ medium [5], swelling 11.0 (±0.6); Cl^- space 52.5 (±1.0); and sucrose space, regardless of time of addition, 43.5 (± 4.6).
††With 5 mM K^+ medium [4], swelling 5.9 (± 4.0). # Inulin space [2] 24.4 (±0.8).
§Incomplete diffusion of sucrose for additions of less than 40 min. duration.
**Inulin space [9] 24.3 (±3.0).
Values tabulated represent means (± S.D.) for the number [n] of experiments indicated.

chloride spaces appearing at this stage could reflect an alteration in accessibility to some compartment(s) by the larger sucrose molecule.

By three months post-natal age, dramatic changes in the behavior of incubated cortical slices are evident. Slice swelling in 27 K medium is double previous values and swelling in 5 K medium is now demonstrable at roughly half the 27 K value. The chloride space is significantly increased, and for the first time the size of the sucrose spaces in 27 K medium differs depending on whether the solute is added initially or at 40 minutes incubation time. Thus, by three months of age the behavior of incubated cortical slices is in general close to, if not identical with, that of adult cortical slices. [At this time the brain and cerebral cortex are very close to maturity in most characteristics with one significant exception. As Brizee and Jacobs have shown, the density of neurons and neuronal volume in kitten cerebral cortex change little after two months post-natal age. At this age, their study showed that the glia/neuron index was 0.834 compared to the adult cortex value of about 1.45. In view of the relatively constant neuron density, this increase of glia/neuron index after two months post-natal age must reflect a significant proliferation and absolute increase of cortical glial cells (Brizee & Jacobs). In the absence of differential counts, we can only speculate that a major portion of the increase may represent astrocytes.]

Accordingly, it seems reasonable to infer that the additional swelling, additional compartment(s) accessible to chloride, and the "subdivision" of sucrose spaces could all be associated with the increased prevalence of glial cells (? astrocytes), which are permeable to chloride, permeable under sub-optimal conditions to sucrose, and prone to swell under in vitro conditions. Any such interpretation must be taken with a great deal of reservation since detailed morphological information about kitten cerebral cortex at this age is not yet available. An objection may be raised regarding the suggested permeability of some cellular membranes to sucrose and, by association (Table 3), to inulin. We believe that normally, under optimal physiological conditions inulin is probably excluded from intracellular loci in cerebral cortex, but there are sufficient instances both from studies summarized here and from reports by others (Ames, et al.; Cotlove) to suggest that cell membranes may become permeable to inulin with time or under less than optimal circumstances. This is even more likely to be the case for sucrose, which in incubated slices from other tissues like liver (Table 5) and kidney gains access to a greater proportion of total tissue fluid than does inulin (Pappius and Elliott; Tower and Bourke).

(b) Adult Corpus Callosum: The behavior of incubated segments of adult cat corpus callosum (of approximately equivalent thickness to cortical slices) is very different than that of cerebral cortex under identical in vitro conditions (Table 5). Swelling is minimal and uninfluenced by the K^+ concentration of the medium. The chloride and sucrose spaces are identical in size and about twice the size of the inulin spaces. Diffusion of sucrose and inulin into such samples is definitely a factor (Tower & Bourke), so that studies of solute additions at different incubation times cannot be carried out.

Since the cellular elements in these samples, exclusive of myelinated axons, are glial cells, it seems obvious that they do not behave as glial cells in cerebral cortex are presumed to behave under these in vitro conditions. If this interpretation be correct, then it follows that we cannot generalize about the properties of glial cells with respect to their possible roles in fluid and solute distribution in brain. Furthermore, the obvious predilection of subcortical white matter for edema following freezing lesions or alkyl tin intoxication (Aleu, et al.; Klatzo, et al.; Pappius & Gulati; Torack, et al.), stands in sharp contrast to the lack of swelling under in vitro conditions which promote swelling in cerebral cortex. This is at least consistent with observations that these forms of white matter edema primarily involve interstitial spaces (freezing lesions) or myelin lamellae (alkyl tin) rather than glial cells (Klatzo, et al.; Torack, et al.).

DISCUSSION

Many specific points relevant to individual observations have been considered above, so that discussion here is limited to more general aspects: the question of discrepancies between morphological estimates and biochemical estimates of extracellular space in cerebral cortex, and the significance of the progressive increase of cortical sucrose-inulin and chloride-thiocyanate spaces with increasing species brain size. In addition the relevance of foregoing findings on cerebral cortex to changes therein following circulatory arrest are considered briefly.

Morphological vs. Biochemical Spaces: The discrepancy between physiological or biochemical estimates of the size of cerebral extracellular spaces and the much smaller estimates based on electron microscopy needs to be resolved. If this is not yet completely feasible, at least several steps toward such a resolution seem possible. One factor which has been overlooked or minimized by electron microscopists is the possibility of artifacts introduced during fixation and dehydration preparatory to embedding and examining brain sections under the electron microscope. Bahr, et al. (1957), called attention to the volume changes which occur to during fixation and dehydration and concluded that gross distortions of tissue samples and presumably of the cells therein occur during these procedures and render difficult any interpretation of the original geometry of the sections. On the basis of our own studies in this context, some of which are summarized in Table 6, we concur with the views and findings of Bahr, et al. (1957).

Even brief (but morphologically adequate) fixation in buffered osmium tetroxide is associated with significant swelling of cat cerebral cortex slices (Table 6). More prolonged fixation produces even greater swelling (Bahr, et al., 1957; Pappius, et al., 1962; Tower, 1965). Subsequent dehydration in graded alcohols is associated first with marked additional swelling followed at higher alcohol concentrations by severe shrinkage to much less than the original unfixed weight of the slices. Such changes during dehydration were not observed by Pappius, et al. (1962), but are clearly shown in studies by Bahr, et al. (1957) and by our own data (Table 6). On the basis of analogous studies on erythrocytes, Bahr, et al. (1958), and Tooze have suggested that much of the swelling during fixation and initial stages of dehydration is intracellular. If this proves to be the case for brain sections, the likelihood of partial or complete obliteration of aqueous interstitial spaces must be considered. Evidence in favor of this view has been recently reported by Van Harreveld, et al. (1965).

On the other hand, the biochemical estimates are based on measurements of spaces accessible to indicator solutes, such as inulin, and these measurements imply nothing a priori about morphological loci. Under normal, optimal circumstances inulin is passively distributed only to extracellular fluid compartments of most tissues, but this is unlikely to apply under all circumstances for all tissues. Phelps has called attention to certain problems inherent in the use of inulin as a fluid space indicator, and our own data as well as those of Ames, et al., and Cotlove indicate that inulin may be able to penetrate some cellular membranes under special circumstances. One has only to consider the distribution of the much larger ferritin molecule in cerebral tissue (Brightman) to appreciate the complexities of this general problem.

Morphology has its limitations as well. On the basis of their studies, Pappius, et al. (1962), concluded that under suitable conditions they ought to be able to observe by electron microscopy the swelling associated with incubation of cerebral cortex slices. Originally we had hoped this would be the case but experience has shown otherwise, since we have failed to visualize such swelling by electron microscopy even under the most rigidly controlled and ideal conditions of fixation and dehydration which we have been able to devise. Doubtless part of the difficulty relates to the volume changes cited in Table 6. But there is also a geometrical factor to

TABLE 6

EFFECTS ON CORTICAL SLICES OF FIXATION AND DEHYDRATION FOR ELECTRON MICROSCOPY*

Conditions	[n]	Total Slice Weight (relative %)	[n]	Slice Solids (relative %)	Specific Gravity
Unfixed		100 (= 1000 mg.)	[7]	100 (= 160 mg.)	1.003
Fixed 5 min. in buffered† 1% OsO_4	[6]	118.8 (±2.6)	[4]	124.4 (±4.3)	1.015
Dehydrated 10 min. each in:					
(a) 10, 25, and 50% ethanol	[3]	184.6 (±7.8)		—	0.928
(b) 70, 80, 90, 95 and 100% ethanol [directly or preceded by (a)]	[5]	79.6 (±3.6)	[5]	65.0 (±8.7)	0.767

Values tabulated represent means (±S.D.) for the number [n] of experiments indicated and have all been corrected for the observed specific gravity differences.

*Taken from Tower (1965), and unpublished studies of Bourke, Wanko and Tower.

†Buffered in 27 mM K^+ incubation medium: see Table 4, footnote, for composition.

be considered. If interstitial spaces are assumed to be cylinders with a diameter of 150 Å, the volume of a 100 μ segment would be 0.0177 μ^3. A 30% increase of this volume as swelling would result in increasing the diameter of the cylinder to 170 Å, a widening too small to be appreciated visually as significant. Similarly if a glial cell is assumed to be a sphere with a diameter of 10 μ, the volume of the cell would be 525 μ^3. A 30% increase of this volume as swelling would result in increasing the diameter of the sphere to 10.9 μ, again a widening which would scarcely be detectable. On the other hand, if the interstitial volume of the above-mentioned cylindrical segment were three times that estimated by microscopic examination (i.e., a difference between a 10% and 30% space), the diameter of the cylinder would then be 260 Å or only about 1.7 times wider than the original figure. The foregoing considerations, crude as they may be, illustrate some of the difficulties of correlating volumes and morphology at the microscopic level. In this connection there is the possibility, originally suggested by Siekevitz, that interstitial fluid may include fluid within the lumina of the cellular endoplasmic reticulum. Certainly these lumina swell under certain circumstances (Birks; Wanko & Tower) and hence must be taken into account in any assessment of fluid and solute distribution.

Inter-Species Relationships: If the inter-species differences observed in vivo (Fig. 1) reflect some morphological or functional characteristic of mammalian cerebral cortex rather than some artifact of the in vivo technique, such interspecies differences ought to be demonstrable for incubated cerebral cortex slices in vitro where quite different experimental conditions prevail. This aspect has not been investigated in a definitive manner, but a comparison of in vitro data for cat and monkey cortex is highly suggestive (Table 7). Similarly, data for inulin spaces in slices of guinea pig cerebral cortex incubated under conditions similar to our own (Keesey, et al.), indicate a difference from comparable values for cat cerebral cortex (Table 3; 5 K, addition at 0 min.) of $\Delta \cong 10$, which is of the same order of magnitude predicted from in vivo data ($\Delta = 8.6$; Table 2). These few data are consistent with the view that the inter-species differences in cortical spaces accessible to indicator solutes are real and reproducible in vitro and hence likely to represent differences characteristic of the species for some fluid compartment(s) of cerebral cortex.

The identity of such compartment(s) may be tentatively suggested from data plotted in Figure 3. Studies by Shariff and by Tower (1954) and Tower and Elliott have demonstrated that there is a significant correlation of neuron density in mammalian cerebral cortex with average species brain weight (Tower, 1954). This correlation (Fig. 3; open circles) indicates a progressive decrease of

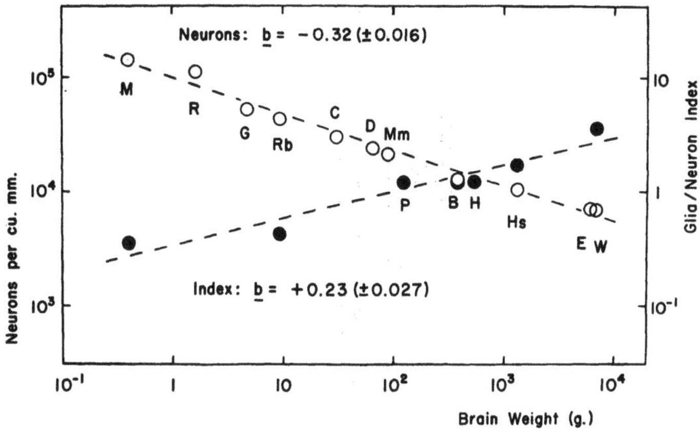

Fig. 3. Correlations of cortical neuron density (left ordinate, log scale) and glia/neuron index (right ordinate, log scale) with total species brain weight (abscissa, log scale) for various mammalian species. Data for neuron densities and brain weights are taken from Tower (1954) and from Tower and Elliott. Data for glia/neuron indices are taken from Friede and from Hawkins and Olszewski. The plotted curves have been calculated from these data by the method of least squares and the respective slopes (b) ±S.D. are given on the figure. In both cases the correlation coefficients are statistically highly significant (P 0.001). See text for discussion. (Key to species: as in Figure 1 plus D, dog; P, pig; H, horse; E, elephant.)

TABLE 7

SUCROSE SPACES *IN VIVO* AND *IN VITRO* IN CAT AND MONKEY CEREBRAL CORTEX

Observations	[n]*	Sucrose Spaces (%) Cat	Monkey (*M. mulatta*)	Δ	*P* Value
In Vivo:†	[4/5]	27.1 (±0.9)	33.6 (±2.45)	6.5	< 0.01
In Vitro:‡					
Sucrose added at:					
(a) 40 min.	[32/2]	29.4 (±2.5)	34.95 (±2.6)	5.55	< 0.01
(b) 0 min.	[33/4]	42.3 (±2.5)	48.5 (±4.2)	6.2	< 0.01
Slice Swelling (%)	[102/6]	32.7 (±4.9)	33.5 (±4.1)	-	-

*Values represent means (± S.D.) for the number of experiments [n] on cat and monkey respectively.

†Taken from Bourke, *et al*.

‡All slices were incubated aerobically at 37° for 1 hour in bicarbonate-saline-glucose medium containing 27 mM K^+. Sucrose was added to incubating slices either at 40 minutes incubation time (a) or was present for the entire incubation period (b).

TABLE 8

EFFECTS OF CIRCULATORY ARREST IN SITU ON CORTICAL FLUID SPACES AND ELECTROLYTES

Observations	[n]*	Control Values	After 30 min. Arrest of Circulation	P Values
Biopsy Samples†				
CSF K^+ (μeq./ml.)	[2/1]	3.8 (±0.55)	29.5	—
Na^+	[1/1]	142.5	143.5	—
Cl^-	[2/2]	130.0 (±0)	136.7 (±3.6)	0.1
Cortex K^+ (μeq./g.)	[6/2]	94.5 (±5.4)	80.5 (±4.6)	0.01
Na^+	[6/2]	54.4 (±2.6)	66.5 (±3.1)	<0.01
Cl^-	[6/2]	44.8 (±1.2)	46.0 (±2.8)	—
Cl^- Space (%)	[5/2]	34.5 (±0.95)	33.7 (±0.8)	—
Solids (%)	[9/4]	16.0 (±0.9)	13.5 (±0.9)	<0 001
Calculated Swelling (%)		0	18.5	
Incubated Cortical Slices‡				
Swelling (%)	[102/8]	32.7 (±4.9)	13.6 (±3 9)	<0.001
Cl^- Space (%)	[19/8]	64.1 (±3.9)	56.2 (±3.6)	<0.001
Sucrose Space (%)				
addition at 0 min.	[33/4]	42.3 (±2.5)	40.1 (±1.8)	—
addition at 40 min.	[32/4]	29.4 (±2.5)	29.5 (±1.4)	—
Slice K^+ (μeq./g.)	[17/8]	99.9 (±8.0)	81.8 (±3.5)	<0.001
Na^+	[17/8]	75.3 (±10.1)	73.1 (±1.9)	—
Cl^-	[19/8]	80.1 (±5.1)	71.8 (±4 1)	<0.001

Values tabulated represent means (±S.D.) for the number [n] of experiments indicated. Control samples were taken immediately after sacrifice; arrest samples were taken in identical fashion 30 minutes after clamping of neck vessels.

†Biopsy control data taken from Bourke, et al.

*Figures in brackets denote number of experiments for control and arrest samples respectively.

‡Incubation aerobically at 37° for 1 hour in 27 mM K^+ medium.

cortical neuron density with increasing species brain size. On the other hand the reverse correlation for glia/neuron index appears to obtain, based on data reported by Friede and by Hawkins and Olszewski, i.e., there is a progressive increase of the index value with increasing species brain size (Fig. 3; solid circles). The calculated slopes of the two curves are sufficiently close to suggest that they may in fact be identical. If this be so, the density of glial cells per unit volume of cortex would be essentially constant from mouse to whale. Such a conclusion must for the present remain subject to considerable reservation, but it does seem that there is no obvious or significant increase of cortical glial density from rabbit to whale, the number per cu. mm. of cortex remaining fairly constant at about 20000 (based on data from Tower, 1954, and from Friede and Hawkins and Olszewski). These two factors, decreasing neuron density and apparently constant glial density, contrast with the progressive increase in size of indicator solutes spaces with increasing species brain size (Fig. 1). Thus, either the cellular volumes must increase to offset the decline or lack of increase in number of cells or the interstitial space between cells must increase in order to account for all three factors. The likelihood is that both explanations obtain in part. In the cerebral cortex of larger mammals the neurons appear on the average to be considerably larger, yet at the same time the space between cells becomes increasingly impressive, at the light microscope level (Tower, 1954). To our knowledge, adequate information on cell volumes, either glial or neuronal, is not available. Hence no final conclusion is permissible at present, but a reasonable, circumstantial case may be made for an extracellular locus for most of the fluid compartment(s) accessible to inulin, sucrose, chloride and thiocyanate in cerebral cortex *in vivo*.

Cortical Edema following Circulatory Arrest: The observations reported by Varon and McIlwain stress the importance of rapid sampling and preparation of cortical slices for incubation. However, studies on human samples may not be possible without an appreciable delay *in situ* after arrest of cerebral circulation, whether sampling is at the time of surgery or at autopsy. For this reason, Dr. R. S. Bourke in our laboratory undertook an experimental evaluation of the problem by comparing the fluid and solute distributions in control samples of cat cerebral cortex, studied after rapid excision following clamping of neck vessels, with the same parameters in samples obtained 30 min. after such circulatory arrest (Table 8). Previously, Rall, *et al.*, and Van Harreveld, *et al.*, have suggested that a major consequence of arrest of cerebral circulation appeared to be intracellular swelling.

As a consequence of circulatory arrest (Table 8), cerebrospinal fluid K^+ concentration rose markedly and appeared to be paralleled by the decrease of tissue K^+ content. No changes of CSF Na^+ or Cl^- were evident, but tissue Na^+ content increased to essentially balance the loss of K^+. Influx of fluid into cerebral cortex *in situ* was clearly indicated by the decrease of tissue dry weight (solids) and was calculated to represent swelling to the extent of about 18.5%. It is noteworthy that the cortical chloride content and space did not differ from those in control brains.

Further comparisons were made on incubated slices from both preparations under identical *in vitro* conditions (Table 8). Swelling of the pathological slices during incubation was markedly reduced, and it seemed likely that the swelling which had already occurred in situ could account for the difference from control slices (i.e., 18.5 + 13.6 = 32.1). The chloride space of the pathological slices was significantly smaller than that of control slices but was of the correct order of magnitude predicted for the degree of in vitro swelling (Bourke and Tower). Sucrose spaces of the pathological slices were indistinguishable from those in control slices, and the electrolyte contents of the two sets of slices differed only in the lower chloride level and the reduced K^+ content (coinciding with in vivo values) for the pathological slices. The in vitro behavior of these slices suggested that the usual in vitro K^+ effects of 27 K medium (Fig. 2; Table 3) had already occurred in vivo and merely persisted in vitro. It is of interest that the fluid bathing these samples of cortex in vivo appeared to have the same K^+ concentration as that employed in the in vitro media.

Clearly a major effect of circulatory arrest on cerebral cortex in situ is the occurrence of swelling or edema in a fluid compartment inaccessible to chloride or sucrose. Hence this compartment must be intracellular, and from the behavior of the incubated slices, it may reasonably be inferred that the intracellular compartment is neuronal and not glial. These observations confirm the interpretations previously reported by Rall, et al., and by Van Harreveld, et al., although the latter group proposed that concomitant with the flux of fluid, chloride also entered the swollen cells. This last conclusion is not supported by the data in Table 8, but the experimental conditions were not entirely comparable in the two studies and evaluation of other factors such as lactic acid and ammonia would be desirable. The data on effects of circulatory arrest illustrate the value and applicability to pathological situations of the techniques and studies reported in the body of this paper. The data also emphasize a complication of studies in which brain sampling cannot be effected until some time after death.

Envoi: Consideration of the distribution of Na^+ and K^+ in the various fluid compartments of cerebral cortex has been deliberately omitted from this presentation. The complexities of fluid compartmentation within the cortex obviously make it difficult to decide on what basis to calculate electrolyte concentrations from data on indicator solute spaces and the gross tissue contents of electrolytes. The problem is somewhat clarified by the recent study by Gibson and McIlwain in which the potential differences across cortical cell membranes were measured with microelectrodes in incubating slices of guinea pig cerebral cortex. These observed values correlated well with those calculated from slice electrolytes, assuming the inulin space (as determined by addition at 0 minutes) to be extracellular. In addition the report presents a valuable discussion of the effects of added K^+ or glutamate and of the numerous factors to be considered in such studies. The assumption that inulin measures extracellular space thus appears to be a good approximation from several standpoints. However, in terms of the numerous fluid compartments which can be measured and inferred and in view of the heterocellular nature of cerebral cortex, any more precise or detailed distribution of electrolytes therein seems unwarranted on the basis of currently available data.

Again it is to be emphasized that the various studies discussed in this paper cannot be considered definitive or complete but merely illustrative of the many problems and complexities to be considered in evaluating the compartmentation of fluids and electrolytes in cerebral tissues. This is difficult enough under experimental conditions where many aspects can be controlled or compensated for; the situation for pathological states especially under clinical conditions can be no less difficult. If the data and discussion have provided more questions than answers, it is perhaps because, as Blaise Pascal so aptly wrote: "Knowledge is like a sphere in space, the greater its volume the larger its contact with the unknown."

SUMMARY

Compartmentation of tissue fluids in cerebral cortex and subcortical white matter is considered on the basis of accessibility to tissue fluids of such indicator solutes as chloride, thiocyanate, sucrose and inulin. For cerebral cortex in vivo, sizes of the respective spaces accessible to representative solutes are closely similar for a given mammalian species, but between any two species, such spaces exhibit significant differences, varying as a function of species brain size. Complementary studies in vitro present additional complexities in terms of tissue swelling, divergent distributions of the respective indicator solutes, and pronounced variations under different conditions of incubation. Contrasts between adult and neonatal cerebral cortex and between cortex and subcortical white matter (corpus callosum) provide the basis for relating the various fluid compartments, as defined by indicator solutes, to tissue and cellular loci. The significance of the various data for interpretation of pathological situations is exemplified by discussion of changes in cerebral cortex following circulatory arrest in vivo.

ACKNOWLEDGMENT

The majority of the data presented in this paper are derived from investigations carried out by or in association with Dr. Robert S. Bourke, and many of the interpretations stem from his investigational ingenuity and keen grasp of the significance of the various findings.

REFERENCES

Ames, A., J. B. Isom and F. B. Nesbett: Effects of osmotic changes on water and electrolytes in nervous tissue, J. Physiol. (London), 177, 246-262 (1965).

Aleu, F. P., R. Katzman and R. D. Terry: Structure and electrolyte analyses of cerebral edema induced by alkyl tin intoxication, J. Neuropath. Exp. Neurol., 22, 403-413 (1963).

Bahr, G. F., G. Bloom and U. Friberg: Volume changes of tissue in physiological fluids during fixation in osmium tetroxide or formaldehyde and during subsequent treatment, Exp. Cell Res., 12, 342-355 (1957).

_____, _____ and E. Johannisson: Further studies on fixation with osmium tetroxide, Histochemie, 1, 113-118 (1958).

Berl, S.: Compartmentation of glutamic acid metabolism in developing cerebral cortex, J. Biol. Chem., 240, 2047-2054 (1965).

_____ and D. P. Purpura: Postnatal changes in amino acid content of kitten cerebral cortex, J. Neurochem., 10, 237-240 (1963).

Birks, R. I.: The effects of a cardiac glycoside on subcellular structures within nerve cells and their processes in sympathetic ganglia and skeletal muscle, Canad. J. Biochem. Physiol., 40, 303-315 (1962).

Brizee, K. R. and L. A. Jacobs: Postnatal changes in volumetric and density relationships of neurons in cerebral cortex of cat, Acta Anat., 38, 291-303 (1959).

_____ and _____: The glia/neuron index in the submolecular layers of motor cortex in the cat, Anat. Record, 134, 97-105 (1959).

Bourke, R. S., E. S. Greenberg and D. B. Tower: Variation of cerebral cortex fluid spaces in vivo as a function of species brain size, Am. J. Physiol., 208, 682-692 (1965).

_____ and D. B. Tower: Fluid compartmentation and electrolytes of cat cerebral cortex in vitro. I. Swelling and solute distribution in mature cerebral cortex. J. Neurochem., 13, 1071-1097 (1966).

Brightman, M. W.: The distribution within brain of ferritin injected into cerebrospinal fluid compartments. I. Ependymal distribution, J. Cell Biol., 26, 99-123 (1965).

Cotlove, E.: Mechanism and extent of distribution of inulin and sucrose in chloride space of tissues, Am. J. Physiol., 176, 364-410 (1954).
Davson, H. and E. Spaziani: The blood-brain barrier and the extracellular space of brain, J. Physiol. (London), 149, 135-143 (1959).
Elliott, K. A. C.: Swelling of brain slices and the permeability of brain cells to glucose, Proc. Soc. Exp. Biol. Med., 63, 234-236 (1946).
_____ and H. H. Jasper: Measurement of experimentally induced brain swelling and shrinkage, Am. J. Physiol., 157, 122-129 (1949).
Farquhar, M. G. and J. F. Hartmann: Neuroglial structure and relationships as revealed by electron microscopy, J. Neuropath. Exp. Neurol, 16, 18-39 (1957).
Flexner, L. B. and J. B. Flexner: Biochemical and physiological differentiation during morphogenesis. IX. The extracellular and intracellular phases of the liver and cerebral cortex of the fetal guinea pig as estimated from distribution of chloride and radiosodium, J. Cell. Comp. Physiol. 34, 115-127 (1949).
Freygang, W. H. and W. M. Landau: Some relations between resistivity and electrical activity in the cerebral cortex of the cat, J. Cell Comp. Physiol., 45, 377-392 (1955).
Friede, R.: Der quantitative Anteil der Glia an der Cortexentwicklung, Acta Anat., 20, 290-296 (1954).
Gerschenfeld, H. M., F. Wald, J. A. Zadunaisky and E. D. P. De Robertis: Funtion of astroglia in the water-ion metabolism of the central nervous system, Neurology, 9, 412-425 (1959).
Gibson, I. M. and H. McIlwain: Continuous recording of changes in membrane potential in mammalian cerebral tissues in vitro; recovery after depolarization by added substances, J. Physiol. (London), 176, 261-263 (1965).
Hawkins, A. and J. Olszewski: Glia/nerve index for cortex of the whale, Science, 126, 76-77 (1957).
Horstmann, E. and H. Meves: Die Feinstruktur des molecularen Rindengraues und ihre physiologische Bedeutung, Z. Zellforsch u. mikroskop. Anat. 49, 569-604 (1959).
Katzman, R.: Electrolyte distribution in mammalian central nervous system, Neurology, 11, 27-36 (1961).
Keesey, J. C., H. Wallgren and H. McIlwain: The sodium, potassium and chloride of cerebral tissues: maintenance, change on stimulation and subsequent recovery, Biochem. J., 95, 289-300 (1965).
Klatzo, I., A. Piraux and E. J. Laskowski: The relationship between edema, blood-brain barrier and tissue elements in a local brain injury, J. Neuropath. Exp. Neurol., 17, 548-564 (1958).

Koch, A., J. B. Ranck and B. L. Newman: Ionic content of the neuroglia, Exp. Neurol., 6, 186-200 (1962).
Koechlin, B. A.: On the chemical composition of the axoplasm of squid giant nerve fibers with particular reference to its ion pattern, J. Biophys. Biochem. Cytol., 1, 511-529 (1955).
Kuffler, S. W. and D. D. Potter: Glia in the leech central nervous system: physiological properties and neuron-glia relationship, J. Neurophysiol., 27, 290-320 (1964).
Leaf, A.: On the mechanism of fluid exchange of tissues in vitro, Biochem. J.,62, 241-248 (1956).
Nichols, J. G. and S. W. Kuffler: Extracellular space as a pathway for exchange between blood and neurons in the central nervous system of the leech: ionic composition of glial cells and neurons, J. Neurophysiol., 27, 645-671 (1964).
Noback, C. R., E. M. Housepian and D. P. Purpura: Development of cat neocortex, Anat. Rec., 139, 260 (1961).
_____ and D. P. Purpura: Postnatal ontogenesis of neurons in cat neocortex, J. Comp. Neurol., 117, 291-307 (1961).
Pappius, H. M. and K. A. C. Elliott: Water distribution in incubated slices of brain and other tissues, Canad. J. Biochem. Physiol., 34, 1007-1022 (1956).
_____ and D. R. Gulati: Water and electrolyte content of cerebral tissues in experimentally induced edema, Acta Neuropath., 2, 451-460 (1963).
_____, I. Klatzo and K. A. C. Elliott: Further studies on swelling of brain slices, Canad. J. Biochem. Physiol., 40, 886-898 (1962).
_____, M. Rosenfeld, D. M. Johnson and K. A. C. Elliott: Effects of sodium-free media upon the metabolism and the potassium and water contents of brain slices, Canad. J. Biochem. Physiol., 36, 217-226 (1958).
Pascal, B.: [Cited by C. Stern: Thoughts on research, Science, 148, 772-773 (1965).]
Phelps, C. F.: The physical properties of inulin solutions, Biochem. J, 95, 41-47 (1965).
Rall, D. P., W. W. Oppelt and C. S. Patlack: Extracellular space of brain as determined by diffusion of inulin from the ventricular system, Life Sci., 1: 2, 42-48 (1962).
Reed, D. J. and D. M. Woodbury: Kinetics of movement of iodide, sucrose, inulin and radio-iodinated albumin in the central nervous system and cerebrospinal fluid of the rat, J. Physiol. (London), 169, 816-850 (1963).
_____, _____ and L. Holtzer: Brain edema, electrolytes and extracellular space, Arch. Neurol., 10, 604-614 (1964).
Schaltenbrand, G. and P. Bailey: Die perivaskuläre Piagliamembran des Gehirns, J. f. Psychol. u. Neurol., 35, 199-278 (1928).

Schultz, R. L., E. A. Maynard and D. C. Pease: Electron microscopy of neurons and neuroglia of cerebral cortex and corpus callosum, Am. J. Path., 100, 369-408 (1957).

Schariff, G. A.: Cell counts in the primate cerebral cortex, J. Comp. Neurol., 98, 381-400 (1953).

Siekevitz, P.: On the meaning of intracellular structure for metabolic regulation, in: Ciba Symposium on Regulation of Cell Metabolism (ed. by G. E. W. Wolstenholme and C. M. O'Connor) Boston: Little, Brown, pp. 17-45 (1959).

Stern, J. R., L. V. Eggleston, R. Hems and H. A. Krebs: Accumulation of glutamic acid in isolated brain tissue, Biochem. J. 44, 410-418 (1949).

Stewart-Wallace, A. M.: Biochemical study of cerebral tissue, and changes in cerebral edema, Brain, 62, 426-438 (1939).

Streicher, E.: The thiocyanate space of rat brain in experimental cerebral edema, J. Neuropath. Exp. Neurol., 21, 437-441 (1962).

Thomas, J. and H. McIlwain: Chloride content and metabolism of cerebral tissues in fluids low in chlorides, J. Neurochem., 1, 1-7 (1956).

Tobias, J. M.: A chemically specified molecular mechanism underlying excitation in nerve: a hypothesis, Nature (London), 203, 13-17 (1964).

Tooze, J.: Measurement of some cellular changes during fixation of amphibian erythrocytes with osmium tetroxide, J. Cell Biol., 22, 551-563 (1964).

Torack, R. M., R. D. Terry and H. M. Zimmerman: Fine structure of cerebral fluid accumulation. II. Swelling produced by triethyl tin poisoning compared with that in human brain, Am. J. Path., 36, 273-287 (1960).

Tower, D. B.: Structural and functional organization of mammalian cerebral cortex: The correlation of neurone density with brain size. Cortical neurone density in the fin whale (Balaenoptera physalus L.) with a note on the cortical neurone density in the Indian elephant, J. Comp. Neurol., 101, 19-52 (1954).

_____: The effects of 2-deoxy-D-glucose on metabolism of slices of cerebral cortex incubated in vitro, J. Neurochem., 3, 185-205 (1958).

_____: Problems associated with studies of electrolyte metabolism in normal and epileptogenic cerebral cortex, Epilepsia, 6, 183-197 (1965).

_____ and R. S. Bourke: Fluid compartmentation and electrolytes of cat cerebral cortex in vitro. III. Ontogenetic and comparative aspects, J. Neurochem., 13, 1119-1137 (1966).

_____ and K. A. C. Elliott: Activity of acetylcholine system in cerebral cortex of various unanesthetized mammals, Am. J. Physiol., 168, 747-759 (1952).

Van Harreveld, A., J. Crowell and S. K. Malhotra: A study of extracellular space in central nervous tissue by freeze-substitution. J. Cell Biol., 25, 117-137 (1965).

_____ and J. P. Schadé: On distribution and movements of water and electrolytes in cerebral cortex, in: Structure and Function of the Cerebral Cortex (ed. by D. B. Tower and J. P. Schadé), Amsterdam: Elsevier, pp. 239-254 (1960).

Varon, S. and H. McIlwain: Fluid content and compartments in isolated cerebral tissues, J. Neurochem., 8, 262-275 (1961).

Vernadakis, A. and D. M. Woodbury: Electrolyte and amino acid changes in rat brain during maturation, Am. J. Physiol., 203, 748-752 (1962).

Voeller, K., G. D. Pappas, and D. P. Purpura: Electron microscope study of development of cat superficial neocortex, Exp. Neurol. 7, 107-130 (1963).

Wanko, T. and D. B. Tower: Combined morphological and biochemical studies of incubated slices of cerebral cortex, in: Morphological and Biochemical Correlates of Neural Activity (ed. by M. M. Cohen and R. S. Snider), New York: Hoeber-Harper, pp. 75-97 (1964)

Weed, L. H. and W. Hughson: Intracranial venous pressure and cerebrospinal fluid pressure as affected by the intravenous injection of solutions of various concentrations, Am. J. Physiol., 58, 101-130 (1921).

_____ and P. S. McKibben: Experimental alteration of brain bulk, Am. J. Physiol., 48, 531-558 (1919).

Welty, J. D., W. O. Reed and E. H. Shaw: Isolation of 2-hydroxyethane-sulfonic acid (isethionic acid) from dog heart, J. Biol. Chem., 237, 1160-1161 (1962).

W. W. OPPELT
D. P. RALL

BRAIN EXTRACELLULAR SPACE AS MEASURED BY DIFFUSION OF VARIOUS MOLECULES INTO BRAIN

There is currently controversy as to the extent of extracellular space (ECS) in the brain. Estimates of brain ECS range from 0-5% as reported from electron micrographs (Farquhar & Hartmann, 1957; Gershenfeld, et al., 1959; Horstmann & Meves, 1959; Maynard, et al., 1957; Schultz, et al., 1957; DeRobertis, 1962), to 50% when one equates in vitro sodium or chloride spaces to brain ECS (Manery & Bale, 1941; Elliott & Jasper, 1949).

In order to understand the transfer of materials between brain cells and capillaries, it is necessary to know the extent of brain ECS. The usual mechanism of such transport between tissue cells and blood is thought to involve diffusion of the various ions and metabolites in tissue ECS, which might be thought of as a highway connecting the tissue cell and the capillary. Most electron micrographs (Maynard, et al., 1957; Schultz, et al., 1957), show brain cells to be tightly packed with intercellular spaces of less than 150Å. Calculations of ECS from such pictures indicate brain ECS of about 3-5%. Should this be the in vivo situation, brain ECS would not be able to function as the transferring medium for various ions and metabolites on their way to and from the cell, and it would be necessary to postulate specific trans-membrane transport mechanisms for every molecule that is involved in brain cell metabolism. One might therefore wonder if the low values for brain ECS in electron microscope (EM) pictures might be the result of artifacts produced during the fixation process. There is indication that anoxia and death results in brain swelling (Varon & McIlwain, 1961; Pappius, et al., 1962). That such brain swelling may represent primarily a swelling of the intracellular space at the expense of the extracellular space is indicated by studies of Van Harreveld concerning electrical impedance and conductance (Van Harreveld & Crowell, 1964; Van Harreveld & Ochs, 1956; Van Harreveld, et al., 1961). Also, recent studies of Schultz and Karlsson indicated that the extent of brain ECS on EM pictures can be varied at will using fixing solutions of varying compositions (Karlsson & Schultz, 1965; Schultz & Karlsson, 1965). It is therefore not surprising that various physiological measurements of in vivo brain ECS (Streicher, et al., 1964; Bourke, et al., 1965; Davson, et al., 1963), indicated it to be considerably larger than indicated in most EM pictures.

Recently we reported preliminary studies on inulin spaces in various parts of the brain (Rall, et al., 1962; Oppelt, et al., 1964). An inulin containing buffer was perfused through the ventricular system of dogs at a steady rate, and the diffusion of inulin from ventricle into brain was measured. Such measurements indicated the inulin space (considered to be equivalent to ECS) to be in the vicinity of 12%. When similar experiments were done in dead dogs, the inulin space shrank about 50%, thus indicating significant decrease in brain ECS with anoxia and death. We have since then studied inulin diffusion into brain in various other animals, have used ECS indicator molecules other than inulin, and have performed a few experiments in which the ventricular perfusate was made hypo- or hypertonic, or where an attempt was made to change osmolarity of the animal's plasma.

MATERIALS AND METHODS

Dogs, cats, green and rhesus monkeys were anesthetized with pentobarbital. A burr hole was made near the mid-parietal area of the skull, and a 22 gauge needle was introduced stereotaxically into one of the lateral ventricles. A larger needle was placed into the cisterna magna. A CSF-like buffer (Rall, et al., 1962), was then perfused for 1-8 hours at 0.2 ml/min. Depending on the experiment, this buffer contained either inulin-C-14, sucrose-C-14, or dextran-C-14. A certain number of animals were killed with an overdose of pentobarbital as soon as ventricular perfusion had been established, and the experiment was continued in the dead animal. In some dogs, the osmolarity of the perfusate was changed by either adding 50% more or decreasing NaCl by 50%. In other dogs, either 0.8% or 33% glucose in water was injected intraperitoneally in an attempt to raise or lower plasma osmolarity. At the end of each experiment the brain was rapidly removed, 5mm coronal sections were taken through caudate nucleus, thalamus and pons, and narrow strips of brain were cut from the coronal sections, from ventricle outward. Accurately measured 1 or 2mm pieces of brain were then cut from the strips, and radioactivity in each piece was determined in a liquid scintillation system. Radioactivity was also determined in ventricular inflow and outflow. Brain indicator molecule concentration relative to perfusate concentration was then plotted as a function of distance from the ventricle, and diffusion coefficients and total indicator molecule spaces were determined. As a check on the methodology, similar experiments were performed allowing the indicator molecules to diffuse into blocks of agar. Diffusion coefficients thus obtained were compared to diffusion coefficients of the same molecules in brain.

THEORETICAL CONSIDERATIONS OF THE METHODOLOGY

The general approach of this method is to perfuse the ventricular system of an animal with a buffer containing a constant concentration of an indicator molecule. The molecule is then allowed to diffuse into the brain, and its concentration profile in the brain is measured as a function of distance from the ventricular surface and is compared to indicator molecule concentration in the perfusate. From this profile, the maximum indicator substance concentration in the brain may be calculated (Maximum concentration = concentration in first mm brain + concentration in first mm − concentration in second mm). This maximum indicator molecule space is assumed to represent ECS. Certain further assumptions must then be made: 1) The ECS is an infinitely long, uniform slab, bathed on one end with the indicator solution. The slab is initially free of the indicator molecule. 2) The diffusion coefficient of the indicator material is constant, independent of concentration. 3) The material diffuses freely in the ECS. 4) The ECS is homogeneous in any one region of the brain. 5) There is no bulk flow or mixing of the solution within the ECS during the experiment. 6) The ependymal layer, lining the ventricle, is completely permeable to the material. 7) The test material does not bind to cell membranes in the brain. 8) The test material remains extracellular. 9) The capillaries of the brain are impermeable to the indicator material. These assumptions will be discussed later.

RESULTS

Inulin spaces: (Table 1)

TABLE 1

INULIN SPACES (%) IN LIVE AND DEAD DOG, CAT AND MONKEY BRAIN

Animal	#	C.N.	Thal.	Pons
live dog	35	12.7 ± 3.9 (SD)	6.1 ± 2.3	11.5 ± 3.9
dead dog	10	5.4 ± 2.4	2.2 ± 1.4	4.3 ± 2.0
live cat	3	11.7 ± 2.3	9.3 ± 1.3	11.9 ± 3.3
dead cat	3	7.2 ± 1.1	4.9 ± 2.0	5.2 ± 1.4
live green monkey	2	8.7 ± 0.7	11.0 ± 3.4	10.6 ± 2.5
dead green monkey	2	7.5 ± 2.6	7.2 ± 4.2	3.8 ± 2.7
live rhesus monkey	2	10.1 ± 1.5	17.5 ± 5.6	10.4 ± 2.0
dead rhesus monkey	2	3.1 ± 1.1	5.8 ± 0.9	8.4 (only sample)

These spaces are maximum inulin spaces in brain as determined from the diffusion profile of inulin in brain. They are thought to represent brain extracellular space. C.N. = caudate nucleus; Thal.= thalamus; SD = Standard deviation.

In live dogs, inulin spaces in caudate nucleus averaged around 13%. In the pons they were about 12%, while in thalamus they were about half that. Similar values were found in cats and in rhesus and green monkeys. When the same experiment was done in dead animals, inulin spaces decreased at least 50%, bringing them very close to values for ECS usually observed in EM pictures. Typical diffusion profiles in live and dead brain may be seen in Figures 1 and 2.

Sucrose spaces: (Table 2)

Somewhat larger sucrose spaces were observed in all animals as compared to inulin spaces. Again, sucrose space decreased about 50% when the same experiment was performed in the dead animal.

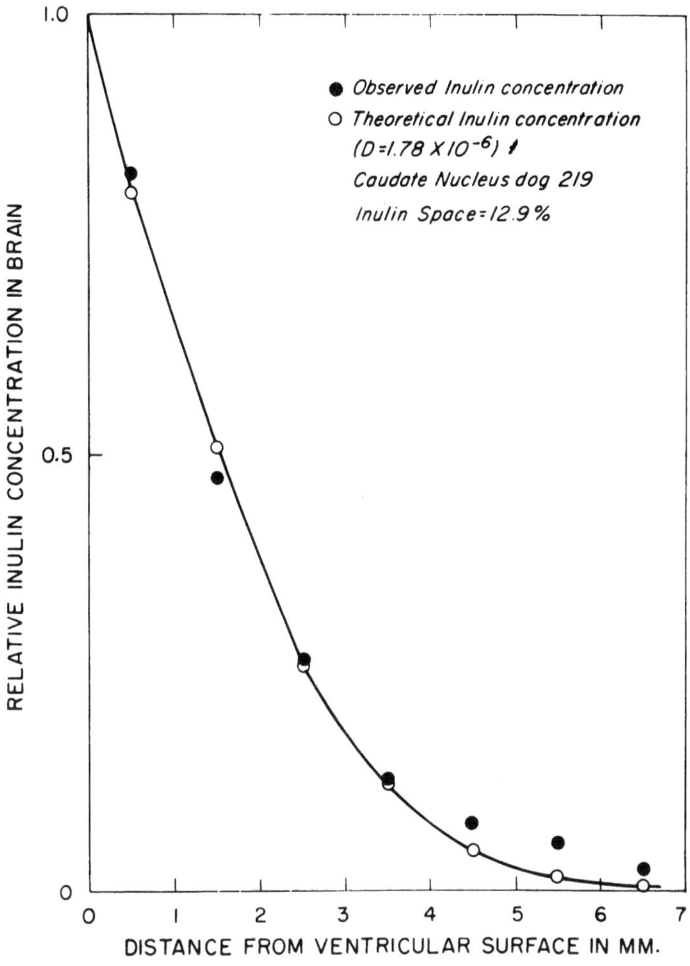

Fig. 1. Inulin concentration in dog brain as related to distance from the ventricle. Note the close parallel between observed inulin concentration and the calculated inulin concentration derived from the diffusion coefficient for that experiment.

Dextran spaces: (Table 3)

Dextran of uniform molecular weight was used in these experiments. Molecular weights in various experiments ranged from 12,500 to 77,700. Dextran spaces were very similar to corresponding inulin spaces. There was no significant difference between experiments using dextrans of varying molecular weight. This is probably due to the relatively small number of experiments.

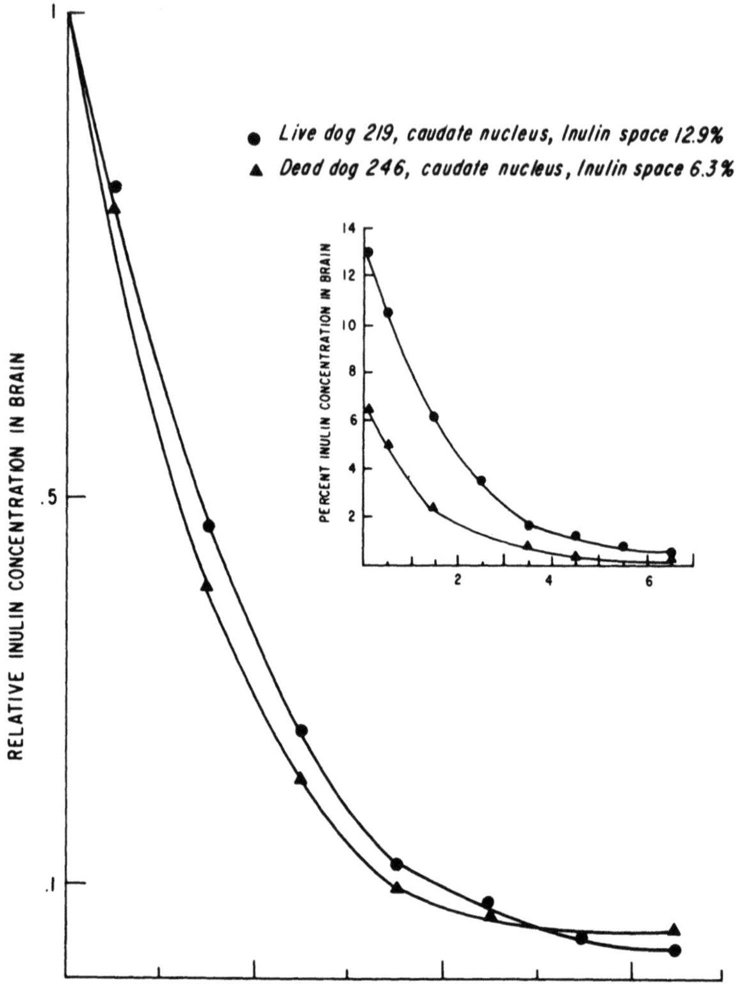

Fig. 2. Absolute and relative inulin concentration in live and dead dog brain as related to distance from the ventricle. It is well shown that the absolute inulin space is decreased about 50% in the dead preparation. However, the close parallelism of the diffusion curves when one plots relative inulin concentration indicates that inulin travels through brain extracellular space in the same manner in dead or live brain.

Inulin spaces during osmotic changes: (Table 4)

When hypotonic buffer was used as the ventricular perfusate, the brain appeared slightly edematous. Inulin spaces, however, were very similar to those found during isotonic perfusion. When hypertonic buffer was used, brain appeared grossly somewhat shrunken, and there was a tendency for inulin spaces to be slightly greater than when isotonic buffer was used. When hypotonic glucose

TABLE 2

SUCROSE SPACES (%) IN LIVE AND DEAD DOG BRAIN

Animal	#	C.N.	Thal.	Pons
live dog	8	18.1 ± 5.9 (SD)	11.2 ± 4.0	22.4 ± 8.2
dead dog	3	6.6 ± 2.5	6.0 ± 3.5	10.6 ± 3.4

These spaces are maximum sucrose spaces as determined from the diffusion profile of sucrose in brain. C.N. = caudate nucleus; Thal.= thalamus; SD = Standard deviation.

was injected intraperitoneally, the gross appearance of the brain was not changed, and inulin spaces in these experiments were similar to those in control experiments. Hypertonic glucose intraperitoneally resulted in a great decrease in plasma volume, occasionally leading to shock in the animal. However, again, neither gross appearance of brain nor inulin spaces were changed from the control situation.

TABLE 3

DEXTRAN SPACES (%) IN LIVE DOG BRAIN

Animal	#	C.N.	Thal.	Pons
live dog	5	10.2 ± 1.1 (SD)	6.3 ± 0.7	10.0 ± 1.2

These spaces are maximum dextran spaces in dog brain as determined from the diffusion profile of dextran in brain. Dextran of uniform molecular weight as used in each experiment. The highest molecular weight used was 77,700, the lowest 12,500. In these few experiments, there was no discernable difference in dextran spaces with varying molecular weights. This is indicated by the small standard deviation (SD) of each result. C.N.= caudate nucleus; Thal.= thalamus.

TABLE 4

INULIN SPACES (%) IN LIVE DOG BRAIN EXPOSED TO HYPO- OR HYPERTONIC ENVIRONMENTS

Environment	#	C. N.	Thal.	Pons
Control (Table 1)	35	12.7 ± 3.9 (SD)	6.1 ± 2.3	11.5 ± 3.9
hyper perf.	4	15.6 ± 1.4	10.5 ± 2.0	14.1 ± 3.7
hypo perf.	4	10.8 ± 1.3	6.4 ± 1.0	11.8 ± 2.2
hyper I. P. gluc.	5	13.0 ± 0.6	9.4 ± 1.1	17.5 ± 5.1
hypo I. P. gluc.	3	12.8 ± 0.7	6.5 ± 1.9	9.8 ± 1.1

Inulin spaces were determined as in Table 1. Hypertonic or hypotonic ventricular perfusates (hyper perf., hypo perf.) were produced by either increasing or decreasing perfusate NaCl concentration by 50%. 33% glucose in water (hyper I.P. gluc.) or 0.8% glucose in water (hypo I.P. gluc.) was injected intraperitoneally at the beginning of the experiment. C.N. = caudate nucleus; Thal.= thalamus; SD = Standard deviation.

Diffusion coefficients: (Table 5)

Diffusion coefficients for inulin in live or dead brain ranged from 2.0 to 3.4 X $10^{-6}cm^2$/second. Similar values were obtained for the other indicator substances. Calculation of diffusion coefficients of inulin and sucrose in agar shows them to be very similar to those found in brain. There is also close agreement between these diffusion coefficients and those reported in the literature (Schantz & Laufer, 1962).

TABLE 5

DIFFUSION COEFFICIENTS CALCULATED IN BRAIN OR AGAR FOR INULIN, SUCROSE AND DEXTRAN

Substance	Medium	#	diffusion coefficient X 10^{-6} (cm^2/sec.)
inulin	live dog brain	24	3.3 ± 1.6 (SD)
inulin	dead dog brain	5	3.4 ± 1.7
inulin	live cat brain	3	2.8 ± 1.6
inulin	dead cat brain	3	2.7 ± 1.8
inulin	live green monkey brain	2	2.1 ± 1.9
inulin	dead green monkey brain	2	2.1 ± 1.2
inulin	live rhesus monkey brain	2	2.0 ± 1.0
inulin	dead rhesus monkey brain	2	2.4 ± 1.6
inulin	agar	3	3.2 ± 0.2
sucrose	live dog brain	7	4.4 ± 2.4
sucrose	dead dog brain	3	3.5 ± 2.7
sucrose	agar	5	4.9 ± 1.5
dextran	live dog brain	5	3.5 ± 1.6

Diffusion coefficients were calculated from the diffusion profile of each substance in brain or agar.
SD = Standard deviation.

DISCUSSION

Assumptions which have to be met to make this method a valid one in determining brain ECS will now be discussed.

1. The requirement that the system be an infinitely long slab

is satisfied by the fact that the diffusing substance concentration farthest from the bathing surface is negligible. Even at a distance of 1 cm from the ventricular surface, diffusing substance concentration was less than 1% as compared to ventricular surface concentration. As the indicator substances used were of a type not naturally occurring in the body, the system was initially free of the indicator material.

2. Because of the very low concentration of the diffusing substance in the brain, it can safely be assumed that its diffusion coefficient will remain constant.

3. The close agreement of the experimental diffusion constants found in brain, the diffusion constants in agar and the theoretical diffusion constants in an aqueous medium as found in the literature indicates that the indicator molecules moved through brain ECS by simple diffusion.

4. The requirement that ECS in brain be homogeneous is only partially satisfied. Regions such as caudate nucleus or pons probably have a relatively homogeneous ECS, however the thalamus, with its mixture of gray and white matter would not be expected to have such a homogeneous ECS. What is therefore determined, in these experiments, is average ECS.

5. Should there be bulk flow or mixing of the indicator material in brain ECS the diffusion profile of each substance in the brain would be expected to be distorted; and diffusion constants calculated from such a profile would be expected to vary from theoretical ones for simple diffusion. As the constants were very close to theoretical ones for simple diffusion, one can safely assume that no significant mixing or bulk flow of indicator material occurs in brain ECS.

6. If there were a significant barrier at the ependymal surface, the ratio of indicator substance concentrations in the ependyma (C_s) to concentration in the ventricle (C_v), i.e., C_s/C_v, would increase with increasing length of the experiment. In our method, C_s = ECS. Thus, the calculated ECS in our experiments should increase with increasing length of the experiment. In performing experiments lasting from one to eight hours, no such change in value for ECS was found, thus suggesting that there is no significant barrier at the ependymal surface.

7 and 8. The primary indicator substance used in these experiments, inulin, has been a common indicator of ECS in other tissues. There is no evidence to our knowledge that it either binds to, or enters cells. Again, should this occur in the brain, the diffusion profile of inulin in the brain should not be consistent with simple diffusion. Thus, it is likely that inulin in the brain neither binds to cell membranes, nor enters cells to any significant degree.

9. It is well known that inulin, given intravenously, enters the brain in very small quantities, presumably because of difficulty in

crossing of the blood-brain barrier. It thus seems very unlikely that significant quantities of inulin will passively diffuse from brain ECS into capillaries. The other possibility to be considered concerns an active transport mechanism for inulin from brain ECS to blood. There is no evidence for an active transport mechanism for inulin in any biological system, thus it would be unlikely that such a system should be present in the brain capillary. Again, if significant amounts of inulin should leave the brain ECS, the typical diffusion profile of inulin in the brain should be distorted. It is likely that very small amounts of inulin or the other test substances leave brain ECS via the capillaries. This error would result in an underestimation of brain ECS by our method. It could thus be considered that these experiments put a lower limit on the extent of brain ECS.

It thus appears that the assumptions necessary to the validity of the experiments are satisfied, and that it is possible to determine brain ECS fairly accurately by allowing various indicator molecules to diffuse from ventricle into the brain.

In the past, information concerning the extent of brain ECS has been primarily derived from three types of studies: 1) diffusion of ECS indicators from plasma to brain; 2) incubation in vitro of brain slices with various electrolytes and ECS indicators; 3) electron miscroscopy of brain. In the first type of study (sulfate, inulin), only about 5% of plasma concentration of ECS indicators were found in the brain, and this was thought to represent ECS (Woodbury, 1958; Barlow, et al., 1961). Present evidence indicates that such low values were due to slow and limited passage of such ECS indicating molecules across the blood-brain barrier, and thus are not a valid indication of brain ECS.

In vitro incubation of brain slices seemed to indicate larger extracellular spaces, at times in the range of 50% (Manery & Bale, 1941; Elliott & Jasper, 1949). Interpretation of such studies, however, is difficult. The brain slices were most certainly anoxic, many dendritic processes and cells were ruptured in such preparations, and swelling and water uptake, indicating a non-physiological state, can easily be demonstrated in such preparations (Varon & McIlwain, 1961; Pappius, et al., 1962).

The obviously very small amount of ECS seen in most EM pictures is more difficult to explain. Fixation of tissue has been rapid, and most authors claim that this preserves normal cell relationships. However, recent studies by Van Harreveld's group (Van Harreveld & Crowell, 1964; Van Harreveld, et al., 1961) concerning the electrical behavior of brain indicate extremely rapid fluid and electrolyte shifts when brain is made anoxic. These authors noted an almost immediate shift of water and electrolytes from ECS into cells, resulting in an up to 300% increase in cell volume. Other studies

(Karlsson & Schultz, 1965; Schultz & Karlsson, 1965), show that the appearance of the extent of ECS on EM pictures can be varied by altering the composition, pH or osmolarity, of the EM fixing medium.

It therefore seems likely that the usual estimate of brain ECS of 3-5% from EM pictures is an underestimate of ECS, and is due to post-mortem and fixation artifact.

There have been other recent studies that suggest that brain ECS is in the vicinity of 10-15%, sufficient for diffusion of various molecules. Streicher, et al. (1964), measured thiocyanate spaces in brain after intravenous injection, and found them to be around 15%. Bourke, et al. (1965), measured inulin and sucrose spaces in cortex after single intracisternal injections and found them to be between 18 and 32%. This may be somewhat of an overestimate, as the indicator substance concentration in the subarachnoid CSF was constantly falling. Davson, et al. (1963), performed a similar study, and estimated ECS in whole cord to be around 12%.

It thus seems likely that brain ECS occupies about 10-15% of whole brain. Our studies using inulin and dextran in dog, monkey and cat indicate that such is the case. Sucrose space in our studies was consistently somewhat larger than inulin space. This may well be due to the smaller molecular size of sucrose, allowing it to penetrate into the more remote and smaller extracellular spaces to which the larger inulin molecule has no access. The inulin spaces can thus be considered a minimum ECS, the true ECS probably being closer to that found with sucrose.

It is very interesting to note that both inulin and sucrose spaces decrease at least 50% when the experiments are being performed in the dead animal. This lends support to the contention that anoxic and dead brain cells swell at the expense of ECS. It is interesting that under these conditions, ECS is very similar to that found in most EM pictures.

Not many conclusions can be drawn from the preliminary studies involving change of osmolarity of the perfusate or plasma. One has to remember that these were rather short-term studies of only four hours, probably not enough time for significant total fluid changes to take place in the brain. Under the conditions of the study, there was probably no change in inulin space when hyper- or hypotonic glucose was injected intraperitoneally. We also do not have microscopic pictures of brain to indicate the presence or absence of brain edema during these experiments. If there would be brain edema, it would have to involve both extra- and intracellular spaces in equal proportions. Extension of these studies is necessary to draw firm conclusions.

During hypo- or hypertonic ventricular perfusion there was some gross evidence of cerebral swelling or shrinkage. There was a tendency for inulin spaces to be larger than control values during hypertonic perfusion, and smaller during hypotonic perfusion. More experiments are necessary to be certain of the validity of this finding. Should this prove to be true, it would indicate that such brain edema involves both the extra- and the intracellular compartment, more so the intracellular compartment. It would be very interesting to study inulin spaces during other edematous states, such as the edema produced by tin salts.

SUMMARY

The diffusion of inulin, sucrose and dextran from ventricular space into brain was measured by ventriculo-cisternal perfusion in live and dead dogs, cats, rhesus monkeys and green monkeys.

The concentration of these substances was measured in brain and ventricular perfusate, and the space which each of these substances occupies in the brain was determined. It was found that these substances move through the brain by simple diffusion, and that diffusion constants of the substances in brain were similar to diffusion constants in agar and as obtained from the literature.

Inulin, dextran and sucrose spaces thus calculated were thought to represent brain extracellular space (ECS). In caudate nucleus and pons, ECS thus calculated was about 12-15% in the live animal, while it decreased by 50% in the dead animal. Somewhat smaller values were found for thalamus.

Inulin spaces were also measured in dog brain exposed to hypo- or hypertonic perfusate, as well as after intraperitoneal injection of hypo- or hypertonic glucose. There was no change in ECS after the intraperitoneal injections, while there was a suggestion of an ECS increase with hypertonic, and an ECS decrease with hypotonic perfusate. It is suggested that any brain edema produced by such manipulations involved both extra- and intracellular fluid shifts

REFERENCES

Barlow, C. F., N. S. Domek, M. A. Goldberg and L. J. Roth: Extracellular brain space measured by S^{35} sulfate, Arch. Neurol. 5, 102-110 (1961).

Bourke, R. S., E. S. Greenberg and D. B. Tower: Variation of cerebral cortex fluid spaces in vivo as a function of species brain size, Am. J. Physiol., 208, 689-692 (1965).

Davson, H., C. F. Kleeman and E. Levin: The blood-brain barrier, in: Proceedings of the First International Pharmacology Meeting, Vol. 4: Drugs and Membranes (ed. by C. A. M. Hogben), Pergamon Press (1963).

DeRobertis, E.: Some old and new concepts of brain structure, World Neurol., 3, 98-111 (1962).

Elliott, K. A. C. and H. Jasper: Measurement of experimentally induced brain swelling and shrinkage, Am. J. Physiol., 157, 122 (1949).

Farquhar, M. G. and J. F. Hartmann: Neurological structure and relationships as revealed by electron microscopy, Neuropath. Exp. Neurol., 16, 18-39 (1957).

Gershenfeld, H. M., F. Wald, J. A. Zadunaisky and E. D. P. DeRobertis: Function of atroglia in the water-ion metabolism of the central nervous system, Neurology, 9, 412-425 (1959).

Horstmann, E. and H. Meves: Die Feinstruktur des molekularen Rindengraues und ihre physiologische Bedeuting, Z. Zellforsch. Mikroskop. Anat., 49, 569-604 (1959).

Karlsson, U. and R. L. Schultz: Fixation of the central nervous system for electron microscopy by aldehyde perfusion. I. Preservation with aldehyde perfusates versus direct perfusion with osmium tetroxide with special reference to membranes and the extracellular space, J. Ultrastruct. Res., 12, 160-186 (1965).

Manery, J. F. and W. F. Bale: Penetration of radioactive sodium and phosphorus into the extra- and intracellular phases of tissues, Am. J. Physiol., 132, 215 (1941).

Maynard, E. A., R. L. Schultz and D. C. Pease: Electron microscopy of the vascular bed of rat cerebral cortex, Am. J. Anat., 100, 409-433 (1957).

Oppelt, W. W., C. S. Patlak and D. P. Rall: Extracellular space in brain exposed to hypo- or hypertonic environments, Clin. Res., 12, 197 (1964).

Pappius, H. M., I. Klatzo and K. A. C. Elliott: Further studies on swelling of brain slices, Canad. J. Biochem. Physiol., 40, 885-898 (1962).

Rall, D. P., W. W. Oppelt and C. S. Patlak: Extracellular space of brain as determined by diffusion of inulin from the ventricular system, Life Sci., 2, 43-48 (1962).

Schantz, E. J. and M. A. Laufer: Diffusion measurements in agar gell, Biochem., 1, 658-663 (1962).

Schultz, R. L., E. A. Maynard and D. C. Pease: Electron microscopy of neurons and neuroglia of cerebral cortex and corpus callosum, Am. J. Anat., 100, 369-408 (1957).

_____ and U. Karlsson: Fixation of the central nervous system for electron microscopy by aldehyde perfusion. II. Effect of osmolarity, pH of perfusate and fixative concentration, J. Ultrastruct. Res., 12, 187-206 (1965).

Streicher, E., D. P. Rall and J. R. Gaskins: Distribution of thiocyanate between plasma and cerebrospinal fluid, Am. J. Physiol., 206, 251-254 (1964).

Van Harreveld, A. and J. Crowell: Extracellular space in central nervous tissue, Federation Proc., 23, 304 (1964).

_____ and S. Ochs: Cerebral impedance changes after circulatory arrest, Am. J. Physiol., 187, 180-192 (1956).

_____, N. K. Hooper and J. T. Cusick: Brain electrolytes and cortical impedance, Ibid., 201, 139-143 (1961).

Varon, S. and H. McIlwain: Fluid contents and compartments in isolated cerebral tissue, J. Neurochem., 8, 262-275 (1961).

Woodbury, D. M.: in: Biology of Neuroglia (ed. by W. F. Windle). Springfield: Charles C. Thomas, pp. 120-128 (1958).

_____, P. S. Timiras, A. Koch and A. Ballard: Distribution of radiochloride, radiosulfate and inulin in brain of rats, Fed. Proc., 15, 501 (1956).

H. DAVSON
M. BRADBURY
L. BITO

KINETICS OF CEREBROSPINAL FLUID EXCHANGES

In this paper I propose to review very briefly the main factors concerned in the exchanges of materials within the central nervous system; other authors will be dealing with specific aspects in more detail, so that here I shall only draw a simple sketch for the assistance of those whose interests do not lie specifically in this direction.

Essentially, then, we are dealing with the passage of dissolved substances and of water to and from three principal compartments, namely the blood, cerebrospinal fluid (CSF), and central nervous parenchyma. The last named is often referred to loosely as "brain" but of course includes the spinal cord, and it may be subdivided into an extracellular fluid, or space, and an intracellular compartment constituted by the internal milieu of the neurons and glial cells. If certain glial cells, possibly the astrocytes, are concerned with transport of material from one region of the parenchyma to another, as has often been suggested, then it will become desirable to subdivide the intracellular compartment on this basis.

The blood comes into relation with the CSF primarily in the choroid plexuses, which may be regarded as outpouchings of the pial vasculature into the lumens of the ventricles, retaining the ependymal covering which is here called the choroidal epithelium. This juxtaposition of epithelium and capillary network probably constitutes an arrangement whereby water and solutes may be transported from blood into the ventricles in the form of a characteristic secretion, the "primary CSF." In other regions of the pia it is generally accepted now that there is no capillary system, the pia or pia-arachnoid merely acting as a framework through which the larger blood vessels are conducted (Millen & Woollam, 1961).

THE BLOOD-CSF BARRIER

When we inject a substance into the blood we find usually that it appears in the CSF, and when different substances are compared we find quite large differences in rate of appearance, i.e., in the rate of build-up of concentration. This experimental observation is the basis of the concept of the blood CSF barrier. An example is provided by Figure 1 where a number of different substances, of

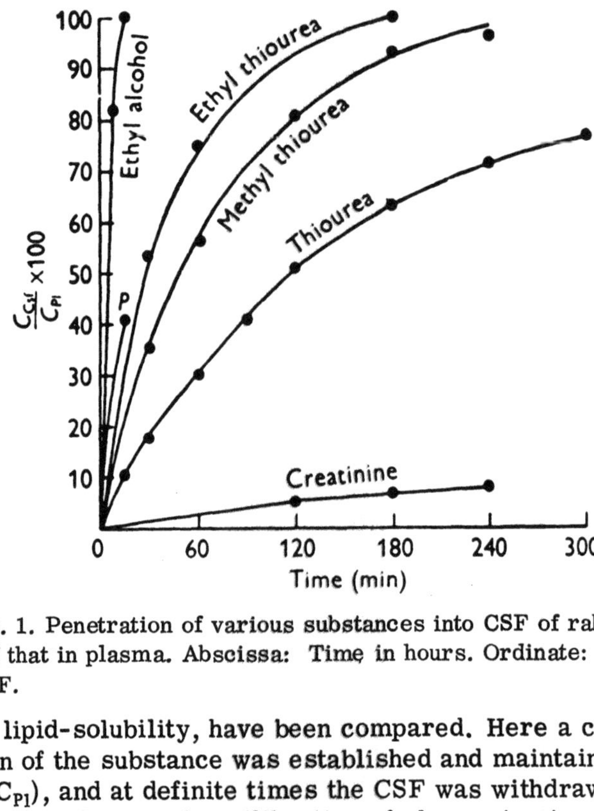

Fig. 1. Penetration of various substances into CSF of rabbit as percentage of that in plasma. Abscissa: Time in hours. Ordinate: Concentration in CSF.

different lipid-solubility, have been compared. Here a constant concentration of the substance was established and maintained in the plasma (C_{Pl}), and at definite times the CSF was withdrawn and analysed. The degree of equilibration of plasma is given by the ratio of the concentrations in CSF (C_{csf}) and plasma (C_{Pl}), which may be converted into a percentage.

In general, the more lipid-soluble the substance the more rapidly equilibrium is attained. With a relatively lipid-insoluble substance, such as creatinine, the rate of equilibration is slow and the concentration in the CSF shows no indication that it will reach that in the plasma even at "infinite time."

The mechanism whereby the concentration in the CSF builds

up towards that in the blood plasma must now be examined. If the substance is highly lipid-soluble it will rapidly enter the secretory cells of the choroid plexuses and emerge in the new secretion probably with the same concentration as that in the plasma. With the passage of time this new secretion, containing the substance, replaces the original fluid in the ventricles and subarachnoid spaces, so that the concentration eventually builds up to that in the plasma. If we know the rate at which CSF is replaced by new fluid, i.e., the rate of turnover of CSF, we can estimate how long such a process of equilibration would take. Experimentally the "turnover constant" for CSF can be determined with some precision; in the rabbit, to which the results of Figure 1 refer, this is on the average .005 min^{-1}. This means that 99% equilibration would be achieved in 15 hours. This is a very long time compared with the few minutes required for equilibration of ethyl alcohol with plasma as shown in Figure 1, so that there must be an additional mechanism of passage from blood to CSF apart from that involved in the replacement of CSF. This additional mechanism could be given by passage from blood to the extracellular fluid of brain and thence across the ependyma and pia-glia to the CSF in the ventricles and subarachnoid spaces respectively. Clearly this passage would be independent of the flow of CSF and would accelerate equilibration; furthermore, if passage into the extracellular fluid from blood was favored by lipid-solubility of the molecules, we would be able to account for the marked influence of lipid-solubility on rate of equilibration revealed by Figure 1.

THE BLOOD-BRAIN BARRIER

To demonstrate the possibility of this additional route for equilibration we must measure the simultaneous passage into brain parenchyma and CSF. If passage into the parenchuma is markedly influenced by lipid-solubility, and if the concentration in the extracellular fluid is, at any time, higher than in CSF, we may assume that the gradient for diffusion from brain to CSF is present, and this will be good prima facie evidence for the existence of this route of exchange. In Figure 2 the penetration of ethyl thiourea and thiourea into both brain and CSF have been plotted against time. It will be seen that the more lipid-soluble ethyl thiourea passes more rapidly into brain than thiourea, and also that for both substances rate of equilibration with brain-water is more rapid than equilibration with CSF. Since a high percentage of the brain-water is intracellular, the actual concentration in the extracellular fluid may be higher, so that there is no doubt at all that the necessary concentration gradient for passage from parenchyma to CSF is always present.

Thus, to examine fully the exchanges between blood and CSF we must examine the exchanges between blood and the central nervous parenchyma, i.e., we must examine the blood-brain barrier as well as the blood-CSF barrier. Furthermore, we must appreciate that it is virtually impossible to examine the one in isolation

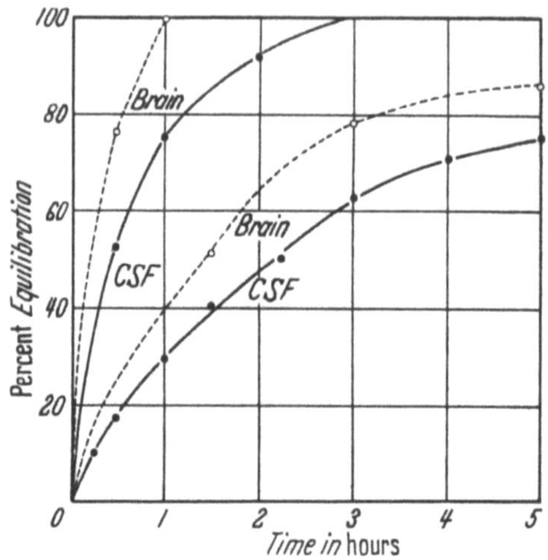

Fig. 2. Penetration of ethyl thiourea (upper curves) and thiourea (lower curves) into cerebrospinal fluid and brain.

from the other. For example, if we are concerned with the passage of ethyl alcohol from blood to brain, we may measure the rate at which the alcohol accumulates in the brain but we must make allowance for the losses that will necessarily take place from brain to CSF. Under other conditions it is conceivable that the concentration in the brain may rise secondarily to a rise in concentration in the CSF. A further example of the complexity of the relationships between the three compartments of the central nervous system, and of the difficulties in studying exchanges in isolation, is given by the study of the passage from CSF to brain. For example, we may perfuse the ventricular system with an artificial CSF containing the substance in which we are interested, and we may measure the rate of accumulation in the brain, and it might be argued that under these conditions we were measuring the permeability of the ependymal lining of the ventricles. In fact, however, the limiting factor for accumulation in the brain is usually the ability of the blood to wash the substance away into the general circulation, i.e., it is a function of the brain-blood barrier. Thus it is quite likely that inulin would accumulate more rapidly in brain than ethyl alcohol, because the brain-blood barrier to inulin is very high indeed, so that practically all the inulin passing out of the perfusion fluid remains in the brain; by contrast, the passage of ethyl alcohol across the blood-brain barrier is very rapid indeed, so that the reverse passage will also be very rapid, and the chances of an alcohol molecule remaining in the brain are very small compared with those of an inulin molecule.

An excellent example of this inter-relationship of the exchanges between compartments is given by the study of ^{131}I. When a steady concentration of this isotope is maintained in the blood, the concentration in the brain after some hours is only a small fraction of that in the blood; the concentration in the CSF is very low, too (Davson, 1955; Davson & Spaziani, 1959; Reed & Woodbury, 1963). As a result of the pioneering study of Pappenheimer and subsequent workers (Pappenheimer, et al., 1961; Davson & Pollay, 1963; Welch, 1962; Becker, 1961), it has become clear that the low rate of appearance in the CSF, and the very low steady-state levels reached at "infinite time," can be attributed to an active transport mechanism in the choroid plexuses that "pumps" iodide outwards from CSF to blood. This is demonstrated by perfusing the ventricular system with artifical CSF containing ^{131}I and measuring the concentration of the effluent fluid emerging from the cisterna magna as a fraction of the inflowing concentration. As Figure 3 shows, the concentration in the effluent builds up to a steady value of about 25 per cent of the inflowing concentration; this is partly due to dilution of the inflowing fluid by newly formed CSF, but mainly due to diffusion into the blood of the choroid plexuses and also into the brain. The figure shows that when the concentration of non-radioactive iodide is increased, the concentration of ^{131}I in the effluent rises, indicating the inhibition of a large part of the absorptive process. It is for this, and other reasons, that the absorption is considered to involve an active process which is saturable by high concentrations of iodide; much more effective is perchlorate, a concentration as low as 0.02 mM having a marked inhibitory action.

The question now arises as to how much the low rate and extent of accumulation of ^{131}I in the brain, when this isotope is maintained at a steady concentration in the plasma, are a consequence of the low concentration maintained in the CSF by this active process that causes the iodide ion to move more easily out of the CSF than into it across the choroid plexuses. In other words, is the high blood-brain barrier to ^{131}I a consequence of the high blood-CSF barrier?

That losses to the CSF are, indeed, a significant factor in the slow accumulation of ^{131}I in brain may be shown by studying the passage of the isotope under three separate conditions as follows:

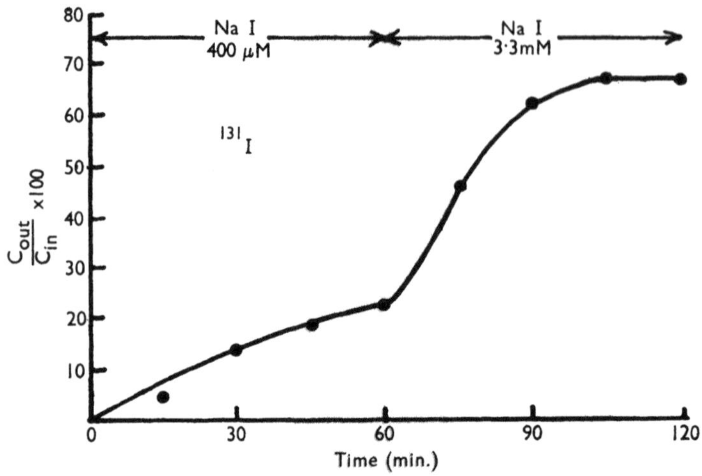

Fig. 3. Active transport of ^{131}I by choroid plexuses as demonstrated by ventriculo-cisternal perfusion. At 60 min. the concentration of inactive iodide was raised to 3.3 mM, with the result that absorption of ^{131}I was reduced. Ordinate: Outflow concentration as percentage of inflow concentration. Abscissa: Time in minutes after beginning perfusion.

a) A steady concentration is maintained in the blood plasma while the ventricles are perfused with ordinary artificial CSF containing no ^{131}I. After a given period the brain is analyzed. b) The ventricles are perfused with an artificial CSF containing ^{131}I and after a given period the brain is analyzed. c) The ventricles are perfused with an artificial CSF containing ^{131}I while a steady concentration of ^{131}I is maintained in the blood plasma. The concentrations in plasma and perfusion fluid are adjusted so as to be approximately equal. After a given period the brain is analyzed.

The results have been plotted in Figure 4, where the ^{131}I uptake of brain has been plotted against time from beginning of the perfusion or infusion. The uptake of isotope has been expressed in terms of the concentration in the appropriate reference fluid. Thus for simple intravenous infusion the uptake is expressed as C.p.m. per gram of brain/C.p.m. per gram of plasma water; for simple ventriculo-cisternal perfusion the reference fluid is the perfusion fluid; for the combined infusion-perfusion the ventriculo-cisternal fluid was used as reference fluid since the uptake is more sensitive to this than to the plasma; usually the difference of concentration between plasma and perfusion fluid was only a few per cent. The figure shows that with intravenous infusion alone, Curve A, the ratio: Activity in Brain/Activity in Plasma H_2O reaches a value of 0.052, so that one might refer to an "^{131}I-space" of 5.2 per cent achieved by intravenous infusion alone. With cisternal perfusion (Curve B)

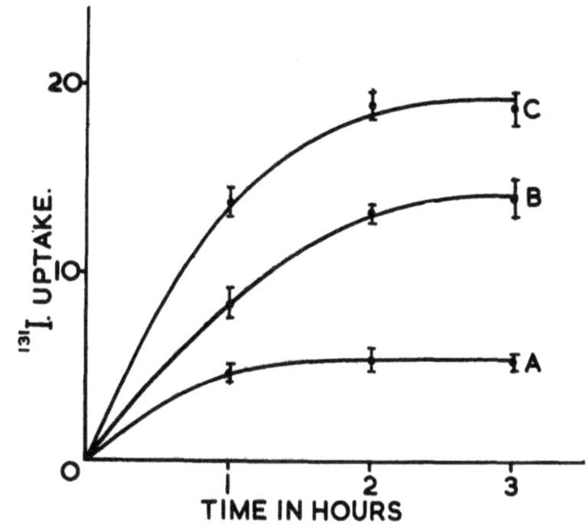

Fig. 4. Penetration of ^{131}I into brain of rabbit under three different conditions as described in text. In all cases active transport by choroid plexuses was inhibited by chlorate in perfusion fluid. Ordinate: Activity per unit wt. brain as percentage of that in unit wt. of plasma. Abscissa: Time in hours after beginning of infusion or perfusion.

the ratio becomes much higher, namely 0.14, so that by this technique one might say that an "^{131}I-space" of 14 per cent had been reached. With combined intravenous infusion and ventriculo-cisternal perfusion (Curve C) the ratio becomes 0.22 and the "^{131}I-space" may be said to be 22 per cent. This may well represent the true iodide-space of brain but is probably, even under these conditions, a low estimate since the computed spaces for different parts of the brain varied. The curves emphasize the significance of the blood-brain barrier in an unequivocal fashion; thus Curve B is below Curve C because of the escape of ^{131}I from brain into blood, and it is simple to show, by simple kinetic analysis, that the difference in ordinates of Curves C and B should be equal to the ordinates of Curve A, and this is very nearly the case. The experiment emphasizes, too, the importance of maintaining both plasma and CSF levels constant when it is proposed to estimate the "space" or percentage volume of distribution of a given substance. Thus merely maintaining a constant blood level for a long period of time, as for example has been done with $^{35}SO_4$ (Barlow, et al., 1961; Kibler, et al., 1964), and computing the sulphate-space by the formula: Activity per gram of brain/Activity per gram of Plasma × 100, would give a gross under-estimate of the true sulphate space since escape into the CSF would be ignored (Davson, 1963). A nearer estimate would have been given by ventriculo-cisternal perfusion with $^{35}SO_4$ in the perfusion fluid, but even then it would have ignored losses to blood. It is very clear indeed, that merely giving a single intraventricular injection and analysing brain and CSF after a period of time could lead to the most misleading estimates of space.

The curves of Figure 4 emphasize, too, the importance of the "sink action" of the CSF. With plain intravenous infusion the accumulation by brain is small and the cause is obviously the escape into the CSF since simultaneous perfusion of the ventricles allows accumulation to increase markedly. In these experiments active transport of ^{131}I was inhibited by perchlorate, otherwise the uptake by brain with simple blood infusion, represented by Curve A, would have been even less; and this brings us back to our original question: Can we explain the barrier phenomenon entirely on the basis of this "sink action", i.e., is transport across the blood-brain interface relatively unrestricted, the small uptake being completely accounted for by the escape into CSF In fact, however, it is possible to analyse the curves of Figure 4, and to deduce a constant for passage across the blood-brain barrier that makes allowance for any escapes into the CSF. If this is done, a value of 7.10^{-3} min^{-1} is obtained for ^{131}I in the perchlorate-treated animal. This may be compared with 5.10^{-3} min^{-1} for the turnover of ^{24}Na; in this case a possible sink action by the CSF is ruled out by the finding that passage into CSF keeps pace with passage into brain (Davson, 1955). This turnover constant for ^{24}Na in brain is indicative of a relatively slow passage across the blood-brain barrier, hence the finding that the constant for ^{131}I is of the same order of magnitude leaves one in little doubt that there is a blood-brain barrier to both sodium and iodide ions.

The difference between Curves A and B of Figure 4, emphasizing as it does the importance of escape of material from brain to CSF, raises the question as to the nature of the membrane separating these compartments, namely the ependymal lining to the ventricles. The fact that even the large molecule of inulin can apparently pass from CSF to brain (Rall, Oppelt Patlak, 1962), and the apparent lack of selectivity shown by the ependyma when other small molecules are examined, might indicate that the ependyma was a highly permeable membrane. It is possible, with some approximations, to calculate the flux of ions across the ependyma under appropriate conditions; Bito and Davson (1966) have done this for ^{24}Na and have obtained a figure of 1.65 $\mu mole/cm^2/min$; the experimental measurements involved in making Curve A of Figure 4 permitted the computation of a value of 0.5 $\mu mole/cm^2/min$ for iodide. These fluxes are very high indeed, and greatly in excess of the value of 0.004 $\mu mole/cm^2/min$ obtained for Na across the capillary membrane, a membrane that is generally recognized to be unselective. It is difficult to believe, therefore, that the ependyma exerts significant restraint on the passage of molecules from CSF to brain or vice versa.

In conclusion, we may ask whether the slow passage of iodide across the blood-brain barrier revealed by the analysis of the curves in Figure 4 is due to an active process that pumps iodide from brain tissue to blood, analogous with the active process acting across the choroid plexuses. This point has been examined recently by the present authors (Bito, et al., 1966), and it would seem that, if there is an active process, it is not very significant, so that most of the phenomena associated with the kinetics of exchange of iodide in the central nervous system are explicable in terms of the active process in the choroid plexuses plus slow passive exchanges across the blood-brain barrier.

REFERENCES

Barlow, C. F., N. S. Domek, M. A. Goldberg and L. J. Roth: Extracellular brain space measured by S^{35} sulphate, Arch. Neurol., 5, 102-110 (1961).

Becker, B.: Cerebrospinal fluid iodide, Amer. J. Physiol., 201, 1149-1151 (1961).

Bito, L. Z., M. W. B. Bradbury and H. Davson: Factors affecting the distribution of iodide and bromide in the central nervous system, J. Physiol., 185, 323-354 (1966).

_____ and H. Davson: Local variations in cerebrospinal fluid composition and its relationship to the composition of the extracellular fluid of the cortex, Exp. Neurol., 14, 264-280 (1966).

Davson, H.: A comparative study of the aqueous humour and cerebrospinal fluid in the rabbit, J. Physiol., 129, 111-133 (1955).

_____ and E. Spaziani: The blood-brain barrier and the extracellular space of brain, Ibid., 149., 135-143 (1959).

_____: The cerebrospinal fluid, Ergebn. Physiol., 52, 20-73 (1963).

Kibler, R. F., R. P. O'Neill and E. D. Robin: Intracellular acid-base relations of dog brain with reference to the brain extracellular volume, J. clin. Invest., 43, 431-443 (1964).

Millen, J. W. and D. H. M. Woollam: On the nature of the pia mater, Brain, 84, 514-520 (1961).

Pappenheimer, J. R., S. R. Heisey and E. F. Jordan: Active transport of Diodrast and Phenosulfonphthalein from cerebrospinal fluid to blood, Amer. J. Physiol., 200, 1-10 (1961).

Pollay, M. and H. Davson: The passage of certain substances out of the cerebrospinal fluid, Brain, 86, 137-150 (1963).

Rall, D. P., W. W. Oppelt and C. S. Patlak: Extracellular space of brain as determined by diffusion of inulin from the ventricular system, Life Sciences, 2, 43-48 (1962).

Reed, D. J. and D. M. Woodbury: Kinectics of movement of iodide, sucrose, inulin and radio-iodinated serum albumin in the central nervous system and cerebrospinal fluid of the rat, J. Physiol., 169, 816-850 (1963).
Welch, K.: Active transport of iodide by choroid plexus of the rabbit in vitro, Amer. J. Physiol., 202, 757-760 (1962).

K. FLEISCHHAUER

REGIONAL DIFFERENCES IN TRANSPORT OF SUBSTANCES OUT OF THE CEREBROSPINAL FLUID*

Feldberg and Fleischhauer (1960) have found that on perfusion of the cerebral ventricles with bromophenol blue the uptake of dye varies in different regions of the ventricular walls. These studies, the results of which agreed with observations on the uptake of histamine from the cerebrospinal fluid (CSF) into the brain tissue (Draskoci, Feldberg, Fleischhauer & Haranath, 1960) were carried out with the naked eye because for technical reasons it was impossible to detect the bromophenol blue at the cellular level.

In order to obtain information at the cellular level and to exclude possible artifacts due to the high concentration of bromophenol blue required for the earlier experiments, a technique was developed for studying the fluorescence of 3.6-diaminoacridinetrihydrochloride in paraffin sections. This strongly fluorescent substance of low toxicty was perfused in cats from the left lateral ventricle to the aqueduct in a concentration of 1:5000 for 30 minutes before the animal was killed by perfusion of Bouin's fluid via the aorta. The brain was embedded in paraffin and serial sections of equal thickness (5 μ) were cut from various regions. Alternate sections were then studied unstained by means of fluorescence microscopy or stained so as to reveal the histological structure of the ventricular walls (Fleischhauer, 1960).

With this method it was possible to compare different regions of the ventricular walls under identical conditions, and as the fluorescent dye stains the cell nuclei, regional differences in its uptake

*With grateful appreciation for the support given by Deutsche Forschungsgemeinschaft.

could be detected and related to the histological structure of the respective regions of the ventricular wall.

As described in detail elsewhere (Fleischhauer, 1964), it was found that deep penetration occurs in those regions of the ventricular wall which consist of grey matter mainly, e.g., hypothalamus, septum pellucidum, hippocampus and periaqueductal grey. On the other hand, shallow penetration occurs in those regions of the ventricular wall which consist of white matter, e.g., corpus callosum, fimbria, and lateral wall of the lateral ventricle. It was further found that hypophysis and pineal gland behave differently with regard to the uptake of 3.6-diaminoacridinetrihydrochloride: there was no penetration into the posterior lobe of the hypophysis, whereas the tissue of the pineal gland was deeply stained. There was also deep penetration into the subcommissural and into the subfornical organ.

The results of the experiments with 3.6-diaminoacridinetrihydrochloride thus confirm and extend the previous studies with bromophenol blue and histamine, and they are in agreement with the observations of Roth, Schoolar and Barlow (1959) on the uptake of radioactive acetazolamide from the CSF into the brain tissue. The similar distribution of these four substances within the brain is of particular interest because chemically they are of quite different character. The question therefore arises whether there are some topographically defined pathways for the perferential transport of substances out of the CSF. Further experiments are required to prove this assumption and to elucidate the cellular mechanisms involved in the transport of substances across the ventricular walls and into the depth of the brain.

REFERENCES

Draskoci, M., W. Feldberg, K. Fleischhauer and P. S. R. K. Haranath: Absorption of histamine into the blood stream and its uptake by brain tissue on perfusion of the cerebral ventricles, J. Physiol. (London), 150, 50-66 (1960).

Feldberg, W. and K. Fleischhauer: Penetration of bromophenol blue from the perfused cerebral ventricles into the brain tissue, J. Physiol. (London), 150, 451-462 (1960).

Fleischhauer, K.: Fluorescenzmikroskopische Untersuchungen an der Faserglia, Z. Zellforsch., 51, 467-496 (1960).

_____: Fluorescenzmikroskopische Untersuchungen über den Stofftransport zwischen Ventrikelliquor und Gehirn, Z. Zellforsch., 62, 639-654 (1964).

Roth, L. J., J. C. Schoolar and C. F. Barlow: Sulphur-35 labelled acetazolamide in cat brain, J. Pharmacol. exp. Ther., 125, 128-136 (1959).

T. BROMAN
O. STEINWALL

MODEL OF THE BLOOD-BRAIN BARRIER SYSTEM

The term blood-brain barrier (BBB) denotes the fact that in the brain there is an extraordinary impediment to blood-tissue passage of most plasma solutes, in comparison with such passage in other organs. We know today that this simple definition covers a very intricate biological mechanism and the rapidly increasing literature has provided a very large amount of observations and also many controversial hypotheses. The old idea of a structurally and functionally unitary barrier is now generally abandoned, but the BBB concept is still useful as a heading for the various factors that contribute to the restricted permeation from blood to brain. Among these factors biological transport mechanisms have attracted particular interest in the last years. In the following we will sketch a necessarily much simplified picture of the interrelationship between such transport and certain blood-brain barrier phenomena. (For extensive reviews of recent trends in this field, see, e.g., Tschirgi, 1960; Lajtha, 1962; Davson, 1963; Dobbing, 1963; Edström, 1964; Broman & Steinwall, in press.)

As pointed out by Krogh (1946), Becker and Quadbeck (1952) and later many others, important BBB characteristics seem to be basically analogous to general transfer-controlling properties of cell membranes. Adopting this idea we would like here to characterize the blood-brain interface as a membraneous (cellular) system where a lipid phase is supplemented with specific mechanisms for directed transfer of lipid-insoluble material for the entrance of nutrients and the disposal of waste products. Our concept of transfer conditions and barrier effects in this interface is outlined in Table 1.

From a strict barrier point of view, the lipid-soluble mate-

TABLE 1

HYPOTHETICAL INTERPRETATION OF BLOOD-BRAIN EFFECTS IN RELATION TO TRANSFER MECHANISMS (See Text)

I. LIPOPHILIC SUBSTANCES	Passive diffusion	No barrier effect
II. HYDROPHILIC SUBSTANCES		
1. "Nutrients" (glucose, amino acids, etc.)	Specific transfer* blood → CNS	Barrier effect above max. transport capacity
2. "Waste products," organic ions (conjugates, indicator dyes, PAH, etc.)	Specific transfer* CNS → blood	Barrier effect linked to "counter transport"
3. Non-metabolizable and non-charged solutes (inulin, sucrose, mannitol, etc.)	No specific transfer	Barrier effect "passive"

* carrier mediated – saturable (limited transport capacity) – inhabitable by competitive overloading or by toxic influences.

rial can be briefly described as permeating without appreciable hindrance through the lipid phase. It will not be discussed here how factors influencing the oil/water partition quotient determine the blood-brain passage (see, e.g., Brodie, Kurz & Schanker, 1960). The free passage of water will just be mentioned as a well-known fact of central significance in brain edema pathogenesis.

The barrier effects principally concern the predominantly hydrophilic plasma solutes. Among them we would like to discuss three categories, two of them involved in cell metabolism as nutrients and waste products respectively, the third metabolically inert.

As to nutrients, such as glucose, certain amino acids, etc., we adopt the interpretation that they are able to pass from blood to brain mainly by specific transfer mechanisms (see, e.g., Crone, 1961; Lajtha, 1962). Accordingly, a barrier effect here will appear at plasma concentrations above the limit determined by the maximum capacity of the transport concerned. It will be discussed later how certain pathological stimuli may at the same time depress the transport of nutrients and facilitate the passage of compounds like acid dyes.

The next group, aromatic organic ions, attracts special interest. Besides compounds like p-aminohippuric acid (PAH), Diodrast and various dyes for the indication of BBB damage, this group also represents metabolic waste products like glucuronic-acid conjugates. In general, their configuration seems to make them available for active one-way transport in an excretory direction: from the cerebrospinal fluid (CSF) and aqeous humor to the blood, from the blood to the tubular urine or the bile. That such an excretion takes place also at the blood-brain interface has been proposed by Steinwall (1961) on the basis of inhibition experiments. As regards CSF-blood transfer, thiocyanate and iodide ions seem to behave in much the same manner (see Davson, 1963).

Finally, a number of non-charged and non-metabolizable solutes (e.g., inulin, sucrose, mannitol) are grouped together. Their highly restricted blood-brain passage does not seem to be linked to any transport activity of the types discussed above. In the absence of better explanations we have proposed for them a "passive" barring.

This interpretation of different BBB phenomena has served as a working hypothesis in our experimental work on various pathological conditions of the BBB system. We have been especially interested in the possibilities to inhibit transport components selectively without causing a generalized breakdown of the barrier. This can be illustrated by the following examples.

Controlled chemical influence on the BBB can be produced in one hemisphere of the brain of the living rabbit by short perfusion via the internal carotid artery. Afterwards, the circulation is fully restored and the effect of the noxious stimulus can thus be studied by giving one or more suitable tracers intravenously in order to determine their passage into the injured hemisphere as compared with the control side (see Steinwall, 1958). Using this technique, it was shown (in experiments of short duration) that a very weak BBB damage induced by mercuric ions can cause a decreased passage of a tracer of the nutrient type, such as C14-glucose, concomitant with a minimal or slight increase in the passage of an acid dye (Steinwall & Hansson, unpublished). Similar results were obtained with the non-metabolized nutrient analogs methyl-0-glucose (Steinwall & Klatzo, 1965) and cycloleucine (Steinwall & Snyder, to be published). On the other hand, when C14-inulin (or sucrose) was used together with sodium fluorescein in corresponding experiments, both types of tracers passed into the tissue of the damaged hemisphere. Some differences in distribution, however, indicated a more widespread extravasation of the carbohydrate than of the dye (Steinwall & Klatzo, 1965, 1966).

This may suffice to illustrate a general statement that the analysis of dysfunctional states of the BBB system may call for sets of tracer compounds chosen in accordance with the specific experimental purposes. This is roughly sketched in Table 2.

TABLE 2

PROPOSED CHOICE OF TRACERS FOR INDICATION OF DIFFERENT TYPES OF BLOOD-BRAIN BARRIER INJURY

I. INJURIES	causing free diffusion or flow (mechanical, necrotizing or otherwise rupturing)
INDICATORS:	all normally barred native or foreign blood constituents
II. INJURIES	causing functional alteration of specific transfer mechanism(s)
INDICATORS:	substances presumed to be specifically handled by the actual mechanism(s)
Examples	a) general transport inhibition: decreased CNS uptake of glucose, abnormal ("increased") blood-CNS passage of acid dyes
	b) selective (overloading) inhibition of CNS-blood extrusion of organic acids: abnormal blood-CNS passage of acid indicators only

And now a few remarks as to the structural background of the BBB. Even here more than one component may be engaged in the system. The functional view of BBB effects as analogous to events in cell membranes or special transport cells seem to fit neatly with the statement of many electron microscopists that the brain is virtually without extracellular space as discussed by Lumsden (1955), Edström (1958), Hager (1961). The same functional effect may, however, be exerted by a transfer-controlling glia sheath apposed to the capillaries even in the presence of an appreciable extracellular space. Irrespective of these extravascular conditions, the possibility of specific permeability (transfer) properties of the endothelial layer of the cerebral vessels has to be considered. Certain ionized dyes seem to be unable to permeate the intima of cerebral and pial vessels but are seen to stain locally the mesenchymal structures of the vascular wall after injury from a passing air embolus, as observed under direct microscopy (Broman, et al., 1965), thus showing the staining pattern of arteries outside the brain. The observations by Rodriguez (1955) that a quarternary acridine dye did not penetrate the luminal side of the endothelium but entered from the tissue side when given in the subarachnoidal space, is interesting with regard to the proposed one-way transfer as partaking in the barring of the aromatic organic ions. Recently Klatzo, et al. (1964), have shown that albumin-conjugated fluorescein behaves in a corresponding manner. As to the choroid plexus it is now an established fact that the barrier phenomena as well as unidirectional ion transports reside in the epithelial layer while the capillaries here show leakage even to protein-bound tracers (see Davson, 1963).

Of considerable interest is the observation that BBB damage is demonstrable postmortem by perfusion with, e.g., trypan blue, a procedure that can be used for investigation on human brains (Broman, 1944). Some small differences between the postmortem and the intravital staining characteristics, observed at perfusion with dye-saline solution, are eliminated when the dye is dissolved in plasma (Broman, Klatzo & Steinwall, unpublished data). Furthermore, in a newly killed animal, chemical or air emboli damages can be induced in just the same way as in vivo (Broman, Gröntoft & Steinwall, 1965; Broman, et al., 1965). This "survival" of the BBB to acid dyes as well as its resistance against ischemic anoxia is intriguing in comparison with the considerable vulnerability to certain metabolic inhibitors. It may be that anaerobic metabolism, proceeding also some time after death, is sufficient for the maintenance of this BBB function.

The significance of the BBB system as to the pathogenesis of brain edema is not clear in all details. Edematous states may occur without any disturbance of the BBB demonstrable with dyes or protein tracers; this does not exclude, however, dysfunction of other components of the system. Experimental observations have indicated that even slight chemical BBB impairment, persisting for some hours, gives rise to progressive sequelae such as a gradual deterioration of the electrical activity (as seen in EEG) and a manifest edematous swelling (Flodmark & Steinwall, 1963). As regards edema-producing disease in the human brain, many of them are characterized by a BBB damage that is most likely to be a factor of primary importance for the development of the edema.

SUMMARY

Recent functional and morphological research has added support to the 20-year-old idea that the BBB system in many respects acts as a cell membrane. Analogies with plasma membranes or transport cells may serve as a first approximation, but further research necessitates systematic studies of those special attributes which characterize the BBB.

Leaving aside the controversial question concerning the role of various structural compartments, the "blood-brain interface" may be looked upon as a membraneous (cellular) system where the lipid phase is supplemented with specific mechanisms for the transfer of lipid-insoluble material, serving for the uptake of nutrients as well as the disposal of waste products.

Some consequences of these interpretations in relation to pathological states of the BBB are discussed and illustrated with recent observations on differentiated behavior of simultaneously applied blood-borne tracers.

The "survival" of some barrier effects and the techniques of postmortem assay of BBB damage are briefly mentioned.

REFERENCES

Becker, H. and G. Quadbeck: Tierexperimentelle Untersuchungen über die Funktionsweise der Blut-Hirnschranke, Z. Naturforsch. Vol. 7, 493-497 (1952).

Brodie, B. B., H. Kurz and L. S. Schanker: The importance of dissociation constant and lipid-solubility in influencing the passage of drugs into the cerebrospinal fluid, J. Pharmacol. exp. Ther., 130, 20-25 (1960).

Broman, T.: Supravital analysis of disorders in the cerebral vascular permeability in man, Acta med. scand., 118, 79-83 (1944).

_____, S. I. Branemark, B. Johansson and O. Steinwall: Intravital and postmortem studies on air embolism damage of the blood-brain barrier tested with trypan blue, Acta Neurol. Scand. (in press) (1965).

_____, O. Gröntoft and O. Steinwall: Comparative intravital and postmortem studies on chemically induced blood-brain barrier damage tested with trypan blue, Ibid.

_____ and O. Steinwall: Blood-brain barrier, in: Neuropathology, (ed. by J. Minckler), New York: McGraw-Hill, Ch. 33 (in press).

Crone, C.: Om diffusionen af nogle organiske non-elektrolyter fra blod til hjernevaev, Ejnar Munksgaard (1961).

Davson, H.: The cerebrospinal fluid, Ergebn. Physiol., 52, 20-73 (1963).

Dobbing, J.: The blood-brain barrier: Some recent developments, Guy Hosp. Rep., 112, 267-286 (1963).

Edström, R. F. S.: An explanation of the blood-brain barrier phenomenon, Acta psychiat. scand., 33, 403-416 (1958).

Edström, R.: Recent developments of the blood-brain barrier concept, Int. Rev. Neurobiol., 7, 153-190 (1964).

Flodmark, S. and O. Steinwall: Differentiated Effects on Certain Blood-Brain Barrier Phenomena and on the EEG Produced by

Means of Intracarotidally Applied Mercuric Dichloride, Acta physiol. scand., 57, 446-453 (1963)
Hager, H.: Elekronenmikroskopische Untersuchungen über die Feinstruktur der Blutgefässe und perivasculären Räume im Säugetiergehirn, Acta Neuropath., 1, 9-33 (1961).
Klatzo, I., J. Miquel, P. J. Ferris, J. D. Prokop and D. E. Smith: Observations on the passage of the fluorescein labeled serum proteins (FLSP) from the cerebrospinal fluid, J. Neuropath. Exp. Neurol., 23, 18 (1964).
Krogh, A.: The active and passive exchange of inorganic ions through the surfaces of living cells and through living membranes generally, Proc. roy. Soc. B, 133, 140-200 (1946).
Rodriguez, L. O.: Experiments on the histologic locus of the hematoencephalic barrier, J. comp. Neurol., 102, 27-39 (1955).
Steinwall, O.: An improved technique for testing the effect of contrast media and other substances on the blood-brain barrier, Acta Radiol., 49, 281-284 (1958).
_____: Transport mechanisms in certain blood-brain barrier phenomena — a hypothesis, Acta Psychiat. Neurol. Scand., 36, suppl. 150, 314-318 (1961).
_____ and I. Klatzo: Double tracer methods in studies on blood-brain barrier dysfunction and brain edema, Acta Neurol. Scand., 41, suppl. 13, 591-595 (1965).
_____ and _____: Selective vulnerability of the blood-brain barrier in chemically induced lesions, J. Neuropath. Exp. Neurol., 25, 542-559 (1966).
Tower, D. B.: Molecular transport across neural membranes, in: Properties of membranes and diseases of the nervous system, New York: Springer, 1-40 (1962).
Tschirgi, R. D.: Chemical environment of the central nervous system, in: Handbook of Physiology, vol. III, 1865-1890 (ed. by Field, Magoun, and Hall), Baltimore: Amer. Physiol. Soc. (1960).

ABEL LAJTHA
GIVLIO LEVI
RONALD BLASBERG

SPECIFICITY OF CEREBRAL AMINO ACID TRANSPORT

Recent work in a number of laboratories has shown that the passage of metabolites into and out of the brain occurs through a mechanism that differs from the mechanism governing the passage of foreign substances, including most drugs and dyes. It seems that diffusion, which plays a major role in the passage of foreign substances, has only an insignificant role in the passage of metabolites, which enter, and perhaps leave, the brain through mediated transport. It has been emphasized that these transport mechanisms, which determine the permeability properties of the brain towards metabolites, cannot be localized in a single membrane or in a single anatomical structure, but are most likely present in all membranes, with some differences existing between the properties of these membranes (Lajtha). Therefore, metabolite transport in the nervous system is considered a part of the brain barrier system. Although quantitative differences undoubtedly exist between brain and other organs, our knowledge is not sufficient to permit us to decide whether transport mechanisms present in brain are peculiar to this organ and are not present in other organs.

The properties of the mediated transport can be studied in the living brain and also in simplified systems such as brain slices.

In a recent study a number of similarities were found between brain slices and the living brain (Lajtha, et al.), among them that those amino acids that are at high levels in the free amino acid pool of the living brain (glutamic acid, GABA, etc.), are also accumulated to high levels by brain slices, whereas those amino acids which are at low physiological concentrations in the living brain (leucine, phenylalanine, etc.), are also accumulated by brain slices only to low levels. The similarities between the observations made in vivo and in vitro support the assumption that mechanisms that can be better observed in an isolated system such as brain slices are also operative in the living brain. In this report we want to briefly summarize our findings concerning the substrate specificity of amino acid transport in the central nervous system.

Previous studies of factors which control cerebral amino acid levels (Lajtha, et al.; Levi, et al.), showed that a number of processes participate in determining the level of a compound in the brain such as influx, efflux, and exchange; therefore, for a complete under standing of the nature of the transport system, the properties of all these processes have to be known. In the present paper we will discuss the substrate specificity of influx (initial rate of uptake), of exit, of steady state accumulation and of exchange, and compare the findings in brain slices with those made in the living brain. The aim of this study is to establish the number of transport sites involved in amino acid transport and the requirements of these sites.

SIGNIFICANCE OF THE DIFFERENT APPROACHES TO THE STUDY OF SUBSTRATE SPECIFICITY OF AMINO ACID TRANSPORT

When brain slices are incubated in a medium containing amino acids, they accumulate amino acids to levels above that in the incubation medium. This concentrative accumulation is energy-requiring and can be inhibited if analogs of the amino acid are present in the incubation medium. Inhibition studies have, therefore, been utilized to establish the specificity of transport, since it has been shown that inhibition of transport by an analog is competitive. It is assumed that compounds transported by the same site influence each other's transport, while compounds transported by different mechanisms do not influence each other's transport.

A number of studies demonstrated inhibition of amino acid accumulation in brain slices by related compounds (Neame, 1961, 1964 Abadom & Scholefield; Blasberg & Lajtha, 1965a). These studies mostly used long incubation periods during which accumulation was approaching a steady state value. Since steady state accumulation is determined by the net results of the fluxes occurring at the membrane, the properties of unidirectional fluxes must be studied in order to understand the properties of the processes that together regulate the passage of cerebral metabolites.

Studies in other systems (Christensen, 1962, 1964; Wilson, Rosenberg, et al.), and also in brain (Blasberg & Lajtha, 1965a) indicated that the amino acids can be grouped into several transport classes. Amino acids chosen for our experiments were representative of four classes, and the results are arranged according to classes to facilitate discussion of the emerging specificity patterns. The effect of each compound on the accumulation of other amino acids can be seen by moving vertically in the tables, and a comparison of the inhibitors on the passage of each amino acid can be seen by moving horizontally in the tables.

SPECIFICITY OF AMINO ACID INFLUX IN BRAIN SLICES

To illustrate the specificity patterns, the measurements on only a few amino acids are presented here. Those chosen — α-aminoisobutyric acid, leucine, lysine, and D-glutamic acid — are representative of small neutral, large neutral, large basic, and acidic amino acids, respectively. In our studies (Blasberg & Lajtha, 1965b) which are briefly summarized here, the transport of many other amino acids was also investigated, and some of these results will also be briefly discussed. Influx specificity is summarized in Table 1, where it can be seen that the inhibition pattern of the four amino acids is different and that the inhibitors, in turn, can also be grouped in different classes according to their effects. These classes will be discussed separately.

Neutral amino acids: The substrate specificity of α-aminoisobutyric acid (AIB) is different from that of leucine; AIB influx was inhibited more by neutral α-amino acids with short side chains (glycine and alanine) than by those with long side chains (leucine and phenylalanine). The opposite pattern was observed for leucine; its influx was inhibited more by the large neutral than the small neutral amino acids. A further distinction was seen in the inhibitory effect of diaminopropionic acid and the acidic amino acids on AIB but not on leucine influx. These patterns cannot be explained if the neutral α-amino acids are accumulated at a single transport site. A more likely explanation of these results is that there are at least two sites which mediate neutral α-amino acid transport, one serving predominantly for small neutral amino acids and another predominantly for large neutral amino acids. A similar observation in Ehrlich ascites cells has been made by Oxender and Christensen, who described separate but overlapping transport systems. Their A (alanine-preferring) and L (leucine-preferring) sites would correspond to our small neutral and large neutral sites.

As mentioned above, a more detailed study on inhibition of accumulation of other amino acids revealed other groups in addition to those described here; for example, a rather unique specificity pattern was described for γ-aminobutyric acid (GABA) accumulation by brain slices (Blasberg & Lajtha, 1965a and 1965b). The transport of this amino acid seems to occur at a site specific for its particular molecular structure, to which α-amino acids have little or no affinity. The study of proline and betaine influx suggested that these amino acids may also have affinity to a transport site which is separate from those of AIB and leucine.

Basic amino acids: The specificity of basic amino acid influx differed from that of the neutral amino acids; the basic amino acids could be further divided into two groups, since the inhibition pattern of small diamino acids seemed to be different from that of large diamino acids. Lysine influx was inhibited considerably more by arginine and ornithine than by diaminobutyric acid and diaminopropionic acid; that is, large basic amino acid influx was inhibited more by large basic than by small basic amino acids (Table 1). In contras small basic amino acids were inhibited more by small basic than by large basic amino acids (Blasberg & Lajtha, 1965b). Differences between small and large basic amino acids were shown also with AIB and glutamate, which were inhibited more by diaminopropionic acid than by lysine (Table 1). A difference in the specificity pattern of diaminopropionic acid would be expected, since its α-amino group is not significantly protonated at physiological pH.

A unilateral interaction between large diamino acids and large neutral amino acids was observed: lysine influx was inhibited by leucine and phenylalanine, whereas lysine and arginine had no effect on leucine influx. The specificity pattern of basic amino acids in the brain is similar to the pattern in Ehrlich ascites cells established by Christensen (1964) and suggests the existence of two distinct transport systems capable of accommodating a cationic side chain, one predominantly utilized by large diamino acids and another predominantly utilized by small diamino acids. Neutral amino acids apparently have an affinity to the site mediating large diamino acids, whereas the site mediating the transport of large neutral amino acid cannot accommodate the cationic side chain of diamino acids.

Acidic amino acids: Acidic amino acids strongly inhibited acidic amino acid influx, but the basic amino acids and the large neutral had no significant effect. It seems that the anionic side chain of the acidic amino acids prevents their interaction with the transport site of basic and neutral amino acids, although a slight interaction betwe glutamic acid and the small neutral α-amino acids, β-alanine, and diaminopropionic acid was observed.

When the acidic side chain of glutamic acid was modified by decreasing the negative charge on the γ-carboxylic group by amide

TABLE 1

SUBSTRATE SPECIFICITY OF AMINO ACID INFLUX IN BRAIN SLICES

	Per cent change from control influx			
Amino acid analog	AIB	L-leucine	L-lysine	D-glutamate
Glycine	−55	−28	−20	−5
Alanine	−67	−28	−32	−11
AIB		−16		
Leucine	−34		−41	−2
Isoleucine		−41		
Phenylalanine	−34	−46	−28	−1
Histidine	−26	−29	−37	
Diaminopropionic acid	−34	−1	−18	−36
Diaminobutyric acid	0	−7	−27	0
Ornithine		0	−34	
Lysine	−6	−3		0
Arginine	0	−8	−46	
Aspartic acid	−17	−8	0	−93
D-glutamic acid	−30		0	

(From Blasberg & Lajtha, 1965b)

Mouse brain slices were preincubated for 30 min. in Krebs-Ringer medium at 37 C, then C^{14} amino acid and C^{12} amino acid analog were added to the medium to give the following final concentrations: C^{14} amino acid 2mM, C^{12} amino acid 10mM. The incubation time was 3 min. The control values of influx expressed as M/ml tissue intracellular water/min. are: AIB 1.51, Leucine 1.23, Lysine 0.56 D-glutamate 3.48.

formation or by esterification (glutamine and glutamic acid γ methylester, respectively), the altered molecule no longer behaved in its specificity as glutamic acid did. When using glutamine or glutamic acid methylester as inhibitors instead of glutamic acid, the inhibition of AIB influx remained about the same, the inhibition of glutamic acid influx decreased, and an inhibition appeared of leucine and lysine influx. The inhibition pattern of glutamine and glutamic acid methyl ester was therefore similar to that of neutral amino acids. These findings indicated that dicarboxylic amino acid influx in brain slices predominantly occurs at a specific site capable of accommodating an anionic side chain. Although there is a slight interaction between acidic and small neutral amino acid transport, the sites mediating neutral and basic amino acid transport apparently cannot accommodate the anionic side chain of acidic amino acids.

SPECIFICITY OF AMINO ACID EXCHANGE

It has been demonstrated that the influx of an amino acid across the cell membrane is increased by the presence of an amino acid analog on the other side of the cell membrane. For example, the influx of amino acid from the medium was increased by preloading ascites cells with an amino acid analog (Heinz & Walsh). This effect was explained as the flow of the preloaded amino acid from the cell driving a counterflow of another amino acid into the cell fro the medium (exchange diffusion). We examined the specificity of exchange in brain slices by studying the effect of the extracellular amino acid analogs on the exit of AIB, leucine, lysine, and D-glutamic acid from brain slices. The greatest effects were obtained with amino acids belonging to the same class: AIB and the small neutral amino acids had the greatest effect on AIB exit, leucine and the larg neutrals on leucine exit, lysine and large basic amino acids on lysine exit, and the acidic amino acids on D-glutamate exit (Table 2). Other classes of amino acids had little or no effect. These findings emphasize the fact that if an amino acid analog is on the outside of the membrane it may influence not only the influx from the outside but also the efflux from the inside; that is, a compound on one side of a membrane can have an influence on another compound on either side of the membrane. In any experimental condition in which amino acids belonging to the same class are present on both sides of the cell membrane, the effect of heteroexchange, as well as any effect on influx and efflux, must be taken into consideration in the evaluation of the results.

SPECIFICITY OF AMINO ACID EXIT

The grouping of amino acids into the various transport classes is further strengthened by the substrate specificity of amino acid exit in that compounds of the same class preferentially affect each other exit. If the amino acid analogs used are grouped into classes, as with influx and exchange measurements, it can be seen (Table 3) that the small neutral amino acids inhibit mostly AIB and D-glutamate exit, and have less effect on leucine and lysine exit. The large basic amino acids inhibit significantly only within their own class, and the small basic amino acids, diaminopropionic acid, diaminobutyric acid, and histidine strongly inhibit all the amino acids studi the acidic amino acids strongly inhibit the exit of D-glutamate, and have a small effect on AIB, leucine, or lysine.

In the experiments described in Table 3, brain slices were first preloaded with the amino acid and the analog and then put into

TABLE 2

SUBSTRATE SPECIFICITY OF AMINO ACID EXCHANGE IN BRAIN SLICES

	Per cent change from control			
Amino acid analog	AIB	L-leucine	L-lysine	D-glutamate
Glycine	+65	+3	-4	-7
Alanine	+77			-7
AIB	+108	+5	+5	
Leucine	+38	+7	+13	-5
Isoleucine		+9		
Phenylalanine	+36	+9	+5	-1
Histidine	+20	+1	+3	
Diaminopropionic acid	+41	0	+2	-11
Diaminobutyric acid	+4		+11	
Ornithine			+35	
Lysine	+23	+2	+43	-6
Arginine	+27		+46	
Aspartic acid	+23	-1	+2	+28
D-glutamic acid	+27		+6	+35

(From Levi, et al.)

Mouse brain slices were preincubated for 30 min. in a Krebs-Ringer medium containing one of the following C^{14} amino acids: AIB 5mM, Leucine 10mM, Lysine 9mM, D-glutamate 1.5mM. The intracellular concentrations after preincubation were: AIB 32mM, Leucine 18mM, Lysine 20mM, D-glutamate 27mM. The slices were then incubated for 10 min. in a Krebs-Ringer medium containing 1mM C^{12} amino acid analog.

The control exit in 10 min. incubation in amino acid-free medium expressed as per cent loss was AIB = 16; leucine = 77; lysine = 27; glutamate = 17. Although changes with leucine are small because of the very rapid exit of this amino acid, the values reported in the table are significant.

a medium free of both to avoid any exchange between the analog present in the medium on the outside and the amino acid in the intracellular compartment of the slice, so that only exit should be measured. These experimental conditions resulted in the exit of both the amino acid and its analog from the slice and, since in most cases the exit rates differed in a change in the ratio of their concentrations. Although the change in ratio may explain some of the differences between the pattern in the first and in the second ten-minute period, nevertheless, it cannot account for the small inhibition of AIB exit by glycine and alanine and the lack of inhibition of lysine exit by ornithine and arginine during the first ten-minute period. A possible explanation is the following: Even though the slices are put into an amino acid-free medium, nevertheless, at the begin-

TABLE 3

SUBSTRATE SPECIFICITY OF AMINO ACID EXIT

	Per cent change from control exit							
	AIB		L-Leucine		L-Lysine		D-Glutamate	
Amino acid analog	0-10 min	10-20 min	0-10 min	10-20 min	0-10 min	10-20 min	0-10 min	10-20 min
Glycine	-23	-49	-29	-12	-20	+6	-29	-43
Alanine	-9	-32					-21	-36
AIB			-17	-19	-12	-10		
Leucine	+221	+45			+77	+54	+34	+18
Isoleucine			+17	+12				
Phenylalanine	+160	+48	+21	+17	+55	+35	+29	+11
Histidine			-64	-61	-50	-20		
Diaminopropionic acid	-76	-51	-51	-39			-82	-72
Diaminobutyric acid					-34	-34		
Ornithine					0	-39		
Lysine	+3	-5	-4	-7			-4	+8
Arginine	+2	+2			+2	-35		
Aspartic acid			-29	-21	-18	-3	-72	-57
D-glutamic acid	-11	-19						

(From Levi, et al.)

Mouse brain slices were preincubated for 30 min. in a Krebs-Ringer medium containing C^{14} amino acid and C^{12} amino acid analog. A portion was taken as control (zero time exit) and other portions were incubated in amino acid-free medium for different lengths of time. The concentrations of C^{14} amino acid in the preincubation medium were chosen to give an intracellular concentration between 1 and 10mM during the exit period. The concentrations of C^{12} amino acid analog were chosen to give an initial intracellular concentration several-fold higher than that of the labeled amino acid.

ning of the measurement of exit the extracellular concentration of the analog within the slice may still be significant; therefore an exchange can occur within the slice between the extracellular and intracellular amino acids. Since in the study of exchange it was shown (Table 2) that extracellular alanine and glycine significantly increased the exit of AIB and that extracellular ornithine and arginine exerted the same effect on the exit of lysine by heteroexchange, it seems likely that the lower inhibition of AIB exit by glycine and alanine and the lack of inhibition of lysine exit by ornithine and glycine in the first period of exit incubation was due to a heteroexchange of the extracellular analog, which by increasing exit counteracts the inhibitory effect of the intracellular analog.

The inhibitory pattern of small neutral, large basic, and acidic amino acids on the exit of AIB, leucine, lysine, and D-glutamate, is similar to the inhibitory pattern of these classes of amino acids on initial amino acid accumulation, showing a similar specificity in efflux and influx.

Although the specificity pattern of exit is not as clear as the pattern of influx, the finding that an analog can influence the exit of an amino acid is a very important one, and it strongly suggests the involvement of a carrier-mediated process in the exit of amino acids from brain slices. Evidence for mediated efflux of amino acid in vivo was reported previously, when it was found (Lajtha & Toth) that the exit of intracerebrally administered amino acids can occur against a concentration gradient even when plasma levels are above brain levels.

Although in our in vitro experiments with brain slices no study of competitive inhibition was done, the inhibition of amino acid exit by closely related analogs is likely to occur through a competition for the exit carrier site; however, this is probably not the only mechanism of exit inhibition. For example, the strong inhibition of exit of all four amino acids studied by small basic amino acids (diaminopropionic and diaminobutyric acid) and histidine would be hard to explain on the basis of competition for a carrier site, in view of the large differences in structure and polarity of the side chains of these compounds.

Whereas in influx experiments amino acid analogs either had no effect or were inhibitory, in exit not only inhibition but also activation could be observed. This effect also seemed to depend on the structure of the amino acid, as the large neutral amino acids (leucine, phenylalanine) were unique in that they increased (activated) the exit of all four amino acids studied. A possible explanation for this phenomenon, as discussed in more detail elsewhere (Levi, et al.), is that leucine and phenylalanine may activate the membrane carrier responsible for their own transport as well as for the transport of other classes of amino acids. The exit activation would be more evident for amino acids having lower exit rates (AIB has lower exit rate than lysine, and lysine than leucine), and would also have some degree of specificity as shown by the fact that D-glutamate exit is only slightly activated, in spite of its low exit rate.

SPECIFICITY OF STEADY STATE AMINO ACID ACCUMULATION AND ITS PREDICTABILITY

The overall pattern of the substrate specificity of steady state amino acid accumulation by brain slices (Table 4) is similar in mar ways to that observed for initial amino acid accumulation (Table 1).

TABLE 4

SUBSTRATE SPECIFICITY
OF AMINO ACID STEADY STATE ACCUMULATION

	Per cent change from control accumulation			
Amino acid analog	AIB	L-leucine	L-lysine	D-glutamic acid
Glycine	−41	−19	−24	+28*
Alanine	−59	−24	−37	+11*
AIB		−25	−15	
Leucine	−57		−64	−6
Isoleucine		−55	−42	−7
Phenylalanine	−56	−55	−49	−7
Histidine	−28	+83	+54	−34
Diaminopropionic acid	−11	+36	+14	+54*
Diaminobutyric acid	−14	−3	+50	−9
Ornithine	0	0	−21	−3
Lysine	0	−3		0
Arginine	0	−15	−33	−1
Aspartic acid		−5	−3	−19*
D-glutamic acid	−10*			

(From Blasberg & Lajtha, 1965a)

Mouse brain slices were incubated for 70 min. in a Krebs-Ringer medium containing 2mM C^{14} amino acid and 10mM C^{12} amino acid analog. The amount of incubation medium was varied to giv similar amino acid concentrations in the medium at the end of the incubation time. The control value for steady state accumulation (μM/ml tissue water) were: AIB = 14.5; Leucine = 4.84; Lysine = 5.18; D-glutamate = 40.9. Experiments marked with * were run at lower amino acid concentration to reduc the swelling due to acidic amino acid accumulation: amino acid conc.0.1mM. Analog conc.0.5mM.

Nevertheless, since the substrate specificity of steady state and of initial accumulation were measured under similar conditons, a number of important differences must be emphasized. The most apparent difference is that certain amino acids appear to stimulate amino acid accumulation at steady state, whereas they either inhibit or have no effect on initial accumulation (Tables 1 and 4). Also, the magnitude of the inhibitory effect in the two types of accumulation experiments differs significantly.

As already discussed in this publication, the initial rate of amino acid accumulation is not sufficient to explain the extent of accumulation at steady state. For example, AIB and leucine have similar initial rates of accumulation, whereas the steady state accumulation level of AIB is considerably higher. The reason that initial uptake rates do not always parallel steady state levels is that there are differences in exit rates. The higher steady state level of AIB is due not to its uptake rate being higher but to its exit rate being lower than that of leucine (Lajtha, et al.).

Obviously, in experiments where the substrate specificity of steady state amino acid accumulation is studied, the effect of the analog present will be not only on amino acid influx, but also on amino acid exit and exchange.

An inhibitory effect of the analog on amino acid exit will result in a higher amino acid level at steady state than that predicted by influx alone. The analog effect on exchange, both into and out of the cell, may magnify or diminish the effect on exit. On the basis of these considerations, knowing the specificity of amino acid influx, exit, and exchange, it is possible to predict the specificity of steady state amino acid accumulation. An exact steady state level, however, cannot be predicted from the data presented, since the experimental conditions in which the specificity of exit and heteroexchange was measured are not in all respects comparable with those of steady state.

The steady state accumulation of leucine and lysine is increased to levels above control by the presence of histidine in the incubation medium (Table 4), whereas histidine was shown (Table 1) to inhibit the initial accumulation of these amino acids. The difference between the two accumulation experiments is explained by the strong inhibition of leucine and lysine exit by intracellular histidine. The effect of exchange in this case is probably small, as shown in Table 2. The stimulation of D-glutamate steady state accumulation by glycine and diaminopropionic acid, and the stimulation of leucine and lysine accumulation by diaminopropionic acid and diaminobutyric acid, respectively, have most likely a similar explanation: in each case the analog produced a strong inhibition of amino acid exit.

A comparison of the inhibition of AIB accumulation by the neutral amino acids in the two experimental approaches also demonstrates significant differences (Tables 1 and 4). These apparent differences are resolved by the effects of the small and large neutral amino acid analogs on AIB exit (Table 3). The small neutral amino acids inhibited AIB exit and therefore increased the steady state level above that expected from influx alone. In contrast, the large neutral amino acids activated AIB exit and therefore decreased the steady state level below that expected from influx alone. The effect of large neutral amino acids on AIB exchange is likely to be small in comparison to their effect on AIB influx and efflux; AIB exchange with the small neutral amino acids was shown to be significant. The differences between the inhibition of initial and steady state accumulation for the other amino acids can be similarly explained. The inhibition of lysine, leucine, and D-glutamate exit by the large basic, small neutral, and acidic amino acids, respectively, explains why the steady state accumulation of these amino acids is inhibited less by the respective analogs than is their influx. Similarly the activation of lysine and leucine exit by the large neutral amino acids explains why the steady state accumulation of lysine and leucine is inhibited more than their influx.

These results clearly demonstrate the complexity of amino acid transport in brain slices at steady state condition. The substrate specificity patterns of steady state accumulation are determined by the specificity patterns of the various processes involved. It is therefore not sufficient to relate the inhibition of steady state accumulation to the inhibition of amino acid influx; the specificity patterns of amino acid exit and exchange play an equally important role in determining the extent of amino acid accumulation in the presence of an amino acid analog.

SPECIFICITY OF CEREBRAL AMINO ACID EXCHANGE IN VIVO

The complexity of the problems related to the specificity of amino acid transport in a relatively simple system such as brain slices emphasizes the much greater complexity of amino acid transport in the living brain, where many other factors have to be considered. The basic mechanisms and properties of transport are likely to be the same in brain slices as they are in the living brain, just as the basic biochemical mechanisms, such as the pathways of carbohydrate metabolism or protein systhesis, are the same in vivo and in vitro. The properties of the transport mechanisms in the living brain are the composite of the properties that can be observed in isolated systems; in the living brain, however, factors in addition to those that can be observed in brain slices are likely to be operative. The rate of metabolism of energy supply is different in the living brain, and other control mechanisms, such as hormones, may also be operative. We found that the rates of amino acid exchange in slices are considerably higher than they are in the living brain (Lajtha, et al.).

Our initial observations about specificty of cerebral amino acid exchange in vivo support the similarities of the metabolite transport mechanisms in vivo and in vitro. The in vivo experiments are more difficult to interpret since the cerebral distribution of the analog is heterogeneous and its level changes during the experimental period, in contrast to the influx measurements with slices, where the level of the analog in the incubation medium is constant throughout the experiment. The in vivo results with leucine and lysine indicate a specificity pattern similar to that observed in slices. The pattern appears to be that the large neutral analogs have a greater effect on leucine than lysine exchange, while the basic analogs have a greater effect on lysine than leucine exchange (Table 5). These and other preliminary observations did not reveal differences in substrate specificity between brain slices and the living brain.

TABLE 5

SUBSTRATE SPECIFICITY OF AMINO ACID EXCHANGE IN VIVO

	Per cent change from control exchange	
Amino acid analog	L-leucine	L-lysine
AIB	+29	
Leucine	+45	+15
Isoleucine	+72	+26
Valine	+58	+2
Phenylalanine	+18	+8
Histidine	+53	+35
Lysine	+13	+50
Arginine	+15	+37
Aspartic acid	+12	+21

(From Lajtha & Toth, in preparation)

Mice were injected intracerebrally with 0.02 ml saline containing 2μmoles of the amino acid analog at the beginning of the experiment. At 5 min. C^{14} leucine or lysine was injected intravenously and the animals were sacrificed at 10 min.; that is, 5 min. exchange was measured.

CONCLUSIONS

a.) It is clear from the specificity pattern of cerebral amino acid fluxes that not only one site serves for the transport of amino acids, but that several sites can be distinguished.

b.) There is not, however, a separate transport site for each amino acid; each site is used by several amino acids. Those sharing a site have similar structures, and therefore the site can be distinguished according to the amino acids which use it: 1) small neutrals, 2) large neutrals, 3) small basics, 4) large basics, and 5) acidics.

c.) Most likely several other sites exist in addition to the five mentioned under (b). We obtained evidence for at least three more sites that participate in the transport of such amino acids and analogs as γ-aminobutyric acid, proline, betaine, and taurine.

d.) Each amino acid group has primary (high) affinity to its own transport site and is most likely transported chiefly by this site. Some of the groups, however, have some affinity also to other sites (lower than to their own), and therefore members of one group may interact with the transport site of another group.

e.) Amino acids having affinity to the same transport site interfere with each other's transport by competition for the site. Such competitive inhibition of transport may have an important role in pathological alterations. Increasing the level of an amino acid will interfere with the movements of related compounds. If the specificity of amino acid fluxes and the affinities are known, these interferences can be predicted and explained.

f.) The effect of a compound on influx may be different from its effect on efflux and on exchange; there are, therefore, differences in the specificity patterns of these processes. Exit of amino acids, but not influx, could be activated by the presence of amino acid analogs on the same side of the membrane.

g.) In slices the fluxes determine the steady state levels of amino acids; compounds with high influx and low efflux accumulate to a higher degree than compounds with low influx and high efflux. If the flux of an amino acid in the two directions is known, its steady state level can be predicted. If an analog has an effect on the transport of an amino acid, with knowledge of the effects on influx and efflux and exchange, the extent of alteration of the steady state level of the amino acid can also be predicted. Thus by altering fluxes amino acid levels will be altered.

h.) The substrate specificity pattern of an amino acid seems to be similar in brain slices and in the living brain. Transport processes contribute to determining the level of cerebral metabolities and, possibly, alterations in the level of these metabolities under physiological and pathological conditions.

ACKNOWLEDGMENTS

This investigation was supported in part by Public Health Service Research Grants NB 03226 and NB 04360 from the National Institute of Neurological Disease and Blindness. The valuable help of Dr. J. Kandera, Mr. Z. Ronay, and Mr. A. Mazeika is gratefully acknowledged.

REFERENCES

Abadom, P. N. and P. G. Scholefield: Amino acid transport in brain cortex slices. II. Competition between amino acids, Can. J. Biochem. Physiol., 40, 1591-1602 (1962).

Blasberg, R. G. and A. Lajtha: Substrate specificity of steady state amino acid transport in mouse brain slices, Arch. Biochem. Biophys. 112, 361-377 (1965a).

_____ and _____: Heterogeneity of the mediated transport systems of amino acid uptake in brain, Brain Research 1, 86-104 (1965b).

Christensen, H. N.: Biological Transport, W. A. Benjamin, Inc.: New York (1962).

_____: A transport system serving for mono-and diamino acids, Proc. Natl. Acad. Sci. U. S., 51, 337-344 (1964).

Heinz, E. and P. M. Walsh: Exchange diffusion, transport, and intracellular level of amino acids in Ehrlich carcinoma cells, J. Biol. Chem., 233, 1488-1493 (1958).

Lajtha, A. The brain barrier system, in: Neurochemistry (ed. by K. A. C. Elliott, I. H. Page, and J. H. Quastel), Springfield: Charles C. Thomas; pp. 399-430 (1962).

_____ and J. Toth: The brain barrier system. II. Uptake and transport of amino acids by the brain, J. Neurochem., 8, 216-225 (1961).

Levi, G., R. G. Blasberg and A. Lajtha: Substrate specificity of amino acid exit from mouse brain slices (in preparation).

Neame, K. D.: Phenylalanine as inhibitor of transport of amino acids in brain, Nature, 192, 173-174 (1961).

_____: Effect of amino acids on uptake of L-histidine by rat brain slices, J. Neurochem., 11, 67-76 (1964).

Oxender, D. L. and H. N. Christensen: Distinct mediating systems for the transport of neutral amino acids by the Ehrlich cell, J. Biol. Chem., 238, 3686-3699 (1963).

Rosenberg, L. E., S. J. Downing and S. Segal: Competitive inhibition of dibasic amino acid transport in rat kidney, Ibid., 237, 2265-2270 (1962).

Wilson, T. H.: Intestinal Absorption, Philadelphia: W. B. Saunders Co. (1962).

G. QUADBECK
O. HESS

BRAIN EDEMA AND GLUCOSE TRANSPORT ACROSS THE BLOOD-BRAIN BARRIER

When, in order to study the blood-brain barrier (BBB) permeability under varying conditions we only use one indicator substance, we are running the risk of erroneous conclusions. Experiments with one BBB indicator are valuable only when the BBB is damaged or destroyed so that its specific barrier function has become ineffectual. In order to recognize smaller changes of the BBB we have to use several chemical barrier indicators simultaneously. Glucose, being in vivo under normal conditions the sole source of energy for the brain, must be transported across the BBB by a special transport process. So far we know that only a small part of the glucose needed by the brain comes from the blood into the brain by a simple diffusion process. The greater part of glucose is transported by a liver-dependent process. The relation between liver and glucose metabolism has been demonstrated by Geiger and his group in animals (1) and by Bermsmeier in humans (2). There are many arguments that a polysaccharide-containing structure, located at the borderline between the capillaries and the brain tissue, is involved in this glucose transport as an intermediate stage. Relying on the results of Geiger we can assume that this polysaccharide is built up continuously on the BBB's blood side and broken down at the same time and in the same measure on the brain side. This mechanism may explain the large glucose uptake by the brain without opening the BBB for other substances.

This being correct, we could expect a steady state between the blood's and this polysaccharide's radioactivity shortly after an intravenous injection of radioactive glucose. We succeeded in isolating a fraction of the mouse brain characterized by this behavior. This fraction is not precipitated by 20% of trichloracetic acid (TCA) and gives a positive PAS-reaction. Figure 1 shows this fraction coming into steady state with the blood activity after a short interval, but not with the water soluble or the lipid soluble fraction or the TCA precipitate. Under experimental conditions the brain glucose uptake can be markedly reduced in deep anesthesia. A reduction of glucose uptake to half of normal values has been shown in patients by Gottstein, et al. (3). This finding has been confirmed recently by Hoyer and Becker (4). In accordance with Gottstein they found in most patients with the clinical diagnosis "cerebral arteriosclerosis" the glucose uptake much more reduced than the oxygen uptake. We, therefore, assume the reduced blood flow through the brain in many cases to be a consequence of reduced glucose uptake by the brain.

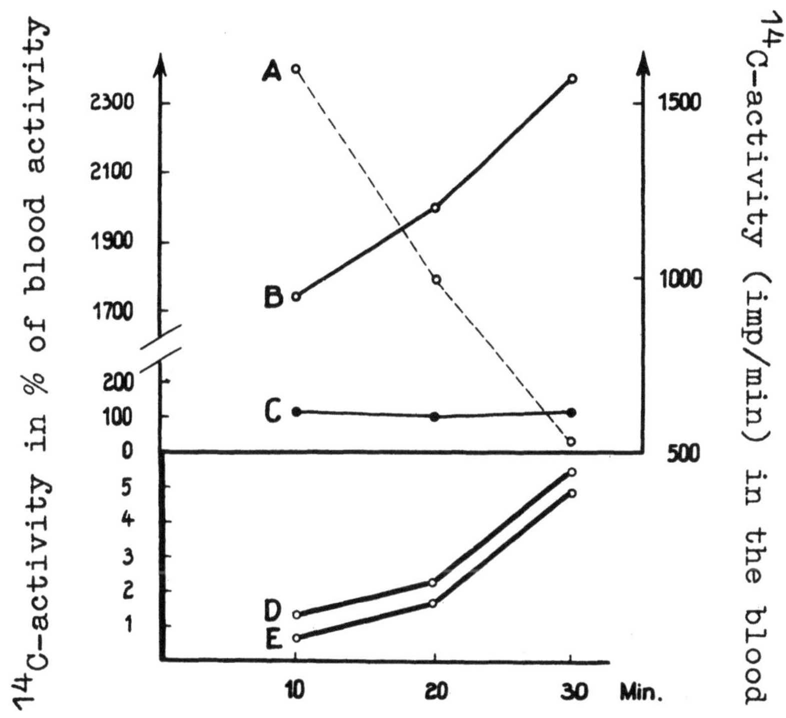

Fig. 1. Different fractions in the mouse brain. Fraction C is in a steady state with the blood activity. A: blood; B: water soluble (high mol weight); C: water soluble (low mol weight); D: lipid soluble; E: precipitate.

In animal experiments we could show that some drugs effective in geriatrics increase the brain glucose uptake without influencing the BBB-permeability for other substances (5). Furthermore, we could demonstrate that drugs increasing the brain glucose uptake also increase the resistance of the brain against oxygen deficiency (6). The greater glucose supply to the brain caused by these drugs may intensify the energy production via the glycolytic metabolism. The effect on the brain glucose uptake can be shown with several drugs, e.g., with nicotinic acid immediately after a single administration or with pyrithioxine after prolonged administration.

Hoyer and Becker could show that in patients with reduced cerebral glucose uptake a pyrithioxine treatment increased this uptake and the patients improved clinically at the same time. Hence, we may interpret the disturbed glucose transport from blood to brain as being a more important reason for cerebral dysfunction than cerebral blood flow reduced by arteriosclerosis. Currently we do not know how these drugs increase the cerebral glucose uptake.

The osmotic pressure of brain tissue is higher than that of plasma. Therefore, the water influx from the blood into the brain must be a downhill transport and conversely the water efflux out of the brain must be an energy dependent uphill transport. Therefore the brain continuously needs energy to maintain its water balance. Brain edema and its therapy, seen under a dynamic aspect, is shown in Figure 2 a-f;

From a theoretical point of view we have three ways of treating brain edema: 1) reduction of the osmotic pressure difference between plasma and brain tissue by osmotherapy or desiccation; 2) sealing of the traumatically disturbed BBB (by flavonol-glycosides and related compounds); 3) increase of the cerebral energy supply by a drug increasing the glucose transport to the brain. To study these possible methods of therapy, we produced brain edema in rats by cold injury without opening the skull. After two hours the rats were killed and the water content of the brain was measured by the dry-freezing technic. Figure 3 demonstrates that all these theoretically postulated therapeutic methods are effective in our experimental brain edema of the rat. As shown in Figure 4, Persantin (C. H. Boehringen Sohn, Ingelheim/Rh.) in normal rats increases the BBB permeability for glucose but not significantly for other indicator substances. So we assume its effect on the brain edema is related to this mechanism. In the same way Solcoseryl (A. G. Solco, Basel) (Actihaemyl) has a therapeutic effect on this kind of edema. This substance has been shown to increase the glucose supply to the brain and its resistance against oxygen deficiency (7).

The treatment of an experimental brain edema by osmotherapy reduces the traumatically increased porosity of the BBB. To be effective, the BBB needs energy. When the blood supply is reduced by a compressing brain edema the BBB will be less effective. After improvement of the brain edema the blood supply is normalized and

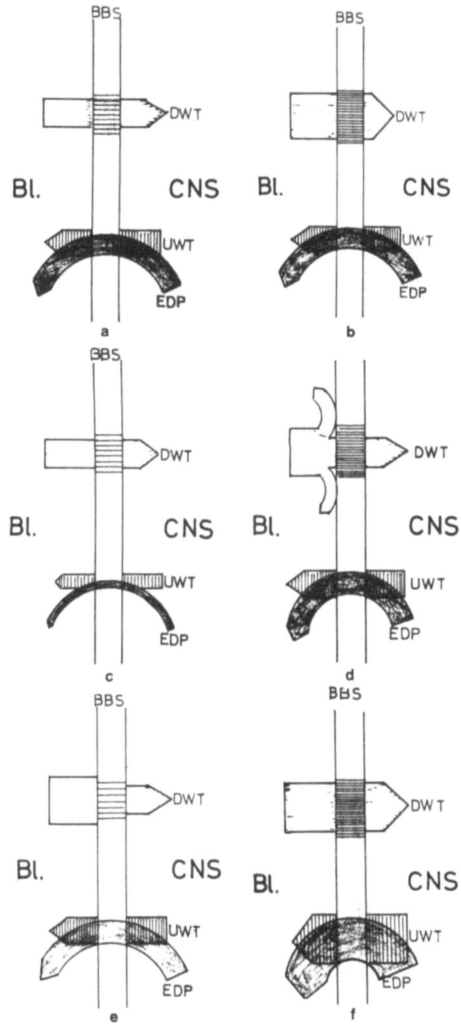

Fig. 2. Bl = blood; CNS = central nervous system; DWT = downhill water transport; UWT = uphill water transport; EDP = energy depending process; BBS = blood-brain-barrier system. 2a) the normal condition with a steady state of water exchange; 2b) brain edema, increased water influx by increased porosity of the BBB; 2c) brain edema, decreased water efflux by decreased energy supply; 2d) osmotherapy, decreased water influx by increased osmotic pressure of the plasma; 2e) decreased water influx by sealing of the BBB; 2f) increased water efflux by increased energy supply.

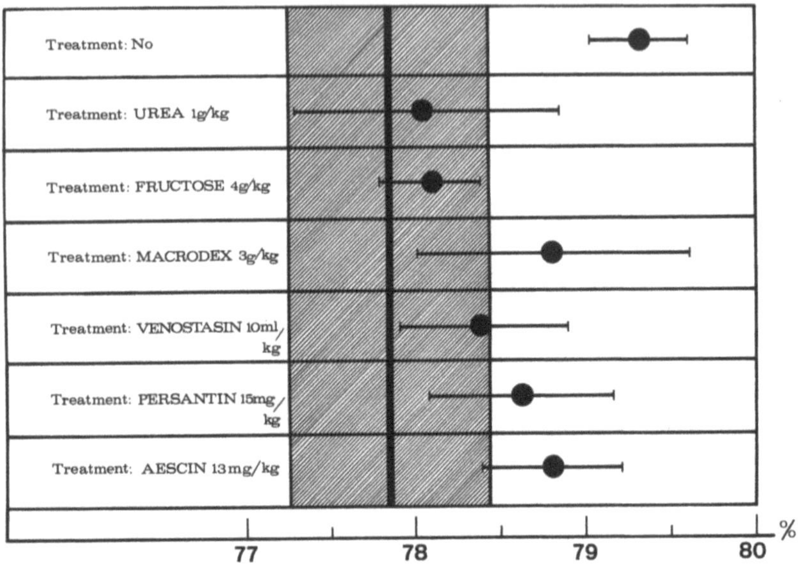

Fig. 3. Effect of several treatment methods on the experimental brain edema in the rat, measured by the water content of the brain in % of fresh weight; black space = controls.

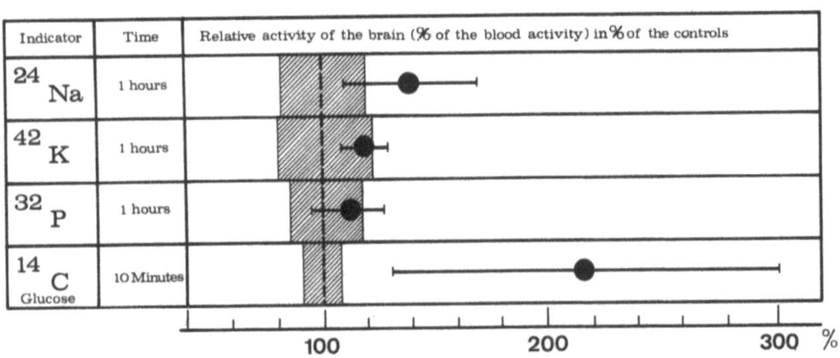

Fig. 4. Effect of Persantin on the BBB permeability for several indicators; significant increase in only glucose uptake.

the traumatically increased permeability of the BBB will be partly improved.

REFERENCES

1. Becker, K. and S. Hoyer: Hirnstoffwechseluntersuchungen unter der Behandlung mit Pyrithioxin, Dtsch. Ztschr. f. Nervenheilk., 188, 200 (1966).
2. Erbslöh, F., A. Bernsmeier and H. R. Hillesheim: Der Glucoseverbrauch des Gehirns und seine Abhängigkeit von der Leber Arch., Psychiatr. u. Nervenkr., 196, 611 (1958).
3. Geiger, A.: Correlation of brain metabolism and function by the use of brain perfusion method in situ., Physiol. Rev., 38, 1 (1958).
4. _____, J. Magnes, R. M. Taylor and M. Versalli: Effects of blood constituents on uptake of glucose and on metabolic rate of the brain in perfusion experiments, Am. Journal Physiol., 177, 138 (1954).
5. Gottstein, U., A. Bernsmier and J. Sedlmeyer: Der Kohlenhydratstoffwechsel des menschlichen Gehirns II. Klin. Wschr., 42, 310 (1964).
6. Quadbeck, G. and J. Nickel: Über den Glucosetransport aus dem Blut ins Gehirn., Bull. Soc. Chim. Biol., 46, 206 (1964).
7. _____: in: D-Glucose und verwandte Verbindungen in Medizin u. Biologie (ed. by H. Bartelheimer, W. Heyde and W. Thorn), Stuttgart (1966).

B. K. SIESJÖ
J. BRZEZIŃSKI
Å. KJÄLLQUIST
U. PONTÉN

CARBON DIOXIDE AND ACID-BASE EQUILIBRIA IN BRAIN TISSUE*

In discussions of brain swelling or brain edema, terms like "tissue hypercapnia" and "tissue pH" are often used. Work in our laboratory has dealt more with relations covered by these terms than with the actual conditions of tissue swelling or edema. However, it is felt that a discussion of some basic principles related to the normal acid-base regulation of brain tissue will be helpful when considering the even more intricate problems of a tissue with disturbed water and electrolyte metabolism.

A useful quantitative approach to the acid-base metabolism of a tissue will require that respiratory mechanisms are strictly separated from non-respiratory ones. This is an elementary requirement but it has not always been fulfilled. Thus, a quantitative analysis of acid-base changes in any tissue must be preceded by an evaluation of the CO_2 tension, not in the blood, but in the tissue itself. This parameter will, therefore, be considered in some detail before turning to the non-respiratory component, and to some interesting acid-base effects observed in hypoxia and in carbonic anhydrase inhibition.

*Supported by contract N62558-4288 between the Office of Naval Research, Department of the U.S. Navy; the University of Lund; and by the Swedish Medical Research Council.

THE TISSUE CO_2 TENSION

The metabolic CO_2 produced by the cells of the central nervous system is responsible for about a 10 mm Hg increase in the CO_2 tension of the blood flowing through the tissue (e.g., from 40 to 50 mm Hg). The CO_2 molecules thus leave the cells and end up in capillary blood, and, by all that is known, this occurs solely by diffusion. Diffusion depends upon concentration gradients, and it is easy to realize that the gradients of CO_2 tension in the tissue will depend on the rate of CO_2 production, on the diffusion coefficient for CO_2, and on the capillary geometry of the tissue. In the tissue model originally proposed by August Krogh (1918-1919), the tissue was considered as a series of cylinders, each supplied by a central capillary. This procedure has proved very fruitful since it allows suitable boundary conditions to be defined for solving the appropriate diffusion equations (Thews, 1953, 1960; Kety, 1957), and since it leads to the definition of a physiologically useful mean tissue tension.

The tissue model is by necessity a simplification, and the calculation of a mean tissue tension must be accompanied by a number of assumptions, but the analysis has given promising results. In Figure 1, an attempt has been made to visualize the mean tissue tension. To the left, a tissue cylinder is shown from the side with the arterial end of the capillary on the left-hand side. When blood flows through the tissue, CO_2 is added, and the total CO_2 content of the flowing blood increases continuously. If it is assumed that the CO_2 is produced at the same rate everywhere in the cylinder, and that it diffuses radially into the capillary, it follows that the CO_2 content of the capillary blood increases linearly from the arterial to the venous end. There are reasons to believe that for physiological ranges a linear increase in total CO_2 means a linear increase in P_{CO_2} from the arterial towards the venous end of the capillary (Gleichmann, Ingvar, Lübbers, Siesjö and Thews, 1962), whence it follows that the mean capillary tension is the arithmetic mean of the arterial and the venous tensions (indicated by a filled circle in the lower part of the figure).

If we now regard the cross section of the tissue cylinder at the point where the CO_2 tension of the blood equals the mean capillary tension, i.e., halfway between the arterial and the venous ends, we can visualize the tension gradients within the tissue itself (right side of Fig. 1). It is clear that the lowest tissue CO_2 tension (in the radial direction) will be found just at the capillary border, and the highest at a point which is equidistant to two capillaries. The mean CO_2 tension within the tissue cylinder (and thus by assumption also within the tissue proper) will apparently fall in between these two

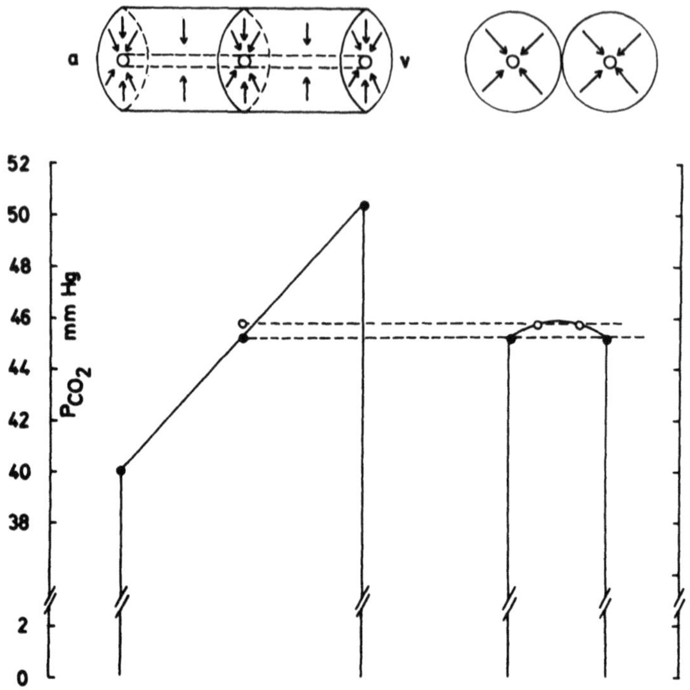

Fig. 1. Schematic diagram of two Krogh tissue cylinders, viewed from the side (left) and from the short ends (right), together with the corresponding longitudinal and radial CO_2 tension gradients (below). CO_2 is assumed to be produced at a uniform rate everywhere in the cylinder (arrows), leading to a linear increase in the CO_2 tension from the arterial towards the venous ends (illustrated by unbroken straight line below). The radial increase in the CO_2 tension in the tissue (i.e., between the capillaries is shown below (right) and the integrated mean tissue CO_2 tension is indicated (open circles) Note that the mean tissue tension is less than 1 mm Hg higher than the mean capillary CO_2 tension.

values and will be obtained from the expression

$$\Delta P_{CO_2} = \frac{A}{K}\left[\frac{R_2^4}{2(R_2^2 - R_1^2)} \ln \frac{R_2}{R_1} - \frac{1}{8}(3R_2^2 - R_1^2)\right] \qquad (1)$$

where ΔP_{CO_2} (in atm.) is the difference between the mean tissue and the mean capillary CO_2 tension (i.e., the increase in CO_2 tension in the radial direction from the mean capillary to the mean tissue CO_2 tension), A the CO_2 production in $cm^3/g/min$, K the diffusion coefficient for CO_2 in the tissue in $cm^3/cm/min/atm.$, R_1 the diameter of the capillary, and R_2 half the intercapillary distance, both in cm. Plausible values for the cat cerebral cortex would be a

CO_2 production of $5 \cdot 10^{-2}$ $cm^3/g/min$, a diffusion coefficient of 5.4 $\cdot 10^{-4}$ $cm^3/cm/min/atm.$/ (Siesjö and Thews, 1962), a cylinder radius of 30 and a capillary radius of 2.5 micron. If these values are inserted into the equation, ΔP_{CO_2} calculates to near 0.6 mm Hg. This means that the theoretical mean tissue CO_2 tension in a case with an arterial CO_2 tension of 40 mm Hg, and a cerebral venous CO_2 tension of 50 mm Hg, would be slightly less than 46 mm Hg.

The calculation of a mean tissue CO_2 tension from the Krogh model is obviously an oversimplification. Thus, apart from the assumptions regarding the spatially and temporally uniform CO_2 production, and the linearity of the in vivo dissociation curve, very sweeping assumptions are introduced by considering the tissue capillaries as running in strict parallelity with a unidirectional flow. There is evidence that a counter-current prevails with a reversed flow in adjacent brain capillaries (Diemer, 1965), in what case the radial and longitudinal tension gradients would be asymmetrical (cf. Lübbers, 1965). However, these objections are only of potential importance and far more important is the useful concept of a mean tissue CO_2 tension, introduced by the original Krogh model, and the agreement obtained between the calculated values and the values obtained in direct experiments using different approaches. Thus, in a large series of cat experiments (Pontén & Siesjö, 1966), it was found that if the arterial and the cerebral venous CO_2 tensions were measured simultaneously with the CO_2 tension in cerebrospinal fluid (CSF) from the suboccipital cistern, the relations of Figure 2 (open squares) were obtained.

At an arterial CO_2 tension of 40 mm Hg, it was found that the cerebral venous tension was 50.3 mm Hg. From these tensions, and from Equation 1 above, a theoretical mean tissue CO_2 tension of 45.8 mm Hg could be calculated. The agreement between this value and that actually measured in the CSF (45.7 mm Hg) is striking and must lead to the working hypothesis that under normal conditions the CSF CO_2 tension is a measure of the mean tissue CO_2 tension.

In a corresponding number of experiments the blood CO_2 tensions were measured simultaneously with those obtained from the surface of the tissue with the tissue electrode (Fig. 2, open circles). In this case a significantly larger mean arteriovenous CO_2 tension difference was obtained (12.6 mm Hg), indicating that the mere exposure of the tissue gave some impedement of the cortical circulation. In spite of this, however, there was a good agreement between the theoretical mean tissue CO_2 tension (6.9 mm Hg above the arterial P_{CO_2} when the latter was 40 mm Hg) and the CO_2 tension measured on the surface of the tissue (7.8 mm Hg above the arterial tension). It was found that even in animals with a low blood pressure the expected P_{CO_2} gradients were found, although the arteriovenous P_{CO_2} differences in such cases could increase even further (Fig. 2, open triangles). These results indicate

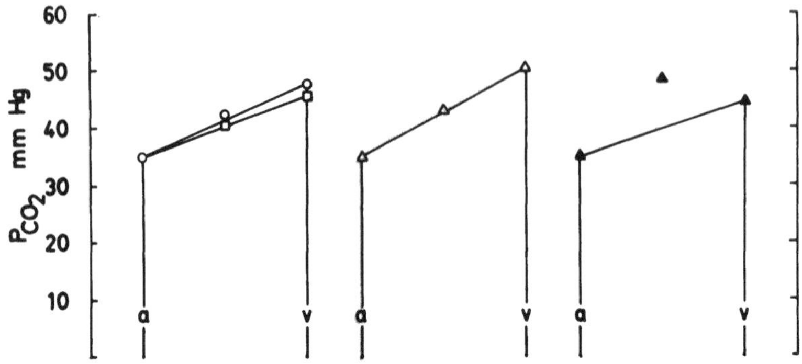

Fig. 2. Relation between the arterial (a), the cerebral venous (v) and the mean tissue CO_2 tension (symbols in the middle). The different groups were corrected for variations in arterial P_{CO_2} in order to facilitate comparisons. In the figure are shown the normal relations between the blood CO_2 tensions and that measured in cerebrospinal fluid (open squares), as well as on the surface of the tissue (open circles), (Pontén & Siesjö, 1966 . Two abnormal situations are illustrated. In one (open triangles) there was a large arterio-venous P_{CO_2} difference in a cat with a critically low blood pressure but the CSF CO_2 tension showed the normal relation to the blood CO_2 tensions. In the other case (closed triangles) the mean tissue CO_2 tension was measured with a CO_2 electrode over an area which was visibly damaged and the P_{CO_2} measured was disproportionally high when compared to the corresponding arterial and venous CO_2 tensions.

that both the CSF CO_2 tension, and the CO_2 tension measured with a tissue CO_2 electrode, can be used to indicate the mean tissue CO_2 tension, as defined by integration along the capillary and across the cross section of the tissue cylinder in the Krogh model.

It must be clearly pointed out that calculation of the mean tissue CO_2 tension from the corresponding arterial and venous CO_2 tensions is a valid procedure only if the venous blood sampled is representative of the tissue under study. The same objections evidently apply to conclusions regarding the mean tissue tension, drawn from measurements on the CSF. In Figure 2 (closed triangles) are shown the relations obtained in an experiment where the tissue surface was damaged with the visible subpial extravasations. In this case the CO_2 tension measured with the tissue electrode markedly exceeded the mean capillary CO_2 tension. It is clear that in similar conditions of vascular damage or local edema, neither calculation from blood CO_2 tensions, nor measurements on CSF from the great cisterns, will be a reliable procedure for obtaining a relevant mean tissue CO_2 tension.

THE BICARBONATE CONCENTRATION OF BRAIN TISSUE

There are several ways of expressing the non-respiratory component of an acid-base system, but the most unequivocal one is based on a consideration of the bicarbonate concentration. Any biological system, irrespective of the number of compartments, can be expected to give a curve like the middle one in Figure 3 when the CO_2 tension

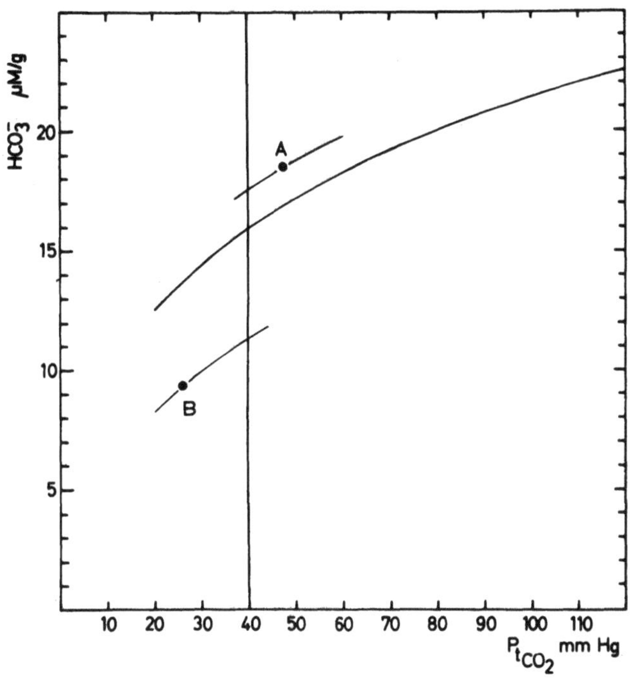

Fig. 3. CO_2 binding curve for brain tissue, determined by exposing rats to different CO_2 concentrations or to varying degrees of hyperventilation (Pontén, 1964, 1966). The filled circle along curve A denotes parameters measured under carbonic anhydrase inhibition and is equivalent to a non-respiratory increase in the bicarbonate concentration. The corresponding point B was obtained from an experiment in which sodium cyanide was administered to a rat, leading to a large increase in the tissue concentration of lactate. The position of the curve shows that bicarbonate ions have disappeared from the system.

is varied. Thus, here it is assumed that at a CO_2 tension of 40 mm Hg, the bicarbonate concentration equals 16 mE/kg, and since the tissue is composed of both an aqueous and a solid phase, where the ion HCO_3^- is presumably entirely confined to the aqueous phase, the concentration has been expressed per unit weight of water. It follows from the curve, and theoretically from a consideration of the sequential reactions when CO_2 is dissolved in an aqueous buffer, that the bicarbonate concentration increases with the CO_2 tension, and decreases when the CO_2 tension is lowered.

If we now envisage a situation where a few milliequivalents of a non-volatile base is added to the system we may get a new point along the curve A in Figure 3. In this new situation the bicarbonate concentration has increased, partly due to the addition of base ($OH^- + CO_2 = HCO_3^-$), and partly due to the increased CO_2 tension. However, if the CO_2 tension is varied we can expect to get a "dissociation curve" which is very nearly parallel to the original one in the physiological P_{CO_2} range. Accordingly, we may follow the curve down to a CO_2 tension of 40 mm Hg, and the difference in bicarbonate concentration at this tension will be an expression of the amount of base added to the system. Theoretically, this situation might arise if there was a net passive influx of bicarbonate ions into the tissue from the outside (or an efflux of hydrogen ions), or if in the tissue a hydrogen ion pump was turned on, extruding the ions to the surroundings.

Opposite changes would ensue if hydrogen ions were added to the system, as described by the point along curve B in Figure 3. Again, we would get an expression for the amount of hydrogen ions added if we titrated the system back to the original 40 mm Hg in CO_2 tension. This situation could be expected to arise in tissue hypoxia if a certain amount of a non-volatile acid (e.g., lactic acid), was formed.

The quantitative relations depicted by Figure 3 can equally well be obtained from a plot of the logarithm of the CO_2 tension against pH which is routinely used in clinical acid-base chemistry. However, the term pH as applied to a collodial system like a tissue is a subject of controversy, and there are theoretical objections to using it for a system with heterogeneous compartments (Siesjö & Pontén, 1965a, b). This can be avoided by plotting log $(HCO_3^-/P_{CO_2} \cdot S)$ instead of pH, as has been done in Figure 4. Certain advantages are obtained by using this plot as compared to the simple diagram of Figure 3. Thus, when the CO_2 tension is varied the system is titrated along a very nearly straight line, and the slope of this line is an expression of the buffer capacity of the system to carbon dioxide, defined as

$$\beta_{CO_2} = \frac{d \log P_{CO_2}}{d \log (HCO_3^-/P_{CO_2} \cdot S)} \qquad (2)$$

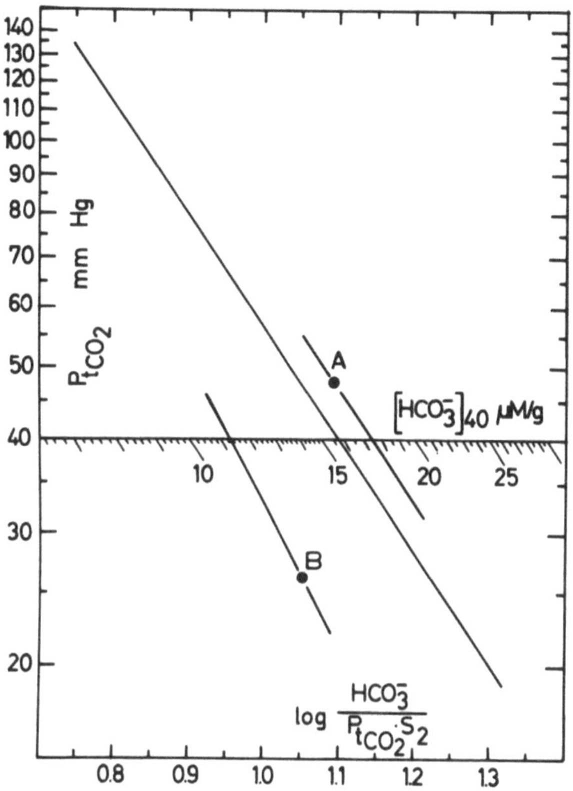

Fig. 4. The same curve and points as in Figure 2 but the curves have been plotted in a semilogarithmic diagram. The buffer curve of the tissue is now a nearly straight line and the slope of the line is an expression of the buffer capacity $\beta_{CO_2} = \frac{d \log P_{CO_2}}{d \log (HCO_3^-/P_{CO_2} \cdot S)}$. The buffer capacity can be calculated to about 1.5, i.e., the buffer capacity of brain tissue in vivo approximates that of whole blood in vitro.

Moreover, the change in bicarbonate concentration at constant CO_2 tension ("standard bicarbonate") is found from the intersection of the buffer line with a standard bicarbonate scale at the 40 mm Hg horizontal, and the change in log $(HCO_3^-/P_{CO_2} S)$, which should be identical to the "pH" change, is read directly on the x-axis (see further discussion below).

The lines and points given in Figures 3 and 4 are not chosen at random but represent actual conditions. Thus, the full lines in Figures 3 and 4 represent the buffer curve for rat brain tissue, determined by exposing the animals in vivo either to different CO_2 concentrations or to varying degrees of hyperventilation (Pontén, 1964, 1965). The slope of the line corresponds to a buffer capacity of about 1.5, and it can be shown theoretically that this buffer capacity requires that the tissue contains a minimum buffer concentration of 35 mE/kg of water (Siesjö & Pontén, 1966b). The point on curve A represents a group of animals given a carbonic anhydrase inhibitor (Diamox, see below), and the point on the curve B corresponds to a state of hypoxia where a rat was given sodium cyanide in a dose of 50 μE/kg prior to freezing the brain in situ.

The conditions of tissue hypoxia and carbonic anhydrase inhibition have been chosen to exemplify non-respiratory changes in the tissue acid-base metabolism. It has previously been shown that the administration of cyanide affects the tissue concentrations of labile constituents like lactic acid and phosphocreatine (Albaum, Tepperman & Bodansky, 1946; Olsen & Klein, 1947), and the procedure is a convenient way of liberating a non-volatile acid within the tissue. In the experiment illustrated as point B in Figures 3 and 4, sodium cyanide was given intravenously in repeated doses until the EEG disappeared or remained seriously depressed for about ten minutes, after which time the tissue was frozen and subsequently analyzed for bicarbonate, water and lactic acid. The lactic acid concentration was found to have increased to 20.8 mEq/kg of wet tissue, or about 26 mEq/kg of tissue water (normally, the value is about 1 mEq/kg of wet tissue under barbiturate anaesthesia), and the standard bicarbonate concentration was calculated to 11.3 mEq/kg of tissue water, which is a decrease of about 5 mEq. The results show that the liberation of a non-volatile acid within the tissue markedly affects the bicarbonate concentration.

The carbonic anhydrase inhibitor acetazolamide (Diamox), which has been used in the management of both epilepsy, hydrocephalus and brain edema, has interesting effects on the central nervous system. Thus, the drug leads to a marked reduction of the CSF production, it increases the threshold for experimentally induced convulsions, and it affects the HCO_3^-/Cl^- ratio between blood and CSF (Davson & Luck 1957; Maren & Robinson, 1960; Wistrand, Nechay & Maren, 1961; Oppelt, Patlak & Rall, 1964). Its effect on the acid-base metabolism of the brain tissue is unknown, although some of its physiological effects have been ascribed to an increase in the molecular CO_2 of the tissue (Koch & Woodbury, 1960). However, since carbonic anhydrase seems to be localized to cells in the choroid plexus, and to glia cells (Giacobini, 1961), it has been assumed that it is involved in active transport of ions.

In order to clarify the effect of Diamox on acid-base parameters in the brain, we have investigated its effect on the bicarbonate concentration and on the CO_2 tension gradients in rat and cat brain tissue (Brzeziński, Kjällquist & Siesjö, 1967; Kjällquist & Siesjö, 1966). When the animals were given Diamox in two doses of 50 mg/kg each and analyzed three hours after the first dose the values depicted in Figures 3 and 4 were found (point A). The curve has been shifted to the right, meaning that bicarbonate ions have accumulated in an amount which roughly corresponds to a 2 mE change in the standard bicarbonate of the tissue phase. However, it cannot be immediately assumed that this is a purely non-respiratory effect. It is well-known that Diamox interferes with the elimination of CO_2 from the tissues, including the lungs (Carter & Clark, 1958; Mithoefer & Davis, 1958), and that the CO_2 tensions measured in arterial and venous blood samples are not the same as those existing in vivo (Cain & Otis, 1960). In other words, when we measure the arterial CO_2 tension and use the experimentally derived relation between the arterial and the mean tissue tensions (Pontén & Siesjö, 1966a) in order to calculate the mean tissue CO_2 tension after Diamox administration, we might underestimate the tissue tension grossly. If this were so, the increase in bicarbonate concentration in the brain could perhaps be entirely respiratory, in what case the only effect of the drug would be to interfere with the CO_2 elimination from the tissue, i.e., simply to increase the CO_2 tension in the tissue. However, there are several reasons to believe that the calculation of the mean tissue tension from the measured arterial tension is not far from being right. Thus, it has been reported that the arterial CO_2 tension measured under carbonic anhydrase inhibition is an overestimation of the actual in vivo tension (Carter & Clark, 1958; Mithoefer, 1959). Moreover, measurements of the CSF CO_2 tension after administration of Diamox to cats (Brzeziński, Kjällquist & Siesjö, 1967), show that the latter tension initially increases above the measured venous CO_2 tension, but that the CSF CO_2 tension is found to fall in between the measured arterial and cerebral venous CO_2 tensions within 1-2 hours after the first dose of Diamox. Finally, if the CSF CO_2 tension is measured in the rats at the time when the bicarbonate concentration is significantly increased, it is found that it approximates the value found by calculation from the apparent arterial CO_2 tension.

In the preceding account, CSF has been used as an in vivo tonometer for evaluating the mean tissue CO_2 tension. The conclusions drawn are, of course, valid only if the mean tissue CO_2 tension agrees with the CO_2 tension of the tissue in direct contact with the CSF. If there are inhomogenities in the CO_2 tension between different brain areas after Diamox, the interpretation of the results will be another, but if no such inhomogenities exist, the experiments must be interpreted to show that inhibition of carbonic anhydrase leads to a non-respiratory increase in the bicarbonate concentration in brain tissue. This is an entirely unexpected result, but its interpretation must await a further validation of the mean tissue CO_2 tension under the experimental conditions.

"Intracellular pH"

So far we have only discussed the CO_2 tension and the bicarbonate concentration. These terms give us a possibility to define respiratory changes (changes in the CO_2 tension) as well as non-respiratory ones (changes in the bicarbonate concentration at constant P_{CO_2}). The situation is analogous to that in clinical acid-base chemistry apart from the fact that the pH term is then used to express the over-all change in the acid-base composition of the plasma while the CO_2 tension and, e.g., the "standard bicarbonate" are used to define this over-all change in terms of a respiratory and a non-respiratory component. In a reasonably homogeneous system like plasma the bicarbonate concentration and the CO_2 tension have an unambigous relation to pH

$$pH = pK_1' + \log \frac{(HCO_3^-)}{P_{CO_2} \cdot S} = pK_1' + \log \frac{(T_{CO_2} - P_{CO_2} \cdot S)}{P_{CO_2} \cdot S} \qquad (3)$$

where pK_1' is the apparent ionization constant for carbonic acid (considered to be equal to CO_2 plus H_2CO_3), and S is the solubility factor (e.g., mMoles carbonic acid/mm Hg/kg at a specified temperature). The second part of equation (3) denotes the fact that the bicarbonate concentration is obtained from a measurement of the total CO_2 concentration (T_{CO_2}) obtained upon acidification. This is not a chemical definition of the bicarbonate concentration but a physiological one since it includes all compounds which would appear as CO_2 upon acidification, e.g., carbamino compounds. This problem can, however, be solved by a determination of an operational pK_1' value, which would then compensate for any non-bicarbonate CO_2 compounds present. Thus, if S is known, and this can be determined separately by equilibrating acidified plasma with known CO_2 tensions and if the acid-labile CO_2 and the pH are determined at a known CO_2 tension, pK_1' can be calculated.

The above equation (3) has not been used to calculate the pH of a plasma sample but rather the CO_2 tension, and this was a standard procedure at a time when tension measurements were technically difficult. In a tissue pH measurements are not easily made, and when such measurements are performed on single cells the values can only be referred to the cytoplasmatic phase of the cells and they can say nothing about pH changes in membrane-confined compartments of the cell interior. It is then easy to understand that the equation has been used for calculation of "intracellular pH." This is, however, a precarious procedure which requires much consideration. We will now show that apart from the mean CO_2 tension, which has been dealt with above, both the solubility factor and the bicarbonate concentration must be critically evaluated before the equation can be used with any form of accuracy.

The CO_2 solubility of a tissue can only be measured in a homogenate, and the true amount of CO_2 dissolved in the tissue must be approximated by means of an extrapolation from the homogenates (Siesjö, 1962a). We will now consider a hypothetically intact tissue, which consists of a 20 per cent solid phase (proteins, lipids, etc.), and an 80 per cent water phase. It is generally assumed that the inorganic ions of the tissue are confined to its aqueous phase and, accordingly, we want to use Equation 3 for that phase. This means that the bicarbonate content of the tissue is expressed as a concentration per g of tissue water, whether this is derived from the cytoplasm or from any other intracellular or extracellular phase. But how should we then express the solubility? It appears as if the routine procedure previously used (Danielson, Chu & Hastings, 1939), stems from a misunderstanding, and the reasons for this are made clear from the following arguments. If we introduce the solubility coefficient γ_1 we will find that γ_1 for brain tissue equals 0.49 ml at 37.5°C, meaning that under a gas pressure of 1 atm. the tissue as a whole dissolves 0.49 ml per g. The question now is if this amount of CO_2 is dissolved only in the aqueous phase or if some of it is dissolved also in the solid phase. Danielson, et al. (1939), proposed that proteins increased the solubility of the gas in the water phase of muscle tissue, i.e., they considered that the total amount of CO_2 dissolved in the tissue was dissolved in the aqueous phase. If we draw the consequence of this argument we would consider the 0.49 ml dissolved in our hypothetical tissue as being confined to the 80 per cent aqueous phase, and the solubility coefficient would then be 0.61 (0.49/0.80) ml/g of tissue water. However, it seems much more plausible that the solids of the tissue dissolve some CO_2 (cf. van Slyke, et al., 1928, and Siesjö, 1962a). We could assume that the water phase approximates a salt solution with an ionic strength of about 0.160 and with a CO_2 solubility of 0.53 ml/g at 37.5°C. The solubility coefficient obtained for the total tissue — 0.49 ml/g — would thus result if the solids dissolved 0.33 ml/g of solid phase. But if this be so, we must use two solubility coefficients, and none of these would correspond to that calculated by Danielson, et al. (1939). Thus, when we subtract the dissolved CO_2 from the total CO_2 of the tissue we must use the coefficient expressing the total solubility (γ_1 = 0.49 ml/g of tissue, S_1 = 0.0292 μMoles/g of tissue/mm Hg), and when we calculate ionic equilibria in the water phase of the tissue we can only assume that the solubility equals that in a salt solution with an ionic strength of 0.160 (γ_2 = 0.53, S_2 = 0.0314 μMoles/g of tissue water/mm Hg).

The bicarbonate concentration calculated approaches the true mean bicarbonate concentration only if negligible amounts of non-bicarbonate compounds are present. It is still unknown why a large part of the acid-labile CO_2 of muscle tissue is not precipitated by barium at alkaline pH (Conway & Fearon, 1944). These authors considered this part to represent non-bicarbonate CO_2, and applied an appropriate correction when calculating "intracellular pH." For brain tissue, pK_1' determinations on tissue homogenates have indicated that no such compounds are likely to be present in significant amounts (Siesjö, 1962b), and it must presently be assumed that calculation according to Equation 3 gives a true mean bicarbonate concentration.

Given reliable measurements of the mean tissue CO_2 tension, the mean bicarbonate concentration, and the $\log \frac{(HCO_3^-)}{P_{CO_2} \cdot S_2}$ (log buffer ratio = log BR), we are in a position to talk confidently about respiratory and nonrespiratory shifts in the acid-base composition of the tissue, but we are still far from being able to translate these parameters into "tissue pH" values. The first obvious reason for this is that we have so far not corrected for the extracellular fluid, but this objection will concern also the bicarbonate and the log BR values. Thus, if we want to express our changes for the cellular phase, such corrections must be made (see below). However, there are other reasons why we had better refrain from using the pH term. Thus, pH is a logarithmic term, and the mean value of two or more pH values does not constitute a "mean pH." Moreover, the steady state distribution of H_2CO_3, or any other buffer acid such as 5,5-dimethyl-2,4-oxazolidinedione (DMO) which has been used on both brain and muscle tissue (Waddell & Butler, 1959; Roos, 1965), will not allow the calculation of a true mean hydrogen ion, or hydroxyl ion, concentration in the tissue (Siesjö & Pontén, 1966a). This follows from the fact that neither the buffer acid, nor the buffer anion, can be expected to exist in a uniform concentration in the tissue (see arguments in Siesjö & Pontén, 1966a). We thus have a situation with a theoretically awkward term ("tissue pH," "intracellular pH," "overall pH") which cannot be measured directly and cannot be calculated properly from actual measurements. What we can measure is the mean bicarbonate concentration (or the mean buffer anion concentration of any buffer system). Under such circumstances we can see no real reason for persisting in the use of the term pH. It seems so much better to use only the terms which we can measure, especially since we end up with the same basic information.

COMPARTMENTATION OF BICARBONATE IONS IN THE TISSUE

The objections raised against the pH term as applied to tissue systems is no real drawback since the scheme outlined above will give the appropriate information about acid-base shifts in the tissue. However, the discussion has hitherto focussed on the tissue as a one-compartment system (if we do not include the blood confined to the tissue, which is easily corrected for). There is still a considerable controversy regarding the size and the composition of the extracellular fluid in the brain. However, recent studies of the in vivo distribution of inulin and of sucrose (Rall, Oppelt & Patlak, 1962; Bourke, Greenberg & Tower, 1965), indicate that the extracellular space is considerably higher than that calculated from electron micrographs (see discussion in this symposium). There are also indications that the CSF and the true extracellular space have similar composition (see Pappenheimer, et al., 1965). There is presently insufficient information for a quantitative appraisal of acid-base changes in the combined extracellular space of brain tissue, as analyzed in the experiments referred to above, but we may introduce certain assumptions in order to allow a semi-quantitative analysis, and to facilitate a discussion of available data.

The main tissue phases are blood, cerebrospinal fluid (CSF), extracellular fluid proper (ECF), and intracellular fluid (ICF). The latter is by necessity inhomogeneous but we will consider only the mean bicarbonate concentration. In order to discuss our findings we must introduce certain assumptions. Thus, we will assume that there is a free diffusion of ions between the CSF and the true extracellular fluid, and that measurements of the bicarbonate concentration in CSF from the suboccipital cistern will indicate the concentration in the combined extracellular fluid (CSF + ECF). In a normal rat material under barbiturate anaesthesia the mean tissue standard bicarbonate is 15.8 mE/kg of tissue water, and the water content is 780 mg/g of wet, blood-free tissue. We can then calculate the mean intracellular bicarbonate concentration at different values for the combined extracellular volume according to the simple equation

$$(HCO_3^-)_t \cdot V_t = (HCO_3^-)_{CSF} \cdot V_{ECF} + (HCO_3^-)_{ICF} \cdot V_{ICF} \qquad (4)$$

where t denotes total tissue water phase, and V_{ECV} the combined extracellular volume. If V_{ECV} is assumed to be 10, 20, and 30 per cent the intracellular bicarbonate concentration is calculated to 14.1, 11.9 and 8.8 mE/kg of intracellular water, respectively. It is thus seen that the uncertainty regarding the extracellular volume (meaning the true extracellular volume plus the volume of the CSF contained in the parts of brain tissue used for analysis), must mean that we are equally uncertain about the true mean intracellular bicarbonate concentration. However, this does not mean that there is a corresponding uncertainty about the nature of the tissue acid-base changes under study. If, for example, the extracellular bicarbonate concentration should increase by 3 mE/kg we would get increases in the tissue standard bicarbonate concentration of 0.4, 0.8, and 1.2 mE/kg of tissue water at a combined extracellular volume of 10, 20, and 30 per cent, respectively. This means that it is difficult to measure small changes in the extracellular bicarbonate concentration by analyses on the total tissue, especially if the extracellular volume were in fact small. However, the extracellular bicarbonate ion concentration is easy to measure directly (as the CSF concentration), and it is far more important that small changes in the extracellular bicarbonate concentration will not seriously disturb the interpretation of intracellular events, even if the extracellular volume would be comparatively large. Thus, in the experiments referred to above where Diamox was given to rats, there were no significant changes in the bicarbonate concentration of the CSF (see Kjällquist & Siesjö, 1966), and the conclusion must be drawn that the changes observed (a standard bicarbonate change of about 2 mE/kg of tissue water) represent predominantly intracellular events.

We can advance similar arguments for intracellular bicarbonate changes. Thus, if we consider a 3 mE decrease in the mean intracellular concentration we will find that the tissue standard bicarbonate concentration will decrease by 2.6, 2.2, and 1.8 mE/kg of tissue water if the combined extracellular space is 10, 20, and 30 per cent, respectively. In other words, the method is very sensitive to intracellular changes and not seriously influenced by the presence of even a relatively large extracellular volume. We can now consider the changes obtained when cyanide was administered to the rats (see above). In the experiment referred to the lactate concentration increased to almost 21 mE/kg of wet tissue or to about 26 mE/kg of tissue water. However, the initial intracellular concentration should have been even higher and presumably at least 30 mE/kg of intracellular water (provided that the extracellular water occupies at least 10 per cent of the tissue weight). This means that the majority of the intracellular bicarbonate ions should disappear, since more than half of the released hydrogen ions will react with bicarbonate (see Siesjö & Pontén, 1966b). This finding suggests that there is one or more compartments, occupying at least 20 per cent of the tissue weight, which are not reached by the initially released lactic acid. It remains for future experiments to show if these compartments are mainly extracellular, or if the results can be explained by the presence of metabolic mechanisms for the regulation of intracellular acidity. However, the results obtained after administration of either cyanide or acetazolamide show that the tissue acid-base metabolism is complex and provides a number of intricate problems for future research. It is imperative that some of these problems will concern derangements in acid-base regulation in clinical conditions of brain swelling and edema.

REFERENCES

Albaum, H. G., J. Tepperman and O. Bodansky: The in vivo inactivation by cyanide of brain cytochrome oxidase and its effect on glycolysis and on the high energy phosphorus compounds in brain, J. Biol. Chem., 165, 45-51 (1946).

Bourke, R. S., E. S. Greenberg and D. B. Tower: Variation of cerebral cortex fluid spaces in vivo as a function of species brain size, Amer. J. Physiol., 208, 682-692 (1965).

Brzezinski, J., Å. Kjällquist and B. Siesjö: Mean carbon dioxide tension in the brain after carbonic anhydrase inhibition, J. Physiol. 188, 13-23 (1967).

Cain, S. M. and A. B. Otis: CO_2 retention in anesthetized dogs after inhibition of carbonic anhydrase, Proc. Soc. Exp. Biol. and Med, 103, 439-441 (1960).

_____ and _____: Effect of carbonic anhydrase inhibition on mixed venous CO_2 tension in anesthetized dogs, J. Appl. Physiol., 15, 390-392 (1960).

Carter, E. T. and R. T. Clark, Jr.: Respiratory effects of carbonic anhydrase inhibition in the trained unanesthetized dog, Ibid., 13, 42-46 (1958).

Conway, E. J. and P. J. Fearon: The acid-labile CO_2 in mammalian muscle and the pH of the muscle fibre, J. Physiol., 103, 274-289 (1944).

Danielson, I. S., H. I. Chu and A. B. Hastings: The pK_1' of carbonic acid in concentrated protein solutions and muscle, J. Biol. Chem., 131, 243-257 (1939).

Davson, H. and C. P. Luck: The effect of acetazoleamide on the chemical composition of the aqueous humour and cerebrospinal fluid of some mammalian species and on the rate of turnover of ^{24}Na in these fluids, J. Physiol., 137, 279-293 (1957).

Diemer, K.: Eine verbesserte Modellvorstellung zur Sauerstoffversorgung des Gehirns, Naturwissenschaften, 19, 617-618 (1963).

Giacobini, E.: A cytochemical study of the localisation of carbonic anhydrase in the nervous system, J. Neurochem., 9, 169-177 (1962).

Gleichmann, U., D. H. Ingvar, D. Lübbers, B. K. Siesjö and G. Thews: Tissue pO_2 and pCO_2 of the cerebral cortex, related to blood gas tensions, Acta Physiol. Scand., 55, 127-138 (1962).

Kety, S. S.: Determinants of tissue oxygen tension, Fed. Proc., 16, 666-670 (1957).

Koch, A. and D. M. Woodbury: Carbonic anhydrase inhibition and brain electrolyte composition, Amer. J. Physiol., 198, 434-440 (1960).

Krogh, A.: The number and distribution of capillaries in muscles with calculations of the oxygen pressure head necessary for supplying the tissue, J. Physiol., 52, 409-415 (1918-19).

Kjällquist, Å. and B, K. Siesjö: Increase in the intracellular bicarbonate concentration in the brain after acetazolamide, Acta Physiol. Scand., 68, 255-256 (1966).

Lübbers, D. W.: Capillary pattern and oxygen tension of the cerebral cortex, in: Regional Cerebral Blood Flow (ed. by D. H. Ingvar and N. Lassen, Acta Neurol. Scand., suppl. 14, 92-93 (1965).

Maren, T. H. and B. Robinson: The pharmacology of acetazolamide as related to cerebrospinal fluid and the treatment of hydrocephalus, Bull. Johns Hopkins Hosp., 106, 1-24 (1960).

Mithoefer, J. C.: Inhibition of carbonic anhydrase: its effect on carbon dioxide elimination by the lungs, J. Appl. Physiol., 14, 109-115 (1959).

_____ and J. S. Davis: Inhibition of carbonic anhydrase: Effect on tissue gas tensions in the rat, Proc. Soc. Exper. Biol. & Med., 98, 797-801 (1958).

Olsen, N. S. and J. R. Klein: Effect of cyanide on the concentration of lactate and phosphates in brain, J. Biol. Chem.,167, 739-746 (1947).

Oppelt, W. W., C. S. Patlak and D. P. Rall: Effect of certain drugs on cerebrospinal fluid production in the dog, Amer. J. Physiol., 206, 247-250 (1964).

Pappenheimer, J. R., V. Fencl, S. R. Heisey and D. Held: Role of cerebral fluids in control of respiration as studied in unanesthetized goats, Ibid., 208, 436-450 (1965).

Pontén, U.: The CO_2-binding capacity of rat brain tissue in vivo, Experientia, 20, 287-288 (1964).

_____: Acid-base changes in rat brain tissue during acute respiratory acidosis and baseosis, Acta Physiol. Scand., 68, 152-163 (1966).

_____ and B. K. Siesjö: Gradients of CO_2 tension in the brain, (to be published).

Rall, D. P., W. W. Oppelt and C. S. Patlak: Extracellular space of brain as determined by diffusion of inulin from the ventricular system, Life Sciences, 2, 43-48 (1962).

Roos, A.: Intracellular pH and intracellular buffering power of the cat brain, Amer. J. Physiol., 209, 1233-1246 (1965).

Siesjö, B. K.: The solubility of carbon dioxide in cerebral cortical tissue from the cat at 37.5°C. With a note on the solubility of carbon dioxide in water, 0.16 M NaCl and in cerebrospinal fluid, Acta Physiol. Scand., 55, 325-341 (1962).

_____: The bicarbonate/carbonic acid buffer system of the cerebral cortex of the cat, as studied on tissue homogenates. II. The pK_1' of carbonic acid and the relation between carbon dioxide tension and pH, Acta Neurol. Scand., 38, 121-141 (1962).

_____ and U. Pontén: Tissue pH – true parameter or misnomer?, Annals N. Y. Acad. Sci., 133, 78-86 (1966).

_____ and _____: The CO_2 buffer capacity of brain tissue and of equivalent systems, Annals N. Y. Acad. Sci., 133, 180-194 (1966).

_____ and G. Thews: Ein Verfahren zur Bestimmung der CO_2-Leitfähigkeit der CO_2-Diffusionskoeffizienten und des scheinbaren CO_2-Löslichkeitskoeffizienten im Gehirngewebe, Pflüg. Arch., 276, 192-210 (1962).

van Slyke, D. D., J. Sendroy, Jr., A. B. Hastings and J. M. Neill: Studies of gas and electrolyte equilibria in blood. X. The solubility of carbon dioxide at 38°C in water, salt solution, serum and blood cells, J. Biol. Chem., 78, 765-799 (1928).

Thews, G.: Über die Mathematische Behandlung Physiologischer Diffuzionsprozesse in Zylinderförmigen Objekten, Acta Biotheoretica, 10, 105-137 (1953).

_____: Die Sauerstoffdiffusion im Gehirn. Ein Beitrag zur Frage der Sauerstoffversorgung der Organe, Pflüg. Arch., 271, 197-226 (1960).

Waddell, W. J. and T. C. Butler: Calculation of intracellular pH from the distribution of 5.5-dimethyl-2.4 oxazolidinedione (DMO). Application to skeletal muscle of the dog, J. Clin. Invest., 38, 720-729 (1959).

Wistrand, P., B. R. Nechay and T. H. Maren: Effects of carbonic anhydrase inhibition on cerebrospinal and intraocular fluids in the dog, Acta Pharmacol Toxicol., 17, 315-336 (1961).

DISCUSSION

FONCIN: Concerning Dr. Towers' presentation, I think that in order to draw conclusions as to the validity of electron microscopic observations versus his kind of observation, it would be instructive to study the slices with the electron microscope after they have been incubated and subjected to various adverse conditions.

TOWER: We have done as Dr. Foncin has suggested. I did not have time to cover completely the material I presented, let alone show a lot of electron micrographs. But our electron micrographs show what you would expect from the data presented. There is a great deal of swelling, particularly of astrocytes. How much of this is due to the swelling which we can measure and how much is due to the fixation artifact which I discussed, I do not know. We had hoped, as Pappius, et al., originally suggested (Canad. J. Biochem. Physiol. 40: 885, 1962), that we could see differences depending on how much swelling we measured. But a little calculation will show that it would be extremely difficult to visualize such differences in the electron micrographs, particularly with fixation artifacts superimposed. I would be happy to show you copies of our pictures, but I don't think they will contribute much to the problems which you raise.

STEINWALL: One question to Dr. Brightman and Dr. Fleischhauer. You have both studied the migration of tracers from the ventricles into the brain tissue. Did you see any of these tracers enter the vessel wall or the lumen of the vessel?

BRIGHTMAN: Very little. The basement membrane around the capillaries trapped most of the colloid. In a few cases a pericyte immediately surrounding the endothelium swept up quite a bit of the marker pinocytotically and segregated it within the usual inclusion bodies; by the time the endothelium was reached, there was very little Ferritin left to be ingested. Occasionally, however, a few micelles were found within pinocytotic pits in the endothelium, but this was uncommon.

SIESJÖ: I was thinking of the papers of Dr. Tower and Dr. Oppelt. They were, as I see it, very convincing demonstrations that there is an appreciable extracellular space, but what is appalling is that there is quite a difference in the results you obtain. Dr. Rall's and Dr. Oppelt's space is about 10 to 15%, but Dr. Tower is getting much higher figures for the inulin space in these large animals. There is one difference. I think Dr. Tower is using the superficial cortical layers and Dr. Oppelt is using the deep layers. Could that explain the difference? Dr. Oppelt, did you also study the cortical layers? Is it possible to perfuse for such a long time that the tagged inulin penetrates all the way through the tissue?

OPPELT: In our usual studies, insufficient inulin reached the cortical subarachnoid space or penetrated all the way through the brain to allow us to estimate accurately the cortical extracellular space. A few preliminary studies using a slightly different perfusion technique allowed inulin to equilibrate in the cortical subarachnoid space and indicated a similar cortical extracellular space as compared to the other tissues we measured. In order to explain the difference between Dr. Tower's and our values for brain extracellular space, we should consider the difference in his and our technique. He used a single inulin injection and was thus dealing with a constantly falling inulin concentration in the subarachnoid space. Our perfusion technique allowed us to maintain a constant inulin concentration in the ventricle, on which we based our space calculations. Dr. Tower's constantly falling reference concentration of inulin may, in part, explain his higher values for brain extracellular space.

I would like to comment again on the relationship between space the indicator molecule occupies in brain and the length of time it is allowed to diffuse into the brain. Theoretically, the total space occupied as calculated from the diffusion profile for each molecule in the brain should be independent of time. As I had mentioned in my paper, this was, indeed, true for inulin, where similar brain spaces were found in experiments lasting from one to eight hours. Another implication of this finding involves the problem of ependymal permeability. Should there be a significant barrier to inulin at the ependyma, inulin spaces in brain should increase with increasing length of the experiment. That this did not occur suggests the absence of such a barrier at the ependyma.

TOWER: I think this is a difficult question to resolve because of the difference in tissue studied, differences in technique, and a number of factors of this sort. Most of us would probably agree that the spaces are likely to be somewhat larger in cerebral cortex than in white matter or in areas of mixed gray and white matter. The absolute values are quite another matter. I believe Dr. Davson's figures, under the best conditions, were intermediate between Dr. Oppelt's and ours. I don't know which species he was using, but the spread indicates that there are still some technical problems to be dealt with. In regard to the falling level of indicator solute, Dr. Oppelt is quite right. This was a condition of our experiments. The solute was injected intracisternally; a period of equilibration, usually about 6 hours, fol-

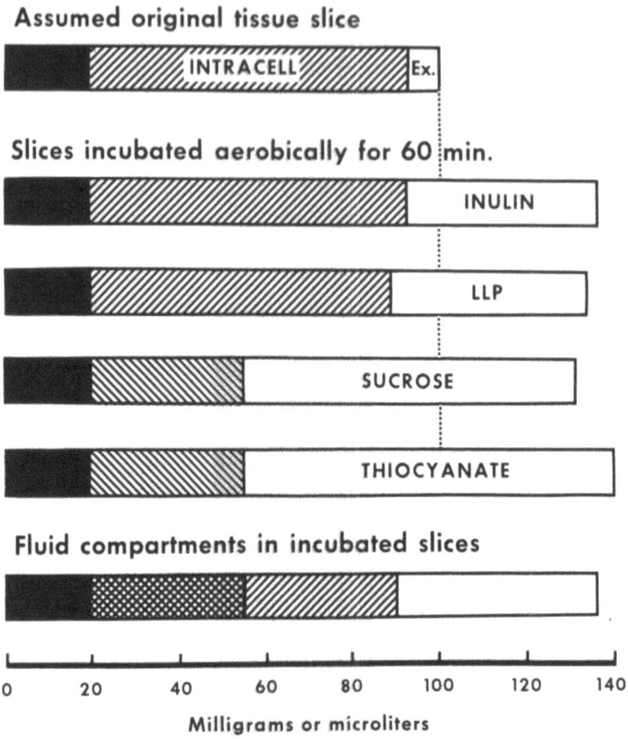

Fig. 1. The distribution of inulin, labelled protein, sucrose and thiocyanate in incubated cerebral cortex slices. The total length of each bar represents the average weight of slices after incubation per 100 mg of initial weight. The portion to the right of the vertical broken line indicates the extent of swelling. The black portion represents the dry weight and the open portion represents the "marker" space. The shaded portion, obtained by difference, gives the water not equilibrated with the "marker" or "non-space."

lowed; and then sampling was begun. However, at any time, from about one hour to 24 hours after injection, the tissue spaces measured the same size regardless of what the absolute solute level in CSF was at the time. Hence, I do not consider this to be a really valid objection in itself. There are some other points which could be raised, so that the only way we can settle the matter is a collaborative experiment with Dr. Rall's group.

PAPPIUS: I have some data on the in vitro distribution of the so-called extracellular substances which Prof. K. A. C. Elliott and I have accumulated during several years of work on this subject (Pappius and Elliott; Pappius, et al.; Pappius). Since our interpretation of what the inulin space repre-

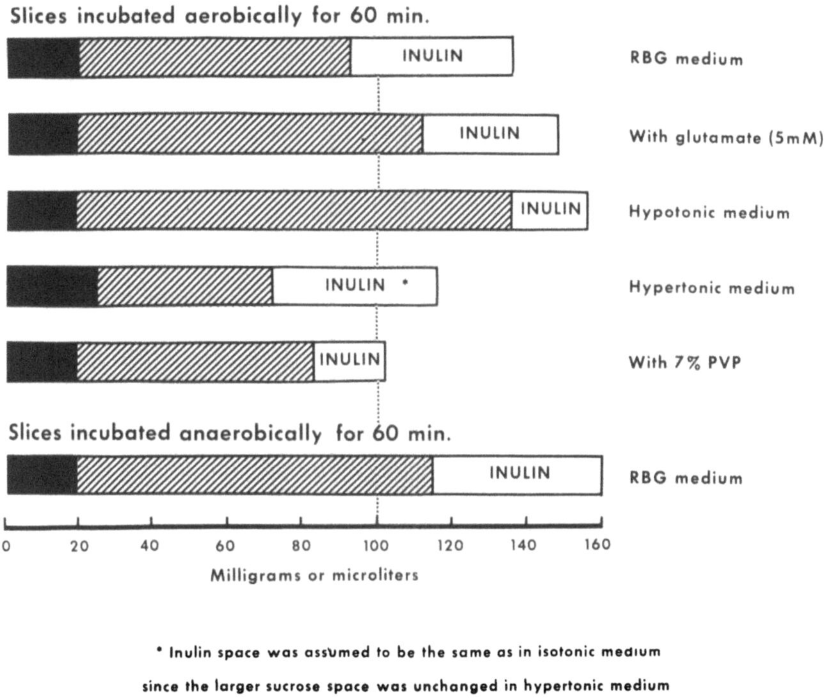

Fig. 2. Inulin space in cerebral cortex slices incubated under various experimental condition. For explanation, see Figure 1. RBG = Ringer–bicarbonate–glucose.

sents in vitro is different from that of Dr. Tower, I feel I must add to the confusion at this stage (Fig.1). In our experiments, rat cerebral cortex slices were incubated in glucose containing Ringer-bicarbonate medium to which was added one of the four markers: inulin, protein labelled with a fluorescent dye, sucrose or thiocyanate. All our results are expressed on the basis of 100 mg of fresh weight of tissue. The increase in weight or swelling after incubation is indicated by the portion of each bar to the right of the vertical broken line. In the unincubated original slice, the extracellular space is assumed to be 7% of the total tissue volume. Figure 1 summarizes a great number of experiments and shows clearly that three fluid compartments exist in the incubated slices. Inulin and labelled protein equilibrated with the swelling fluid and a little bit more with the tissue water. Sucrose and thiocyanate equilibrated with a much larger fraction of the tissue water. (In this respect our results differ from those of Dr. Tower, which showed inulin and sucrose spaces of the same magnitude). In other words, of the three fluid compartments, one equilibrated with sucrose and thiocyanate but not with inulin or protein, and the third did not equilibrate with any of the markers used. We measured the size of the compartment equilibrating with inulin under a variety of experimental conditions (Fig. 2).

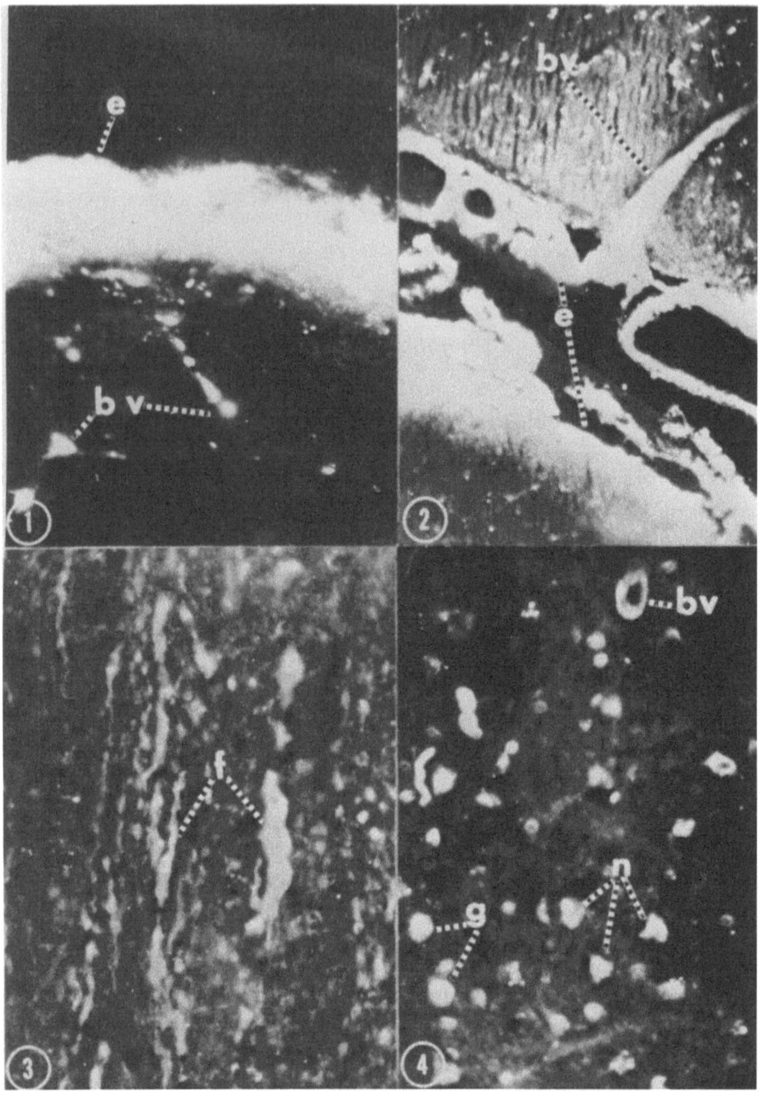

Fig. 3. Fluorescence photomicrographs of cat brain tissue slices incubated aerobically in medium containing 0.3% fluorescein-labelled bovine albumin (FLA). 1. White matter, showing edge (e) of slice. Slices processed by freeze-drying. Intense green fluorescence of the marginal zone and of the blood vessels (bv). White globules and granules scattered in the section are due to the presence of autofluorescent pigments. (X230) 2. Cerebral cortex, showing the edges of two slices (e). Section processed by freeze-drying. Intense green fluorescence of the leptomeninges and of the blood vessel (bv)

penetrating into the cortex. Superficial areas of the cortex showed a diffuse green fluorescence. The granular material in the cortex represents autofluorescent cellular pigment. (X230) 3. White matter. Formaldehyde-saline fixed frozen section. Area next to edge of slice. Green fluorescent nerve fibers (f) show distorted, swollen outlines. (X450) 4. Cerebral cortex. Formaldehyde-saline fixed frozen section. Area next to edge of slice. Neurons (n), glial cells (g), and blood vessels (bv) are green fluorescent. The occasional bright, small granules in the cells represent orange autofluorescent pigment. (X450).

We were impressed by the fact that while the amount of swelling was affected by changing the experimental conditions, the inulin space remained fairly uniform. In other words, the changes in swelling occurred in the non-inulin space while neither metabolic conditions nor osmotic forces seemed to influence greatly the extent of the inulin space. Since the labelled protein and inulin have quantitatively the same distribution in the incubated cerebral cortex slices, we assume that they equilibrate with the same fluid compartment. We were able to visualize this compartment microscopically with the help of Dr. Klatzo. Photomicrographs of cat cerebral cortex and subcortical white matter slices incubated aerobically in fluorescein-labelled albumin solution were prepared and some representative examples are shown in Figure 3. I think it is quite obvious that the labelled protein was restricted to the area of damage on the edge of the slice. Thus protein and, by inference, inulin, equilibrate with the fluid in damaged regions of the slice, and their distribution in vitro is not a measure of a true extracellular space. On the other hand, the non-inulin, non-protein space can be regarded as the intracellular space of undamaged cells. Others, e.g., Levi, et al., have come to a similar conclusion regarding the nature of the inulin space in brain tissue slices in vitro.

REFERENCES

Pappius, H. M.: The distribution of water in brain tissues swollen in vitro and in vivo, in Biology of Neuroglia, Progress in Brain Research, Vol. 15, Elsevier Publishing Co., 1965.

___________ and K. A. C. Elliott: Water distribution in incubated slices of brain and other tissues. Canad. J. Biochem. Physiol., 34, 1007-1022.

___________, I. Klatzo, and K. A. C. Elliott: Further studies of swelling of brain slices. Canad. J. Biochem. and Physiol., 40, 885-898, 1962.

Levi, G., A. Cherayil, and A. Lajtha: Cerebral amino acid transport in vitro. J. Neurochem., 12, 757-770, 1965.

FLEISCHHAUER: Dr. Oppelt, you have measured the concentration of the substance along a line through the caudate nucleus to the outside. This would be a perfect example for uptake in a region with high ependyma and grey matter underneath. Have you ever compared your values in this region with the uptake in a region further back in the lateral ventricle? If you go to about the mid-part of the lateral ventricle and determine the concentration along a line which goes through the corona radiata to the outside, you would obtain values for a region with flat ependyma and white matter underneath. I guess that there would be a tremendous difference.

OPPELT: The only regions we studied extensively were caudate nucleus, thalamus and pons. Gray matter predominates in caudate nucleus, while there is a mixture of gray and white matter in thalamus and pons. Extracellular space was similar in caudate nucleus and pons, while results in thalamus were variable. This variability may be due to differences in cutting thalamic sections and strips in different experiments and not due to differences in extracellular space in this part of the brain. To comment on Dr. Fleischhauer's studies: the molecules he was studying, namely Diamox, fluorescine, acridine and histamine, are all either protein bound or penetrate into the cell. I think this may well account for the difference of his findings as compared to ours. The molecules we studied do not bind and are not known to get into cells and would thus be expected to occupy only extracellular space.

TOWER: I would like to comment on Dr. Pappius's remarks. It is true that the results which she and Dr. Elliott have reported are somewhat at variance with our results and, incidentally, also with those of Varon and McIlwain (J. Neurochem. 8: 262, 1961). I think the studies by Varon and McIlwain have been the most detailed in regard to the various factors and compartments involved in the swelling in vitro of brain slices. Despite the fact that the three groups of investigators are dealing with different species, our results agree, as nearly as I can tell, with those of Varon and McIlwain, if one takes account of species differences, and this would leave the data of Pappius and Elliott somewhat discrepant. There are several technical factors which come to mind. First, in the studies by Dr. Pappius, there was considerably more swelling of slices than either McIlwain's group or our own have encountered. I would guess that this is attributable to what McIlwain has called "preparative" swelling. This is simply a technical problem relating to how long one leaves slices immersed before starting incubation, but this factor could well have something to do with the size of spaces one eventually measures. Secondly, there is certainly a factor of tissue damage. I don't agree with Dr. Pappius's interpretation, but this is only a personal opinion which need not concern us here. However, Varon and McIlwain have shown that if there are two cut surfaces to a brain slice, there is more swelling than with only one cut surface. For this reason and because of greater ease of handling, we have restricted our slices to "pial" slices with only one cut surface. It is also more difficult to work with rat cerebral cortex, which is what Dr. Pappius uses, than with cortex from larger animals. The rat cortex slices are more friable and harder to handle. I feel that it is largely in these technical areas that the source of any discrepancies may lie. From our own studies and from those of Varon and McIlwain and of Keesey, et al. (Biochem. J. 95: 289, 1965), I must conclude that there is considerably more inulin space in incubated cortical slices than Dr. Pappius would allow, and that, in general, inulin and sucrose spaces are similar, if not identical. Rather than prolong the argument, it is probably best to leave this question in the realm of techniques until we can resolve the differences.

KATZMAN: I just wanted to ask Dr. Quadbeck what is the specific evidence that water transport in either direction is energy-dependent. I am unaware in biology of any well-demonstrated water pump. Of course, if you pump ions, water could come along secondarily. Is that what you meant, or did you imply that there was actually direct pumping of water?

QUADBECK: If we inhibit the energy-giving processes, we have in all circumstances an increase of water in the brain. That is the only possibility to demonstrate the active transport out of the brain, but I think that it is permissible to say that the water goes out of the brain without energy. If one inhibits it by inhibiting the energy-giving processes, then an energy-depending process must be responsible.

SIESJÖ: If the primary thing is the transport of sodium, then the water flux is definitely passive, i.e., it is downhill from an energy standpoint; and if you don't have evidence that the water itself is the substance which is being transported, then I wonder if you should use the phrase "uphill transport of water." If the movement of water is secondary to that of the solute, then water transport must be passive.

QUADBECK: Yes, this is a question of definition.

SIESJÖ: But that is downhill for water.

QUADBECK: That is downhill for water, but something must go uphill to transport the water out of the brain, and it is not the transport of sodium or potassium.

SIESJÖ: But if you don't know that the transport of water is uphill, you are confusing the terminology by saying that water is the thing that is being transported actively.

QUADBECK: Yes, but it is a question of definition.

BROMAN: Another question to Dr. Quadbeck. Is it possible to exclude that the variations in the uptake of these indicator substances which you have demonstrated are influenced by changes in the cerebral blood flow and the systemic blood pressure?

QUADBECK: If this transport would be dependent on the blood pressure, all substances would go in the same direction, which they really do not. Some are increased, some are decreased in their transport, and therefore I cannot believe that it is dependent on the blood pressure.

STEINWALL: It is my opinion, too, that the blood flow deserves careful consideration. As far as the blood-brain transfer of nutritive compounds like glucose and many others is concerned, I think that circulatory conditions might be of particular importance for the amount taken up.

QUADBECK: This question has been studied in man, and there no effect of the blood flow on the uptake of glucose can be found. We have some patients with a very high blood flow and a very low uptake of glucose, and in other patients there is normal blood flow and very low uptake of glucose.

CLASEN: May I change the subject? I would like to ask a question of Dr. Steinwall. Did you use an aqueous solution of trypan blue in the postmortem profusions?

STEINWALL: Trypan blue in saline was used in the present experiments. Recently, however, we have started comparative studies on the use of dye in saline and dye in plasma or protein solution in postmortem indication of BBB damage. Both types of tracer solutions appear to be unable to penetrate out of normal brain vessels. As regards the distribution pattern in areas of extravasation, however, they seem to differ in certain respects. Our preliminary impression is that the dye-protein complex spreads easier after extravasation and gives a picture more like that seen in vivo.

CLASEN: It looked from your slides as if there were staining even of normal cortex. Have you ever tried to reproduce this with an inert colored particle in aqueous solution?

STEINWALL: We haven't done it, and as far as I know, it has not been done elsewhere.

CLASEN: I think we should emphasize the point that the role of the blood proteins is here quite important.

STEINWALL: I agree.

CLASEN: I propose that the dyes are bound by albumin.

STEINWALL: Dr. Clasen mentioned that one picture of a postmortem brain gave the impression that also the normal cortex was stained. This might be a result of the technical difficulties of delimiting the application of the BBB damaging solution to one hemisphere under postmortem conditions. Major parts of the control hemisphere, however, generally showed no extravasation of the perfused dye. This was controlled also by microscopical examination.

MIQUEL: I would like to ask Dr. Quadbeck if he has investigated the rate of penetration of glucose in edematous nervous tissue. We have observed that the rate of penetration of methyl glucose in the edema induced by ultraviolet radiation is near normal. We have also measured the penetration rate of methyl glucose in the cat brain one month after inducing edema. At this time, the astrocytes showed fibrous hyperplasia and a very striking increase in the activity of its oxydative enzymes. Nevertheless, the penetration rate of methyl glucose in the altered white matter was near normal. It would be very interesting to know if Dr. Quadbeck has made similar observations.

IV. Experimental Studies on Brain Edema

Chairman: ***K. J. Zülch***

DON M. LONG
J. FRANCIS HARTMANN
LYLE A. FRENCH

ULTRASTRUCTURAL SUBSTRATES OF EXPERIMENTAL CEREBRAL EDEMA*

The developing clinical interest in cerebral edema and its neuropathological definition has been paralled by an increasing number of attempts to produce an adequate experimental model for the study of this process. The entity has been vigorously studied and there is a voluminous literature on the subject filled with conflicting reports and divergent opinions with regard to both reliability of methods and morphological changes produced.

Kocher, as early as 1901, was attempting to produce cerebral edema as a sequel to head injury, and Cannon (1901-02) independently performed similar experiments though it appears that neither was fully successful. The increase in brain volume obtained was secondary to a combination of factors and at present holds no more than historical interest in the study of the subject. Weed and McKibben (1919) discovered that the intravascular infusion of hypotonic solutions gave rise to marked brain swelling and increased cerebrospinal fluid (CSF) pressure. Detailed histological examinations revealed distended perivascular spaces, enlarged intercellular spaces particularly in white matter, and enlarged pericellular spaces with questionable glial nuclear shrinkage. The cells of the choroid plexus were swollen and there was a generalized alveolar appearance of the tissue (Weed, 1923-24). These descriptions are strikingly similar to those later propounded by Greenfield and Scheinker and defined as cerebral edema. Penfield and Buckley (1928) were able to produce satisfactory brain swelling around sterile cerebral puncture wounds. Ferraro (1930) substantiated the observations of Weed in a detailed analysis of the effect of hypotonic fluids upon the brain.

*Aided by research grants MH00388, NB00782, and NB05591 from the National Institutes of Health.

Pilcher (1937) in the course of investigation of cerebral trauma concluded that the production of brain swelling by trauma alone was not possible. He was able to obtain satisfactory experimental edema by exposure of the brain to air (1941). Denny-Brown (1941), in contradistinction to Pilcher, was able to produce edema by graded cerebral trauma. However, from the microscopic description it is apparent that the brain swelling produced did not fully conform to the morphology which has been established for the diagnosis in humans. White, et al. (1943), reviewed the methods then current for the production of brain edema and the methods for its measurement. The importance of the blood volume in brain swelling was stressed and it was established that simply increasing brain volume by an experimental method was not synonymous with the production of cerebral edema, thereby forcing a much more detailed histological investigation of experimental brain swelling than had been previously existant. Reid (1942) produced edema both by the intravenous injection of distilled water and by exposure of the brain to air. Severe swelling was produced by each method; however, no histological changes were evident in the exposed brains. The subsequent infusion of hypotonic fluids caused extreme swelling of the neurons which often progressed to cell rupture. There was marked swelling of the myelin and acute oligodendroglial swelling was very common. Pericellular spaces were increased and perivascular spaces were also enlarged. There was swelling of choroid plexus cells as well. Other elements were not abnormal. These changes were compared with those accepted as diagnostic of cerebral edema in the human and found to be similar. The oligodendroglia were the cells primarily involved in the edematous process, and the majority of the fluid was in an extracellular position and in the perineural and perivascular spaces. White (1943) was able to produce demonstrable brain swelling in cats by experimental concussion but no histological changes in the tissue were identifiable. Obrador (1943) reported immediate brain swelling following placement of lesions in the floor of the fourth ventricle in dogs, and he concluded that a concomitant increase in blood pressure was the primary offender and that an increased vascular volume within the brain was responsible for the swelling. Maintenance of the blood pressure at normal levels resulted in control of the observed brain swelling. Prados, et al. (1945), disputed the observation of Reid that exposure of the brain resulted in no histological changes suggestive of cerebral edema. Swelling and chromatolysis of the neurons was noted. The microgl underwent typical phagocytic reactions. No change was noted in oligodendrogliocytes but the astrocytes proliferated rapidly.

There was a breakdown in the blood-brain barrier around the area exposed as demonstrated by the injection of trypan blue. The edematous reaction was found to be very marked in the hypothalamus. Elliott and Jasper (1949) could determine no edema formation after exposure of the brain in rabbits. Clasen, et al. (1953), described a method for the production of acute closed cerebral lesions by the application of liquid nitrogen in a closed container to the skull. An area of infarction surrounded by a rather predictable area of edema was consistently produced. Edstrom (1955) observed that the brain was capable of appreciable swelling after death. In guinea pigs, 4% of brain volume was gained in 30 minutes after sacrifice, and this increase continued though more slowly for a long period of time. Larger animal brains appeared to swell more slowly than smaller. McGee, et al. (1957), administered triethyl tin compounds in the diet of rats to produce gross swelling of the CNS. The primary change appeared to be an increase in the interstitial space within the white matter. Klatzo (1958) devised a method of cold application to the brain for the production of edema. Diffuse PAS staining was apparent in the interstitial spaces in the area of edema and within astrocyte cytoplasm as well. Astrocytes were markedly enlarged and white matter extracellular space was also increased. Axon sheaths and myelin were swollen but no changes were noted in oligodendroglia or microglia. In an attempt to mimic more closely the clinical situation Chou (1961) produced edema by the intracerebral implantation of carcinoma in rabbits. Both the gross and microscopic appearances of this swelling were quite compatible with the accepted criteria for the diagnosis of edema. Sperl (1959) reviewed the methods for the production of edema and concluded that none available was completely satisfactory to correlate with brain swelling complicating cerebral tumors. In an effort to produce a model which would be easily reproducible and closely correlated with the clinical situation, he employed intracerebral placement of substances calculated slowly to gain volume. The most effective of these was found to be hydrophillic psyllium seed. The intracerebral implantation of a measured mass of these seeds in dogs resulted in a predictable amount of brain swelling, if the seeds did not rupture to the cortical surface or into the ventricle. The swelling was identical grossly and histologically with that encountered surrounding cerebral tumors. Histologically, a marked increase in the extracellular fluid of the white matter was noted to cause an alveolar appearance. Myelin sheaths were swollen and distended, as were axons. There was an increase in the perivascular and pericellular spaces. In the cortex few changes were noted and the glia were thought not to be markedly affected. Mild swelling of the oligodendroglia was evident and clasmatodendrosis of astrocytes was apparent. Gerschenfeld, et al. (1959), produced satisfactory edema by inflicting a sterile stab wound upon the cortex. Kalsbeck and Cumings (1963) reported additional observations upon the brain swelling which followed triethyl tin administration. Clasen and associates (1962) have more recently published a series of articles dealing extensively with cerebral edema produced by the method of focal freezing previously mentioned. Histological examination indicated changes which are quite similar to those accepted as diagnostic of cerebral edema. Blinderman, et al. (1962), revived a technique originally proposed by Edstrom, producing edema by the injection of vegetable oil into the carotid artery of dogs.

The introduction of the electron microscope into the study of cerebral edema did not immediately clarify the experimental situation. Torack, et al. (1960), produced swelling in the brains of mice by the application of solid carbon dioxide directly to the pial surface. The predominant change was found to be tremendous swelling of the clear glial cell. Surprisingly, no evidence of extracellular fluid accumulation was found. Gerschenfeld, et al. (1959), had reported the same intracellular swelling in edema surrounding cortical stab wounds. Luse and Harris (1960, 1961) produced edema by the intravenous infusion of distilled water and by brain exposure. In both instances there was an obvious increase in clear cell cytoplasm, particularly in the pericapillary region. Torack, et al. (1960), examined brain swelling secondary to triethyl tin administration and compared this to human edema surrounding brain tumors. The processes were thought to be morphologically similar. Glial swelling was demonstrated, but no extracellular fluid was discovered. The first inkling that these observations might be incomplete came with presentations by Evans and Raimondi (1961) and by Long, et al. (1962). The former authors described edema developing after subdural balloon inflation in cats. A definitely enlarged extracellular space was evident in the white matter in addition to the glial swelling previously described. Long, et al., reported similar findings in human cerebral edema and in edema surrounding implanted psyllium seeds in dog cerebrum. Obvious difficulty came from the lack of descriptions of white matter in early investigations. Observations concerning cortical changes in edema were transposed to characterize the entire process. The intracellular theory of edema was at obvious variance with physiological and light microscopic data, and an interdisciplinary controversy arose (De Robertis & Gerschenfeld, 1961).

Raimondi, et al. (1962), amplified their original report concerning edema in white matter following subdural balloon inflation. The occurrence of extracellular fluid was well documented. Gonatas, et al. (1963), produced edema in the rat by implantation of cryptococcal polysaccharide. Extracellular fluid accumulation in the white matter was observed, and subsequent reports by the same group have substantiated this contention (Hirano, 1965). Bakay and Haque (1964) have studied edema arising from cold lesions and supported earlier studies demonstrating an increased white matter extracellular space. Herzog, et al. (1965), utilized intracerebral tumors in rabbits to produce edema. The characteristics of this edema correlated well with the features of human and experimental brain swelling recently reported.

It is entirely possible that all or at least most of the methods described are successful in producing a brain swelling. However, it has not been established that the morphological characteristics of all these forms of brain swelling are the same. Those types of swelling which result primarily from an increase in CSF or blood volume within the cranium may be discarded. Clearly, the use of a method which closely mimics the clinical situation is desirable. For this reason those methods which employ the use of an expanding intracranial mass for the production of cerebral edema have been deemed most suitable, but it is likely that less exacting methods produce an experimental edema of equal quality (Hauser, et al., 1960).

The light microscopic characteristics of cerebral edema are well established from the study of human cases. It is immediately apparent that no experimental brain swelling can be defined as edema unless it fully conforms to that established morphologically. The ultrastructure of human cerebral edema has been reported recently. An important consideration then becomes the review of the more popular methods of experimental edema production with the electron microscope and their comparison with those characteristics accepted as diagnostic of the condition in the human.

METHOD

In order to make the observations of this investigation clinically applicable and to allow correlation with the studies on human material it seemed imperative to approximate as closely as possible the pathological process as it exists in the human. Accordingly, the method of Sperl, which involves intracerebral psyllium seed implantation, was utilized. This method allows the development of edema around the slowly expanding intracranial mass and in addition is easily reproducible. From the literature review it seems likely that the edema of the brain noted after variety of other insults is of constant gross and microscopic characteristics. In order to test this supposition and for purposes of comparison of the present study with other published reports the most popular of the procedures earlier described were duplicated. Some of these such as triethyl tin poisoning and the application of cold to the brain have been very extensively studied and excellent reports concerning them are already in the literature. For this reason these techniques were not repeated. Several of the others mentioned have been proven previously to be ineffective in the production of cerebral edema and no attempt was made to repeat them.

The animals utilized in this study were male and female albino rabbits weighing from 2 to 4 kg and adult male and female mongrel dogs weighing from 10 to 24 kg.

The control material consisted of brain removed from three normal rabbits and two normal dogs. Edema was produced in a variety of ways. In three rabbits psyllium seeds were placed in the extradural space while in three subdural placement was utilized. In three additional animals the seeds were inserted into the cerebrum. Two dogs underwent psyllium seed placement and in two others a small subdural balloon was slowly inflated. In one dog an extradural balloon was utilized. Two rabbits were subjected to the intravenous infusion of distilled water and in two animals the fluid was administered intra-arterially. In four rabbits the cortex was widely exposed to air for from one to four hours and in two additional rabbits a sterile cortical stab wound was inflicted.

To obtain control material, three rabbits and two dogs were lightly anesthetized with pentobarbital given intravenously and then allowed to breathe spontaneously. A linear midline incision along the sagittal suture was made and skin retracted laterally. An incison was made through the periosteum and the periosteum scraped away from the bone with a periosteal elevator. A hand trephine was utilized to remove a quarter-inch button of bone. In the rabbits this button of bone was removed in the midline while in the dogs it was placed laterally to avoid the sagittal sinus. The dura was opened in a cruciate fashion and care taken to avoid manipulation of the tissue or electrocoagulation of the dura. A 5×5 mm^2 of cortex and subcortical white matter was incised with a sharp knife and quickly removed. A pituitary ronguer was then utilized to remove a specimen of deep white matter in the case of the dogs. The tissue was then rapidly transferred to 1% buffered osmium tetroxide for fixation.

For the experimental production of edema the intracranial placement of psyllium seeds in rabbits was predominantly utilized. The technique of anesthesia and exposure of the brain was identical with that described in the normal controls. With the dura exposed the procedure varied according to the proposed site of placement of the seeds. In three animals the dura was opened in a curvilinear fashion and a 2 mm linear cortical incision made with a sharp knife blade. Eight sterile psyllium seeds were then introduced into the cortical incision. This corresponds to about 0.15 ml of seed. The dura was sutured and the bone button replaced. The bone button was sealed in place with a combination of methyl methacrylate cement and an experimental adhesive available from the Minnesota Mining & Manufacturing Co. The skin was closed with metal clips and the animals returned to their cages without special postoperative care. If the psyllium seed placement was to be in the subdural space, the same type of linear dural incision was made and 0.25 ml of seed gently placed in the subdural space through the dural incision. The dura was closed and the bone cemented into position as previously described. If the seeds were to be in the extradural space the unopened dura was dissected away from the overlying bone and 0.25 ml of seed was placed in the extradural space. The bone button was demented in position as described. Three animals were utilized in each category. At 24, 48 or 72 hours the animals were re-anesthetized with intravenous sodium pentobarbital and the incision widely opened. Samples of cortex and white matter were removed from directly under the site of the lesion and 0.5 and 1.0 cm from it in the manner described for the removal of control tissue. The animals were then sacrificed by the intracarotid injection of 200 cc of formalin in 10% saline, the brain removed, and immersed in the same solution for subsequent processing for light microscopy.

In two dogs similar operative procedures were performed. Both the animals underwent the intracerebral placement of 1.2 ml of psyllium seed. They were sacrificed after 48 and 72 hours respectively and samples of edematous brain taken 0.5, 1.0, 2.0 and 4.0 cm from the lesion in a radial fashion.

Three additional dogs underwent the subdural or extradural placement of a Number 8 Foley catheter through a small trephine opening. After placement of the catheter the opening was sealed with methyl methacrylate cement. In one animal the balloon was rapidly inflated to a pressure of 60 mm Hg. In two others the inflation took place gradually over 24 or 48 hours. The final volume of the balloon was about 4 ml. Forty-eight hours after the final inflation of the balloon the animals were sacrificed and tissue obtained at regular radial distances in a manner identical to that which has been described.

In the final phase of the experiment reproduction of some of the other methods of edema production reported in the literature was accomplished. Again, all the rabbits were anesthetized lightly with penobarbital given intravenously. In two animals the right jugular vein was isolated and 20 cc of distilled water slowly injected. The cranium was then rapidly opened and samples of cortex and white matter obtained. In a second pair the same volume of distilled water was injected directly into the right common carotid artery shortly after the right cerebral hemisphere had been exposed by extensive craniectomy. Four rabbits underwent exposure of the cerebrum bilaterally for one, two, three and four hours respectively. In these animals a midline incision was made and as much of the cranium superiorly removed as possible. The dura was opened widely exposing both hemispheres to air. The animals were allowed to revive and ambulate in a padded cage until the prescribed time had elapsed. In all cases the brain was noted to herniate through the cranial defect markedly rising as much as 1 cm above the level of the bone. Multiple samples of both gray and white matter were obtained. Two rabbits were subjected to sterile cortical stab wounds after a small craniectomy had been performed. Skin was closed after the injury and 48 hrs later the area was again exposed and tissue samples excised from the proximity of the wound.

After the tissue had been obtained it was immediately immerse in 1% buffered osmium tetroxide. After one to two minutes of immersion the tissue was cut into 1 mm squares and immersion continued until fixation was complete. In the early part of the study the tissue was then embedded in methyl methacrylate in the manner standard for electron microscopy. All of the later samples were embedded in Epon 812 rather than methacrylate because of the superior qualities of this agent for brain tisue preservation. Sections were obtained by the use of a glass knife in the Serval Port-Blum Ultramicrotome MT2 or the LKB Ultramicrotome. Section thickness was about 600 Å. The majority of the tissue was unstained though a few sections were stained with uranyl acetate. Sections were examined in the RCA EMU 3F electron microscope or the Siemens Elmiskop I.

The tissue obtained for light microscopy was fixed <u>in situ</u> by perfusion as described, and the brain then totally removed. The brains were then immersed in a 10% formalin in saline solution and fixed for a minimum of two weeks. Areas selected for microscopic examination were prepared in the routine manner for light microscopy and stained with hematoxylin and eosin. Sections were then examined with a standard light microscope. None of the preparations was accepted as representing cerebral edema unless both the gross and light microscopic characteristics considered pathognomic of the process were found to be present.

RESULTS

In the sections of normal rabbit brain no abnormalities were noted. This appearance of the tissue resembled that described in the literature. Neither did the examination of normal dog brain reveal any variation from the accepted structure in this animal.

The intracranial placement of psyllium seed resulted in cerebral edema of decreasing radial severity surrounding the mass of the seeds. Since there were no qualitative differences in the appearance of this edema, whether the result of intracerebral, subdural or extradural placement of the psyllium seeds in rabbits or dogs, all of these groups will be described together.

In the cortex the astrocytes evinced the most obvious change. There was enlargement of these cells with decreased cytoplasmic electron density. Compression of surrounding tissue by the enlarged astrocytes or their processes was common. The cell nuclei did not change appreciably and intracytoplasmic inclusions did not vary significantly from their normal appearances or numbers as could be judged without quantitation (Fig. 1).

The astrocyte cytoplasm increase in the pericapillary region was quite marked. The perivascular extensions of the astrocytes were swollen and of great clarity. In an occasional tissue sample increased numbers of intracytoplasmic vacuoles and mitochondria were noted. The capillary basement was unchanged and no space ever appeared between the basement membrane and the astrocyte processes. There was no notable change in the capillary endothelial cells though increased vacuolization was occasionally noted (Fig. 2). Compression of tissue surrounding capillaries was quite common secondary to the increase in size of the glial-capillary complex. The rarely seen oligodendroglial vascular processes were of essentially normal appearance.

There was no increase in the cortical extracellular space in most of the preparations. Enlargement of this space (and that in white matter) could be obtained by rapid hypotonic fluid infusion.

The oligodendroglia were for the most part unchanged though a slight increase in the volume of perinuclear cytoplasm and a slight decrease in its density were discovered. Endoplasmic reticulum ballooning was occasionally seen.

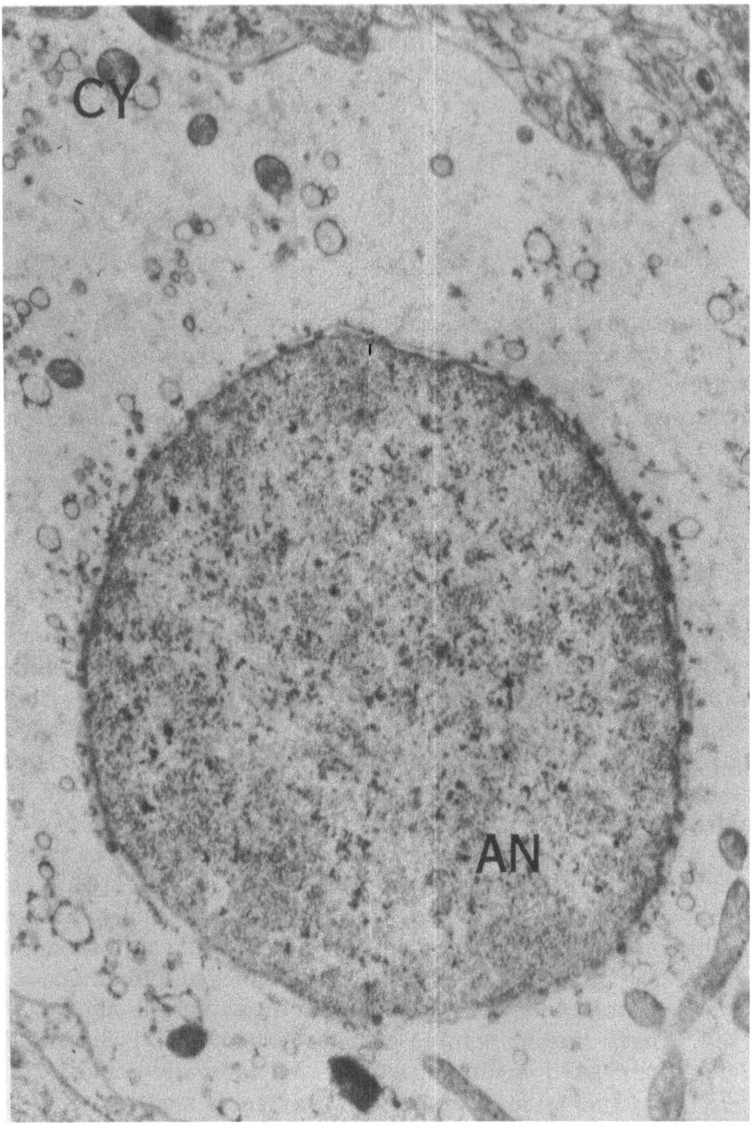

Fig. 1. Within the cortex remarkable enlargement of the astrocytes occurs. The nucleus (AN) is normal, but the cytoplasm (CY) is increased in volume and of decreased electron density. Intracytoplasmic formed elements are unchanged in appearance. Rabbit. Subdural psyllium seeds. X16,300 (reduced).

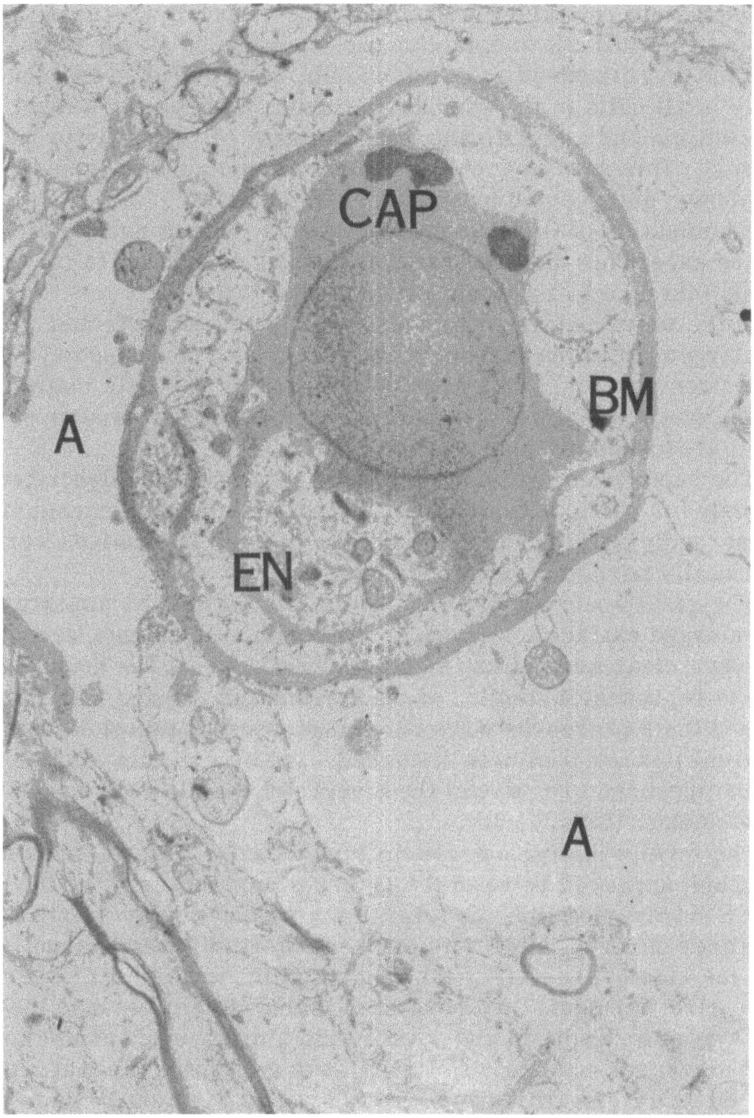

Fig. 2. A cortical capillary (CAP) is completely surrounded by clear, swollen astrocyte processes (A). The basement membrane (BM) is preserved, and the endothelium (EN) appears normal. Dog. Subdural balloon. X9,740 (reduced).

The microglia were not changed except in areas immediately underlying the seed mass where tissue necrosis was common. In this area the common reactive cell forms were seen.

Nerve cells were consistently normal except for occasional ballooning of the endoplasmic reticulum. Since the preservation of the endoplasmic reticulum is one criterion of excellent tissue preservation, it is difficult to establish the significance of this finding in neurons and oligodendroglia. Such enlargement was seen occasionally in all cells in the edematous tissue. That this is a facet of brain swelling and a significant finding cannot be definitely proven at present. This swelling could frequently be obtained by rapid fluid infusion and seemed proportional to the rate.

Examination of the neuropil revealed it to be of normal appearance except for the compression changes secondary to the tremendous increase in astrocyte process size (Fig. 3).

In the white matter astrocytes were again most affected. There was enlargement of the astrocyte cytoplasm with decreased cytoplasmic electron density. The astrocyte swelling in the white matter, however, was less impressive because of the smaller number of cells and cell processes present (Fig. 4).

The capillaries presented the same abnormalities described previously for cortical capillaries. Astrocyte vascular extensions were markedly swollen and clear but the vessels themselves were of essentially normal appearance.

The great abnormality in the white matter was the appearance of an enlarged extracellular space. The cellular elements were separated by a clear area of low electron density which has been assumed to represent distention of the extracellular space with fluid. Cells and their processes were not compressed by this fluid but their usual juxtaposition was disturbed. The size of this extracellular space appeared to parrallel the severity of the edema as measured by other means (Figs. 4, 6).

The myelin lamination was disrupted early. Spaces, seemingly fluid-filled, appeared between the layers of myelin, splitting the myelin at the intraperiod line. Between the axon and myelin sheath larger fluid spaces occured, often with marked deformation and vacuolization of the axis cylinder (Fig. 6). The significance of these observations is hard to judge. They have been included here because the changes were widespread and severe, and similar changes did not appear in control material. However, it is quite possible that a portion of these abnormalities represents artifact inherent in immersion fixation of edematous tissue. Perfusion techniques should settle this question.

Oligodendrogliocytes exhibited endoplasmic reticulum swelling, but the cytoplasm volume was not enlarged. Microgliocytes were little changed unless tissue necrosis appeared (Fig. 5).

The progression of the severity of the edema process followed the same general outline in all instances. Remarkable cellular distention first appeared, followed by evidences of impending cell death, rupture of plasma membranes with creation of a "pseudoextracellu-

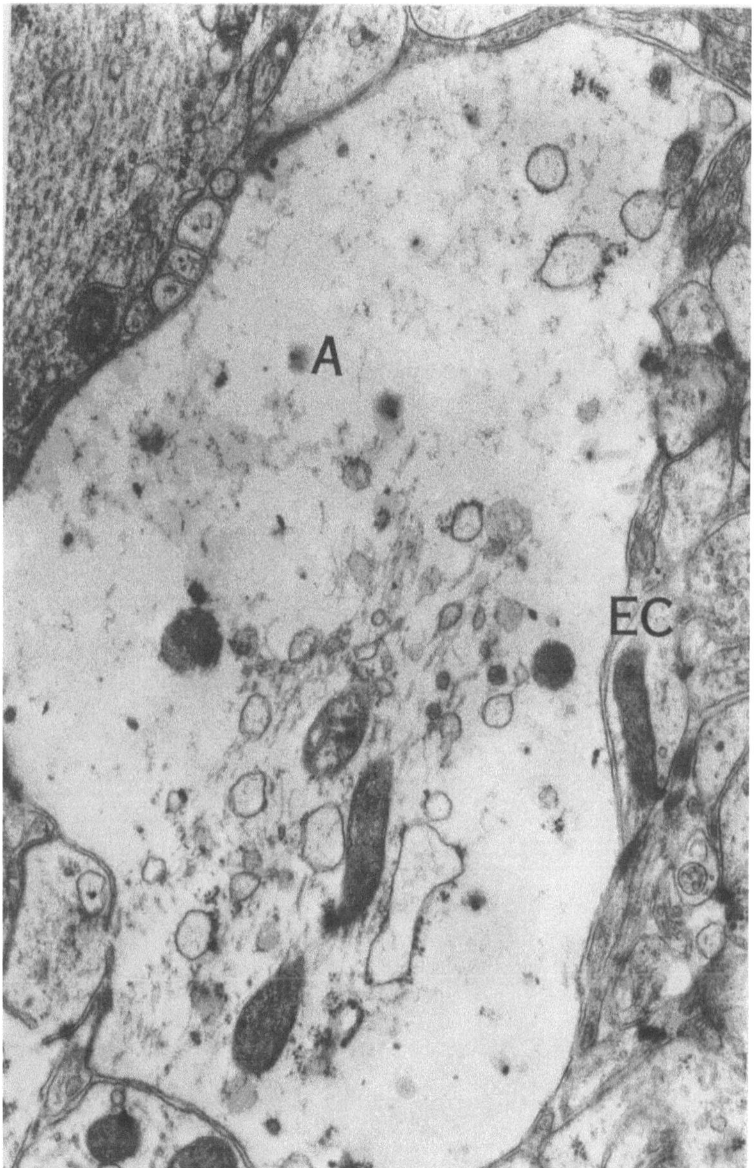

Fig. 3. A single clear, enlarged cortical astrocyte process (A) occupies most of the field. The cortical extracellular space (EC) is normal. Dog. Intracerebral psyllium seed implantation. X16,100 (reduced).

lar" space, enlargement of the white matter extracellular space, and finally the appearance of actual tissue necrosis (Fig. 7). If the

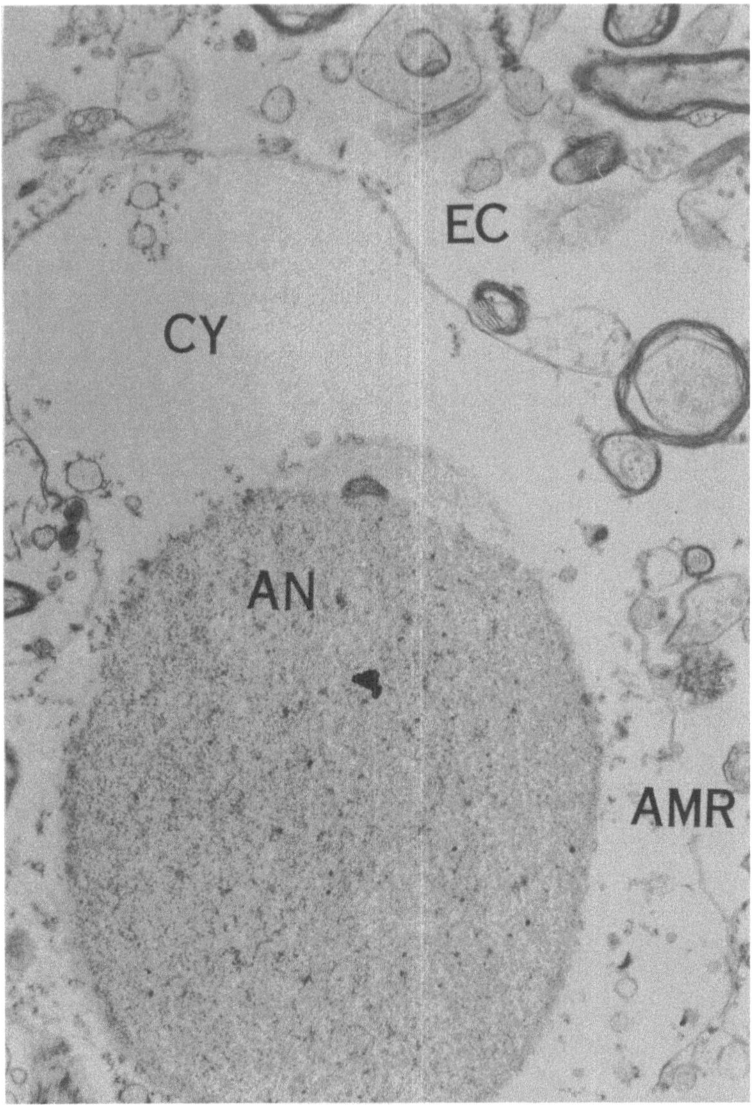

Fig. 4. In the white matter astrocyte swelling is also apparent. The nucleus is preserved (AN). Cytoplasm (CY) is also enlarged in volume, and membrane rupture (AMR) may occur. Concomitant increase in extracellular space (EC) is seen. Rabbit. Extradural psyllium seed placement. X10,180 (reduced).

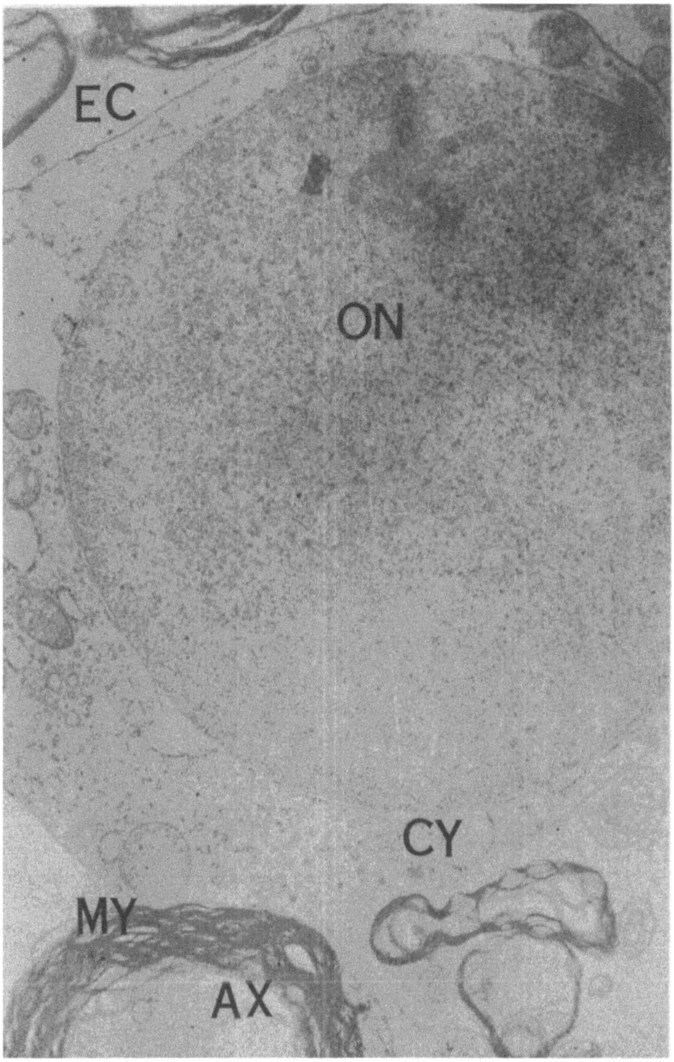

Fig. 5. Oligodendrogliocytes are little changed in either cortex or white matter. Nucleus (ON). Cytoplasm (CY). Myelin (MY). Axon (AX). The extracellular space (EC) is obviously enlarged. Rabbit. Subdural psyllium seed implantation. X24,950(reduced).

process was severe enough there was eventually complete loss of viable-appearing nervous tissue.

The animals were sampled in the following manner: One tissue block was removed from directly beneath the mass of the seeds.

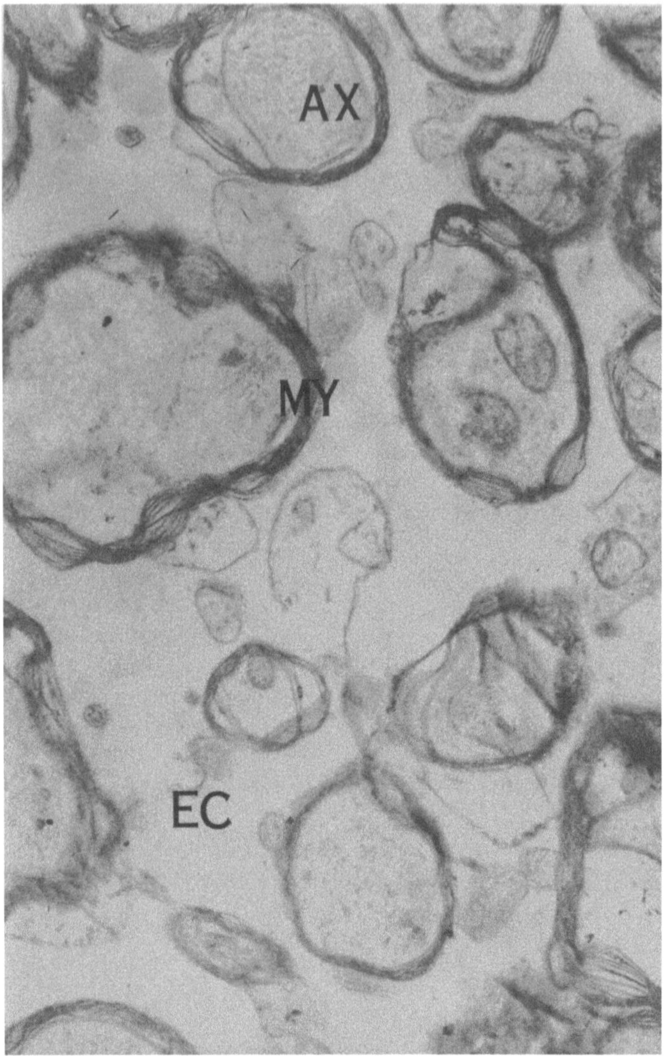

Fig. 6. The consistently enlarged white matter extracellular space (EC) is demonstrated. Preservation of axons (AX) and myelin (MY) is poor, a characteristic of immersion fixed, edematous white matter. Dog. Intracerebral psyllium seed placement. X16,480(reduced).

The edema process was most severe in this area and many of these specimens were necrotic. A second sample was removed from swollen brain tissue at the margin of the seed mass. The edema present in this

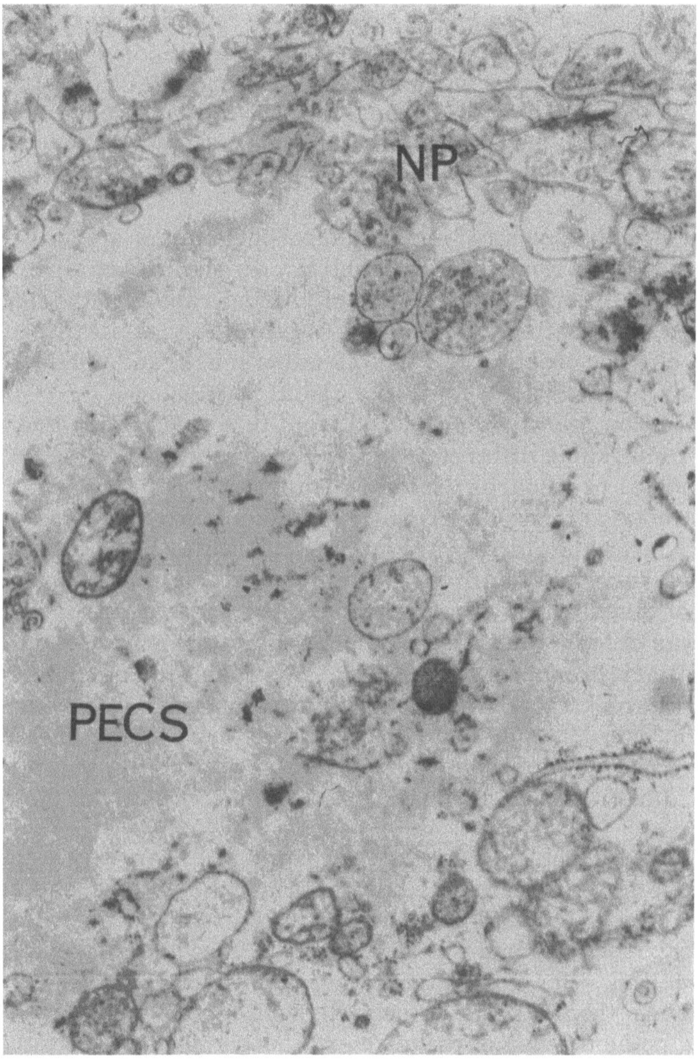

Fig. 7. Severe edema eventually merges with tissue necrosis. Plasma membranes rupture with creation of a "pseudoextracellular space" (PECS). Tissue elements (NP) gradually lose their characteristics. Rabbit. Four-hour exposure. X24, 100 (reduced).

region was usually of less degree than that seen in the first sample and evidence of tissue necrosis was rare. A third sample was then removed from the frontal or occipital pole in the rabbit or at a distance of 1, 2 or 4 cm from the mass of the seed in the dog. The edema features were consistently less in these samples and decreased in severity in a radial fashion. Both the white matter and cortex were more or less parallel in edema development. The clinical state of the animal, the assessment of brain edema at the time of the craniectomy and the light microscopic appearance correlated well with the severity indicated in the ultrastructural picture.

In dogs the subdural or extradural inflation of a small balloon was also utilized for edema production. No significant differences in this tissue when compared with either the rabbit or the dog psyllium seed preparations were noted. Again, the most severe changes were in closest proximity to the offending mass, and the severity of the edema process decreased in a radial fashion.

It can be readily appreciated from this description that there was no remarkable difference in the edema seen following any of the experimental procedures already described.

In those animals undergoing the miscellaneous edema-producing procedures the changes were also generally similar to those which have been recorded. Following the intra-arterial or intravenous injection of distilled water a tremendous increase in astrocyte cytoplasm was discovered. This was particularly remarkable in the pericapillary processes. Artifactual increase in both cortical and white matter extracellular space could be obtained by an excessive rate of infusion, a high perfusion pressure or volume. The endoplasmic reticulum of the neurons and oligodendroglia was often ballooned but no other abnormalities of these cells or of the microg: were noted.

Exposure of the cortex to air resulted in changes which were similar to those described in edema. The severity of these abnormalities correlated well with the length of exposure time, i.e., thos brains exposed for longer periods of time showed more evidence of brain swelling. However, a moderate amount of hemorrhage occurred in these preparations. Tissue disruption was much more common and petechial hemorrhages were found routinely throughout the cortex and white matter. A number of red cells were seen free within the disrupted neuropil, particularly in the pericapillary regic

Simple stab wounds of the brain were found to be surrounded by an area of typical cerebral edema in 24 to 48 hours. This swelling had no special characteristics.

DISCUSSION

The problem of cerebral edema, recognized since the time of Rokitansky and Virchow, has lately been the subject of extensive investigation (Long, 1964). In this voluminous literature there are many divergent opinions concerning the histology of the process. Multiple unrelated methods of experimental edema production are found and morphological studies are frequently in disagreement. Electron microscopic observations have been, in many instances, difficult to reconcile with light microscopic concepts. The first step in the investigation of cerebral edema has been the correlation of the multiple descriptions of the process available in print. A composite morphology has been abstracted and serves to define cerebral edema for the purposes of this investigation. This composite includes, grossly: increase in brain volume, often focal; flattening of gyri and narrowing of sulci; enlargement of white matter volume; loss of gray-white demarcation; decrease in ventricular size; and shift of midline structures if the process is unilateral. Histologically the characteristics which define cerebral edema are: reticulation or alveolar appearance of tissue, distention of perivascular and pericellular spaces with fluid, venous congestion, capillary endothelial-cell proliferation, swelling and pallor of axons and myelin, subpial rarefaction, glial swelling (thought by most investigators to be astrocytic) and protein-rich extracellular fluid accumulation (Greenfield, 1939).

Recently the electron microscopic appearance of human cerebral edema has been detailed. The morphological characteristics of cerebral edema as seen with the electron microscope are as follows: There is pericapillary enlargement of astrocyte processes with decrease in electron density and rarely with increased process vacuolization. Generalized swelling and increased clarity of astrocyte processes appears throughout the neuropil. There is great increase in astrocyte cell body size without nuclear change. The white matter extracellular space increases remarkably. Disruption of myelin lamination and axonal compression by submyelin fluid accumulation occurs but may be partly an artifact. In more severe cases there is rupture of plasma membranes with the creation of a "pseudoextracellular space," particularly within the cortex. Obvious signs of tissue damage and ischemic cell changes eventually occur and frank tissue necrosis may appear as well. The cortical extracellular space does not increase. Neurons show ischemic changes only. Microglia undergo reactive change if tissue necrosis has occurred. Oligodendroglia are minimally swollen. Capillary endothelium is occasionally increased in volume and increased vacuolization may occur. The intracytoplasmic inclusions are not changed, at least as far as can be determined without a quantitative method (Long, 1964).

It is obvious that these changes correlate very well with the accepted light microscopic abnormalities in cerebral edema and that the ultrastructural studies both substantiate and supplement the earlier findings.

It is equally apparent that the descriptions of edema resulting from the various methods utilized in this study are quite similar with the descriptions of brain swelling complicating a variety of intracranial lesions in the human. This lends credence to the supposition that morphologically cerebral edema is a specific reaction of brain though biochemical differences exist.

Even though a variety of edema-producing methods are available to produce brain swelling which is morphologically quite similar to human cerebral edema, it does not follow that all of these methods are of equal value in the study of edema, or its response to therapy. From the literature review it is appreciated that certain of the procedures which have been utilized in the past are ineffectual or cause brain swelling secondary to increase in blood or CSF volume. These techniques are not related to the problem under consideration and these methods may be deleted from the study of cerebral edema (Arutynov, 1962). Methods which most closely mimic the clinical situation of a slowly or rapidly expanding intracranial mass would seem to be most desirable. There are several techniques available which attempt to create such a situation and one of these techniques serves as the basis for this investigation and as the standard against which other techniques have been compared. Certain other procedures have been so adequately studied and reported that it did not seem necessary to repeat them in the present investigation and comparisons have been drawn on the basis of the previously published material.

Direct or indirect brain trauma has been a popular method for edema production for many years. Ultrastructural analysis of this type of edema reveals it to be quite similar to that obtained by nearly any other method. However, the techniques are both unreliable and difficult to reproduce (Raimondi, et al., 1959). In addition the accompanying hemorrhage and the evidence of direct tissue injury make the structural interpretations more difficult. The intravascular infusion of hypotonic solutions also produces brain swelling but this is a highly artificial type of lesion and cannot be closely correlated with the clinical situation. While of value in hydration and dehydration studies of brain tissue, these methods can scarcely be recommended for edema production in the present context. Exposure of the brain to air for varying periods of time also results in brain swelling which has the morphological characteristics of cerebral edema. At least a portion of this apparent brain swelling is secondary to vascular stasis and an increase in blood volume in the venous circulation of the exposed hemisphere, and the morphological picture is clouded by the presence of numerous pericapillary petechial hemorrhages.

The use of several CNS poisons, notably the alkyl tin derivatives, to produce cerebral edema has recently been studied in detail

(Katzman, et al., 1963). While there are some descrepancies between the light and electron microscopic descriptions of the resulting edema, it has been generally accepted that the brain swelling which results from the administration of these compounds consists of astrocytic volume enlargement and intralaminar myelin fluid accumulation, ontogenetically but not anatomically, extracellular. The morphological characteristics of this type of swelling are not similar to those seen in vascular edema and it must be considered that this type of brain swelling is not completely analogous to human cerebral edema of the usual type.

The application of cold to the intact calvarium or directly to brain substance has been well studied and has been shown to be an excellent method for the reproducible production of cerebral edema (Clasen, et al., 1953; Klatzo, et al., 1958). The published morphological characteristics of this edema conform in every way to those accepted as diagnostic of the conditions. The area of tissue necrosis and hemorrhage which immediately underlies the area of the site of cold application is minimal and the method appears to be quite effective and quite acceptable for the experimental evaluation of cerebral edema.

The intracerebral production of brain tumors is perhaps the most closely analogous to the human situation. These tumors have been produced by the direct implantation of neoplastic cells, by the use of carcinogenic agents, and by virus inoculations (Herzog, et al., 1965). These methods are mechanistically satisfactory. However, they are somewhat unpredictable in their results and frequently hard to duplicate. In addition, they are cumbersome and in general require a greater period of time and greater numbers of animals in order to obtain adequate material.

The intracerebral implantation of hydrophilic substances calculated to slowly gain water and, so, slowly gain volume also produces brain swelling which is similar to human cerebral edema (Sperl, 1959). The light microscopic characteristics of this edema have been previously proven to be those described for the human, and the ultrastructural characteristics of this swelling have been presented in this investigation. The method has the virtue of being simple and is easily reproducible. In addition, it mimics the clinical situation quite closely. However, it is difficult to adapt to small animals.

Previously a number of studies of cerebral edema have dealt with rodents and other small animals. The study of such preparations has been of value but their structural differences from human brains are many and it is suggested that the study of cerebral edema is best carried out in larger animals, with brain structures more strictly comparable to the human both grossly and microscopically.

At least a portion of the controversy over the presence or absence of an enlarged white matter extracellular space in cerebral edema probably arose from the early descriptions of edema dealing with rodent brains. In these small animals the white matter volume is small, and adequate samples of white matter are difficult to obtain. The preliminary descriptions of edema which appeared in the literature dealt primarily with cortex and subcortical white matter and it is probably here that the descrepancies remarked upon arose.

In conclusion it can be stated that there are a number of excellent methods for the production of cerebral edema in the experimental animal. The experimental edema thus produced correlates well with human cerebral edema grossly, microscopically and ultrastructurally, if certain peculiarities of the various animal brains are taken into consideration. Those procedures which most closely mimic the human situation are considered to be the most desirable for the establishment of an experimental model. There are a number of miscellaneous techniques which are effective in producing a brain swelling which is similar to human edema, but these techniques have no strict clinical correlates and seem to be inferior to those procedures which do.

It is suggested that the further study of experimental cerebral edema is best performed upon the larger experimental animals with brain structures similar to the human. The application of cold to the brain, the intracerebral growth of experimental tumors, intracranial balloon inflation, or the intracerebral implantation of hydrophilic substances all appear to be adequate methods of edema production and the most valuable of the multiple procedures described within the literature for correlation with human edema.

SUMMARY

A review of the literature concerning the experimental production of cerebral edema reveals a multiplicity of techniques which have not been adequately correlated with one another or with recent ultrastructural concepts. In order to categorize these various procedures a composite morphology has been abstracted from the literature to define the edema process. The ultrastructural morphology of cerebral edema has been the subject of interdisciplinary conflict until recently. Initial observations indicated only intracellular swelling. However, this controversy has been largely resolved following the subsequent demonstration of extracellular fluid accumulation. These recent observations correlate light and electron microscopic findings and prove them to be compatible. Review of the ultrastructure of edema produced by cold, tumor implantation and artificial mass lesions indicates that similar edema occurs after each insult. Other methods in the literature for production of brain swelling are not strictly analogous to the human conditions.

TABLE 1

TISSUE SOURCES FOR ELECTRON MICROSCOPY OF EDEMA

Edema Preparations	Dogs	Rabbits
Normal	2	3
Psyllium seeds		
Intracerebral	2	3
Subdural		3
Extradural		3
Balloon inflation		
Extradural	1	
Subdural	2	
Intravascular distilled water		
Intra-arterial		2
Intravenous		2
Brain exposure		4
Brain puncture wound		2

REFERENCES

Aleu, F. P., R. Katzman and R. D. Terry: Fine structure of cerebral edema induced by alkyl tin intoxication, J. Neuropath. Exp. Neurol., 22, 403-413 (1963).

Arutyunov, A. I.: Cerebral edema and the problem of raised intracranial pressure, Abs. 7, Excerpta Medica: Internat. Cong. Series: Second Internat. Cong. Of Neurol. Surg., 36 (1962).

Bakay, L. and I. U. Haque: Morphological and chemical studies in cerebral edema, J. Neuropath. Exp. Neurol., 23, 393-418 (1964).

Blindermann, E. E., C. Graf and T. Fitzpatrick: Basic studies in cerebral edema, J. Neurosurg., 19, 319-325 (1962).

Cannon, W. B.: Cerebral pressure following trauma, Am. J. Physiol. 6, 91-121 (1901-02).

Chou, S. N.: Experimental brain tumors in rabbits and associated cerebral edema, Journ.-Lancet, 81, 78-82 (1961).

Clasen, R. A., D. V. L. Brown, S. Leavitt and G. M. Hass: The production by liquid nitrogen of acute closed cerebral lesions, Surg. Gyn. Obst., 96, 605-616 (1953).

_____, P. M. Cooke, S. Pandolfi, D. Boyd and A. J. Raimondi: Experimental cerebral edema produced by focal freezing, J. Neuropath. Exp. Neurol., 21, 579-596 (1962).

Denny-Brown, D. and W. R. Russel: Experimental cerebral concussion, Brain, 64, 93-164 (1941).

De Robertis, E. and H. M. Gerschenfeld: Submicroscopic morphology and function of glial cells, Int. Rev. Neurobiol., 3, 1-65 (1961).

Edstrom, R. and H. E. Essex: Swelling of damaged brain tissue, Neurology, 5, 490-493 (1955).

Elliott, K. A. C. and H. Jasper: Measurement of experimentally induced brain swelling and shrinkage, Am. J. Physiol., 157, 122-129 (1949).

Evans, J. E. and A. Raimondi: Presented to Surgical Forum, Am. Coll. Surg. (1961).

Ferraro, A.: The reaction of the brain tissue to intravenous injection of hypotonic solutions, J. Nerv. Ment. Dis., 71, 129-144 (1930)

Gerschenfeld, H. M., F. Wald, J. A. Zadunaisky and E. De Robertis: Function of astroglia in the water-ion metabolism of the central nervous system, Neurology, 9, 412-425 (1959).

Greenfield, J. G.: The history of cerebral edema associated with intracranial tumors, Brain, 62, 129-152 (1939).

Gonatas, N. K., H. M. Zimmerman and S. Levine: Ultrastructure of inflammation with edema in the rat brain, Am. J. Path., 42, 455-469 (1963).

Hauser, H. M., B. F. McKenzie, H. J. Svien and N. P. Goldstein: Experimental cerebral edema in dogs: a new technic for objective measurement, Surg. Forum., 10, 760-763 (1960).

Herzog, I., W. A. Levy and L. C. Scheinberg: Biochemical and morphological studies of cerebral edema associated with intracerebral tumors in rabbits, J. Neuropath. Exp. Neurol., 24, 244-255

Hirano, A., H. M. Zimmerman and S. Levine: The fine structure of cerebral fluid accumulation. VII Reactions of astrocytes to cryptococcal polysaccharide implantation, J. Neuropath. Exp. Neurol., 24, 386-397 (1965).

Kalsbeck, J. E. and J. N. Cumings: Experimental edema in the rat and cat brain, J. Neuropath. Exp. Neurol., 22, 237-247 (1963).

Katzman, R., F. Aleu and C. Wilson: Further observations on triethyl tin edema, Arch. Neurol., 9, 178-187 (1963).

Klatzo, I. A., Piraux and E. Laskowski: The relationship between edema, blood brain barrier, and tissue elements in local brain injury, J. Neuropath. Exp. Neurol., 17, 548-563 (1958).

Kocher, T.: Hirnerschütterung, Hirndruck, und Chirurgische Eingriffe bei Hirnkrankheiten, in: Northnagel: Specielle Pathologie und Therapie, 5, Wien. A. Holder. (1901).

Long, D. M., J. F. Hartmann and L. A. French: Presented to The Society of Neurological Surgeons. (1962).

_____: The ultrastructure of cerebral edema and its response to glucosteroid administration, Ph. D. Thesis, University of Minnesota (1964).

Luse, S. A. and B. Harris: Electron microscopy of the brain in experimental edema, J. Neurosurg., 17, 436-439 (1960).

_____ and _____: Brain ultrastructure in hydration and dehydration, Arch. Neurol., 4, 139-152 (1961).

Magee, P. N., H. B. Stoner and J. M. Barnes: The experimental production of edema of the central nervous system of the rat by triethyl tin compounds, J. Path. Bacteriol., 73, 107-124 (1957).

Obrador, S. and J. Pi-Suñer: Experimental swelling of the brain. Arch. Neurol. Psychiat., 49, 826-830 (1943).

Penfield, W. and R. Buckley: Punctures of the brain, Ibid., 20, 1-13 (1938).

Pilcher, C.: Experimental cerebral trauma (The fluid content of the brain after trauma to the head), Arch. Surg., 35, 512-527 (1937).

_____: Experimental cerebral trauma, Surg. Gyn Obst., 72, 755-757

Prados, M., B. Stowger and W. Feindel: Studies on cerebral edema; I – Reaction of the brain to air exposure: pathologic changes, Arch. Neurol. Psychiat., 54, 163-174 (1945).

Raimondi, A. J., R. A. Clasen, E. J. Beattie and C. B. Taylor: The effect of hypothermia and steroid therapy on experimental cerebral injury. Surg. Gyn. Obst. 108, 333-338 (1959).

_____, J. P. Evans and S. Mullan: Studies of cerebral edema. III Alterations in the white matter, Acta Neuropath., 2, 177-197 (1962).

Reid, W. L.: Cerebral edema, Aust. New Z. J. Surg., 13, 11-36 (1942).

Sperl, M. P.: Experimental production of local cerebral edema, M. S. Thesis, University of Minnesota (1959).

Torack, R. M., R. D. Terry and H. M. Zimmerman: The fine structure of cerebral fluid accumulation. I Swelling secondary to cold injury, Am. J. Path., 35, 1135-1147 (1959).

_____, _____ and _____: The fine structure of cerebral fluid accumulation. II Swelling produced by triethyl tin poisoning and its comparison with that of the human brain, Ibid., 36, 273-287 (1960).

Weed, L. H.: The effects of hypotonic solutions upon the cell morphology of the choroid plexus and central nervous system, Am. J. Anat., 32, 253-275 (1923-24).

_____ and P. S. McKibben: Experimental alterations of brain bulk, Am. J. Physiol., 48, 531-558 (1919).

White, J. C., J. R. Brooks, J. C. Goldthwait and R. D. Adams: Changes in brain volume and blood content after experimental concussion, Ann. Surg., 118, 619-634 (1943).

HANNA M. PAPPIUS

BIOCHEMICAL STUDIES ON EXPERIMENTAL BRAIN EDEMA

Various methods have been used to measure cerebral edema. From the biochemical point of view measurement of changes in water content seems to be the most rational approach to the study of a process which by definition involves changes in volume brought about primarily by changes in water content.

In the experiments to be described changes in the percentage dry weight of cerebral cortex and of white matter have been used as a measure of cerebral swelling. The sodium and potassium contents in cerebral tissues under study have also been determined to characterize other changes occurring in the tissues and to throw some light on the origin of the fluid involved in edema.

Two types of studies will be summarized. The first consists of experiments in which cerebral edema was induced in cats by local freezing through the exposed dura. In the second group of experiments changes in water content of cerebral tissues were induced osmotically, when uremic dogs were hemodialyzed against standard physiological bath fluid and when normal dogs were dialyzed against hypotonic bath solution.

METHODS

Details of all methods used have been described (Pappius & Dayes; Pappius & Gulati; Pappius, et al.). Briefly the freezing lesions were produced in the brains of cats by a modification of the apparatus originally described by Klatzo, et al. (1958). The area of the end plate with which the lesion was made on the surface of exposed dura was 50 mm^2, the temperature at the moment of application was $-50°$

and duration of application was 20 seconds. The lesions were always made on the right side, so the right hemisphere is designated as experimental hemisphere, the left the control hemisphere.

White matter and cerebral cortex tissue samples were dissected from both hemispheres. In the experimental hemisphere samples of white matter were taken from areas grossly edematous or when edema was not visibly obvious from the region immediately under the lesion. Cortex samples were taken from tissue surrounding the lesion area and overlying grossly edematous white matter but not from the area of cell necrosis at the actual site of the freezing. It must be stressed that these sampling procedures allow measurement of changes in water and electrolyte content of the tissues studied but give no information about the total volume of tissue involved in edema.

In the dialysis experiments the Kolff twin-coil artificial kidney was used. Dogs were made uremic by ligation of both ureters two or three days before hemodialysis and the urea content of the plasma was further increased by a slow infusion of urea solution at least 24 hours before the dialysis. Uremic dogs were dialyzed against physiological salts solution containing 140 m.eq. sodium per liter. When normal dogs were to be dialyzed with hypotonic bath fluid the bath solution contained 90 m.eq. sodium per liter. In these experiments CSF pressure was measured by needle puncture in the cisterna magna.

RESULTS AND DISCUSSION

Cerebral edema induced by local freezing

Changes observed in the dry weight and sodium and potassium content of cerebral tissues 24 hours after a local freezing lesion was made are summarized in Table 1.

No difference in percentage dry weight and sodium and potassium content of white matter was observed between the control hemisphere and the tissue from normal, unoperated animals. In the white matter of the experimental hemisphere there was a sharp decrease in the percentage dry weight, or conversely, an increase in the water content. This change in the dry weight represents about 45% swelling of the tissue (calculated according to formula of Elliott & Jasper). At the same time there was a rise in sodium concentration and a fall in potassium concentration in the white matter with a sharp rise in Na/K ratio.

These changes in the electrolyte content of the edematous tissue indicate that the fluid taken up has a high sodium and low potas-

TABLE 1

THE PERCENTAGE DRY WEIGHT AND SODIUM AND POTASSIUM CONTENTS OF BRAIN TISSUES OF CATS 24 HOURS AFTER LOCAL FREEZING

	Cerebral Cortex				White Matter			
	Dry Weight	Na	K	Na/K	Dry Weight	Na	K	Na/K
Normal (9)	19.2 ± 0.7	57.5 ± 3	102 ± 4	0.56 ± 0.05	31.8 ± 1.2	58 ± 6	82 ± 2	0.70 ± 0.07
Following local freezing (11)								
Control hemisphere	19.3 ± 1.3	66 ± 7†	98 ± 6	0.67 ± 0.09†	31.9 ± 1.7	60 ± 6	80 ± 5	0.74 ± 0.07
Experimental hemisphere	18.3 ± 1.0*	74 ± 8*	88.5 ± 7**	0.84 ± 0.12**	21.4 ± 2.4**	90 ± 8**	57 ± 6**	1.65 ± 0.42**

Averages ± standard deviation. Number of animals in brackets.
Freezing lesion: 50 mm^2; 20 sec.
Dry weight: mgms. per 100 mgms. fresh weight of tissue.
Na and K: m.eq. per kg. fresh weight of tissue.
Significantly different from the control hemispheres.
Significantly different from normal ($p<0.01$). *$p<0.05$ **$p<0.01$

sium concentration. This is compatible with the assumption that the edema fluid is derived from the circulating blood. The decrease in the potassium content of the edematous white matter reflects a dilution of the tissue content of this electrolyte by a fluid low in potassium. This becomes evident when the electrolyte results are calculated on the basis of dry weight (see Table 2) and the difference between the control and the experimental hemisphere with respect to the potassium content of the white matter becomes insignificant (254 and 265 m.eq. per kg. dry weight respectively).

When cerebral cortex tissue in the control hemisphere was compared to tissue from normal animals there was no change in the percentage dry weight or potassium content. However, a statistically highly significant increase in the sodium content of the control cerebral cortex was observed. In the experimental hemisphere a small but significant decrease in the percentage dry weight was found, equivalent to about 5% swelling of the tissue. There was also a rise in the sodium content and a highly significant decrease in the potassium content of the cerebral cortex of the experimental hemisphere. These latter changes produced a small but significant change in the Na/K ratio. In contrast to the findings in the white matter, the decrease in the potassium content of cerebral cortex of the experimental hemisphere represents a net loss of potassium from the tissue. This is seen when the results are calculated per unit of dry weight as in Table 2 (510 and 484 m.eq. per kg. dry weight, in the control and experimental hemisphere respectively; p of difference < 0.05).

It must be pointed out that in a previously published (Pappius & Gulati) smaller series of experiments the decrease in percentage dry weight in the experimental hemisphere was restricted to the white matter with none demonstrable in the cortex. The reason for the discrepancy between the two series of experiments is not clear, although it is possible that in the present experiments the cortical tissue was sampled closer to the lesion than previously. The limited swelling demonstrated in cerebral cortex tissue in the present series of experiments does not invalidate the earlier conclusion that when edema is induced by trauma due to local freezing the bulk of the fluid accumulates in the white matter. Recent chemical studies of Bakay and Haque on cold induced edema lead to the same conclusion.

In previous studies (Pappius & Gulati) it was also shown that the changes in water and electrolyte content of cerebral tissues observed 24 hours after local freezing persisted for three days, with a return to normal values evident five days after a lesion was made. Surgical removal of the occipital lobe resulted in the same pattern of changes as was observed after local freezing. Pretreatment of

TABLE 2

EFFECT OF HYPERTONIC UREA INFUSION ON POTASSIUM AND SODIUM CONTENTS OF CEREBRAL TISSUES OF NORMAL CATS AND 24 HOURS AFTER LOCAL FREEZING

		Potassium		Sodium	
		m. eq. per kg. dry weight of tissue			
		Cerebral Cortex	White Matter	Cerebral Cortex	White Matter
Normal	(9)	533 ± 31	258 ± 11	299 ± 23	182 ± 20
Normal, after urea[1]	(6)	502 ± 22*	235 ± 26*	301 ± 35	179 ± 15
24 hours after freezing lesion[2]					
Control hemisphere	(11)	510 ± 31	254 ± 27	343 ± 52	189 ± 26
Control hemisphere, after urea[1]	(8)	560 ± 34**	282 ± 20*	334 ± 36	192 ± 29
Experimental hemisphere	(11)	484 ± 26	265 ± 31	404 ± 54	430 ± 80
Experimental hemisphere, after urea[1]	(8)	497 ± 29	286 ± 23	395 ± 46	440 ± 35

Averages ± standard deviation. Number of animals in brackets.
(1) 90 min. after infusion of 1.5 g. urea per kg. in 30% solution.
(2) Freezing lesion: 50 mm^2; 20 sec.
Significantly different from corresponding value without urea. $*p<0.05$ $**p<0.01$

the animals with cortisone did affect the water and electrolyte content of either normal or traumatized cerebral tissues.

Changes in water and electrolyte content of cerebral tissues similar to these associated with edema induced by local freezing were described by Katzman, et al., in rat brain with focal inflammatory edema.

The effects of intravenous infusion of a hypertonic urea solution on cerebral tissues have been studied in normal animals and in those in which edema was induced by local freezing (Pappius & Dayes). It was shown that the extent and duration of dehydration of cerebral tissues produced in normal animals by infusion of hypertonic urea correlates well with the extent and duration of a concentration gradient for urea between plasma and tissue water. Thus the changes in the water content of both the cerebral cortex tissue and the white matter brought about by the infusion of urea can be explained as osmotic effects. No secondary swelling of cerebral tissues was noted and no osmotic basis for the occurance of such swelling could be demonstrated.

In animals with freezing lesions the effects of urea have been studied 90 minutes after the start of the infusion since maximum dehydration had been found to occur between 60 and 120 minutes. (Significant dehydration was demonstrated in the cerebral cortex between 15 and 120 minutes and in the white matter between 15 minutes and three hours: [Pappius & Dayes]).

It will be seen from Table 3 that in normal animals and in the control hemispheres of animals in which a freezing lesion had been made 24 hours earlier, there was a significant increase in the percentage dry weight, that is, dehydration, of both the cerebral cortex and the white matter after administration of hypertonic urea. There was also a significant effect on the dry weight of the cerebral cortex tissue of the experimental hemisphere surrounding the lesion area. However, the percentage dry weight of the edematous white matter beneath the freezing lesion was not significantly changed by the administration of hypertonic urea.

The failure of hypertonic urea infusion to change the water content of edematous white matter significantly though it appreciably dehydrates tissues in the control hemisphere and the slightly swollen cerebral cortex tissue in the experimental hemisphere, is not surprising in view of the now well documented extracellular distribution of edema fluid in the white matter (Raimondi, et. al; Gonatas, et al.), and the gross increase in vascular and tissue permeability in the area of the lesion (Klatzo, et al.,1962; Katzman, et al.). Under these conditions there is no membrane across which the osmotic withdrawal of water from the edematous tissue in response to urea infusion would be expected to occur.

TABLE 3

THE EFFECT OF HYPERTONIC UREA INFUSION ON THE PERCENTAGE DRY WEIGHT OF BRAIN TISSUES OF CATS 24 HOURS AFTER EDEMA WAS INDUCED BY FREEZING

		Dry weight mgms. per 100 mgms. fresh weight of tissue	
		Cerebral cortex	White matter
Normal	(9)	19.2 ± 0.7	31.8 ± 1.2
Normal after urea[1]	(6)	21.1 ± 1.5**	34.3 ± 2.2*
24 hours after local freezing[2]			
Control hemisphere	(11)	19.3 ± 1.3	31.9 ± 1.7
Control hemisphere, after urea[1]	(8)	20.7 ± 1.1**	33.4 ± 1.4*
Experimental hemisphere	(11)	18.3 ± 1.0	21.4 ± 2.4
Experimental hemisphere, after urea[1]	(8)	19.9 ± 1.1**	22.4 ± 1.3

Averages ± standard deviation. Number of animals in brackets.
(1) 90 min. after infusion of 1.5 g. urea per kg. in 30% solution.
(2) Freezing lesion: 50 mm^2 20 sec.
Significantly different from corresponding value without urea *$p<0.05$ **$p<0.02$

Clasen, et al., have also demonstrated that infusion of hypertonic urea solution has a dehydrating effect on normal but not on edematous brain.

In the course of the studies on the dehydrating effects of hypertonic urea an unexpected difference in the response to urea infusion between normal and traumatized cerebral tissues became evident. The pertinent data on the effect of hypertonic urea infusion on the sodium and potassium content of cerebral tissues are summarized in Table 2. In normal animals and in animals with freezing lesions infusion of hypertonic urea had no effect on the sodium content of cerebral tissues, per unit of dry weight. This indicates that dehydration was brought about by the withdrawal of sodium-free water.

The potassium content of cerebral tissues changed in response to the infusion of hypertonic urea. In normal animals there was a significant decrease in the potassium content of both the cerebral cortex and the white matter per kg. of dry weight of tissue. Thus there was a net loss of potassium from the tissue. In contrast, when hypertonic urea was administered to animals in which a freezing lesion had been made 24 hours earlier there was a net increase in the potassium content of all cerebral tissues. In the control hemisphere the increase in the ratio of potassium to dry weight was statistically highly significant. In the experimental hemisphere where the effects of urea infusion are superimposed on changes associated with edema the increase was evident but was not statistically significant.

Thus there is a striking difference in the effect of urea on the potassium contents of cerebral tissues of animals with cerebral edema as compared with normal animals. From results summarized in Table 2 it appears that this difference affects the whole brain and is not restricted to areas grossly affected by the edema.

This accumulation of potassium in response to urea administration may not be of special importance per se, but it is of particular interest because it seems to indicate a generalized effect of trauma on the brain. This response obviously involves mechanisms controlling the distribution of electrolytes in cerebral tissues and thus may represent a generalized change in various aspects of cerebral metabolism and possibly of function.

In an effort to further characterize the processes involved, the effects of urea infusion on potassium content of cerebral tissues were studied shortly after a lesion had been made and also in animals with cerebral edema, but pre-treated with cortisone. Results of these experiments are summarized in Table 4. These effects of urea were evident in both hemispheres. However, only the data obtained in cerebral cortex from the control hemisphere are presented in Table 4 since the changes were most clear-cut in this tissue. The dry weight data show that under all the conditions studied a fairly uniform degree of dehydration was achieved by the infusion of hypertonic urea solution.

When urea was administered 30 minutes after a freezing lesion had been made, thus soon after trauma to the experimental hemisphere but before edema developed, the potassium content of the cerebral cortex in the control hemisphere was the same as in normal tissues after urea. Thus it appears that some time (between two and 24 hours) must elapse for the abnormal potassium response to urea administration to develop in the traumatized brain. These results do not indicate whether trauma itself or the consequent edema are the triggering mechanism for the general increase of potassium in cerebral tissues in response to urea administration.

As mentioned earlier, studies have shown that in the cat cortisone has no effect on the gross changes in water and electrolyte content of cerebral tissues associated with edema. It will be seen from results presented in Table 4 that cortisone pre-treatment also failed to influence the distribution of potassium after infusion of hypertonic urea.

TABLE 4

EFFECT OF HYPERTONIC UREA INFUSION ON POTASSIUM CONTENT OF CEREBRAL CORTEX TISSUES OF CATS

		Dry Weight mgms. per 100 mgs. fresh weight	Potassium millimoles per kg. dry weight
Normal	(9)	19.2 ± 0.7	533 ± 31
Normal, after urea[1]	(6)	21.1 ± 1.5**	502 ± 22*
		Control left hemispheres	
2 hours after local freezing[2], after urea	(4)	20.9 ± 0.6	508 ± 37
		Control left hemispheres	
24 hours after local freezing	(11)	19.3 ± 1.3	510 ± 31
24 hours after local freezing, after urea	(8)	20.7 ± 1.1**	560 ± 34**
24 hours after local freezing after urea, with cortisone pre-treatment[3]	(8)	21.3 ± 0.8**	540 ± 28*

Averages ± standard deviation. Number of animals in brackets.
(1) 90 minutes after infusion of 1.5 g. urea per kg. in 30% solution.
(2) Freezing lesion: 50 mm^2 ; 20 sec; right hemisphere.
(3) Cortisone pre-treatment: 25 mg. cortisone acetate per kg per day i.p. for four days prior to infusion of urea.
Significantly different from corresponding value without urea. *$p<0.05$ **$p<0.01$

Osmotically induced changes in cerebral tissues and cerebrospinal fluid

Data on what can be described as osmotically induced cerebral swelling were accumulated in the course of studies in the dog on effects of hemodialysis (Pappius, et al.). In these experiments dogs were subjected to rapid hemodialysis for 60 minutes after which brain biopsy was taken.

In uremic dogs dialysis against physiological salt solution caused a sharp decrease in the urea content of the serum which was accompanied by a considerable but slower decrease in the urea content of both the white and gray cerebral tissue and a relatively smaller decrease in the urea content of the cerebrospinal fluid. As a consequence, at the time of the brain biopsy a significant concentration gradient for urea existed, in a decreasing order of magnitude, between the CSF, the white matter and the cerebral cortex on the one hand and the serum on the other. The ratios of urea concentration in the tissues and the CSF to the concentration of urea in the serum before and after dialysis of uremic dogs are presented in Table 5.

From results summarized in Table 6 it will be seen that when normal dogs were dialyzed against hypotonic, low-sodium (90 m.eq/: bath fluid, serum sodium decreased sharply. There was also a smaller, but still significant, fall in the sodium content of the cerebral tissues and of the CSF. Thus, on hypotonic dialysis of normal dogs a concentration gradient for sodium developed between the central nervous system and the plasma. As with the concentration gradient for urea in the case of hemodialyzed uremic dogs, the gradient for sodium was greatest between the CSF and the plasma, smaller between the white matter and the plasma and least between the cerebral cortex tissue and the plasma.

The dry weight and sodium and potassium content of brain tissues of dogs subjected to rapid hemodialysis are presented in Table 7. Hemodialysis of uremic dogs resulted in a decrease of the average dry weight of both the white matter and the cerebral cortex. In both tissues the difference from pre-dialysis values was statisticall highly significant. However, when results of the individual experiments were considered it became clear that cerebral swelling was not present invariably under these conditions. A percentage dry weight within normal limits was found in cerebral cortex of nine of the 18 dialyzed uremic dogs and in white matter of six of the 18. In animals in which percentage dry weight results were below the normal range the average swelling was 14% in the white matter and 11% in the cerebral cortex (calculated from average dry weight by the formula of Elliott and Jasper). In neither tissues was there any

TABLE 5

THE RATIO OF THE CONCENTRATIONS OF UREA IN CEREBRAL TISSUES AND IN CEREBROSPINAL FLUID TO THE CONCENTRATION IN THE SERUM BEFORE AND AFTER 60 MINUTES OF HEMODIALYSIS OF UREMIC DOGS

	CSF/serum	White matter/serum	Cerebral cortex/serum
Pre-dialysis	0.86 ± 0.05 (6)	0.97 ± 0.09 (18)	0.97 ± 0.08 (18)
Post-dialysis	1.83 ± 0.42**(13)	1.53 ± 0.42**(18)	1.27 ± 0.30**(18)

Averages ± standard deviation. Number of animals in brackets.
**Statistically different from pre-dialysis figures. ($p<0.01$).

TABLE 6

SODIUM CONTENTS OF SERUM, CSF AND CEREBRAL TISSUES OF DOGS BEFORE AND AFTER 60 MINUTES OF HYPOTONIC[1] HEMODIALYSIS

	Sodium: m. eq. per liter		Sodium: m. eq. per kg. fresh weight	
	Serum	CSF	White Matter	Cerebral Cortex
Pre-dialysis	146 ± 4 (25)	152 ± 5 (8)	57 ± 3 (15)	60 ± 4 (15)
Post-dialysis	110 ± 4** (7)	142 ± 5**(6)	52 ± 3** (7)	51 ± 4** (7)
Decrease	25%	7%	9%	15%

Averages ± standard deviation. Numbers of animals in brackets.
(1) bath fluid contained only 90 m.eq. of sodium per liter.
**Significantly different from pre-dialysis figure. ($p<0.01$).

TABLE 7

THE PERCENTAGE DRY WEIGHT AND SODIUM AND POTASSIUM CONTENTS OF BRAIN TISSUES OF DOGS SUBJECTED TO HEMODIALYSIS

		Cerebral Cortex					White Matter			
		Dry Weight	Na	K	Na/K		Dry Weight	Na	K	Na/K
Uremic animals										
pre-dialysis	(16)	19.6 ± 0.7	54 ± 5	88 ± 7	0.61	(16)	33.4 ± 1.6	52 ± 6	77 ± 5	0.68
post-dialysis[1]										
total group	(18)	18.4 ± 1.4**				(18)	30.8 ± 2.0**			
edematous[3]	(9)	17.6 ± 1.3**	51 ± 7	85 ± 4	0.60	(11)	29.2 ± 2.1**	52 ± 7	76 ± 7	0.68
Normal animals										
pre-dialysis	(15)	19.9 ± 0.8	60 ± 4	98 ± 6	0.61	(15)	33.9 ± 1.0	57 ± 3	78 ± 6	0.73
post-hypotonic dialysis[2]										
total group	(7)	18.4 ± 0.9**				(7)	31.3 ± 1.1**			
edematous[3]	(4)	17.8 ± 0.9**	48 ± 2**	90 ± 5**	0.52	(5)	30.9 ± 1.2**	52 ± 4**	78 ± 4	0.67

Averages ± standard deviation. Number of animals in brackets.
Dry weight: mgms per 100 mgms fresh weight of tissue.
Na and K: m.moles per kg. fresh weight of tissue.
(1) After 60 min. dialysis against physiological bath solution. (140 m.eq. Na/1).
(2) After 60 min. dialysis against hypnotic bath solution. (90 m.eq. Na/1).
(3) Only animals with dry weight outside the normal range.
**Significantly different from pre-dialysis figures. ($p<0.01$).

significant change in the electrolyte content and thus the Na/K ratio remained unchanged.

Dialysis of normal dogs against low-sodium bath fluid also resulted in a significant decrease in the average dry weight of cerebral tissues. Again, however, the incidence of swelling was not invariable. The decrease in Na/K ratio under these conditions reflects the loss of sodium from cerebral tissues in response to the fall in the sodium concentration in the serum.

On the basis of these experiments it can be concluded that osmotically induced edema affects both the white matter and the cerebral cortex to about the same extent. Further, this type of swelling involves uptake of fluid which does not greatly change the electrolyte content of the tissues, hence does not contain high amounts of sodium and is not a plasma filtrate.

Thus osmotically induced swelling of cerebral tissues is a basically different phenomenon from cerebral edema resulting from trauma.

It is of interest that an increase in the CSF pressure was invariably observed when uremic animals were hemodialyzed against physiological salt solution and when normal dogs were dialyzed against hypotonic, low-sodium solution. When normal dogs were dialyzed against physiological salt solution the CSF pressure remained within normal limits. The CSF pressure in a number of representative experiments is shown graphically in Figure 1.

Changes in CSF pressure in the two experimental groups could not be correlated with either the presence or the degree of swelling of cerebral tissues. In view of the fact that after 60 minutes of hemodialysis a considerable concentration gradient between the CSF and the plasma was demonstrated for urea in uremic dogs and for sodium in normal dogs on hypotonic dialysis, it is likely that direct osmotic effects on CSF volume are responsible for the invariably observed increase in the CSF pressure.

CONCLUSION

When cerebral edema is induced by local freezing the bulk of the fluid accumulates in the underlying white matter while only minimal, though significant, swelling occurs in the cerebral cortex surrounding the lesion and overlying the swollen white matter. The fluid taken up in the white matter has a sodium content in the range of that of the serum. There is no net loss of potassium from the edematous white matter, only dilution of tissue potassium by edema fluid low in this electrolyte. In the cortex the slight swelling is also accompanied by an increase in sodium content and must involve up-

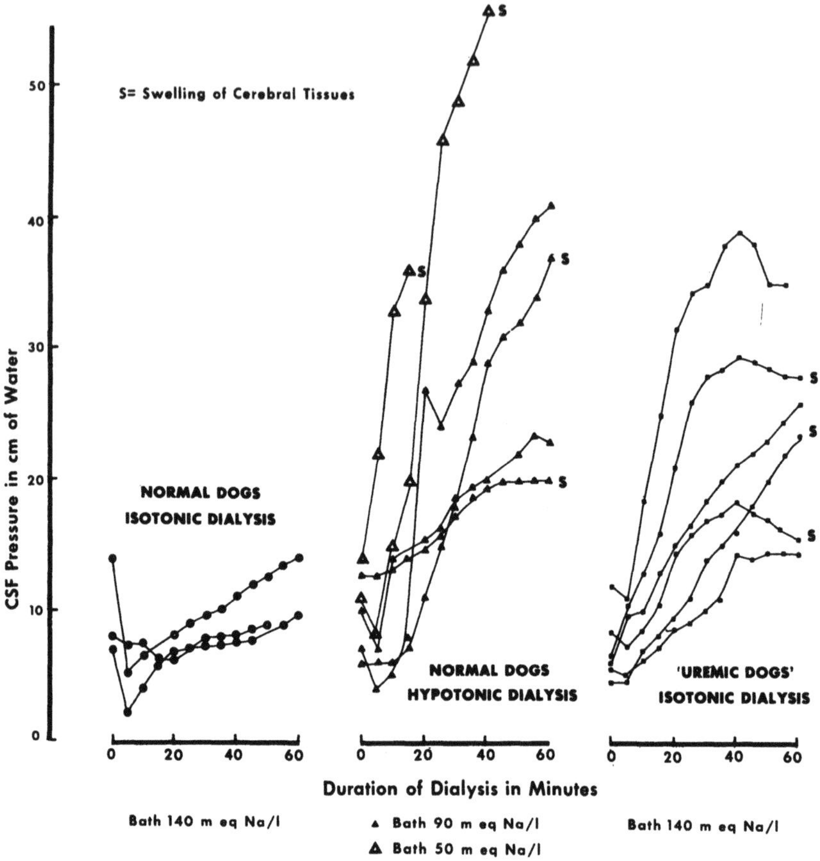

Fig. 1. The cerebrospinal fluid pressure during hemodialysis.

take of sodium-containing fluid. There is however, a significant net loss of potassium from the cerebral cortex tissue surrounding the lesion.

In contrast, cerebral swelling induced osmotically by hemodialysis against relatively hypotonic bath fluid affects both the white matter and the cerebral cortex tissue to the same extent. There is no change in the Na/K ratio of the tissue, indicating that the fluid taken up does not contain high amounts of sodium and probably consists of water only.

This biochemical definition of the two types of edema investigated in these studies shows clearly that the two methods of inducing cerebral swelling produce basically different results.

A difference in the way in which potassium content of cerebral tissues is affected by the administration of hypertonic urea solution was observed in traumatized brain, as compared to normal. This change is interpreted as indicating a generalized effect of trauma (or edema) on the brain. The mechanisms involved are not known.

When osmotic inbalance exists between the central nervous system and the blood, changes in CSF pressure are not well correlated with changes in water content of cerebral tissues, hence are not a reliable measure of cerebral swelling. Direct osmotic effects on the volume of CSF are most probably involved.

ACKNOWLEDGMENTS

I am grateful to Professor K. A. C. Elliott for his continued interest in this work and for his criticism of the manuscript.

I also wish to acknowledge the helpful suggestions of Dr. M. Spence during the preparation of the manuscript.

REFERENCES

Bakay, L. and I. U. Haque: Morphological and chemical studies in cerebral edema, J. Neuropath. and Exptl. Neurol., 23, 393-418 (1964).

Clasen, R. A., P. M. Cooke, S. Pandolfi, G. Carnecki and G. Bryar: Hypertonic urea in experimental cerebral edema, Arch. Neurol., 12, 424-434 (1965).

Elliott, K. A. C. and H. H. Jasper: Measurement of experimentally induced brain swelling and shrinkage, Amer. J. Physiol., 157: 122-129 (1949).

Gonatas, N. K., H. M. Zimmerman and S. Levine: Ultrastructure of inflammation with edema in the rat brain, Amer. J. Path., 42: 455-469 (1963).

Katzman, R., N. Gonatas and S. Levine: Electrolytes and fluids in experimental focal leucoencephalopathy, Arch. Neurol., 10: 58-65 (1964).

Klatzo, I., J. Miquel and R. Otenasek: The application of fluorescein-labeled serum proteins (FLSP) to the study of vascular permeability in the brain, Acta Neuropathol., 2: 144-160 (1962).

_____, A. Piraux and E. J. Laskowski: The relationship between edema, blood-brain barrier and tissue elements in a local brain injury, J. Neuropath. exp. Neurol., 17, 548-564 (1958).

Pappius, H. M. and L. A. Dayes: Hypertonic urea. Its effect on the distribution of water and electrolytes in normal and edematous brain tissues, Arch. Neurol. 13, 395-402 (1965).

_____ and D. R. Gulati: Water and electrolyte content of cerebral tissues in experimentally induced edema, Acta Neuropathol., 2, 451-460 (1963).

_____, J. Oh and J. B. Dossetor: The effects of rapid hemodialysis on brain tissues and cerebrospinal fluid of dogs, Can. J. Physiol. Pharm. 45, 129-147 (1967).

Raimondi, A. J., J. P. Evans and S. Mullen: Studies of cerebral edema. 111. Alterations in the white matter: an electron-microscopic study using ferritin as a labelling compound, Acta Neuropathol., 2, 177-197 (1962).

ROBERT KATZMAN

BIOCHEMICAL CORRELATES OF CEREBRAL EDEMA

Although cerebral edema may be produced by a multitude of agents, the biochemical responses are limited in number. Chemically defined, cerebral edema is manifested by an increase in the water of the brain, usually accompanied by a corresponding increase in salt. This increase in water and salt characteristically occurs in white matter to a greater degree than in gray matter. We have had the opportunity of measuring other parameters in cerebral edema and will summarize these in the present report. In addition, a method for the simultaneous study of biochemical and morphological changes will be described.

TRIETHYLTIN EDEMA

Triethyltin edema was clinically important only when alkyl tin compounds were used as medicinal agents, and it is not anticipated that there will be any future epidemics of this disorder such as those that occurred in France in the mid-1950's (Magee, et al., 1957). Nevertheless, this form of edema is of considerable interest, because of the unusual morphological and biochemical pattern observed.

In gray matter, swelling of astrocytic processes is found on electron micrographs along with a modest increase in water and salt. In white matter, the striking intramyelinic swelling or myelin blebs appear as reported by Aleu, et al. (1963) (Fig. 1). This is accompanied by a very marked increase in water content; when referred to the dry weight of the tissue, the water content is increased

*Supported by grants NB-01450, NB-03356, and NB-K3-17044, U.S. Public Health Service.

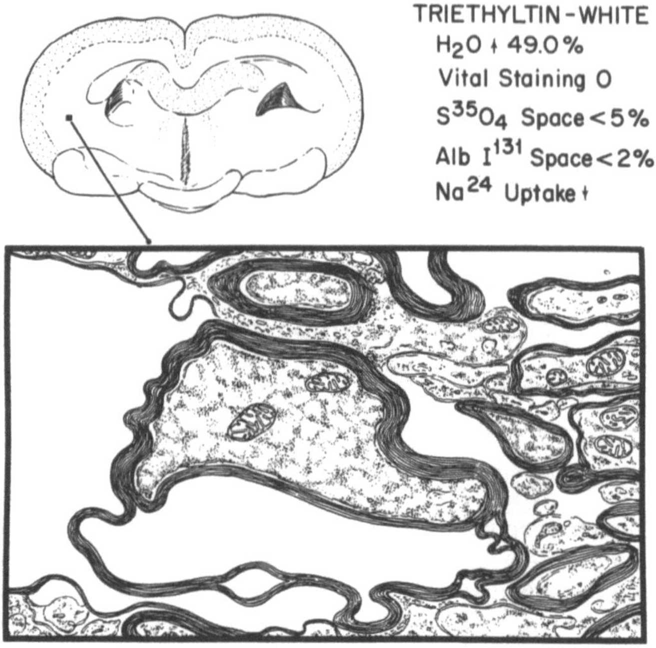

Fig. 1. The ultrastructural changes in white matter in triethyltin edema are shown in an artist's rendering of previously published electron micrographs (Aleu, et al., 1964). Note accumulation of fluid within myelin blebs These blebs are found throughout the central nervous system white matter. The water content of tissue, referred to dry weight, was markedly increasec but there was no breakdown of the blood-brain barrier. The exchange of Na^{24} between blood and brain is depressed.

50%. There is a correlated increase in Na and Cl such that the concentration of the additional Na and Cl in the extra water constitutes an ultrafiltrate of plasma reasonably well.

Aside from this rather remarkable degree of swelling, few changes are observed. There is no alteration of the blood-brain ba: rier as studied with trypan blue. There is no increase in the rate o uptake in a six hour period of $S^{35}O_4$ or albumin I^{131}. There is no increase in total soluble protein nor any increase in albumin as measured by acrylamide gel disc electrophoresis.

A most interesting finding is the change in the uptake of Na^{24} (Katzman, et al., 1963). Unlike other forms of edema where Na^{24} uptake is normal or increased, it appears to be reduced in triethyltin edema, when the specific activity of the brain as compared to plasma (relative specific activity) is measured as a function of tim

However, further analysis of this kinetic data indicates that there is not an actual decrease in the rate of uptake of Na^{24}, but rather a large fraction of brain Na that no longer exchanges, presumably representing the Na within the myelinic blebs.

Because of this finding, we attempted to measure the Na dependent ATPase activity of white matter, postulating that the defect might reside in the inability of the myelin to extrude Na. However, the Na-Mg dependent ATPase activity was within normal limits. Torack (1965) reported that a specific Na dependent ATPase was inhibited by the triethyltin, but Novikoff (1965) has been unable to confirm this observation. Thus, the mechanism producing this edema remains unknown: it does not appear to reside in the breakdown of blood-brain barrier; it does not reside in an abnormality in protein metabolism that led to a small soluble osmotically active protein, nor does it reside in inhibition of the ATPase system.

The development of triethyltin edema is prevented or slowed in animals given steroids according to Taylor, et al. (1965). Again, the mechanism of this effect is unknown.

FOCAL EDEMA

In focal edemas produced by the implantation of purified protein derivative pellets in the frontal lobes of rats (Katzman, et al., 1964) (Figs. 2 and 3) and in the edema surrounding implanted glial tumors in mice (Fig. 4), similar biochemical changes have been observed (Aleu, et al., 1964). These include an increase in salt and water in the adjacent tissues of a marked degree, greater again in white matter than in neuropil. In remote areas of the brain, a small degree of edema may or may not develop. These changes are correlated at the ultrastructural level with astrocytic swelling in cortex and the formation of true extracellular space in white matter However, when the uptake of trypan blue, $S^{35}O_4$, albumin I^{131} or I^{125}, or tritiated albumin, or the uptake of iodinated mercuhydrin are measured, it is found that the uptake of all these substances is increased in the brain adjacent to the focal lesion in both gray and white matter. Thus, whereas the $S^{35}O_4$ space in normal brain is less than 5%, it may reach 26 - 30% in edema. Na^{24} uptake in the experimental animals is more rapid than in control animals. These changes could be accounted for in white matter by the increase in extracellular space; but in cortex no corresponding increase in extracellular space occurs, the morphologic changes being confined to astrocytic swelling. Hence, the increased amounts of $S^{35}O_4$ and albumin in the cortex must represent intracellular accumulation, perhaps within the swollen astrocytes.

In these forms of edema there is then a marked change in protein content of the tissue with rapid accumulation of serum albumin

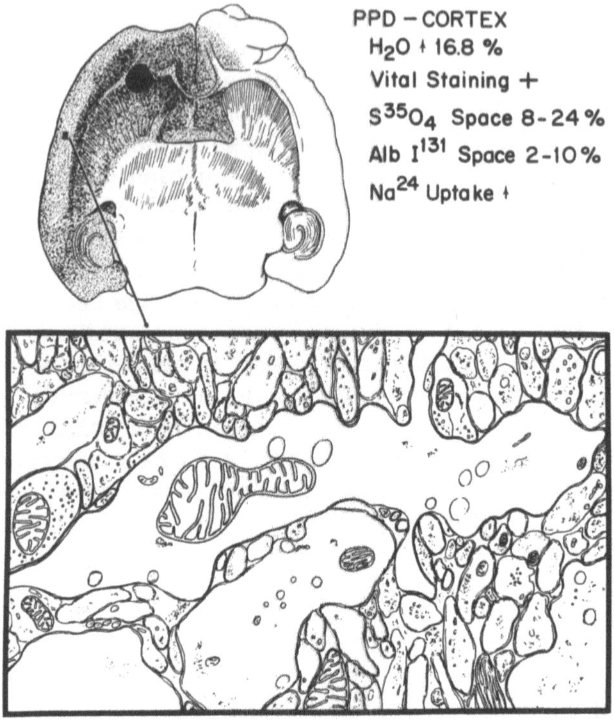

Fig. 2. The ultrastructural changes in rat cortex in edema secondary to implantation of pellets of purified protein derivative are shown in an artist's rendering of previously published electron micrographs (Gonatas, et al., 1963). Note the enlargement of glial cell processes. This is accompanied by moderate accumulation of water but a marked breakdown of the blood-brain barrier and increased permeability to Na^{24}. These changes are in area contiguous to the pellet but may spread to quite distant regions.

which can be counted as iodinated albumin or measured on acrylamide gel disc electrophoresis. The accumulation of these serum proteins in the involved tissue has been previously noted (Klatzo, et al., 1958; Cumings, 1961; Raimondi, et al., 1962; and Lowenthal, 1965).

USE OF GLUTERALDEHYDE PERFUSION FOR COMBINED BIOCHEMICAL AND ULTRASTRUCTURAL STUDIES

In an attempt to find a method which would permit the study of structure and electrolytes in deeper regions of the brain in the same

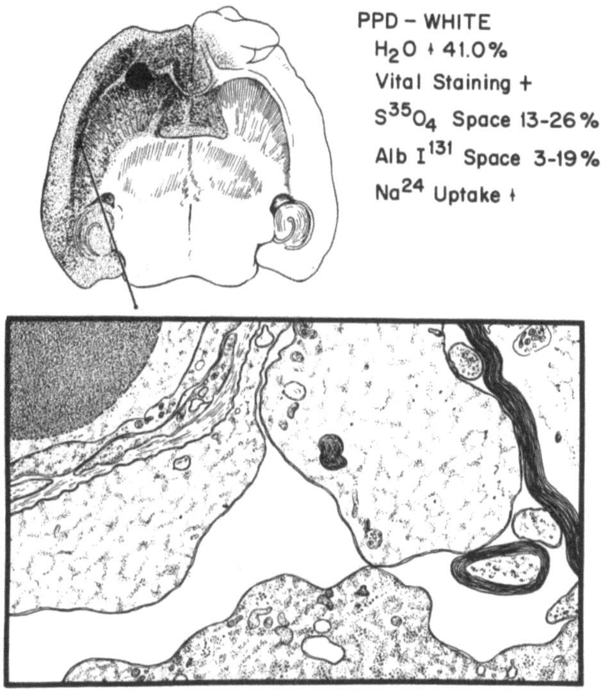

Fig. 3. The ultrastructural changes in white matter of rats in edema secondary to implantation of pellets of purified protein derivative as shown in artist's rendering (Gonatas, et al., 1963). Note the true increase in extracellular space and marked increase in water as well as the breakdown of the blood-brain barrier.

animal, we have studied the effects of brief gluteraldehyde perfusions (Levy, et al., 1965). In mouse, rat, and rabbit such perfusions lasting four to ten minutes are sufficient to harden the brain so that it may be easily handled and, after secondary fixation, used to obtain high quality electron micrographs. There is little alteration in several chemical parameters that we have measured, including per cent dry weight, Na content, and $S^{35}O_4$ space.

The lipid constituents of the tissue appear unaltered, if measured by the total lipid, proteolipids, gangliosides, cholesterol, phosphatides, and cerebrosides. Most surprising of all, little exchange takes place between the ions of the perfusate and those of the brain tissue. The perfusate contains a Na phosphate buffer; when this is labeled with Na^{24}, or if $K^{42}$is added to the perfusate, the uptake by the brain is in the approximate order of magnitude as would be expected in living animal, indicating that the blood-brain barrier may be still intact.

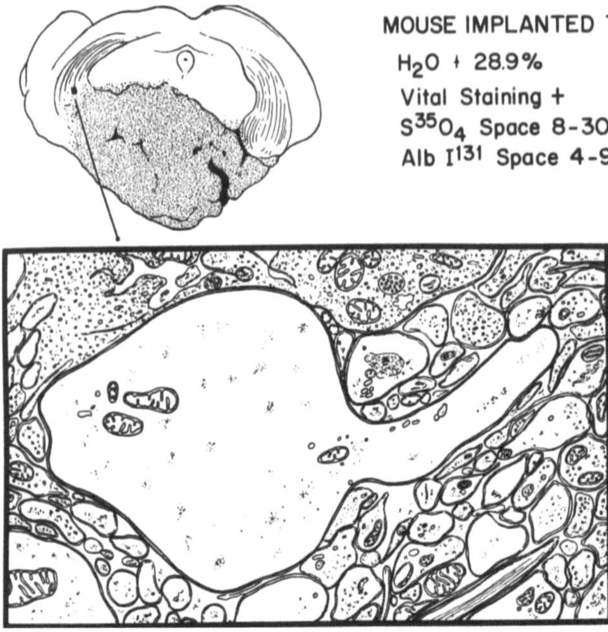

Fig. 4. The neuropil of mice adjacent to implanted glial tumors as shown in artist's rendering (Aleu, et al., 1964). Note the swelling of glial cell processes in area contiguous to the tumor. Both moderate increase in water and increased permeability are seen.

This finding raises an interesting issue as to what happens to membranes after fixation. It may be argued that in contrast to membranes in tissue slices which are very leaky, that membranes may have decreased permeability after fixation. Thus, it is well known that the lipid backbone of the membrane by itself has an exceedingly high resistance which is reduced by the presence of proteins and transport processes. A fixative such as gluteraldehyde does not dissolve the lipid portion of the membrane, but it might denature the protein structures or enzymes which normally act to reduce membrane resistance. Hence, after fixation or death, membrane resistance may actually increase. This, in fact, has been observed in frog skin studied as an ion pump and subjected to anoxia (Finkelstein, 1964).

ACKNOWLEDGMENT

I wish to thank my colleagues whose work is summarized herein.

REFERENCES

Magee, P. N., H. B. Stoner and J. M. Barnes: J. Path. Bact., 73, 107 (1957).
Aleu, F. P., R. Katzman and R. D. Terry: J. Neuropath. Exp. Neurol., 22, 403 (1963).
Katzman, R., F. Aleu and C. Wilson: Arch. Neurol., 9, 178 (1963).
Torack, R. M.: Am. J. Path., 66, 245 (1965).
Novikoff, A.: (unpublished data).
Taylor, J. M., W. A. Levy, I. Herzog and L. C. Scheinberg: Neurology, 15, 667 (1965).
Katzman, R., N. Gonatas and S. Levine: Arch. Neurol., 10, 58 (1964).
Aleu, F. P., F. L. Edelman, R. Katzman and L. C. Scheinberg: J. Neuropath. Exp. Neurol., 23, 253 (1964).
Klatzo, I., A. Piraux and E. J. Laskowski: Ibid., 17, 548 (1958).
Cumings, J. N.: J. Clin. Path., 14, 289 (1961).
Raimondi, A. J., J. P. Evans and S. Mullan: Acta Neuropath., 2, 177 (1962).
Van Bogaert, L., J. Radermecker, J. Hozay and A. Lowenthal: Proceedings of a Symposium on the Neuropathology, Electroencephalography and Biochemistry of Encephalitides, Antwerp, 1959, Amsterdam: Elsevier Press (1965).
Levy, W. A., I. Herzog, K. Suzuki, R. Katzman and L. C. Scheinberg: J. Cell Biol. (in press).
Finkelstein, A.: J. Gen. Physiol., 47, 545 (1964).
Gonatas, N. K., H. M. Zimmerman and S. Levine: Am. J. Path., 42, 455 (1961).

WOLFGANG ZEMAN
JOHN KALSBECK

HISTOCHEMICAL ASPECTS OF BRAIN EDEMA*

INTRODUCTION

The study of experimental cerebral edema is being actively pursued in many laboratories. Experiments have been concerned with the electron microscopic demonstration of the site of fluid accumulation and such observations have contributed importantly towards an understanding of problems associated with fluid exchange as well as with the interstitial and cellular fluid compartments of the mammalian brain. Histochemical studies on brain edema have been primarily concerned with the reactive responses of the glia and provided valuable information (Rubinstein, et al., 1962). Recently, Torack (1965) designed histochemical and electron microscopic experiments of a heuristic nature, in agreement with biochemical findings. Briefly, triethyltin (TET) inhibits oxidative phosphorylation in brain and liver tissue slices and mitochondria (Aldridge, 1958), and Torack (1965) was able to show a selective inhibition of a glutaraldehyde resistant ATPase in the white matter of rats poisoned with TET.

Our own studies evolved from a different point of departure. We have been concerned with the effects of edema on nervous tissue previously exposed to a focal X-irradiation (Zeman, 1965). In these studies, rats received intraperitoneal injections of 2 mg aqueous TET, or of distilled water (100 ml [kg body weight]$^{-1}$) three months after exposure of spinal segments T2 to T4 to 3,5000 X-rays at 320 min^{-1} (HVL 2.1 min Cu). From previous observations it could be anticipated that delayed radiation necrosis would ensue in

* Supported in part by US PHS Grant R01 NB 02960.

these animals after an additional latency period of three to four months. However, 75% of the rats developed a characteristic delayed radionecrosis within two weeks after the injections, though the animals showed only mild and temporary effects of this treatment. Conceivably, a transient edema had sufficed to injure the previously irradiated tissue in such a way as to accelerate the mechanisms which lead to delayed radionecrosis. In order to exclude interference by radiation-induced histoenzymatic alterations, the histochemistry of the acute phase of water-induced edema, of the preclinical phase of TET poisoning and of X-irradiation was studied comparatively. The investigations were made on brain tissue, rather than on spinal cord, because the former affords greater ease of handling and larger bulks of tissue.

MATERIALS AND METHODS

Adult Carworth female rats, aged 150 to 350 days, matched for age, were randomly assigned to four groups. The first group received one injection of aqueous TET (1.25 mg [100 gr body weight]$^{-1}$) intraperitoneally, the second distilled water (10 ml [100 gr body weight]$^{-1}$). The third group was irradiated over the frontal lobe with a 1 cm^2 beam of 250 KV X-rays (HVL 2.1 mm, 8,600 rads at 320 rads min^{-1}), and the fourth was untreated. The animals were sacrificed by decapitation according to the schedule in Table 1. The brains were quickly removed from the skull. 2-mm slices of brain tissue were taken from the frontal lobes at the level of the anterior commissure and from the cerebellum through the declive, all in a frontal plane. One-half of the section was quenched in liquid nitrogen and the other fixed in calcium formalin. Brains from some animals were fixed in glutaraldehyde. In other instances the entire brain or parts thereof were homogenized and 1:1 aqueous extracts were subjected to agar gel electrophoresis. Whole hemisphere or the frontal lobes or the excised corpus callosum were also homogenized and assayed by biochemical methods for various enzymes.

OBSERVATIONS

On the fresh frozen and calcium formalin fixed tissue a number of dehydrogenases were studied. For slide histochemical studies, the right hemisphere of four animals, i.e., control, treated with TET, with distilled water, and irradiated, respectively, were mounted on the same chuck, cut in a cryostat at 8μ, and mounted on the same coverslip. Formalin fixed frozen sections were likewise cut simul-

TABLE 1

EXPERIMENTAL PROCEDURE

Treatment	Sacrificed by decapitation	Remarks
none		
single dose i.p. dist. H_2O 10 ml (100 gr body weight)$^{-1}$	30 min. after injection	animals invariably stuporous no spontaneous or reactive activity
single dose i.p. TET 1.25 mg (100 gr body weight)$^{-1}$	24 hrs. after injection 48 hrs. after injection	animals usually listless, sometimes normal, occasionally slightly stuporous
single dose 8,600 rads 250 KV X-rays at 320 rads min^{-1}(HVL 2.1 mm Cu)	8 days after irradiation	all animals were clinically unremarkable

taneously. No differences in localization and in staining intensity were uncovered between the animals of the four different groups.

Stimulated by the observations of Torack (1965) a major effort was made to reproduce the selective inhibition of a glutaraldehyde resistant ATPase in TET-poisoned animals. When these experiments yielded questionable results, a major effort was made to demonstrate selectively the four different pH dependent ATPases, using the techniques developed by Wegmann and Bankowski (1960). These studies suggested that the TET poisoning effects a selective inhibition of the ATPase giving maximal reaction at pH 7.4, which is predominantly localized in the capillaries. However, the results were inconsistent and reproducible only in those animals which had developed severe clinical disease and showed massive edema morphologically. The selective techniques for ATPases described by Freiman and Kaplan (1960) also produced inconclusive results and we deduced that slide histochemical demonstration of ATPase was not shedding too much light on the problem. We observed, however, that the edematous white matter, despite loosening of the tissue texture, absorbed methylene blue more intensely than the non-edematous white matter by using the method of Fischer and Zeman (1959). Therefore, the examination of other pH dependent hydrolases appeared indicated. Alkaline phosphatase as demonstrated by the methods of Gomori and of Burstone showed no noticeable differences between the four groups of animals. Methods for the histochemical demonstration of thiamine pyrophosphatase and of several dinucleotide phosphatases likewise produced no differential staining effects. However, the technique for 5′-nucleotidase of Barron and Boshes (1961) yielded a consistently decreased staining intensity of brains of TET treated animals, regardless of their clinical condition and the morphologic appearance of their brains. In particular, the staining of the corpus callosum and the anterior commissure was weak (Fig. 1). The brains from animals of the other three groups did never display this decrease and were considered to give a normal staining reaction (Fig. 2).

Biochemical estimations of the activity of 5′-nucleotidase in comparison to acid and alkaline phosphatase were, however, disappointing as shown in Table 2. Though there was usually some decrease in the activity of this enzyme, this was by no means as significant as was surmised from the slide histochemical findings. Ni^{++} ions did not block the staining reaction but cysteine and 80 per cent ethanol reduced it markedly. No differential staining effect was produced when hexose monophosphates and nucleotide diphosphates were used as substrates. That the staining was not due to lead absorption alone was shown by the blank sections obtained from incubation in solutions without adenosine monophosphate.

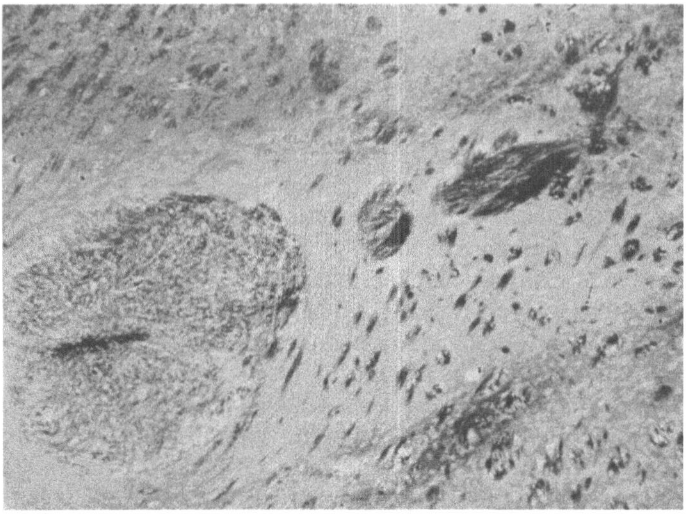

Fig. 1. Rat brain 24 hours after intraperitoneal injection of 2 mg of aqueous TET. Reaction for 5'-nucleotidase after Barron and Boshes. Note the decreased staining of the fibers in the anterior commissure which is about the same size as that shown in Figure 2. No decrease in the staining of the neuropil of the caudate nucleus and nucleus accumbens septi is evident. 80:1.

In order to shed more light on these questionable observations aqueous tissue extracts (1:1) were subjected to slide electrophoresis after Wieme and stained for 5'-nucleotidase using the technique of Barron and Boshes (1961). From tissue extracts of control and water treated animals and from animals exposed to an edema producing dose of ionizing radiation, two distinct cathodal and two less well separated anodal bands were consistently obtained. The tissue extract from TET-poisoned animals yielded a profound reduction of the slow moving cathodal band which, by judiciously employed photography, can be made to disappear completely (Fig. 3). In order to test the possibility that this finding was in any way related to the TET, an unlikely assumption, aliquots of the same tissue extracts were treated for the demonstration of lactate dehydrogenase isozymes which gave identical results for all four groups of animals.

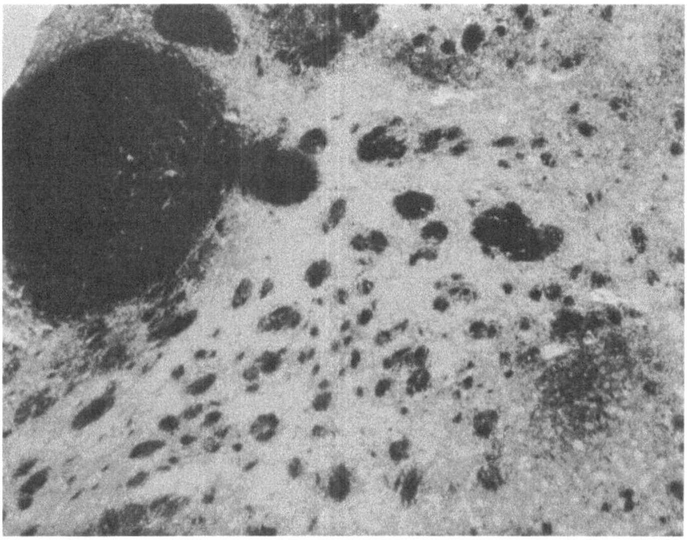

Fig. 2. Rat brain 30 minutes after intraperitoneal injection of 15 ml of distilled water. Reaction for 5'-nucleotidase after Barron and Boshes. The anterior commissure is normally stained. 80:1.

DISCUSSION

It has been the experience of many observers that TET given to rats in doses of about one to two mgs daily, results in brain edema within a period of three to five days. If the injections are discontinued, the animals may completely recover after a period of a few weeks. A single injection of distilled water into the peritoneal cavity in appropriate amounts leads to a rather acute evolution of cerebral edema, the clinical effects of which subside just as quickly. Edema induced by radiation, however, is ultimately followed by a necrosis of the exposed brain tissue. These facts permit the conclusion that different mechanisms are involved in the pathogenesis of edema in these conditions. The decrease of plasma osmolarity which follows the intraperitoneal injection of distilled water probably overtaxes temporarily the physiological membrane transport

TABLE 2

Tissue examined	Treatment	μ mols PO_4 [Gr wet tissue]$^{-1}$ hr^{-1}			Remarks
		5′ nucleotidase	Alk. Pase	Acid Pase	
Frontal lobes only	30 min. after dist H_2O	246	104	302	Animal is stuporous
	24 hrs. after TET i.p.	193	100	303	Animal is listless and displays reduced spontaneous activity
	48 hrs. after 0.2 mg TET i.p.	218	88	269	Animal appears slightly subdued
Right cerebral hemisphere including diencephalon	30 min. after H_2O	333	128	353	Animal is stuporous
	24 hrs. after TET	274	140	354	Animal is listless and moderately stuporous
	48 hrs. after TET	284	107	305	Animal is slightly listless
Corpus callosum and adjacent white matter only	none	145 156 154	76 88 84	320 302 273	
	30 min. after dist H_2O	190 162	85 76	272 282	Both animals are severely stuporous
	24 hrs. after TET i.p.	116 146	63 47	244 196	Both animals are somewhat listless
	48 hrs. after TET i.p.	178 184	68 46	240 257	Both animals are very listless and do not move spontaneously

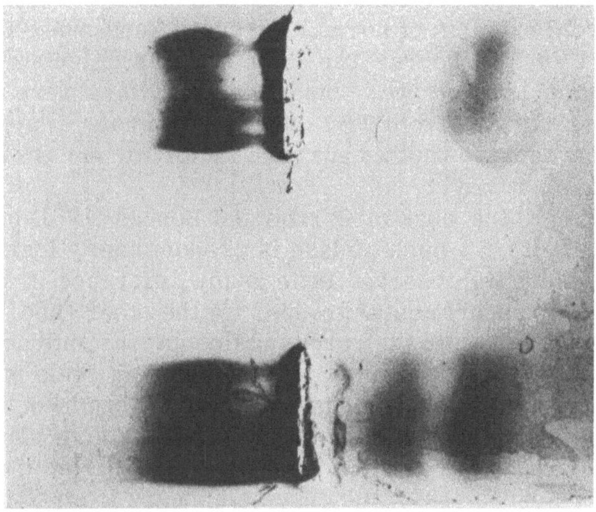

Fig. 3. Electrophoretogram of brain tissue extracts, stained for adenosine-5'-nucleotidase after Barron and Boshes. 22 mA- 110 V, 25 min at 8° C. Lower record from animal treated with water, upper record from animal treated with TET. The intensity of slow moving cathodal band in the extract from the TET-poisoned animal is markedly reduced.

mechanisms. X-irradiation effects edema because of structural membrane changes. TET poisoning appears to produce a transient, yet extended incapacitation of transmembrane transport.

Since the animals in the present experiments were all in a pre-edematous phase, one could expect that reactive enzyme alterations in response to the pathological fluid accumulations were minimal if not absent. Accordingly, the abnormalities in regard to 5'-nucleotidase activity could conceivably be indicative of the biochemical mechanism responsible for TET-induced edema. It could also be speculated that this alteration is related to the long period of reconvalescence in comparison to the short recovery period for water induced edema.

Assuming validity of these conclusions, serious difficulties arise in respect to their interpretation. In the first place, our enthusiasm about the slide histochemical findings was severely dampened by the failure of confirmatory observations by biochemical methods. On the other hand, the consistency of the suppression of the slow moving cathodal band of 5′-nucleotidase may indicate that some change does occur with this enzyme in animals treated with TET before their brains become edematous. It is perhaps worthwhile to add that the first cathodal band of 5′-nucleotidase disappears also from extracts of normal tissues if kept under anaerobic conditions for several hours. The same happens to lactate dehydrogenase isozymes one and two. Since these isozymes were not suppressed in the extracts from TET-poisoned animals, it appears safe to conclude that anoxia is not a causative factor for the alteration of 5′-nucleotidase activity.

According to the work of Barron and Boshes (1961) and of Felgenhauer (1963), 5′-nucleotidase is predominantly localized in the neuropil. Here we observed little if any difference in activity between our four experimental groups. On the other hand, 5′-nucleotidase reactions stain the corpus callosum, the anterior commissure, the fimbria hippocampi, and the centrum ovale particularly deeply and these are precisely the areas where the brains of the TET-treated animals exhibited a markedly reduced staining. The fine localization of 5'-nucleotidase is not well known but from the studies of Barron and Boshes (1961) the enzyme appears to reside predominantly in the myelinated nerve fibers but not in the capillaries. Astrocytes also show considerable activity. Since TET-induced edema leads to a fluid accumulation within the myelin sheaths (Kalsbeck & Cumings, 1962) or in the oligodendrocytes (Torack, Terry & Zimmerman, 1959), a reasonably good topographical correlation is established. On the other hand, the present knowledge of the specific reactions of 5′-nucleotidase does not lend itself to an intelligent explanation of these findings. In particular, it is difficult to provide a satisfactory argument as to how a decreased ability to dephosphorylate a mononucleotide should have any bearing on transmembrane transport mechanisms.

SUMMARY

Slide histochemical studies showed suppression of 5′-nucleotidase activity in the corpus callosum and anterior commissure of rats one day after poisoning with TET (1.25 mg [100 gm body weight]$^{-1}$). No abnormalities of several other hydrolases and oxidases were noted. In brains from animals rendered edematous by the injection of the distilled water into the peritoneal cavity or having received a single exposure to 8,600 rads X-rays, no enzymatic changes were noted by slide histochemistry. Though in some of the TET-poisoned animals depression of 5′-nucleotidase by biochemical methods could be demonstrated, this was not a reproducible finding;

in fact, acid and alkaline phosphatase were more substantially depressed in some animals. On the other hand, electrophoresis of aqueous tissue extracts consistently showed a depression of the slow moving cathodal band of 5'-nucleotidase only in the TET poisoned rats. While it is believed that a suppression of a 5'-nucleotidase isozyme may be causally related to TET-induced edema, no satisfactory biochemical explanation of this finding is presently available.

ACKNOWLEDGMENT

The authors thank Dr. Richard McCaman for performing the biochemical enzyme estimations, Dr. Arland Carsten for the irradiations, Mrs. Dorothy Meyer, Miss Constance Alyea, and Mr. Moises Hernandez for histochemical and isozyme determinations, and Mr. Joe Demma for photography.

REFERENCES

Aldridge, W. N.: The biochemistry of organotin compounds; trialkyltins and oxidative phosphorylation, Biochem. J., 69, 367-376 (1958).

Barron, K. D. and R. Boshes: Histochemical demonstration of 5-nucleotidase in the central nervous system. Effects of magnanous ion and pH, J. Histochem. Cytochem., 9, 455-457 (1961).

Felgenhauer, K.: Die Lokalisation der spezifischen und unspezifischen Phosphatasen im Meerschweinchengehirn, Z. Zellforsch., 60, 518-531 (1963).

Fischer, R. and W. Zeman: Neuronal Dye-absorption as a histochemical indicator of nervous activity, Nature, 183, 1337-1338 (1959).

Freiman, D. G. and N. Kaplan: Studies on this histochemical differentiation of enzymes hydrolyzing adenosine triphosphate, J. Histochem. Cytochem., 8, 159-170 (1960).

Kalsbeck, J. E. and J. N. Cumings: Experimental edema in the rat and cat brain, J. Neuropath. exp. Neurol., 22, 237-247 (1962).

Rubinstein, L. J., I. Klatzo and J. Miguel: Histochemical observations on oxidative enzyme activity of glial cells in a local brain injury, Ibid., 21, 116-136 (1962).

Torack, R. M.: The relationship between adenosinetriphosphatase activity and triethyltin toxicity in the production of cerebral edema of the rat, Amer. J. Path., 46, 245-251 (1965).

_____, R. D. Terry and H. M. Zimmerman: The fine structure of cerebral fluid accumulation. II. Swelling produced by triethyl

tin poisoning and its comparison with that in the human brain, Ibid., 36, 273-287 (1960).
Wegmann, R. and Z. Bankowski: Differenciation histochimique de quatre groupes d'adénosine triphosphatases selon Slater, Ann. Histochim., 5, 121-141 (1960).
Wieme, R. J.: An improved technique of agar-gel electrophoresis on microscope slides, Clin. chem. Acta 4, 317-321 (1959).
Zeman, W.: Zur Pathogenese der Strahlenspätschädigung des Rückenmarks, Sonderbände z. Strahlentherapie 62, 68-76 (1966).

M. WOLMAN
J. J. BUBIS

HISTOCHEMICAL STUDY OF DIFFERENT TYPES OF BRAIN EDEMA

INTRODUCTION

It has been shown previously (Wolman & Wiener, 1965) that one-half of the lipid constituents of myelin can be extracted by water after treatment with Na ions or other agents which increase the hydrophilia of polar lipids, and that such an extraction is prevented by Ca ions or other agents which decrease the hydrophilia. The other half of the lipid constituents are not sensitive to ions or other hydrophilia-increasing agents. These findings indicate that the layer of the plasma membrane which faces the extracellular space might be different from the layer which faces the intracellular space. Evidence favoring this view has been adduced by electron-microscopy (Sjöstrand, 1963) and X-ray diffraction (Finean, 1963). The well-known fact that the inside of cells is electrically negative in respect of the outer surface also favors the notion that the two layers of the plasma membrane differ in structure and composition. It seems reasonable to assume that the two layers also differ in their enzyme content.

Edema in either the white or gray matter in the brain may theoretically be either extracellular, bounded by the outer layers of plasma membranes, or intracellular and bounded by the inner layers of these membranes. Different enzymes will become easily available to their substrates in the one case in comparison to the other. In the present paper experiments designed to test the possible existence of two types of cerebral edema will be described. The results indicate that two types of edema do occur, but that the expansion of the one space or the other depends primarily on factors which affect fixation of membranes. It is suggested that also in vivo the formation of intra- or extracellular edema depends mainly on the nature of phase transitions in the membranes and only secondarily on the nature of the edematogenic factors.

MATERIAL AND METHODS

Adult white mice of either sex were used. Edema of the brain was induced in them by either of the following five procedures: 1) Dry ice was applied for 30 to 60 seconds to the surface of the leptomeninges of the parietal lobe of the brain after trepanation under pentobarbital anesthesia. The mice were sacrificed three days after the operation. 2) Mice were given intraperitoneal injections of triethyl tin sulfate in daily doses of 0.2 ml of 1 mg/ml solution. The animals were killed when obvious signs of paralysis developed (between three to eight days after the beginning of treatment). Only animals in the brains of which obvious signs of white matter edema were seen in H.E.-stained sections were included in the experiment. 3) Mice anesthetized by intraperitoneal pentobarbital had their thoracic cavity opened and 3-5 ml of distilled water were slowly injected into the left cardiac ventricle. 4) Mice anesthetized and operated as above were injected intracardially with 3-5 ml of 0.85% NaCl solution. 5) Mice anesthetized and operated as above were injected intracardially with 3-5 ml of 1.3% $CaCl_2$ solution (approximately isotonic with 0.85 NaCl).

In all these animals and in untreated mice used as controls the cranial cavity was rapidly opened, the brain extracted and coronal sections of the brain, about 1 mm in thickness were fixed in two different fixing solutions. The fixatives consisted of 2% glutaraldehyde in 0.1M veronal buffer pH 7.3-7.4 containing the one 0.01M NaCl, and the other 0.01M $CaCl_2$.

Fixation was done at 4° C and it varied in duration in the various experiments between two hours (in which case often the inner parts of the sections were sometimes incompletely fixed) and 16 hours. The tissues fixed in the NaCl-containing fixative were rinsed in a solution made of equal parts of 0.1M veronal buffer (pH 7.3-7.4) and 0.22M NaCl. The tissues fixed in the $CaCl_2$-containing fixatives were rinsed in a solution made of equal parts of 0.1M veronal buffer and 0.22M $CaCl_2$. The rinsing lasted between 34 and 50 hours with occasional changes of the solutions. Small pieces of such tissues were transferred through graded alcohols and embedded in Epon for future electron microscopical study. The present report deals with a histochemical study done on frozen sections, about 10-15μ in thickness which were cut from each of these tissues and picked up in the same solutions.

The following histochemical procedures were performed on each of the fixed pieces of tissues: 1) Alkaline phosphatase by

Gomori's procedure as in Pearse (1960, p. 868). 2) Acid phosphatase by Gomori's procedure as modified by Holt (1959). 3) Thiamine pyrophosphatase by the procedure of Novikoff and Goldfischer (1961). 4) Tween esterase (Gomori's Tween lipase) as in Pearse (1960, p. 888). 5) Double esterase following the technique of Shnitka and Seligman (1961) for the simultaneous demonstration of inhibitor-sensitive and inhibitor-resistant esterases.

Slides were examined and findings were noted independently by each of the two authors. Sections of edematous tissues fixed with a solution containing Na ions were compared with control sections fixed in a similar solution, and sections of edematous tissues fixed with Ca were compared with control Ca-fixed sections. The experiments were repeated with minor variations four times. Whenever photography was used, the conditions were equal for all slides belonging to any single series.

RESULTS

The experimental results have been summarized in Table 1 and some examples of the findings may be seen in Figures 1-5.

It can be seen in the table that increased enzymatic activities which were not dependent on the treatment with ions were found only in the necrotic tissue damaged by freezing. In all other instances, whenever increases in enzymatic activities occurred, they depended on fixation of tissues in the presence of Ca ions.

DISCUSSION

The present study is based on previously made observations according to which lipoproteic membranes may fold in either direction to form oil in water (o/w) or water in oil (w/o) emulsions when acted upon by excess Na ions or by other hydrophilic agents, or respectively, by excess Ca ions or by other agents which decrease hydrophilia (Wolman & Wiener, 1965). Further studies have shown that enzymes which are attached to various cellular membranes can be either activated by phase transitions, presumably because they have become freely exposed to the continuous aqueous phase and to the substrate, or inhibited, when they have become enclosed in small sacs away from the continuous phase (Wolman & Bubis, 1965).

It was assumed that edema in any compartment bounded by closely apposed charged surfaces may have an activating effect on enzymes situated on such surfaces by allowing a greater number of encounters between enzyme and substrate molecules in the increased

TABLE 1

EFFECTS OF VARIOUS TYPES OF BRAIN EDEMA ON ENZYMATIC ACTIVITIES

Cause of Edema	Enzyme / Ion in Fixative / Structure Affected	Alk. phosph.		Acid phosph.		Thiamine pyrophosph.		Tween esterase		Inhibitor resist. est.		Inhibitor sensit. est.	
		Na	Ca	Na	Ca	Na	Ca	Na	Ca	Na	Ca	Na	Ca
1. Freezing	Lesion Site	+	+	+	+	+	+	++	++	+	+	+	+
2. Triethyl tin	Myelin	0	+	0	+	0	+	0	0	0	0	0	0
	Neuropil	0	0	0	+	+	+	0	0	0	0	0	0
3. Injection of H_2O	Myelin	0	+	0	0	0	0	0	+	0	+	0	+
	Neuropil	0	0	0	0	0	0	0	0	0	0	0	0
4. Injection of NaCl	Myelin	0	+	0	0	0	0	0	+	0	0	0	0
	Neuropil	0	+	0	0	0	0	0	0	0	0	0	0
5. Injection of $CaCl_2$	Myelin	0	+	0	++	0	++	0	+	0	0	0	+
	Neuropil	0	0	0	+	0	+	0	+	0	0	0	0

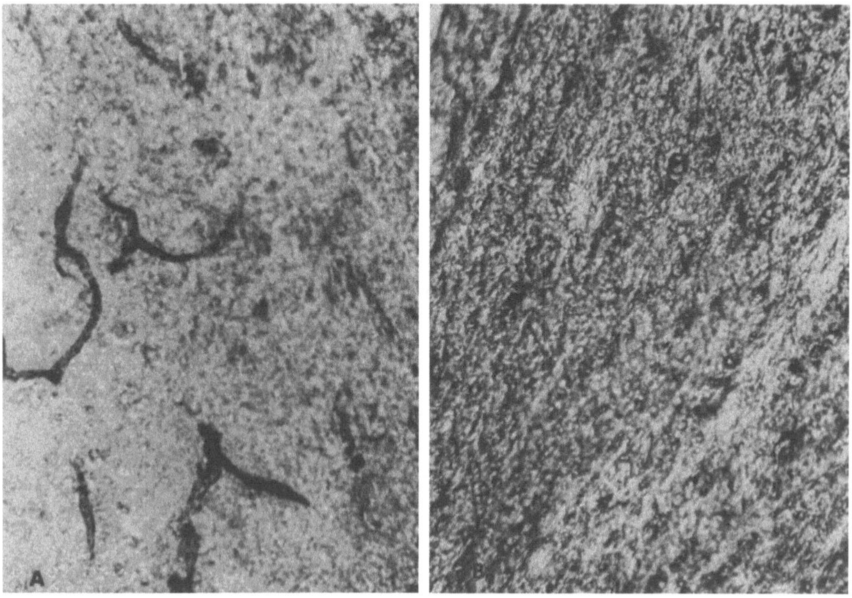

Fig. 1. Cerebral white matter stained for alkaline phosphatase. In A, the mouse was injected with NaCl intracardially and NaCl was added to the fixative. In B, the mouse was injected with $CaCl_2$ intracardially and $CaCl_2$ was added to the fixative. Note the more intense staining in B. X315 (reduced).

space. This assumption is probably correct for both the neuropil and the white matter.

In some preliminary experiments, which were not previously described, it has been found that glutaraldehyde fixation (like formalin fixation, cf. Wolman, 1965) modifies markedly the response of enzymes to the various ions. This observation renders difficult exact determination of the nature of the spaces which are increased in volume after fixation with Ca or with Na ions. In spite of this difficulty it will be shown that the present observations afford the means for comparing the edematogenic effects of various factors.

The only type of lesion associated with increased enzymatic activity which was apparent in both the Na- and the Ca-fixed tissues was the damage caused by local freezing. In this lesion, which consisted of necrosis rather than edema, ions in the fixatives did not have any effect, probably because membranes have disintegrated.

In all other types of edema the nature of the compartment which became expanded appeared to depend partly on the ions present in the fluid used to produce the edema (in the last two experimental setups in the table) and mainly on the ions present in the fixing solutions.

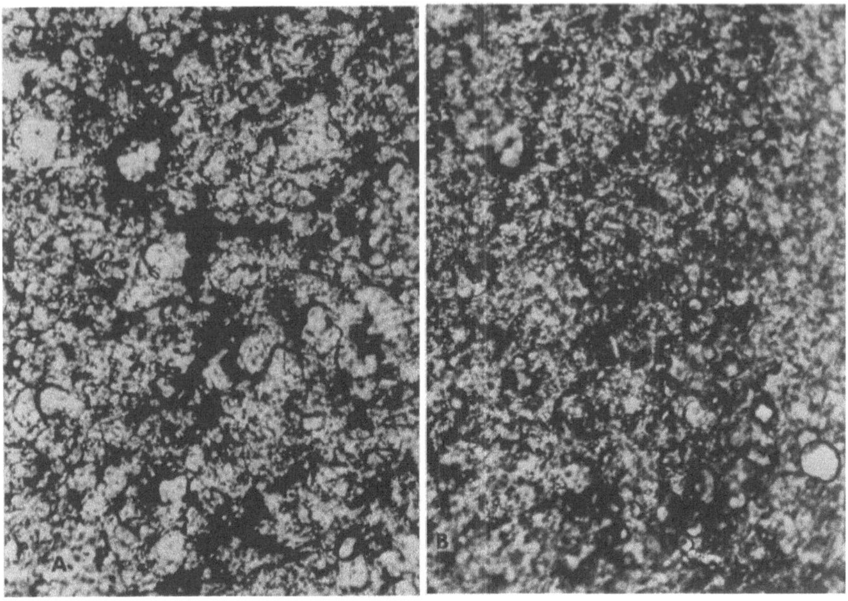

Fig. 2. Cerebral gray matter stained for alkaline phosphatase. A and B as in Figure 1. X315 (reduced).

Comparison of the edema produced by intracardiac injection of NaCl solution and fixed with Na (left side of each column in the fourth row of the table) with the edema caused by injection of the $CaCl_2$ solution and fixed with Ca (right side of each column in the fifth row of the table) shows that no increased enzymatic activities occurred in the first, whereas five of the six enzymes studied showed increased activity in the second. In two instances the effect of the excess Na used in the injection could be reversed to some extent by subsequent fixation in the Ca-containing fixative. It seems, therefore, that the main factor which determines the compartment which becomes swollen by edema in these experiments were the ions.

The present findings may be correlated with available data in the literature in the following way. It has been shown by Luse and Harris (1960) and confirmed by others that edema in the brain of rabbits was mostly intracellular. Other evidence (e.g., Feigin & Popoff, 1962; Aleu, Katzman & Terry, 1963; Hirano, Zimmerman & Levine, 1964) indicates that edema in the white matter is often extracellular and in the gray matter is, in some instances, extracellular in the acute stages. Furthermore, the experiments of Klatzo and Miquel (1960) indicate that extracellular fluid can be absorbed by glial cells.

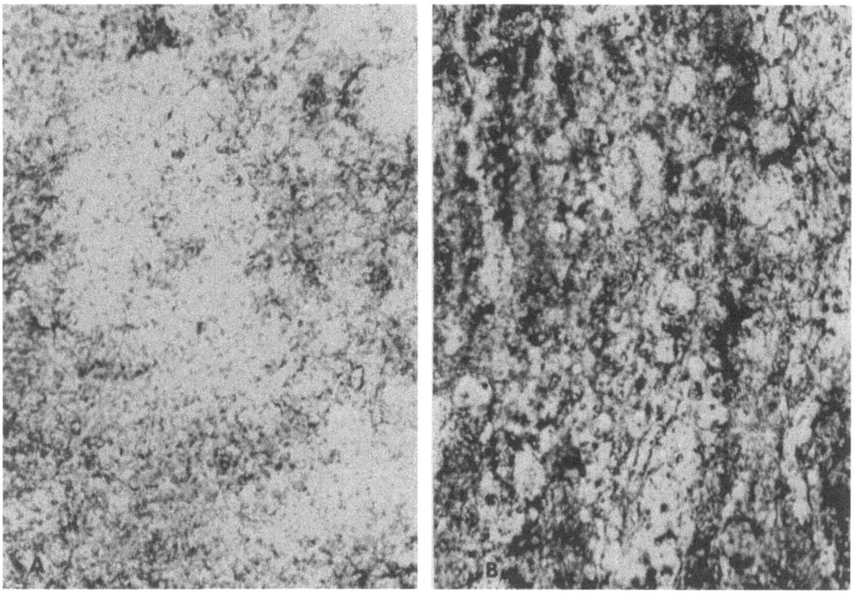

Fig. 3. Cerebral white matter stained for alkaline phosphatase. In both A and B, the edema was caused by intraperitoneal injections of triethyl tin. In A, NaCl was included in the fixing solution. In B, $CaCl_2$ was added to the fixative. Note the more intense staining in B. X315 (reduced).

The presently described experiments indicate that accumulation of fluid inside or outside cells depends to a large extent on fixation and on artificially-induced phase transitions in membranes. It is proposed that similar phase changes may occur in vivo and that the intra- and extracellular compartments exchange fluids in accordance with changes in the degree of hydrophilia of the plasma membrane. Acceptance of the notion that plasma membranes may undergo phase transitions in vivo makes the differentiation of intra- from extracellular edema lose most of its meaning. The metabolic state of the cerebral tissues with consequent changes in the concentration of ions and of other factors affecting the hydrophilia of membranes may determine whether at any given time an accumulation of fluid will be situated on the inside or the outside of plasma membranes.

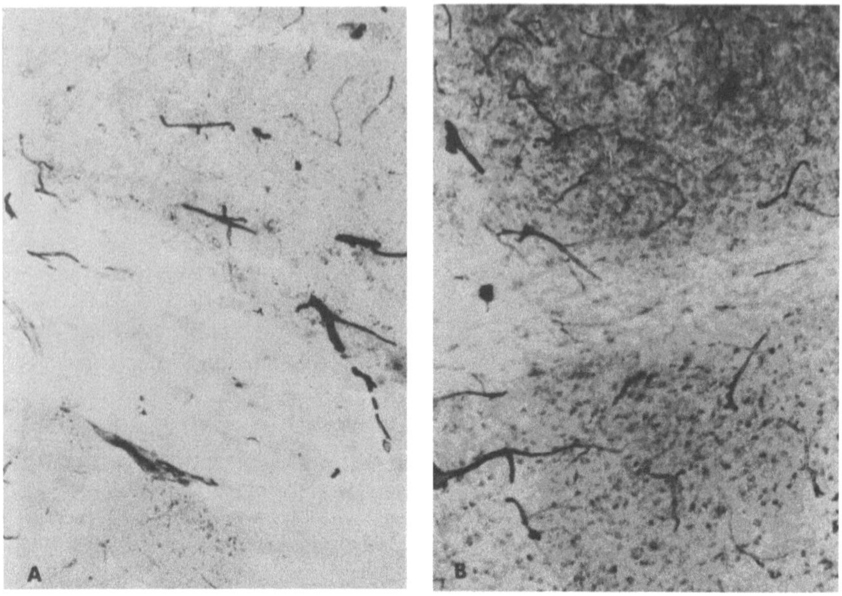

Fig. 4. Bands of cerebral white matter between areas of gray staining for thiamine pyrophosphatase. In A, the mouse was injected with NaCl intracardially and NaCl was included in the fixing solution. B comes from a mouse which was injected intracardially with $CaCl_2$ and $CaCl_2$ was added to the fixative. Note the more intense staining in B in all areas. X105 (reduced).

SUMMARY

Edema of the brain was induced in mice by five different procedures: freezing of the tissues; triethyl tin poisoning; intracardiac injections of large amounts of distilled water, or of isotonic NaCl or of isotonic $CaCl_2$. The damaged brains, as well as control normal brains, were fixed in buffered glutaraldehyde solutions containing either NaCl or $CaCl_2$, and frozen sections were used for the histochemical demonstration of various enzymatic activities. It was found that increases in enzymatic activities, which were presumed to indicate swelling of the compartments adjacent to the surfaces on which the enzymes are located, depended mainly on the nature of the ions included in the fixing solutions. On the basis of these observations and of data available in the literature it is suggested that the nature of the space which is affected by edema depends in vivo on factors affecting the hydrophilia of plasma membranes and that the distinction of intra- from extracellular edema might not be of great importance.

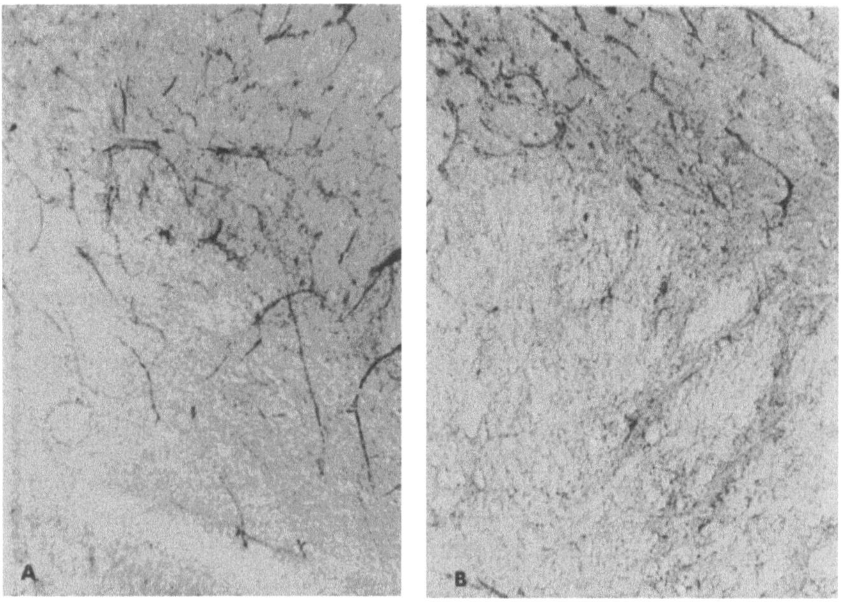

Fig. 5. White and gray matter stained for thiamine pyrophosphatase. Edema in white matter was caused by injections of triethyl tin. In A, NaCl was included in the fixing solution. In B, $CaCl_2$ was added to the fixative. Note the more intense staining in B. X105 (reduced).

ACKNOWLEDGMENTS

This study was supported by grant No. 4X5109 of National Institues of Health, U.S. Public Health Service. The authors are grateful to Mr. J. Gòrski and Miss R. Zelkha for excellent technical assistance and to Mr. J. Aidan for the microphotographs. Thanks are also due to Prof. A. Zilkha and members of the Department of Organic Chemistry of the Hebrew University, Jerusalem, for having put at our disposal the triethyl tin sulfate synthesized by them.

REFERENCES

Aleu, F. P., R. Katzman and R. D. Terry: Fine structure and electrolyte analyses of cerebral edema induced by alkyl tin intoxication, J. Neuropath. Exp. Neurol., 22, 403-413 (1963).

Feigin, I. and N. Popoff: Neuropathological observations on cerebral edema. The acute phase, Arch. Neurol., 6, 151-160 (1962).

Finean, J. B.: Ultrastructural studies on biological membranes, Conference on Permeability, Zwolle: Tjeenk-Willink (1963).

Hirano, A., H. M. Zimmerman and S. Levin: The fine structure of cerebral fluid accumulation. III. Extracellular spread of cryptococcal polysaccharides in the acute stage, Amer. J. Path., 45, 1-19 (1964).

Holt, S. J.: Factors governing the validity of staining methods for enzymes, and their bearing upon the Gomori acid phosphatase technique, Exper. Cell. Res., Suppl. 7, 1-27 (1959).

Klatzo, I. and J. Miquel: Observations on pinocytosis in nervous tissues, J. Neuropath. Exper. Neurol., 19, 475-487 (1960).

Luse, S. A. and B. Harris: Electron microscopy of the brain in experimental edema, J. Neurosurg., 17, 439-446 (1960).

Novikoff, A. B. and S. Goldfischer: Nucleosidodiphosphatase in the Golgi apparatus and its usefulness for cytological studies, Proc. Nat. Acad. Sci. (U.S.), 47, 802-810. (1961).

Pearse, A. G. E.: Histochemistry, Theoretical and Applied, 2nd ed., Boston: Little, Brown (1960).

Shnitka, T. K. and A. M. Seligman: Role of esteratic inhibition on localization of esterase and the simultaneous cytochemical demonstration of inhibitor sensitive and resistant enzyme species, J. Histochem. Cytochem., 9, 504-527 (1961).

Sjöstrand, F. S.: The molecular architecture of cell membrane and cytoplasmic membranes, Proc. First Internat. Pharmacol. Meeting, 4, 1-14 (1963).

Wolman, M.: Study of the nature of lysosomes and of their acid phosphatase, Z. Zellf., 65, 1-9 (1965).

_____ and H. Wiener: Structure of the myelin sheath as a function of concentration of ions, Biochim. Biophys. Acta, 102, 269-279 (1965).

_____ and J. J. Bubis: The relation of various enzymes to cellular membranes. Histochemie 7 105-115 (196).

H. J. COLMANT

SOME REMARKS ABOUT EXPERIMENTAL BRAIN EDEMA

One of the experimental methods of brain edema production is the unilateral ligation of internal carotid artery combined with oxygen deficiency or carbon monoxide inhalation. This technique, originally introduced by Levine, results in infarction and swelling of one of the hemispheres allowing chemical, histochemical or pharmacological comparisons with the uninvolved side. The rate of edema development generally correlates with the extent of infarction and time interval following hypoxia.

Together with Dr. Manweiler from the Pette Institute in Hamburg, we undertook some electron microscopic studies of this preparation applying CO-poisoning, and we observed an enormous swelling of endothelial cells which nearly closed the lumina of capillaries. The edema is closely related to the focal neuronal necrosis; however, in a few cases with longer survival time, we observed a patchy myelin loss with perifocal gliosis but without any evident neuronal depletion. In these cases the succinic dehydrogenase preparations revealed only hyperactive axon swellings without fading of the neuropil. There thus exists a pure focal edema in hypoxidosis, which may or may not be complicated by hypercapnia and other factors.

Another point I would like to discuss is the effect of drugs such as urea on brain edema. This can be evaluated by comparative planimetry of both hemispheres. In untreated rats we have seen relative enlargements of the damaged hemisphere up to 50% and more. The effect of different drugs has been evaluated in this laboratory in collaboration with Fodor and Szücs using as parameters volumetric changes and survival percentage of treated animals. Several drugs, especially 4-chloro N(2 furylmethyl)-5-sulfamoyle-anthranile-acid (Lasix) have remarkable effects on the sequelae of cerebral hypoxemia produced by carbon monoxide intoxication, which, untreated, has about 50% mortality in our experiments. Surprisingly enough, a protective effect also could be shown by extractions of chestnuts (Venostasin) administered before CO-poisoning.

With respect to the paper of Dr. Zeman, I would like to comment upon histochemical findings, especially those concerning the oxidative enzymes. In areas of cellular necrosis, there is a prompt depletion of activity of enzymes such as succinic dehydrogenase, DPN- and TPN-diaphorase and pyrimidine, nucleotide-linked dehydrogenases. On the other hand, the adjacent area of edema shows no fading of enzymatic reactions. Only numerous holes can be seen in the white or gray matter. This indicates that edema by itself does not damage the cellular structures which display enzymatic activities.

Otherwise, preparations for TPN-diaphorase and TPN-linked dehydrogenases demonstrate that in the astroglia the enzyme activities rise very early in the perifocal zone after hypoxic damage. In areas of necrosis, astroglia disappear; on the other hand, early astrocytic reaction can be observed in extensive areas of the damaged hemispheres without any conspicuous pathology demonstra in Nissl-preparations. I think these findings are directly related to discrete or diffuse blood-brain barrier disturbances and represent active defense mechanisms of the cell. I would disagree that these are purely regressive phenomena. This does not exclude alteration of cell membranes in the nervous tissue elements other than astrocytes, as mentioned in Dr. Zeman's paper.

Capillaries and small veins show an increased alkaline phosphatase activity only after several days. Here this increased enzymatic activity must depend largely on elevated resorptive demands in the tissue.

In summary, application of a multiplicity of methods reveals findings in the nervous tissue which cannot be interpreted merely as reaction to tissue damage, e.g., resorption of tissue debris, but they should be assessed as active processes in certain cells direct involved in development of brain edema.

RICHARD M. TORACK
MARY LOU DUFTY
JOEL S. GORDON

SPECIFICITY OF ELECTRON MICROSCOPIC LOCALIZATION OF PHOSPHATASE ACTIVITY TO CEREBRAL FINE STRUCTURE*

INTRODUCTION

The localization of a reaction product formed as a result of enzyme activity to tissue fine structures has promised a new dimension to morphological techniques. In the brain this prophetic viewpoint was enhanced by the demonstration of nucleoside phosphatase activity within various specific components of the blood-brain barrier system of the rat (Torack & Barrnett). These and other membrane bound phosphatases are believed to be involved in membrane permeability (Saw, Schwartz), and ion transfer (Skou, Post, et al.), and their involvement in barrier control mechanisms appeared unlikely. However, a realization of the potential in this method was thwarted because the histochemical demonstration of these enzymes usually lacked the specificity of a biochemical technique. The precise nature of the enzyme or enzyme system responsible for the formation of the final product remained obscure.

The hydrolysis of phosphate esters at acid, neutral and alkaline pH is generally believed to be accomplished by a group of enzymes at each pH rather than a single enzyme (Gomori, 1952a; Kaplan). In order to validly assign enzymatic activity to a specific function such as control of the blood-brain barrier some concept of at

* This investigation was supported by grant (NB-04161-03) from the National Institute of Neurological Diseases and Blindness of the National Institutes of Health.

least the number of these enzymes appeared necessary. Recently a distinction among nucleoside phosphatases in rat brain has been demonstrated following various methods of fixation (Torack, 1965a). This technique was useful in recognizing an inhibition of glutaraldehyde resistant ATP'ase activity by triethyltin intoxication (Torack, 1965b). A biochemical assay of this type of nucleoside phosphatase activity was initiated in order to prove the validity of this finding. Species differences of phosphatase activity have long been recognized (Shimizu, Glick & Fischer). A comparison of the localization of these enzymes in various animals with their response to fluid imbalance could also increase our understanding of these enzymes. Therefore a study of nucleoside phosphatase activity and alkaline phosphatase activity, by means of differential fixation, species variation, biochemical assay and electron microscopy was begun in order to more specifically characterize a histochemical demonstration of these enzyme activities.

MATERIALS AND METHODS

Young adult Sprague-Dawley rats weighing 200-300 grams, guinea pigs weighing 400-600 grams, and New Zealand white rabbits weighing 1 to 1.5 kilograms were used in this study. The brains of these animals were fixed with 4% glutaraldehyde in 0.2 M cacodylate buffer (glutal), 12.5% hydroxyadipaldehyde in 0.2 M cacodylate buffer (HAA) or 10% phosphate buffered formaldehyde, (formalin), either by perfusion or by prolonged immersion according to the technique previously described (Torack, 1965a).

Following fixation the tissue slices were washed in 0.3M sucrose and from them small ($1 mm^3$) blocks and frozen sections (25-50μ) were cut.

Enzyme Incubation

1) Adenosinetriphosphatase (ATP'ase). These tissues were incubated in the Wachstein-Meisel ATP'ase medium (Wachstein & Meisel), at pH 7.0-7.2 for 20-40 minutes at room temperature. The osmolarity of this medium was raised to 280-300 mOs by the addition of sucrose.

2) Alkaline Phosphatase. All tissues were incubated in each of two media to demonstrate phosphatase activity at pH 9.4. The first was a medium using calcium as the capture reagent as reporte by Gomori (1952b). The second technique was recently described by Mitzutani and Barrnet and utilized cadmium as the capture reagent. Both techniques utilized glycerophosphate as the substrate com-

pound and magnesium as an activator ion. Substrate specificity of these media was checked by omitting the substrate and by substituting adenosinemonophosphate as the substrate compound. Inhibition of enzyme activity was studied using adenosinemonophosphate AMP (1×10^{-1}M), potassium cyanide (1×10^{-3}M), nickel (1×10^{-2}M) and cysteine (1×10^{-3}M) in the incubating medium. In these inhibition experiments tissues were preincubated in an aqueous solution of inhibitor at the same concentration for 20 minutes. In all cases control tissues were simultaneously incubated in a medium without the inhibitor compound.

Microscopic Preparation

Those frozen sections which were to be examined with a light microscope were mounted on glass slides with glycerogelatin following conversion of the reaction product to cobalt phosphate and a development in ammonium sulfide to cobalt sulfide. Tissues to be examined with an electron microscope were not treated with cobalt and the reaction product was left as either calcium or cadmium phosphate. These tissues were not immediately osmicated, rather, they were dehydrated in graded alcohols up to 50% alcohol. At this point a mixture containing equal parts of alcohol and 2% osmium tetroxide was used to post-fix the tissue. This method had been previously recommended by Mitzutani and Barrnett in order to avoid removal of the final product by osmium. Following this post fixation the tissues were further dehydrated in alcohol and embedded in epon in the usual manner. Thin sections were cut using an LKB ultrotome and examined with an EMU 3-G electron microscope. These sections were not stained in order to avoid confusion with the reaction product.

Biochemical Assay

Each ATP'ase determination was done on a combination of two cerebral hemispheres from adult 400-500 grams Sprague-Dawley rats, which had been perfused through the ascending aorta with cold isotonic sucrose. The tissue was prepared for assay by homogenization in 2% glutaraldehyde buffered in 1 midazole HCl and dialyzation for 48 hours against deionized distilled water at 4° C. Simultaneous incubation of the homogenates for 20 minutes at 37° C, in ATP'ase medium (Gordon & Torack) with and without (1×10^{-3}M) triethyltin sulfate (TET) preceeded the addition of cold ATP solution for the determination of Mg^{++} – ATP'ase and Na^{+} – K^{+} – Mg^{++} – ATP'ase. The quantity of released phosphorus was determined by the method of Taussky and Shorr. Activity is expressed in μ gm of phosphorus per mgm of tissue per hour, with dry weight being determined on multiple 1 ml. aliquots of the homogenates.

RESULTS

Adenosinetriphosphatase

ATP'ase activity in the rat brain parenchyma following formalin fixation was noted to be present in blood vessels, oligodendrocytes and especially in corpus callosum (Fig. 1a). In the guinea pig there is an absence of the rather dense reaction product seen in the corpus callosum and corona radiata of the rat. Other sites of enzyme activity in the blood vessels and oligodendrocytes appeared similar to the rat but more activity was noted at the cortico-white matter junction (Fig. 1b). The dense fibrillar reaction product in the rat white matter was not seen in the rabbit but the oligodendrocytes of the white matter appear to be much more prominently stained than in either the guinea pig or the rat (Fig. 1c). Following glutal fixation, dense activity could be seen in rat meninges, ependymal lining, corpus callosum and corona radiata (Fig. 2a). However, in the guinea pig no such dense staining of white matter could be observed. Rather, an irregular band of diffuse staining is often present at the bottom of the cortex. Some final product is also present in blood vessels of the cortex (Fig. 2b). In rabbit cerebrum fixed with glutal, activity is only noted on the ependymal lining and meningeal surface. No definite activity is observed within the parenchyma proper (Fig. 2c). In all the brains fixed with HAA blood vessels are reacted. In only the rabbit, however, oligodendrocytes in the white matter appear prominently stained.

Triethyltin (1×10^{-3}M) inhibited the Mg^{++}-ATP'ase in six experiments by an average of 24.6% (Table 1). The control values were within the range previously obtained (Gordon & Torack). Thoug the unexpectedly low values in experiment 5 can be explained by an abnormally high dry weight, the excessive value in experiment 1 can not be explained. However, in all six determinations, despite the absolute values, a consistent relative inhibition of the Mg^{++}-ATP'ase is obtained. In contrast the TET does not inhibit the Na^{+}-K^{+}-Mg^{++}-ATP'ase.

Alkaline Phosphatase

In all species tested, the reaction product was prominently localized in blood vessels following incubation in either the calcium

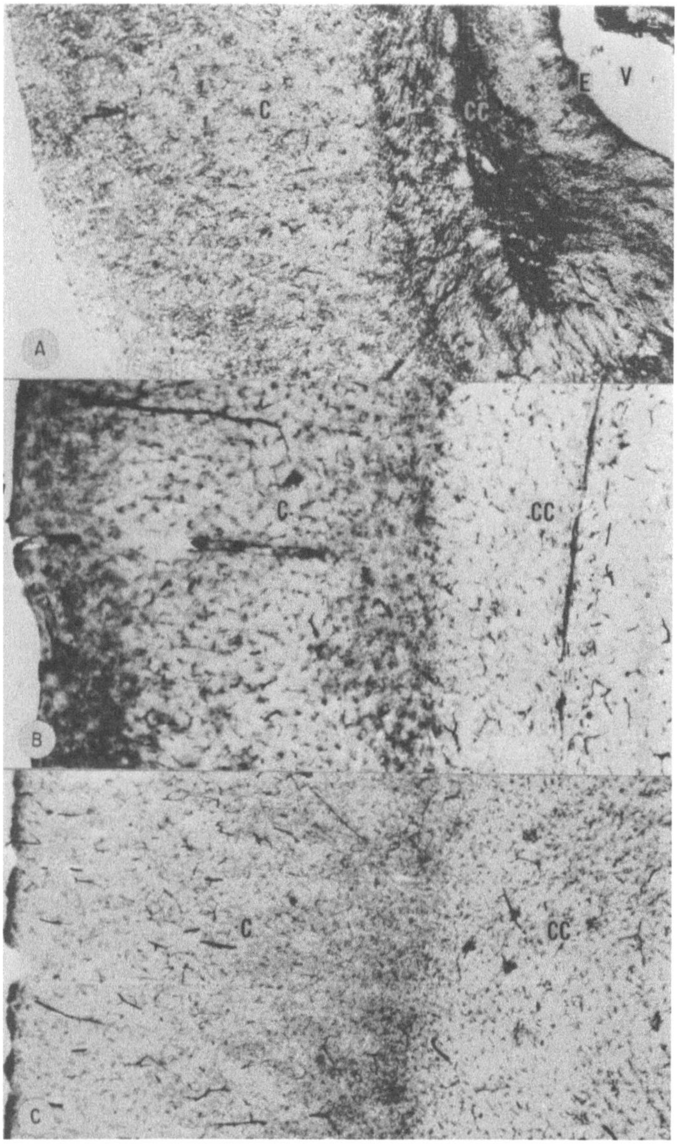

Fig. 1. (a) ATP'ase activity of rat cerebrum following formalin fixation. X25 (reduced). (b) ATP'ase activity of guinea pig cerebrum following formalin fixation. X20 (reduced). (c) ATP'ase activity of rabbit cerebrum fixed in formalin. X20 (reduced). C = cortex; CC = corpus callosum; E = ependymal lining; V = lateral ventricle.

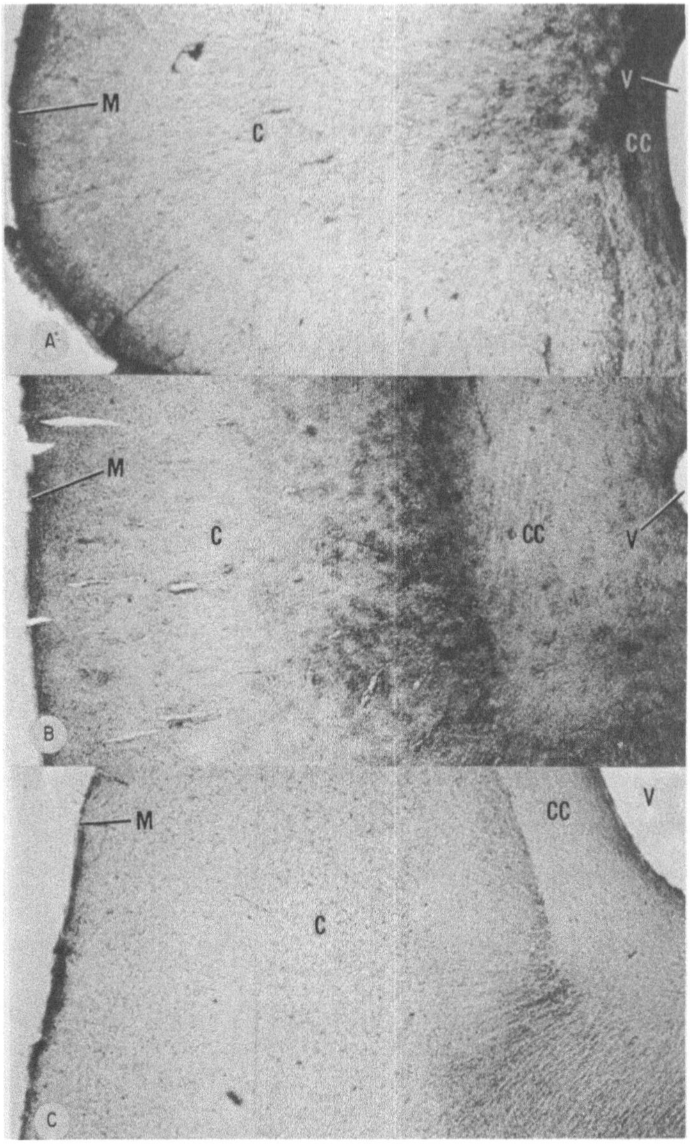

Fig. 2. (a) ATP'ase activity of rat cerebrum fixed in glutal, X25 (reduced). (b) ATP'ase activity of guinea pig cerebrum fixed in glutal. X25 (reduced). (c) ATP'ase activity of rabbit cerebrum following glutal fixation. X25 (reduced). X = meninges; C = cortex; CC = corpus callosum; V = lateral ventricle.

TABLE 1

INHIBITION OF ATP'ase BY 1×10^{-3}M TRIETHYLTIN (TET) IN GLUTARALDEHYDE TREATED RAT CEREBRUM (6 EXPERIMENTS)

	gmP/mg/ 1 hour			% inhibition of Mg
	Without TET	With TET	Difference	ATP'ase (A) by TET
1)	A- 131.0	92.6	−38.4	29.2
	B- 161.8	120.0	−41.8	
2)	A- 86.4	64.4	−22.0	25.5
	B- 124.7	107.2	−16.5	
3)	A- 88.5	64.4	−24.1	27.2
	B- 111.8	95.7	−16.1	
4)	A- 91.0	70.2	−19.8	21.7
	B- 111.2	122.5	+11.3	
5)	A- 62.0	46.4	−11.6	25.0
	B- 71.4	61.4	−10.0	
6)	A- 71.4	57.8	−13.6	19.1
	B- 91.5	71.4	−11.5	

A = Mg^{++} ATP'ase
B = Na^{+}–K^{+}–Mg^{++}–ATP'ase

or cadmium medium. The reaction product of the calcium technique appears to be most dense following HAA fixation and least dense following glutal. Actually a similar variation in the intensity of the final product is also noted in these fixatives utilizing the cadmium technique. For each of these fixatives the use of the cadmium technique resulted in a final product which is less intense than that observed using the Gomori method (Fig. 3). No reaction product is observed in either method when the substrate is eliminated or when AMP is used as the substrate. The inhibition experiments are listed in Table 2, and they indicate the similarity of the enzyme activity demonstrated by either the calcium or the cadmium technique.

Electron Microscopy

Several factors are considered important for the demonstration of a reaction product by means of electron microscopy. When formalin fixation is used, the addition of sucrose to the incubating medium appears to be particularly beneficial in maintaining fine

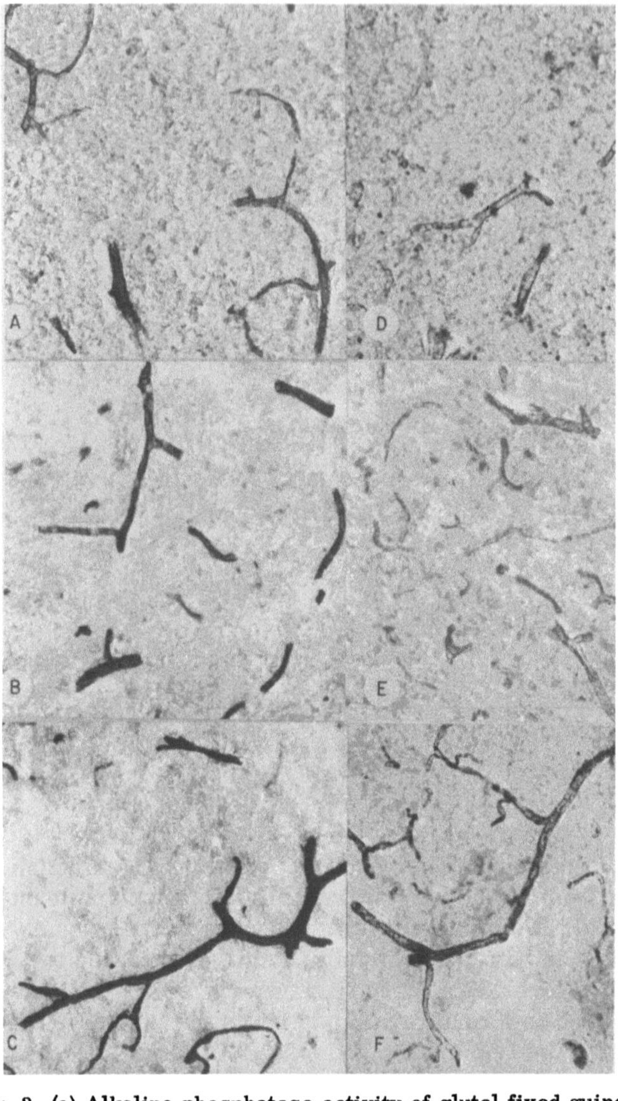

Fig. 3. (a) Alkaline phosphatase activity of glutal fixed guinea pig cerebrum using the Gomori technique. X125 (reduced). (b) Same as (a) but with formalin fixed tissue. X125 (reduced). (c) Same as (a) but with HAA fixation. X125 (reduced). (d) Alkaline phosphatase activity of glutal fixed guinea pig cerebrum using the cadmium technique of Mitzutani and Barrnett. X125 (reduced). (e) Same as (d) but in formalin fixed tissue. X125 (reduced). (f) Same as (d) but following HAA fixation. X125 (reduced).

TABLE 2

INHIBITION CHARACTERISTICS OF ALKALINE PHOSPHATASE IN GUINEA PIG CEREBRUM

	KCN (1×10^{-3}M)		Cysteine (5×10^{-3}M)		Nickel (1×10^{-2}M)		AMP (1×10^{-1}M)	
	Ca	Cd	Ca	Cd	Ca	Cd	Ca	Cd
F	-	-	-	-	-	-	-	-
G	-	-	-	-	-	-	-	-
H	-	-	-	-	-	-	-	-

F = Formaldehyde
G = Glutaraldehyde
H = Hydroxyadipaldehyde

+ = Activity
– = No activity

structure. This did not appear to be necessary following glutal fixation. When the brain was fixed in HAA, the preservation of fine structure during the incubation at pH 9.4 was extremely poor with or without the addition of sucrose. Both calcium phosphate and cadmium phosphate appeared to be removed by prolonged fixation with osmium tetroxide. Therefore, extremely brief osmication in conjunction with 50% alcohol (no longer than 30 seconds) was considered necessary to preserve significant reaction product. However, even utilizing this technique, calcium phosphate could not be visualized in the electron microscope. Rather, holes were noted in blood vessel walls where final product was observed by light microscopy. The final product may have been removed by the action of the electron beam. Therefore, all description of the ultrastructural localization of alkaline phosphatase activity will be of enzyme activity visualized with the cadmium technique.

Following formalin fixation, prominent enzyme activity could be noted on the luminal surface of endothelial cells, in pinocytic vesicles within endothelial cell cytoplasm, and on the basement membrane surface of the endothelial cell (Fig. 4). No activity was observed in the basement membrane area itself. Similar activity could be noted on the plasma membrane and in pinocytic vesicles of perithelial cells. Discrete foci of activity were also identified at the basement membrane attachment of glial end feet. Enzymatic activity was not observed in any other part of glial cell membrane (Fig. 4b). The distribution of enzyme activity on the luminal surface of the endothelial cell did not appear to be uniform but rather it was localized at periodic foci. In particular, final product was noted at indentations

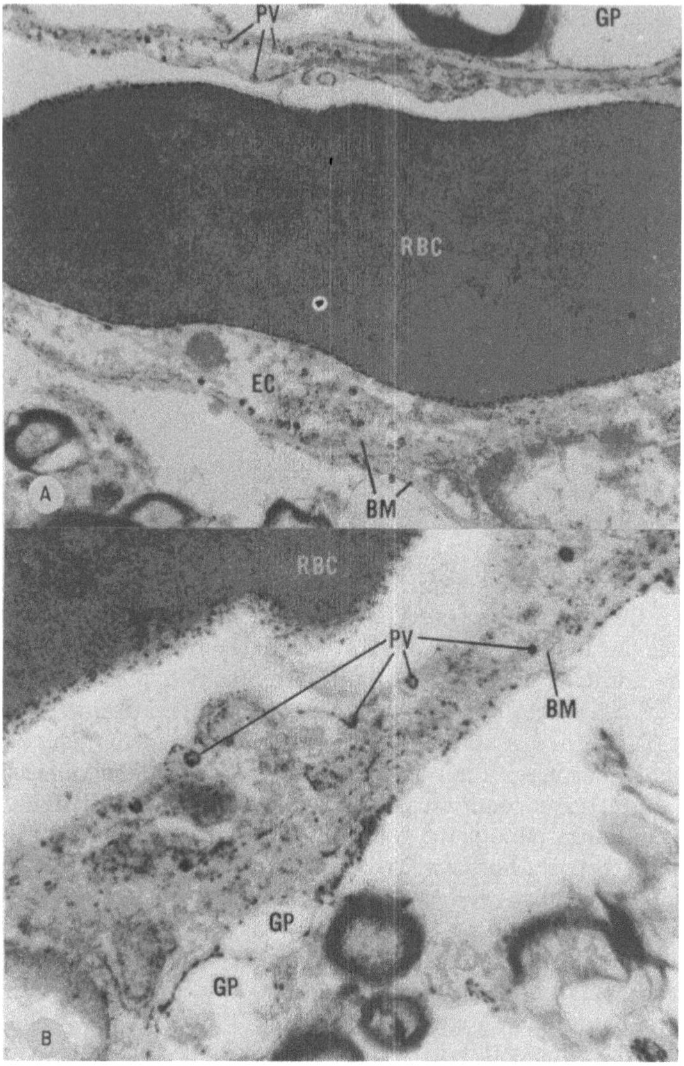

Fig. 4. (a) An electron micrograph of alkaline phosphatase activity in a capillary of guinea pig cerebrum fixed in formalin. Plasma membranes and pinocytic vesicles of endothelial cells, glial end feet and red blood cells contain the reaction product. X15,000 (reduced). (b) Alkaline phosphatase activity after formalin fixation can be seen especially on indentations of the endothelial cells and in pinocytic vesicles. No basement membrane activity is visible. X42,000 (reduced). BM = basement membrane; EC = endothelial cell; GP = glial foot process; PV = pinocytic vesicle; RBC = red blood cell.

of this membrane where pinocytic vesicles appeared to be forming (Fig. 4b). No activity was observed in cellular structures apart from the surface of blood vessels.

Following glutal fixation the localization of enzyme activity was exactly the same as that following formalin fixation (Fig. 5a). However, in general the intensity of the final product was less than that observed following formalin fixation. Following HAA fixation the tissue preservation was extremely poor (Fig. 5b). All that could be said concerning the localization of enzyme activity was that the basement membrane appeared to be devoid of activity and the final product was located in endothelial and perithelial cells.

DISCUSSION

Differential fixation, species variation, biochemical assay and ultrastructural localization contribute to a greater specificity of phosphatase activity at a neutral and alkaline pH. This degree of specificity appears to be essential if enzyme histochemistry is to increase our knowledge of normal and abnormal function at a complex physiological unit as the blood-brain barrier. The distinction in the distribution of nucleoside phosphatases previously observed following differential fixation with formalin, glutal and HAA (Torack, 1965a), was initially çharacterized by means of electron microscopy and later it could also be recognized by means of light microscopy. Although the inhibition of a glutal resistant Mg^{++}-ATP'ase in white matter by triethyltin (1×10^{-3}M) (Torack, 1965b), appears quite definite, the greater amount of reaction product present in formalin fixed or brief glutal fixed tissue masks the reduction in staining intensity due to the TET. Such inhibition by TET has now been confirmed quantitatively. However, preincubation with TET appears to be necessary since preliminary attempts to produce inhibition without preincubation failed. As a result of these findings, the validity of differential fixation as an aid to the characterization of enzyme activity appears enhanced.

A comparison of ATP'ase activity in the brains of the rat, guinea pig and rabbit reveals a marked disparity of the staining pattern. This variation chiefly involves the enzyme activity of the white matter where a dense final product is noted in the rat but not in the guinea pig or rabbit. Felgenhauer has previously noted low activity in unfixed guinea pig white matter. In the guinea pig the glutal resistant activity is at the cortico-white matter junction and not within the white matter proper, whereas the rabbit has virtually no glutal resistant activity at all. The guinea pig oligodendrocytes evince a reaction product that is similar to the rat but the oligodendrocytes

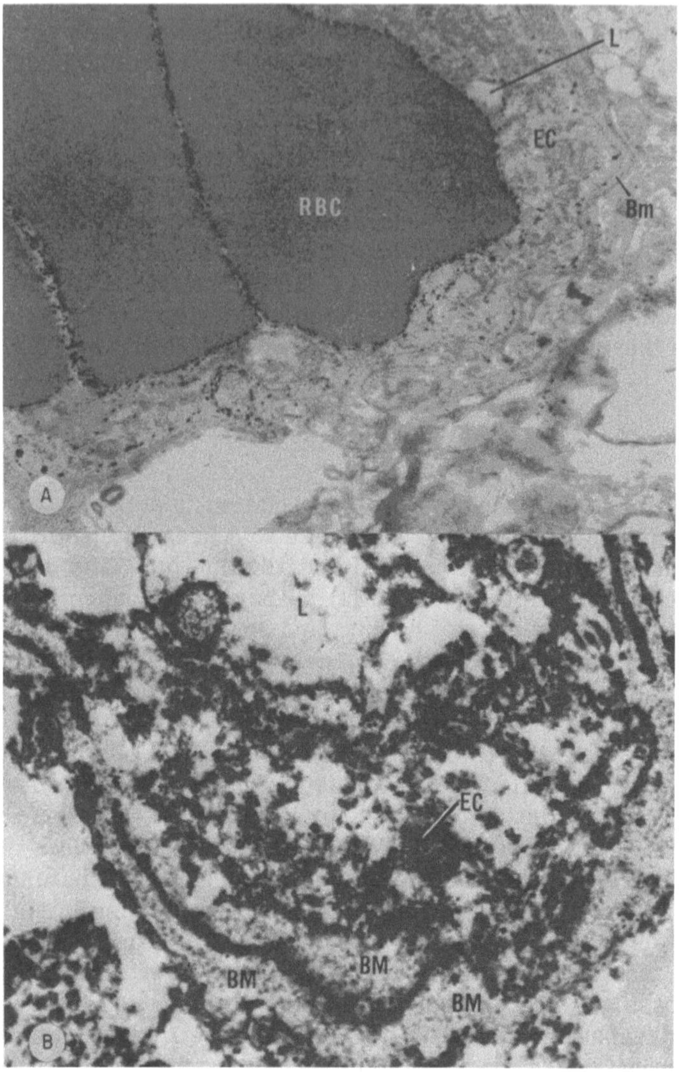

Fig. 5. (a) Alkaline phosphatase activity following glutal fixation appears to be reduced in intensity but is also located on red cells, endothelial cells and perithelial cells. X24,000 (reduced). (b) Alkaline phosphatase activity in a cerebral capillary fixed with HAA. Much activity is present, but because of poor tissue preparation, accurate localization is impossible. X30,000 (reduced). BM = basement membrane; EC = endothelial cell; L = lumen of blood vessel; RBC = red blood cell.

of the rabbit especially in the white matter appear more prominently stained. If these enzymes are involved in the blood-brain barrier system, these variations suggest either a different basis of control in these animals, a different pathway of transfer or both. Therefore when we study barrier systems in various species we may be studying control mechanisms which are peculiar to that animal and not applicable to other species, particularly the human.

An investigation of alkaline phosphatase activity by means of light microscopy reveals the reaction product of the cadmium method to be less dense than that seen using the calcium technique of Gomori. This suggests some inhibition of enzyme activity by cadmium. A variation in the intensity of the final product is also related to fixation, and in this regard glutal appears to inhibit most enzyme activity. However, since the distribution of the reaction product is always similar and since substrate specificity and inhibition characteristics are identical, a single enzyme is believed to exist at this site. In the cerebrum, this enzyme activity has been noted to be largely in blood vessels (Tewari & Bourne; Flegenhauer), and especially in endothelial cells (Bannister & Romanul; Becker, et al.).

Variation of alkaline phosphatase activity in different species has been noted previously by Shimizu. In the present study, only the guinea pig evinces a final product after all methods of fixation. Vascular staining in the rat is observed after HAA and formalin fixation, but not with glutal. Since glutal appears to inhibit more activity than the other fixatives, this probably indicates that the rat has less activity than the guinea pig. No activity is noted in the rabbit after any method of fixation. In all species, the enzyme activity is identically localized, i.e., to vascular structures.

The fine structural localization of alkaline phosphatase activity is greatly facilitated by using the technique of Mitzutani and Barrnett. Apparently cadmium phosphate is a more stable compound than calcium phosphate. Glutal appears to be the fixative of choice in the guinea pig, for ultrastructure is better preserved. However, formalin can be used satisfactorily, and appears to be necessary in animals like rats which have no activity after glutal fixation. The distribution of the reaction product is identical after either method of fixation. Unfortunately, at this pH, HAA did not result in adequate tissue fixation. The final product is very dense and poorly localized.

The localization of enzyme activity in pinocytic vesicles was also noted by Mitzutani and Barrnett. The occurrence of reaction product at indentations of endothelial plasma membrane representing sites of pinocytosis is a good indication that this enzyme is involved in membrane synthesis which is consistent with a phosphotransferase concept for this enzyme function (Saw, Schwartz). The final product on plasma membrane of endothelial and perithelial cells as well as glial foot processes suggests that the enzyme also partakes in membrane synthesis at these sites. The integrity of these membranes appears to be essential for the limited permeabil-ity characteristic of the blood-brain barrier and this may be the manner in which alkaline phosphatase partakes in barrier control.

A analysis of the data obtained for alkaline phosphatase activ-ity in the brain indicates that we can distinguish only one enzyme system at the blood-brain barrier by means of these techniques. Following differential fixation, various degrees of activity can be demonstrated but both light and electron microscopic examination reveals that the final product is located in the same place. The sim-ilarity of substrate preferences and inhibition characteristics also enhance this belief. A variation in alkaline phosphatase activity is noted in the different species tested but this probably represents less activity of the same enzyme. In contrast to alkaline phosphatase when ATP'ase activity is studied at this site using these techniques, several enzymes are believed to be responsible for the hydrolysis of ATP at a neutral pH. Conclusive proof of these concepts must be ob-tained from biochemical assay, but if valid, these methods offer a practical method by which hitherto unrecognized properties of en-zyme activity may be elucidated.

Summary

1) Biochemical assay of glutal resistant ATP'ase activity re-veals a significant inhibition by triethyltin (1×10^{-3} M). This en-hances the value of differential fixation as an aid to the recognition of enzymatic change.

2) Species differences of ATP'ase and alkaline phosphatase ac-tivity emphasize the possibility that various control mechanisms or transport pathway may be present in these animals. The application of animal experiments to human problems, therefore, must be done with much caution.

3) The use of cadmium as a capture reagent appears to be a valid method for the demonstration of the same cerebrovascular alkaline phosphatase as the calcium technique. This procedure also is suitable for ultrastructural localization of this enzymatic activity

4) The localization of alkaline phosphatase activity to mem-branous fine structure of brain blood vessels and adjacent glial end feet suggest an involvement in control at the blood-brain barrier. Prominent final product at sites of pinocytosis support the belief that this enzyme is involved in new membrane formation.

5) The study of the vascular alkaline phosphatase by means of differential fixation, species variation and ultrastructural localiza-tion indicates that only one enzyme is present. The use of these con bined techniques to study enzyme characteristics is advocated.

REFERENCES

Bannister, R. G. and F. C. A. Romanul: The localization of alkaline phosphatase activity in cerebral blood vessels, J. Neurol. Neurosurg. Psychiat., 26, 333-340 (1963).

Becker, N. H., S. Goldfischer, W. Y. Shin and A. B. Novikoff: The localization of enzyme activities in the rat brain, J. Biophys. Biochem. Cytol., 8, 649-663 (1960).

Felgenhauer, K.: The localization of specific and nonspecific phosphatases in the guinea pig brain, Z. Zellforsch., 60, 518-531 (1963).

Glick, D. and E. E. Fischer: The histochemical localization of adenosinetriphosphatase in plant and animal tissue, Science, 102, 429-430 (1945).

Gomori, G.: In: Microscopic Histochemistry: Principles and Practice. Chicago: Univ. Chicago Press (1952a).

_____: The complex nature of alkaline phosphatase, Biochim. Biophys. Acta (Amsterdam), 8, 162-172 (1952b).

Gordon, J. S. and R. M. Torack: Inhibition of cerebral adenosine triphosphate (ATP'ase) activity by various aldehyde fixatives, J. Neurochem. (in press).

Kaplan, N. O.: Symposium on multiple forms of enzymes and control mechanisms; I Multiple forms of enzymes, Bact. Rev., 27, 155-169 (1963).

Mitzutani, A. and R. J. Barrnett: Fine structure demonstration of phosphatase activity at pH 9, Nature (London), 206, 1001-1003 (1965).

Post, R. L., C. R. Merritt, C. R. Kinsolving and C. D. Albright: Membrane adenosinetriphosphatase as a participant in the active transport of sodium and potassium in the human erythrocytes, J. Biol. Chem., 235, 1796-1802 (1960).

Saw, G. K.: Some concepts of the intracellular function of alkaline phosphatase based on investigation of the mechanism of their action, Enzymologia, 26, 169-175 (1963).

Schwartz, J. H.: The phosphorylation of alkaline phosphatase, Proc. Acad. Sci. (United States), 49, 871-878 (1963).

Shimizu, N.: Histochemical studies on the phosphatase of the nervous system, J. Comp. Neurol., 93, 201-219 (1950).

Skou, J. C.: Preparation from the mammaliam brain and kidney of the enzyme system involved in the active transport of sodium and potassium, Biochem. Biophys. Acta., 58, 314-325 (1962).

Taussky, H. H. and E. Shorr: A microcolorimetric method for the determination of inorganic phosphorus, J. Biol. Chem., 202, 675-

Tewari, H. B. and G. H. Bourne: Histochemical studies on the distribution of alkaline and acid phosphatase and 5′ nucleoside in the cerebellum of the rat, J. Anat. (London), 97, 65-72 (1963).

Torack, R. M. and R. J. Barrnett: The fine structural localization of nucleoside phosphatase activity in the blood-brain barrier, J. Neuropath. Exp. Neurol., 23, 46-59 (1964).

_____: Adenosinetriphosphatase activity in rat brain following differential fixation with formaldehyde, glutaraldehyde and hydroxyadipaldehyde, J. Histochem. Cytochem., 13, 191-205 (1965a).

_____: The relationship between adenosinetriphosphatase activity and triethyltin toxicity in the production of cerebral edema of the rat, Amer. J. Path., 46, 245-261 (1965b).

Wachstein, M. and E. Meisel: Histochemistry of hepatic phosphatase at a physiologic pH with special reference to the demonstration of bile canaliculi, Amer. J. Path., 27, 13-27 (1957).

DISCUSSION

CLASEN: I would like to second Dr. Pappius's findings that the edema associated with cold lesions is not affected by intravenous hypertonic urea. We obtained similar results (Arch. Neurol. 12: 424-434).

TOWER: I would like to congratulate Dr. Pappius on her studies, which are very clear and nicely done. They confirm part of Dr. Clasen's work, as he has pointed out, and also correlate very well with work done in 1939 by Stewart-Wallace (Brain 62: 426, 1939) on effects of brain tumors in human brain. His findings were very similar, based on techniques which at that time must have been rather formidable.

I would also like to confirm what Dr. Katzman said about the effects of fixation on the maintenance of membrane barriers. We have carried out somewhat analogous studies to determine how much increase in permeability to sucrose or inulin would occur after fixation of slices of cerebral cortex with osmium. It is remarkable how well these molecules are excluded from areas to which you would expect them to have access after fixation. The only means by which we were able to increase markedly the sucrose spaces of osmium-fixed slices of cerebral cortex was to treat them with deoxycholate which solubilizes much of the lipid moieties of the membranes.

One question to Dr. Torack. What is his evidence for the areas of enzyme activity which he calls pinocytotic vesicles actually being pinocytotic vesicles? It seems to me these might represent portions of endoplasmic reticulum or they might be artifacts of fixation. I think it would be helpful to know whether Dr. Torack can be sure about his interpretation.

Finally, I want to encourage Dr. Terry in the work he reported, because we all badly need to be able to accomplish what he is attempting in these studies.

TORACK: As to the problem of vesicles being formed artifactually due to the fixation, perhaps some caution is necessary, but certainly there is a good deal of evidence that these vesicles are real structures. In some vessels, as cardiac capillaries, they are found in much greater profusion in normal unreactive tissue than in similar structures in the brain. We find the enzyme activity distributed in the same numerical relationship, less in the brain and more in cardiac capillaries. The indentation that I demonstrated is compatible with a vesicle forming at the surface membrane as a pinocytotic vesicle should form. In some vesicles a membrane can be clearly distinguished surrounding the reaction product. It is for these reasons that we feel quite strongly that these structures do represent pinocytotic vesicles.

KLATZO: I was greatly impressed by the presentation of Dr. Torack and I would like to ask him whether he observed the enzymatic activity also at the lateral margins of endothelial cells where they are adjacent to each other in enclosing a vascular lumen. My question is related to an exquisite demonstration by Dr. Lampert of thorotrast entrapped between the endothelial cells in its escape from the vascular lumen. Similarly, in experimental damage of the blood-brain barrier we have observed the passage of fluorescein labeled proteins between the endothelial cells and not directly through their cytoplasm.

TORACK: Dr. Klatzo, we did show glutaraldehyde-resistant ATPase activity in tight junctions between glial foot processes. However, I have never seen a similar activity at tight junctions between endothelial cells. Actually, we did not see any nucleoside phosphatase activity on the luminal surface of the endothelial cell. The alkaline phosphatase activity did not appear to extend between endothelial cells into these areas of tight junction. It appeared to be on the luminal surface as scattered foci and also related to pinocytotic vesicles but not at tight junctions between cells.

STEINBEREITHNER: I would like to ask Dr. Pappius some questions from a clinical point of view. Though she has shown that osmotic edema and posttraumatic edema are different clinically, cases of cerebral trauma which have to be dialysed because of crush syndrome, etc., do very badly with hemodialysis. They may become unconscious and show fits or even status epilepticus. Now, some go into acute brain edema, or whatever you may call it, and some do not. Have you at least any suspicion of what may be the reason for this, so that the treatment in endangered cases could be avoided? Isn't there also a time factor involved in this dialysing edema? I remember a case on our intensive care station where we had to stop dialysis after half an hour every time, while, strangely enough, sodium went up from 150 to 170 milliequivalents per liter though another coil was operating in the same dialysing fluid for a uremic case, which made an uneventful course. When we put this patient on gastric dialysis, pouring in 10 liters of distilled water per day and draining off the water, we could deal easily with his hyperelectrolytemia. Have you ever made determinations of chloride in these cases, since we have the impression that hyperchloremic acidosis plays some role?

PAPPIUS: I am not a clinician, so I cannot speak with authority on the clinical aspects of this problem. However, the following observations may be of interest in this respect. In ou experiments we wanted to follow the changes in the water content of cerebral tissues over a period of time. Initially to do this we did not compare groups of dogs before and after hemodialysis, but we took serial biopsies in individual animals. It was our impression that there was a greater tendency for what we call traumatic cerebral edema to develop in the tissues of the uremic dogs. Thus we could take three or four serial biopsies in normal dogs over a period of up to four hours without the development of edema, while in the uremic dogs the incidence of edema due to traumatic damage of the earlier biopsies appeared to be much higher. Thus the uremic condition may be a complicating factor in cases of cerebral edema due to trauma. On the other hand, it is our impression that the changes in water content of the brain during hemodialysis are very transient. This is quite understandable, since, contrary to assumptions made in the literature, urea is fairly rapidly removed from the brain during dialysis, and after dialysis is terminated, it comes back to equilibrium with urea in the plasma within about an hour or so. It may be of interest to you, however, that while we had only about 50% incidence of swelling of cerebral tissues at the end of 60 minutes of dialysis, the incidence of increased CSF pressure was 100%. This was true of both the uremic dogs on ordinary dialysis and of normal dogs on hypotonic dialysis. In normal dogs on isotonic dialysis, no changes in CSF pressure were observed. This leads us to believe that there are some direct osmotic effects on the volume of the CSF, so that the CSF pressure invariably increases although swelling is not as great a factor as one could expect.

We did not do any chloride analyses.

ZÜLCH: I think we must be very careful to deduce from animal experiments which are called traumatic to trauma which happens in man, because what Dr. Klatzo produces is a local necrosis which probably does not affect the brain stem. What happens in man, even in smaller necrotic lesions, is a disorganization of most of the vegetative functions of the brain stem. I wonder if you can compare what was seen by Dr. Steinbereithner and what has been seen by Dr. Pappius with regard to various parameters. You probably have to make a severe contusion in animal in order to be able to compare results. That is my personal impression and I tried to emphasize this yesterday morning.

REULEN: Dr. Pappius, we have done similiar studies with administration of urea in experimental traumatic brain edema and it was interesting to hear that you could find no significant changes in water and sodium content edematous brain tissue 12 to 24 hours after urea administration. From our own experience, I would like to stress the importance of the timing of the determinations. When we measure the water, sodium and potassium content of edematous rat brain tissue at different intervals after urea infusion, we find a sharp decrease of water content of about 2% after 20 to 30 min. Three hours later the water content increased to normal preedematous values, and after 9 to 12 hours we observed a rather pronounced and significant rebound effect. This course can also be seen by the neurosurgeon during operations, when urea is administered previously. I would like to emphasize that the high sodium values of edematous tissue changed less after urea. We think this is a proof of osmotic effect of urea on the brain tissue. Furthermore, we have evidence that this unaltered high sodium, together with the negative osmotic gradient of urea after 9 - 12 hours, is the cause of the rebound effect. (Zbl. Neurochir., 4/5; 1965).

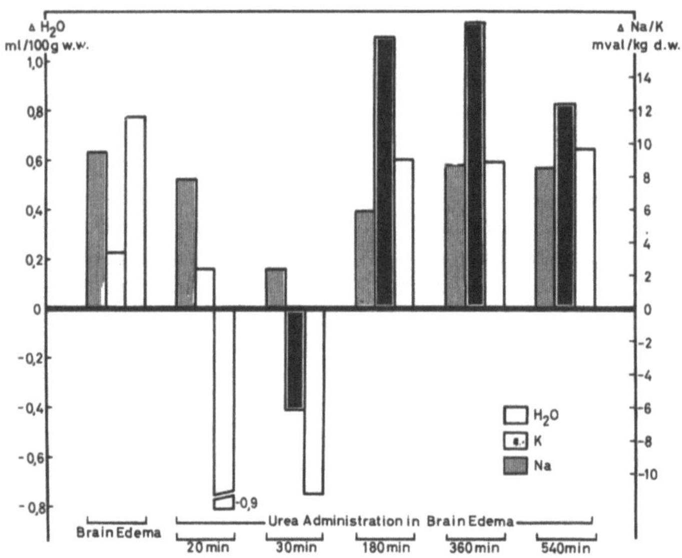

Dr. Steinbereithner, perhaps I may answer your question. If the dialysis is performed very rapidly and the removal of the urea from the blood is faster than the permeability rate of urea from the brain, there is a developing negative osmotic gradient between blood and, depending on the velocity of dialysis, CSF or brain tissue with subsequent osmotic swelling of the brain. When the dialysis is performed at a slow rate, the urea of the brain can equilibrate with the serum urea, or, if serum osmolarity during dialysis is maintained by osmotic substances like Mannitol, such side-effects have never been seen.

PAPPIUS: I am not quite sure that I understand your point. What I would like to say is this: We studied the water content, the urea content and the sodium and potassium content of the brain during 24 hours after urea administration. In our experience there was a significant dehydration of the cortex from about 15 minutes to 2 hours after the administration of urea, and of the white matter up to 3 hours. There was a penetration of urea into both tissues and the urea content of the brain came to equilibrium with that of plasma within 4 and 6 hours. Thereafter there was a loss of urea from the plasma and a concomitant loss of urea from cerebral tissues. I could never demonstrate any osmotic imbalance with regard to urea between tissues and plasma, once equilibrium has been reached at the high concentration, and I could never demonstrate any rebound swelling of the tissues. The dry weight, once it came back to normal from the elevated levels associated with dehydration, always remained within normal limits. Following urea administration in cats, there was no evidence of a rebound phenomenon.

REULEN: The uptake of urea in the brain is much slower in rats than in cats and dogs.

PAPPIUS: I have the impression that the dog is different from the cat and the rat. My studies on effects of urea infusion were done in cats.

FLEISCHHAUER: I should like to ask Dr. Katzman two questions. In your electron micrographs you showed two entirely different types of edema. Are there no differences whatsoever between these two types which could be detected by means of light microscopy after myelin staining? Considering that in one type of edema the myelin sheath is destroyed early, whereas in the other type of edema there is first an extracellular swelling, it seems to me very odd that there should be no differences detectable by light microscopy.

What was the concentration of glutaraldehyde in your fixation experiments and what was the composition of the buffer?

KATZMAN: What I demonstrated today was not electron micrographs but drawings of electron micrographs. The original electron micrographs were done by various collaborators of Dr. Terry, and I'll ask him to answer your first question. However, as to the concentration of the glutaraldehyde, this was a 3% glutaraldehyde in an isotonic sodium-phosphate buffer. The total osmolarity of the buffer was 600 mosm.; that is double the amount of the usual osmolarity of the serum. And yet this high osmolarity did not dehydrate the brain, as, for example, urea would if it had been the osmotic agent. Therefore, one must assume that the glutaraldehyde moves quite freely into the tissue, and, in fact, this is what you see, because fixation takes place almost immediately. Therefore, the effective osmotic pressure of the perfusate is due to the sodium phosphate and not to glutaraldehyde present.

TERRY: First I might just add to Dr. Katzman's comments with regard to concentration of fixative, that we have done extensive experiments as to tonicity as, I think, has Dr. Torack. We find that osmolarities up to 2000 milliosmols make no apparent difference in fixation quality for electron microscopy. Now with regard to light microscopic differences, people who have studied triethyl tin-poisoned animals and human brains have almost concluded that the material was extracellular, simply because the myelin looks somewhat pale and as if it were separated by wide spongy spaces. Obviously this edema is not truly extracellular but rather within myelin lamellae which cannot be seen in the light microscope. In the cold edema there is a somewhat similar appearance in the light microscope, although with more careful examination the individual myelin sheaths appear quite well stained. They are intact but separated from one another.

CUMINGS: May I just comment on that last statement? Kalsbeck and I, in the tin edema, did, in fact, state both from the point of view of histology as well as that of biochemistry that the changes were within the myelin sheath and not extracellular.

ZÜLCH: Didn't you promise us some electron micrographs of Dr. Mair? Are these available?

CUMINGS: We did not report on the electron microscopic studies, but I believe Dr. W. G. P. Mair has some slides. I have not got them here. I have only the ones from the monkey, which I showed.

LEE: I just want to confirm Dr. Terry's statement about the osmolarity of fixatives for electron microscopy. I had measured the osmolarity of 3—5% glutaraldehyde in veronal-acetate buffer with or without $CaCl_2$ and NaCl, being ranged from 600 to 950 milliosmols. I used this fixative of various osmolarities and found no observable differences in the quality of electron micrographs among them.

SIESJÖ: I have two questions to Dr. Pappius and to Dr. Katzman. There are many studies on experimental edema, both on triethyl tin edema and on other types where we have valuable information about the sodium and potassium concentrations in the tissue. Are there corresponding studies on the anion concentrations? This would be interesting to know since, normally, the ions seem to be differentially distributed between the plasma and the CSF, and it appears that the DC potential between these two compartments has got something to do with it. The other thing is that when we speak about ionic concentrations in this context we are, of course, referring to contents. Do you have any information on the concentrations of these ions in CSF? This should be important, since a small concentration change, e.g., of sodium in the CSF, might lead to a marked change in the sodium content of the tissue as a whole.

KATZMAN: The concentration of chloride in these tissues closely parallels the serum concentration of chloride, as you have seen in your own experiments reported today and as Woodbury reported some ten years ago. It seems to follow quite passively in this regard. So far as the concentration in the CSF in those instances in which this has been measured is concerned, the potassium concentration was maintained at its usual level of 3 mosm., which is less than the serum potassium concentration, except where there is gross injury to the adjacent brain. I have not carried out experiments with the water edema, and I had better not comment on that.

PAPPIUS: In uremic dogs dialyzed with isotonic fluid, the sodium in the CSF remained unchanged. Of course, when normal dogs are dialyzed with hypotonic, low-sodium, fluid, the sodium content of the plasma drops sharply and there is a decrease in the sodium content of the CSF, which is, however, much smaller than the drop in the plasma. On the basis of our experiments, it is impossible to say anything about the distribution of the ions within the tissue, whether it is extracellular or not.

HUSZÁK: I would like to ask Dr. Pappius whether the cation binding capacity of protein and lipids plays a role here. A certain quantity of the lipids, those easily hydrolysable, can be split in the brain edema and an increased proteolytic activity may be assumed. I mean the changes in the composition of the lipid and protein components presumably may alter their cation binding capacity.

PAPPIUS: In our experiments, the sodium increase in the edematous brain is very close to what you would expect if the fluid taken up by the tissue was a plasma filtrate. In other words, there is no evidence of any binding of cations, but small amounts of binding would not be demonstrated with our techniques.

IV. Experimental Studies on Brain Edema (Continued)

Chairman: ***H. M. Zimmerman***

LOUIS BAKAY

RADIO-ISOTOPIC STUDIES IN BRAIN EDEMA*

The original source of the tissue fluid of the central nervous system, whether normal or edematous, is the blood plasma. Consequently, the exchange of water and solutes between plasma and normal as well as edematous brain and their distribution within the various intracerebral compartments is of considerable importance. Data available in man in terms of molecular tissue morphology and chemistry are too few for the evaluation of the biological forces involved in the production of edema. This, at the present time, is largely limited to experimental edemas. These experimental, and consequently artificial, conditions are sometimes completely analogous with the conditions affecting man. Other experimental situations are probably similar to, but not identical with, their human equivalent. However, at the present stage of our limited knowledge about the pathophysiology of the different types of cerebral edemas. controlled investigations are indispensable. The application of radioactive and non-radioactive tracers to study the rate of exchange of various compounds between plasma and edematous brain places a heavy emphasis on experimental work.

This review aims to summarize briefly our present knowledge on the dynamic exchange of substances between plasma and edematous brain tissue under various experimental circumstances, with special regard to the author's own experience.

*This study was supported by research grant NB03754 from the U.S. Public Health Service.

TRAUMATIC BRAIN SWELLING

Cold-induced Edema

It is known, particularly since the experiments of Clasen, et al., and Klatzo, et al. (1958), that superficial freezing of the brain is followed by widespread edema of the white matter which reaches its maximum about 24 hours after cold application. Electron microscopic examinations revealed an enlargement of the clear glia cells and their processes, particularly in the vicinity of the blood vessels (Torack, et al.). Lee and Bakay found, in addition to the enlargement of the clear glia cells, an increase in the extracellular space in the white matter. The increased electron density of the content of this space suggested that the fluid is proteinaceous. The electron density decreased in direct proportion with the distance from the frozen lesion. When ferritin was used as a tracer, it spread into the white matter via extracellular as well as intracellular routes.

The expansion of the extracellular space in the white matter, seen by the electron microscope, is in good agreement with recent reports by Streicher, et al. These authors found that at the height of cold-induced edema, the thiocyanate space of the tissue increased from 14% to 33% and the chloride space from 30% to 50%.

The protein and electrolyte concentration (Klatzo, et al., 1958; Bakay & Haque) in cold-induced edema suggests that the fluid resembles plasma. It seems to be well established that the abnormal changes in protein concentration and in ion distribution within the edematous white matter depend on the severity of the edema and on the distance between the primary cortical lesion and the white matter. Consequently, the regional changes in the chemistry of the brain tissue have to be known before the dynamic exchange of labeled substances between plasma and edematous brain tissue can be properly evaluated.

The water content of the edematous white matter directly under the cortical lesion increases by about 20%. The albumin content increases to about 17 times that of normal (Klatzo, et al., 1958; Bakay & Haque) found that radioactive albumin penetrated both lesion and edema from the blood stream. The RISA content of edematous brain and cortical lesion closely followed that of plasma. Radioautography revealed a striking change that occurred with the lapse of time from the time of the injection. One hour after injection, RISA concentrated only in that portion of the edematous white matter that was in closest vicinity to the lesion, although edema had already involved much of the white matter of the ipsilateral hemisphere. At this time radioactivity of remote areas of edema was only slightly higher than normal. The spread of RISA in the edematous brain was seen well at the six-and 24-hour stages, respectively. Microscopic examination revealed that RISA under normal conditions did not penetrate normal cerebral cortex or white matter to any significant degree. The granules representing radioactive albumin, however, could be seen in edematous white matter, although never in such concentration as to equal or even to approximate that of the plasma.

Bakay and Haque found that sodium and potassium values obtained in the severely traumatized frozen part of the cortex were practically identical with that of plasma. This is not surprising considering the appearance of the lesion which is one of a hemorrhagic infarct with little of the original tissue remaining. However, there was a considerable variation in the electrolyte content of various portions of the edematous white matter. The sodium concentration showed definite correlation with the distance of the tissue examined from the lesion in the form of a concentration gradient. The highest concentration only slightly less than that of plasma, was found in the edematous tissue next to the frozen cortex. Sodium decreased in the remote area of edema to 70-80 mM/Kg. It began to approach values for normal brain tissue 45-50 mM/Kg.) in the peripheral areas of edema. Calculations showed that the increased sodium content of edematous white matter exceeded any increments that could be calculated from over-hydration alone. Potassium remained uniformly distributed throughout the edematous white matter. Its concentration, when related to wet weight, was between 60% and 70% of that of normal brain potassium. This was undoubtedly caused by the increase of water content of the tissue rather than by an actual loss of potassium from the cells. Similar values for sodium and potassium and in edematous white matter were obtained by Pappius and Gulati.

After intravenous injection of Na^{24} and K^{42} respectively, the frozen cortical lesion was more radioactive than normal brain tissue, and the Na^{24} and K^{42} content of the lesion more or less paralleled that of the plasma. The declining radioactivity of the lesion indicates a fast exchange of sodium and potassium with that in the plasma and contrasts with the slow exchange between plasma and normal brain tissue which manifests itself by a slowly increasing radioactivity of the latter. The Na^{24}, K^{42} and P^{32} content of edematous white matter followed a course that was halfway between that of the frank lesion and the normal brain. Individual analysis of the various radioactive ions as well as radioautography revealed a wide variety of Na^{24}, K^{42} and P^{32} concentration in the edematous white matter. During the first hour after injection, high isotope concentration was found only in that portion of the edematous area that was immediately adjacent to the cortical infarct. With lapse of time, the wave of increased isotope concentration reached deeper and deeper into the edematous tissue. When expressed in terms of specific activity; equilibrium of Na^{24} between plasma and the cortical lesion is practically instantaneous and is followed by an equilibrium between plasma and edematous white matter.

Although sodium in the edematous brain does not reach an equilibrium with that in the plasma immediately, the exchange between it and the sodium pool of the blood is reasonably rapid and includes all parts of the edematous white matter. Actually, there is a gradual decrease in Na^{24} concentration from the zone adjacent to the cortical lesion to portions of the edematous white matter that are further away from the lesion, but this decrease in radioactivity is in direct proportion to the decrease in Na^+ content of the tissue. The specific activity, therefore, does not change significantly within various parts of the edematous white matter. The exchange of K^+ between blood and the cortical infarct is very rapid, just as it was for Na^+. This is obviously due to the fact that the cold-induced infarct is saturated with plasma and is much closer chemically to plasma than it is to normal cerebral cortex. The specific activity for K^+ in edematous white matter is gradually decreased at increasing distances from the lesion. The discrepancy between specific activity in various parts of the edematous zone does not change significantly with the lapse of time, and an equilibrium with the K^{42} of plasma is not reached in 24 hours. These results indicate that various substances have a definite port of entry to the edematous white matter. This place is the marginal zone of the cortical area of injury. The spread is gradual and rather slow, not only for larger molecules, but also for ions.

Recently, Klatzo, et al. (1962), studied the movement of fluores cein-labeled protein microscopically in cold-induced edema. They came to the conclusion that this substance is extravasated from injured blood vessels and diffuses throughout the extracellular space of the edematous white matter, since its distribution did not appear to be spatially related to any cell. Nevertheless, the relative importance of intracellular transport of the various test substances and their mediation in the extracellular pathway has not been solved and will probably not be known until distribution and movement of various agents can be adequately visualized at the electron microscopic level.

Study of the distribution of radioactive tracers correlated to the chemical changes of the brain tissue rendered edematous by cortical freezing leaves little doubt that the source of this edema is the leakage of fluid from injured blood vessels in the area rendered necrotic by direct freezing. Additional escape of water and Na might occur in areas of edema more remote from the primary lesion, but such secondary factors are probably of not much significance.

Other Traumatic Edemas

An increase in the albumin content of the edematous brain tissue, similar to cold-induced edema, was found by Sperl, et al., in brain swelling produced by the implantation of dried psyllium seeds into the brain substance. Pappius and Gulati studied the water and electrolyte content of edematous brain tissue next to experimental lobectomy. The Na^+ concentration was high and the potassium concentration was decreased. The values are practically identical with those seen in cold-induced edema. In none of these experiments was the dynamic equilibrium of various constituents between plasma and edematous brain tissue studied with tracers. Recently, Cutler, et al., studied the movement of I^{125} -labeled serum albumin in brain tissue rendered edematous by balloon compression. The results of their experiments, and the gross and microscopic radioautograms on the cerebral deposition of radioactive albumin, were in good agreement with the findings of Bakay and Haque obtained with I^{131} -labeled albumin in cold-induced edema. Cutler, et al., raised the question of a possible metabolic breakdown of radioactive albumin within the brain with a subsequent intracellular localization of I^{125} that is not bound to the original albumin. The bulk of the radioactive albumin, however, was obviously intact. The question as to whether intracellular I^{125} represents a metabolic breakdown product or the incorporation of the I^{125} -labeled albumin into the cell by pinocytosis remains unanswered.

INFLAMMATORY EDEMA

Inflammatory edema can be produced in animals by intracerebral injection of various substances. Levine, et al., found that significant cerebral edema followed the intracerebral administration of several agents such as endotoxins, killed and dried micro-organisms, bacterial capsular polysaccharides and purified protein derivative of tuberculin (PPD). Both PPD and endotoxin have chemotactic properties and excite leukocytic diapedesis. This results in a neutrophil exudate which spreads into the white matter while on the other hand the gray matter is relatively unaffected.

Studies of Gonatas, et al., of the ultrastructure of inflammatory edema indicated that the significant changes are in the white matter; the extracellular space was definitely enlarged in the edematous white matter. Hirano, et al., demonstrated that the excess fluid occupies the extracellular space during the acute phase. Their electron microscopic examination indieates that the edema fluid is not uniform but consists of a combination of the polysaccharide solution and plasma exudate.

The exchange of radioactive isotopes between blood and edema fluid produced by the induction of PPD and graphite was studied by Katzman, et al. (1964). Using $S^{35}O_4$, they found in acute experiments that the inorganic sulfate space increased to about 30% of volume in the edematous white matter as compared with a normal value of 2% to 4%. A similar enlargement of the albumin space was also noticed in the edematous tissue when studied with RISA. There is some uncertainty at the present time as to the reliability of the measurement of the inorganic sulfate space with S^{35}, since the possibility exists that some S^{35} leaks into the cerebrospinal fluid and is, therefore, lost from the brain tissue. The strong possibility also exists that some S^{35} partakes in metabolic functions and is deposited within the glial cells.

Katzman, et al. (1964), also found that the edematous white matter showed a greater accumulation of Na^+ and an increased uptake of Na^{24}; however, the uptake of Na^{24} was increased in the entire brain including portions that were not swollen. This suggests that the increase in Na^+ uptake is not entirely related to the accumulation of edema fluid. Among the possible contributing factors, Katzman, et al. (1964), considered an increase in the rate of cerebral blood flow or an alteration in the transport processes involved in the movement of Na^{24} from blood to brain.

TRIETHYLTIN EDEMA

Selective edema of the central nervous system can be produced by the administration of alkyl tin compounds (Magee, et al.). Cerebral edema produced by triethyltin is easily reproducable; it has been extensively studied although the exact mechanism of action of this tin compound is not known at the present time. The subsequent edema is localized almost entirely in the white matter. Electron microscopic examination (Aleu, et al., 1964, and Lee & Bakay, 1965), revealed that the characteristic alteration is a splitting of the myelin sheath in the white matter of the cerebrum, cerebellum and spinal cord. The space enclosed by the split myelin lamellae contains the excess fluid. There is no significant change in the ultra structure of capillaries, glial elements and synapses. The extracellular space of both white and gray matter is not enlarged.

The water content in the edematous white matter increases by as much as 50% or more (Katzman, et al., 1963; Magee, et al.; Bakay). The Na^+ and Cl^- content of the edematous brain tissue increases while the K^+ content decreases. When the electrolytes are calculated to the dry weight of tissue, it becomes obvious that the increase in sodium and chloride is significant in edematous tissue amounting to 60-70% over normal values. Taylor, et al., found an increase of 198% in the white matter following triethyltin intoxication. The decrease of K^+ merely represents the dilution by edema fluid of low K^+ concentration (Magee, et al.; Aleu, et al., 1963; Bakay).

Of all experimental edemas studied so far triethyltin edema is the only one which is consistently lacking vital staining upon the intravascular injection of appropriate vital dyes. Investigations with radioactive isotopes (Katzman, et al., 1963; Bakay), revealed no penetration of I^{131} -labeled serum albumin in the edematous brain tissue from the blood stream at any stage of the edema. The data obtained by Bakay on the exchange of Na^{24} between plasma and normal as well as edematous brain tissue indicate that there is very little difference in the rate of sodium uptake when measured as radioactivity per unit weight of tissue. Consequently, the gross radioautographs revealed no pathological changes in the edematous brains. When related to tissue Na^+, however, and expressed in terms of specific activity, a significant delay was observed in the uptake of Na^{24} by the edematous brains. The delay in Na^+ equilibration became manifest after the first hour and remained consistant through the rest of observations that extended six hours after the injection of Na^{24}. Very similar results were reported by Katzman, et al. (1963), who were able to demonstrate that the slow uptake of Na^{24} from the circulating blood was caused by the edematous white matter, because the cortex did not show any significant alteration from the normal. Variations in the uptake rate of K^{42} by both normal and edematous tissue showed a much wider individual range than the Na^+, accentuated by the slow rate of exchange of K^{42} between the central nervous system and plasma (Bakay).

Reed, et al., studied the effect of triethyltin edema on water content, electrolyte distribution, and the kinetics of Na^{22}, Cl^{36} and C^{14} -sucrose uptake of brain tissue. Unfortunately, "all subcortical tissue was removed," and the results were obtained in the relatively unaffected cortex. The water content of the cortex was increased by about 1.2%. Sodium and chloride increased, but potassium-expressed on a dry weight basis-remained unchanged. "Analysis of the tracer studies suggested that in this edema the cortex is characterized by a reduction in the extracellular space and an increase in glial volume. The analysis further indicates that the increase in glial volume is a result of increased permeability of glial cell membranes to Na^+ and Cl^- rather than a decrease in sodium efflux." Unfortunately, these results could not be applied indiscriminantly to the changes in the white matter which represents the characteristic feature of triethyltin edema.

Katzman, et al. (1963), determined the inorganic sulfate space with S^{35} in triethyltin edema. It was found to be 2.6%, a normal value.

A summary of the ultrastructural and chemical determinations in triethyltin edema seems to suggest that the excess fluid is probably a serum ultrafiltrate which is stored within the vacuoles of the myelin sheath. The possibility that this fluid is actually extracellular, and that it "opens up" and expands embryologically pre-existing extracellular spaces, must be considered. The exact mechanism, however, by which triethyltin and possibly other chemical agents produce edema in the first place, remains unknown. As Katzman, et al. (1963), pointed out, the fluid contained in the sacs within myelin is predominantly saline, but since the salts have seeped into the sacs, it exchanges very poorly, becoming sequestered. They suggested the possibility of an inhibition of the Na^+ pump by enzyme action leading to reduced efflux of Na^+ and accumulation of edema fluid.

EDEMA IN RELATION TO ANOXIA AND HYPERCAPNIA

The effect of a reduction in arterial O_2 concentration on cerebral circulation and on metabolic processes of the central nervous system has been extensively studied in the past; however, information on the relationship between O_2 tension, blood-brain barrier permeability and cerebral edema is scant. Recent experiments by Gunn, et al.; Spector; Hills and Spector revealed beyond doubt that under certain circumstances, hypoxia is followed by brain swelling and is measurable by the increase in the water content of the brain.

Crone demonstrated that anoxia without hypercapnia does not increase the permeability of the blood-brain barrier for relatively large particles. Although hypoxia in his experiments was severe enough to damage the neurons of the cortex and basal ganglia, the blood-brain barrier remained impermeable for inulin and sucrose. Evidence accumulates that factors other than hypoxia alone may be responsible for the increased transfer of substances from blood to brain. Increase in CO_2 concentration, when severe enough, might be an important factor. The experiments of Goldberg, et al., showed that exposure to 25% CO_2 increases the cerebral concentration of a variety of compounds. This increase is not related to changes in blood flow and cannot be brought up by inhalation of 5% CO_2. They found that 25% CO_2 increased the cerebral uptake of S^{35}-sulfate and C^{14}-urea. Their calculations revealed that although the steady-state sulfate space has not changed, the entry of S^{35} was greatly enhanced within a few minutes after injection.

To elucidate some of the factors involved in cerebral edema caused by asphyxiation, Bakay and Bendixen carried out experiments in cats by separating the factors that may be involved in hypoventilation and studying hypoxia, hypercapnia, increased venous pressure, and increased cerebrospinal fluid pressure independently, with the other variables maintained within normal range. These experiments showed that significant cerebral edema could be produced only by a combination of hypoxia and hypercapnia. The combination of severe hypoxia and CO_2 accumulation increased cerebral uptake of Na^+ as well as phosphates; neither hypoxia nor hypercapnia alone produced a similar effect. The increase in Na^{24} and P^{32} concentration involved the cortical and nuclear gray matter more than the white matter, and this pathological increase was clearly related to the degree of cerebral edema. The increased accumulation was most pronounced in the basal ganglia, but it was also evident in the cerebral and cerebellar cortex. An increased concentration of Na^{24} and P^{32} was also observed in the white matter.

I^{131}-labeled serum albumin, given intravenously, did not penetrate the brain tissue when increased venous pressure was applied alone or CO_2 inhalation was given. RISA did not penetrate the capillary wall in hypoxia with unimpaired CO_2 elimination, nor did it in hypoxia with hypercapnia, until the arterial pH fell below 6.75, and the oxygen saturation became less than 20-25%. Above these values, the only excess RISA found in the brains were stored in the dilated and engorged vessels. This seemingly increased uptake of albumin was also seen in the experiments with increased venous pressure and in the vasodilatation caused by CO_2 inhalation; in all of these conditions, the tracer could be easily removed from the brain tissue by vascular perfusion. However, in severe hypercapnic hypoxia that led to pronounced cerebral edema with the O_2 saturation and the arterial pH below the levels just mentioned, true transgression of albumin through the capillary wall into the edematous brain tissue occurred. Perfusion experiments and calculations on the vascular isotope concentration showed that the increase in Na^{24}, P^{32} and RISA in hypoxic edema was caused by a true absorption of these tracers by the nervous tissue rather than by a mere increase in cerebral blood content.

Van Harreveld, et al., related cerebral asphyxia to electrical impedence. They found a marked increase in the impedence of the cortex and other parts of the gray matter within a few minutes after occlusion of the cerebral circulation. Since tissue impedence is mainly determined by the amount of extracellular electrolytes, this observation could be related to the pathogenesis of anoxic edema. Histochemical studies performed by Van Harreveld and Schade indicate that the tissue swelling, under ischemic conditions, is caused by a swelling of the cellular elements rather than that of the intercellular space. They found that following asphyxiation and at the time of increase of impedence, the volume of the apical dendrites increasec and there was an influx of chlorides into the swollen dendrites. It was assumed that the cell membrane in asphyxia became markedly permeable for three of the principal ions of the cortex, namely, Na^+, Cl^-, and K^+. This would be accompanied by increasing hydration of the cells under the influence of osmotic forces.

The results emerging from these experiments seem to indicate that the role of hypercapnic hypoxia in the production of cerebral edema is twofold. Hypercapnic hypoxia damages the cells to such an extent that they cannot maintain their normal ionic homeostasis. In addition, this condition results in a leakiness of the small blood vessels which results in the flow of plasma constituents into the brain tissue.

EDEMA ASSOCIATED WITH BRAIN TUMORS

Aleu, et al. (1964), found that edema surrounding experimental brain tumors in animals is manifested mainly by intracellular fluid accumulation. However, some extracellular edema also develops, perhaps due to the secondary rupture of the plasma membrane of inflated glial cells (Aleu, et al., 1964). The increase in water content of the edematous tissue goes hand in hand with an increase in sodium content. The edematous tissue showed an increased uptake of I^{131}-albumin and of $S^{35}O_4$ from the blood stream. This was in excess over the visible enlargement of the extracellular space. As a result of these findings, Aleu et al. (1964), suggested that altered membrane or transport processes lead to the accumulation of S^{35}, I^{131}-albumin within the cytoplasm of the edematous glial cell processes.

Various radioactive isotopes are administered in humans to detect brain tumors or other pathological foci in the central nervous system by means of external scanning. Although repeated scanning with sophisticated equipment might supply valuable data on the temporal and spatial accumulation of certain isotopes in tumor, peritumoral edema, and normal brain tissue respectively, little effort has been made with this aim in mind. The importance of such investigations was emphasized by Planiol and by Bakay and Lee. Recently, Tator, et al., noticed that, following the injection of RISA in man, the edematous brain, particularly the white matter, was often more radioactive than the adjacent tumor. On other occasions, peri tumoral edema was characterized by a decreased uptake of radioactive isotopes, similar to the situation that is seen occasionally in the case of non-hemorrhagic infarcts (Bakay & Lee).

SUMMARY

The results of the experiments described in this review indicate that the exact mechanism of edema formation in the central nervous system is still unknown. The relative importance of the permeability of the blood-brain barrier and that of the exchange of water and solutes between intracellular and extracellular compartments in the production of brain edema cannot be assessed at the present time.

However, enough evidence accumulated to conclude with certainty that different types of cerebral edema exist. This difference is profound and basic; it involves not only the etiological agent and morphological changes in the central nervous system, but also a wide variation in the exchange of labeled macro- and micromolecules between blood plasma and edema fluid. In traumatic, inflammatory, and peritumoral edemas, a protein-rich exudate or transudate leaks out through the damaged capillaries, mostly in the gray matter, and gradually seeps into the adjacent white matter where it extends over a large area. In triethyltin edema, and perhaps in other toxic edemas, the excess fluid accumulates in intramyelinic vacuoles that are produced by the splitting of the myelin lamellae; there is no evidence of capillary damage, and the edema fluid, at least in its initial composition, resembles plasma ultrafiltrate. The combination of hypoxia and hypercapnia, if severe enough, results in edema. The nature of this swelling is little known, but tracer experiments indicate that increased exchange of water and electrolytes is the main feature while, on the other hand, leakage of the capillaries for large molecules such as protein does not occur unless the condition is severe.

REFERENCES

Aleu, F. P., F. L. Edelman, R. Katzman and L. C. Scheinberg: Ultrastructural and biochemical analysis in cerebral edema associated with experimental mouse gliomas, J. Neuropath. Exp. Neurol., 23: 253-263 (1964).

_____, R. Katzman and R. D. Terry: Fine structure and electrolyte analysis of cerebral edema induced by alkyl tin intoxication, Ibid., 22: 403-413 (1963).

Bakay, L.: Morphological and chemical studies in cerebral edema. Triethyltin induced edema, J. Neurol. Sci., 2; 52-67 (1965).

_____ and H. H. Bendixen: Central nervous system vulnerability in hypoxic states: Isotope uptake studies, in: Selective Vulnerability of the Central Nervous System in Hypoxaemia (ed. by

W. H. McMenemey and J. F. Schade), Oxford: Blackwell Scient. Publ., p. 63-78 (1963).
_____ and I. ul Haque: Morphological and chemical studies in cerebral edema. I. Cold-induced edema, J. Neuropath. Exp. Neurol., 23; 393-418 (1964).
_____ and J. C. Lee: Cerebral Edema, Springfield, Ill.: Charles C. Thomas Publ. (1965).
Clasen, R. A., D. V. L. Brown, S. Leavitt and G. M. Hass: The production by liquid nitrogen of acute closed cerebral lesions, Surg., Gyn. Obst., 96; 605-616 (1953).
Crone, C.: The permeability of capillaries in various organs as determined by use of the indicator diffusion method, Acta Physiol. Scand., 58; 292-305 (1963).
Cutler, R. W. P., G. V. Watters and C. F. Barlow: I^{125}-labeled protein in experimental brain edema, Arch. Neurol., 11; 225-238 (1964).
Goldberg, M. A., C. F. Barlow and L. J. Roth: The effects of carbon dioxide on the entry and accumulation of drugs in the central nervous system, J. Pharm. Exp. Therap., 131, 308-318 (1961).
Gonatas, N. K., H. M. Zimmerman and S. Levine: Ultra-structure of inflammation with edema in the rat brain, Amer. J. Path., 42; 455-469 (1963).
Gunn, C. G., G. R. Williams and I. T. Parker: Edema of the brain following circulatory arrest, J. Surg. Res., 2; 141-143 (1962).
Hills, C. P. and R. G. Spector: Anoxia and cerebral water content in the adult rat, Nature (London), 199; 393 (1963).
Hirano, A., H. M. Zimmerman and S. Levine: The fine structure of cerebral fluid accumulation, III: Extracellular spread of cryptococcal polysaccharide in the acute state, Amer. J. Path., 45; 1-19 (1964).
Katzman, R., R. Aleu and C. Wilson: Further observations on triethyl tin edema, Arch. Neurol., 9, 178-187 (1963).
_____, N. Gonatas and S. Levine: Electrolytes and fluids in experimental focal leucoencephalopathy, Ibid., 10; 58-65 (1964).
Klatzo, I., J. Miquel and R. Otenasek: The application of fluorescein labeled serum proteins (FLSP) to the study of vascular permeability in the brain, Acta Neuropathol., 2; 144-160 (1962).
_____, A. Piraux and E. J. Laskowski: The relationship between edema, blood-brain barrier and tissue elements in a local brain injury, J. Neuropath. Exp. Neurol., 17; 548-564 (1958).
Lee, J. C. and L. Bakay: Ultrastructural changes in the edematous central nervous system, I: Triethyltin edema, Arch. Neurol., 13; 48-57 (1965).
_____ and _____: Ultrastructural changes in the edematous central nervous system, II: Cold-induced edema, Ibid., 14, 36-49 (1966).

Levine, S., H. M. Zimmerman, E. J. Wenk and N. K. Gonatas: Experimental leukoencephalopathies due to implantation of foreign substances, Am. J. Path., 42, 97-117 (1963).
Magee, P. N., H. B. Stoner and J. M. Barnes: The experimental production of edema in the central nervous system of the rat by triethyltin compounds, J. Path. Bact., 73; 107-124 (1957).
Pappius, H. M. and D. R. Gulati: Water and electrolyte content of cerebral tissues in experimentally induced edema, Acta Neuropath., 2; 451-460 (1963).
Planiol, T.: Diagnostic des Lesions Intra-Craniennes par les Radio-Isotopes (Gammaencephalographie), Paris: Masson & Cie. (1959).
Reed, D. J., D. M. Woodbury and R. L. Holtzer: Brain edema, electrolytes and extracellular space. Effect of triethyl tin on brain and skeletal muscle, Arch. Neurol., 10; 604-616 (1964).
Spector, R. C.: Water content of the brain in anoxic-ischaemic encephalopathy in adult rats, Brit. J. Exp. Path., 42, 623-630 (1961).
Sperl, Jr., M. P., H. J. Svien, N. P. Goldstein, J. W. Kernohan and J. H. Grindlay: Experimental production of local cerebral edema by an expanding intracerebral mass, Proc. Mayo Clin., 32; 744-749 (1957).
Streicher, E., P. J. Ferris, J. D. Prokop and I. Klatzo: Brain volume and thiocyanate space in local cold injury, Arch. Neurol., 11, 444-449 (1964).
Tator, C. H., T. P. Morley and J. Olszewski: A study of the factors responsible for the accumulation of radioactive iodinated serum albumin (RISA) by intracranial tumors and other lesions, J. Neurosurg., 22, 60-76 (1965).
Taylor, J. M., W. A Levy, I. Herzog and L. C. Scheinberg: Prevention of experimental cerebral edema by corticosteroids. Biochemical and Ultrastructural studies, Neurology, 15; 667-674 (1965).
Torack, R. M., R. D. Terry and H. M. Zimmerman: The fine structure of cerebral fluid accumulation. I. Swelling secondary to cold injury, Am. J. Path., 35; 1135-1147 (1959).
Van Harreveld, A.: Water and electrolyte distribution in central nervous tissue, Fed. Proc., 21; 659-664 (1962).
_____ and P. J. Schade: On the distribution and movements of water and electrolytes in the cerebral cortex, in: Structure and Function of the Cerebral Cortex Amsterdam: Elsevier Publ. Co., p. 253-256 (1960).

F. W. KOLKMANN
G. ULE

TIN POISONING EDEMA

The experimentally induced tin poisoning edema has already been mentioned in the previous discourses several times; therefore, we would like to give only a short summary of our experimental results. We intend, further, to point out some parallels between the morphological changes of tin poisoning edema and some diseases of human pathology.

Twenty young rabbits were examined both histologically and with the electron microscope. Triethyl tin (TET) was administered intraperitoneally to the animals at a dose of 1 mg/kg body weight daily for two to eight days. The rabbits in our experimental procedures showed a similar clinical symptomatology as those described in the literature but with one difference: the completely developed clinical aspects did not subside, and when the administration of TET was discontinued, the animals did not recover but died of intoxication. Our electron microscopic preparation of the tissue followed the methods of Sabatini. The material was fixed in glutaraldehyde and embedded in Araldite.

The first picture (Fig. 1) shows the typical changes of TET intoxication on the third day of experiment. Only a few myelin sheaths show the characteristic splitting and vacuolization of myelin lamellae. Most of the myelin sheaths are unaffected. Even on the seventh day of treatment many myelin sheaths are not changed, yet the vacuoles and clefts within the abnormal myelin sheaths already reach grotesque degrees.

The following picture (Fig. 2) out of the optic tract of the same animal stresses this observation. Despite the excessive damage of the myelin sheaths, a remarkable part of myelin sheaths is unaffected, and the pericapillary astroglia processes are inconspicuous. There is relatively little change in the cerebral cortex (Fig. 3). Except for some myelin clefts in the myelin sheaths which are

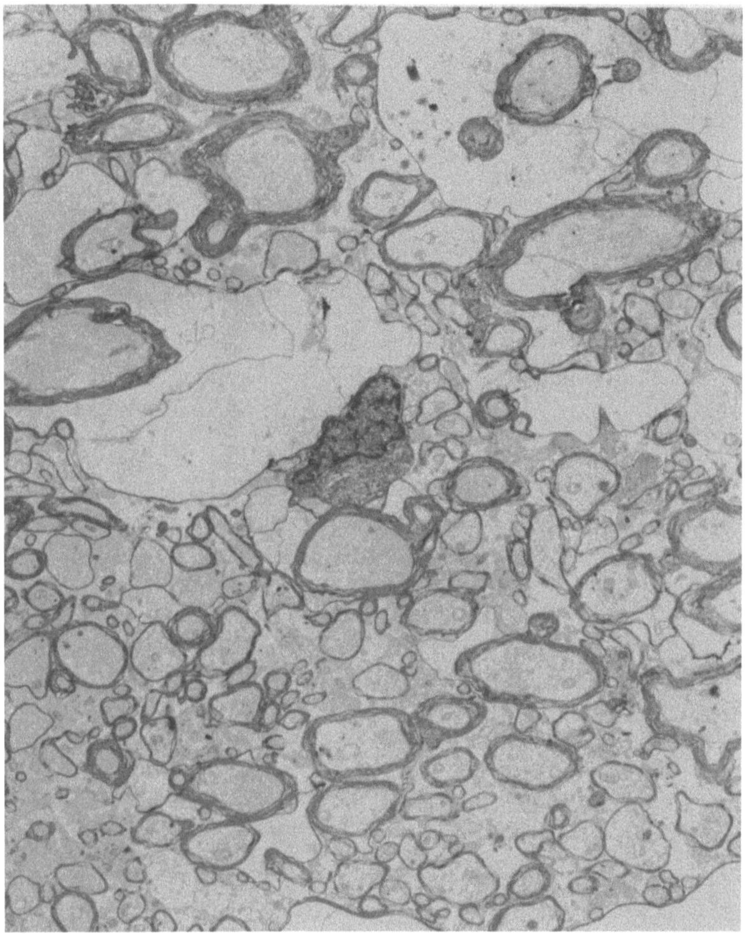

Fig. 1.

diffusely scattered in the gray matter, no other structures are affected.

The splitting and dissociation of the myelin lamellae occurs, as Aleu and co-workers and others have already demonstrated, in the region of the so-called intraperiod line (Fig. 2a). This intraperiod line takes the place of the transitory myelogenetic extracellular space which disappears by apposition of the external surfaces of the oligodendroglial plasma membranes during myelogenesis. This transitory myelogenetic extracellular space is reopened by TET edema.

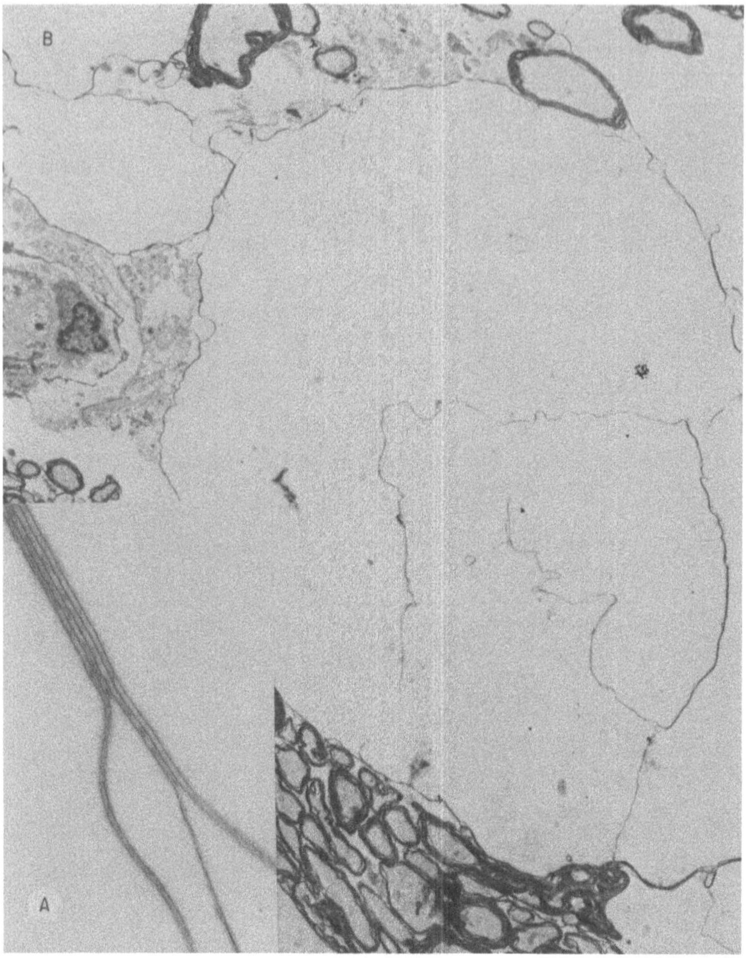

Fig. 2.

The real intercellular space, as has been measured and demonstrated by Gonatas, Ben Shmuel, Brambring, et al., is not markedly increased. This observation seems for us to be important concerning the pathogenetic effect of TET on the myelin, because we did not see the typical splitting of myelin lamellae after we administered diethyltin dichloride to some animals instead of TET. Using this diethyltin, we observed only non-specific edema of the white matter with dispersing of myelin sheaths and widening of the intercellular gap.

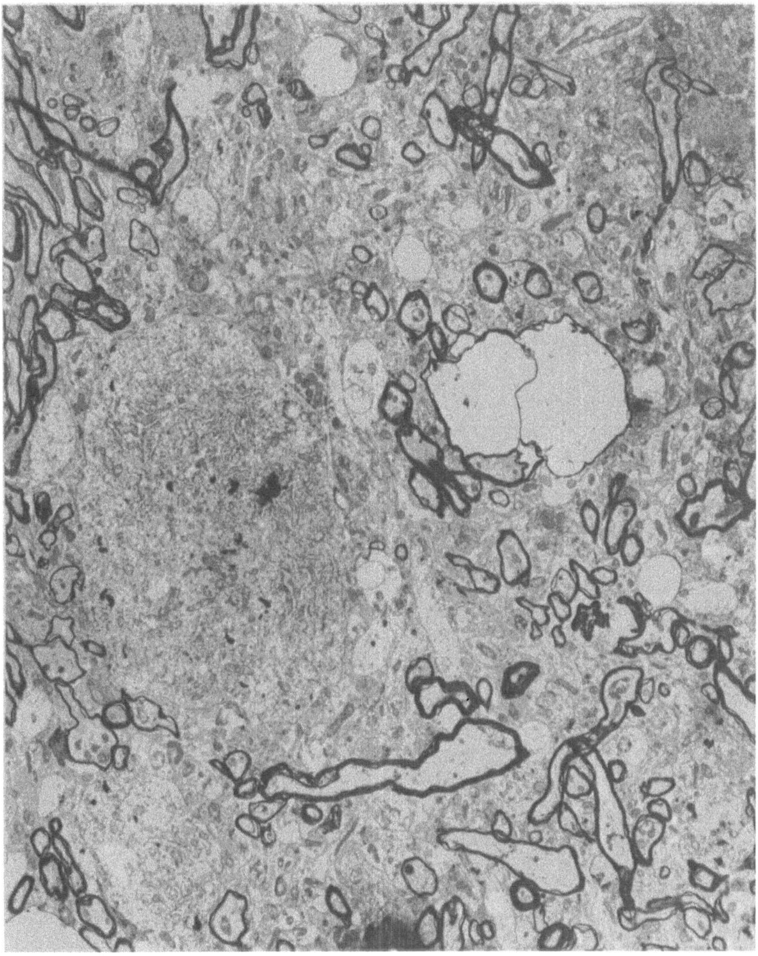

Fig. 3.

We consider the TET edema to be very important for neuropathology, because this pattern of lesion of the white matter presents a simply reproducible experimental model of a myelin damage, that obviously occurs as a widespread phenomenon in neuropathology. Some years following the first electron optical studies of edema in the cerebral cortex, we learned to interpret the conventional histological observations a great deal better and to draw from them conclusions about the ultrastructural relations. We are reminded of a

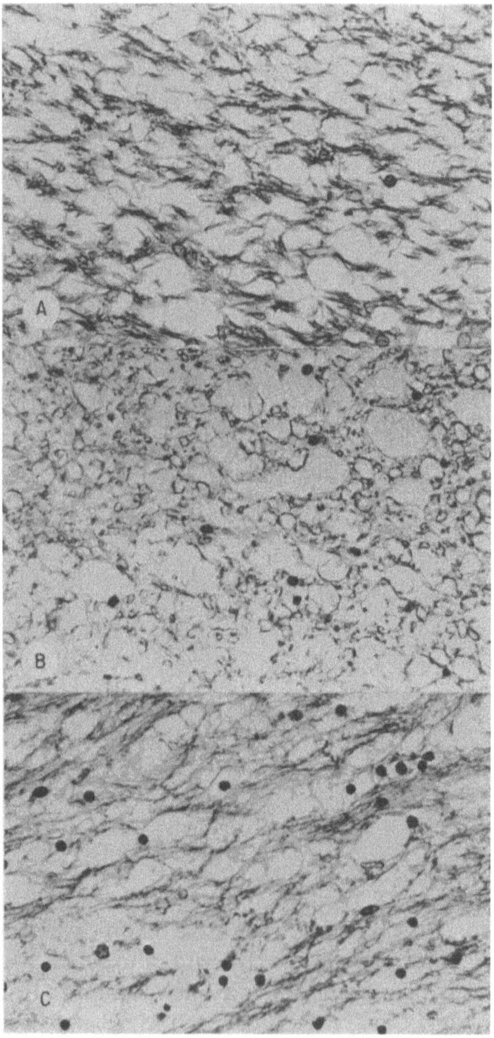

Fig. 4.

term, the so-called "enlargement of Held's glial chambers" in light microscopic studies of brain edema. This term has been carried over to the present on the ultrastructural level as hydropical swelling of pericapillary astroglia processes.

A similar possibility exists in TET intoxication (Fig. 4a). The vacuolated loosening and splitting of the myelin sheaths at the intraperiod line with separation of single or multiple myelin lamellae is also recognized by the experienced investigator by the light microscopical appearance of fine irregular septation and vacuolization of the white matter. This histological picture shows brain tissue of an animal suffering from TET intoxication for eight days. This finding resembles strikingly the disseminated spongy degeneration of white matter in the so-called funicular myelopathy (Fig. 4b).

A group of human diseases showing similar histological changes are the infantile spongy degenerations that may be demonstrated by a picture of a familiar case. It concerns a seven-month-old boy. A brother of this boy died at the age of six months with similar clinical and anatomical appearances. This picture (Fig. 4c) demonstrates a section of the optical nerve with the typical fine septation and irregular vacuolization of the myelin sheaths.

Also in cases of maple syrup disease and hyperglycinemia we observed similar histological changes. An example may be taken from a case published by Diezel. It concerns a female infant suffering from hyperglycinemia, who died on the ninth day of her life. Although most of the nerve fibers of the optic tract of this new-born infant are not completely myelinated, the lesion of the white matter is well recognized. We have examined tissue of the optic tract also by the electron microscope. It is difficult, of course, to reach conclusions from this picture because the tissue has been stored in formalin since 1962. Autolytic changes are quite obvious. Nevertheless there are some structures visible, which could be attributed to the histological disorders of the white matter and to our interpretation above.

Considering the evident relation between the histological and ultrastructural features of TET edema, we assume that also in cases of human pathology associated with the typical light microscopic myelin disorders, the lesion in the white matter must appear similar on the ultrastructural level to TET intoxication of the rabbit.

The demonstrated group of spongy degenerations of the white matter must be differentiated as a special pattern of lesion of the white matter from other types of spongy state, for instance from generalized astroglia hydrops in the gray matter of the edematous loosening and extracellular widening of white matter.

RAYMOND A. CLASEN
HOWARD H. SKY-PECK
SYLVIA PANDOLFI
IRIS LAING
GEORGE M. HASS

THE CHEMISTRY OF ISOLATED EDEMA FLUID IN EXPERIMENTAL CEREBRAL INJURY*

Focal areas of hemorrhagic necrosis were produced in the brains of anesthetized dogs by a freezing technique which has been described in previous publications (Clasen, et al., 1953). Briefly, this consisted of the application of a freezing instrument cooled by liquid nitrogen to the exposed intact skull. The instrument was left in place for five-ten minutes. This resulted in a circumscribed lesion involving both gray and white matter in the underlying brain. In the first hour after injury, cellular damage was restricted to the lesion. Four hours after injury, histologic evidence of edema was seen both in the lesion and in the adjacent white matter. Both areas showed positive staining by the periodic acid-Schiff (PAS) technique (Clasen, et al., 1957).

In continuation of these studies, animals were given intravenous Trypan blue or Evan's blue in a dose of 1 ml. per kilogram body weight of a 2.5% solution prior to production of the lesion. Staining was found in the lesion and edematous areas with both dyes (Fig. 1), but the degree of staining was far more intense with the Evan's blue. This may be appreciated by comparing the above figure with previously published photographs from experiments with Evan's blue (Clasen, et al., 1962). The greater efficiency is probably related to the fact that Trypan blue is more rapidly lost from the blood stream than Evan's blue (Gregersen & Rawson, 1942). It was empirically established for the dog and monkey that, in the firs

* This work was supported by a grant (NB-03677) from the National Institute of Neurological Disease and Blindness, National Institutes of Health, USPH, and from the Otho S. A. Sprague Memorial Institu

24 hours after injury, the vital staining corresponded exactly with those areas which were histologically edematous provided that the dye was given prior to production of the lesion (Clasen, et al., 1962). Gross vital staining could, therefore, be used as a label for edematous white matter.

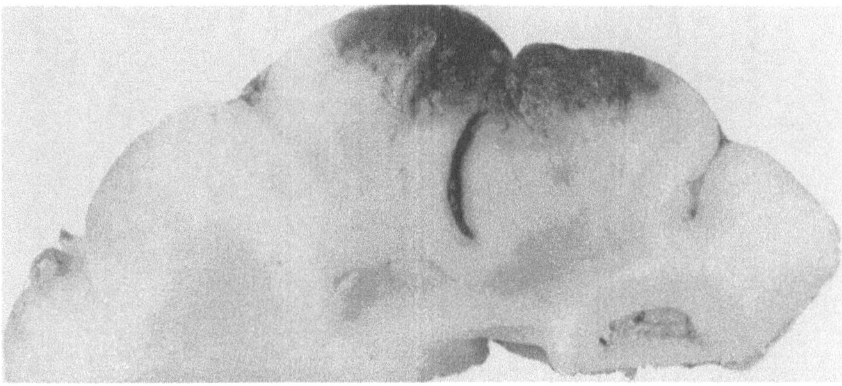

Fig. 1. Dog brain four hours after injury; Typan blue given prior to injury.

Early studies of freezing lesions in the rodent using electron microscopy suggested that the edematous process associated with these lesions was intracellular in nature (Torack, et al., 1959). Since the study of our own material by conventional techniques had indicated that the process was extracellular in nature, tissue obtained by biopsy in the dog four hours after injury was studied. This included white matter from the undamaged hemisphere and blue-stained white matter from the damaged hemisphere. The necrotic lesion was avoided. This material was fixed by immersion in Dalton's solution and, after dehydration, embedded in epon. Sections for microscopy were stained by hot azure-methylene blue. Normal white matter showed no apparent extracellular space on the light microscope level. In edematous white matter, on the other hand, there was an abundant extracellular space (Fig. 2). Examination of this material with the electron microscope revealed no evidence of cellular or fiber necrosis. This was also the case with conventional histologic methods. Whatever may be the nature of the edema associated with freezing lesions in the rodent, it is clear that in higher animals with proportionately more white matter, the fluid accumulation is overwhelmingly extracellular at this time interval.

A squash preparation of fresh normal white matter viewed under a metallurgic microscope by direct light consists of closely

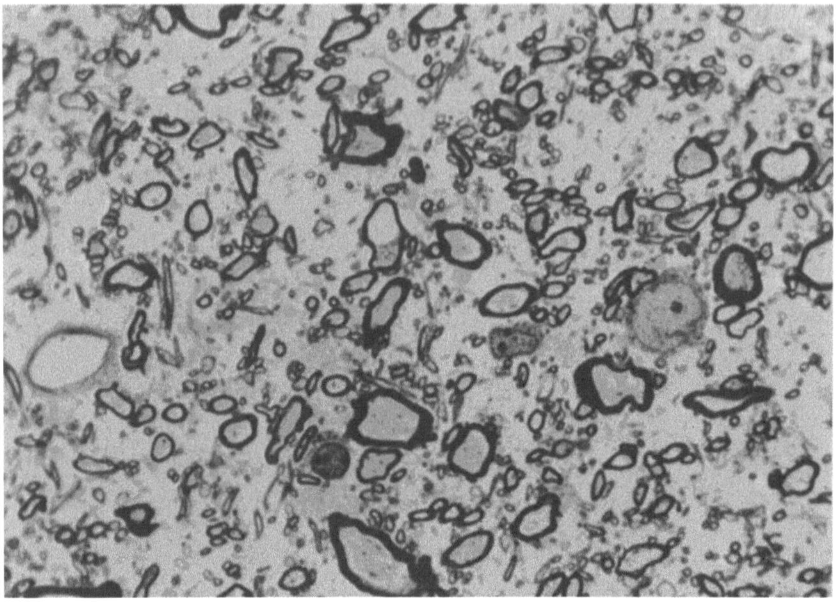

Fig. 2. Edematous white matter fixed by immersion in Dalton's solution followed by embedding in epon and staining with Azure-methylene blue. X1400(reduced).

packed cells and fibers (Fig. 3). With labelled edematous white matter, on the other hand, these structures are rather widely separated. When the temperature of this material is lowered by means of a freezing microscope stage, the fluid in these areas forms ice crystals. When the stage is rewarmed, the ice crystals melt forming sma pools of fluid which then coalesce giving a picture indistinguishable from that seen prior to freezing. An attempt was made to determine the osmolarity of this fluid by quantitatively measuring its freezing point. Widely different figures were obtained for different samples of tissue from the same animal and from different determinations on the same specimen. The attempt was therefore abandoned. It was, however, quite apparent that fresh edematous tissue contained a considerable amount of extracellular fluid and efforts were then made to obtain this in pure form.

Fresh edematous white matter was collected by gross dissection of labelled tissue. Again, the necrotic lesion was avoided. This tissue was placed in a refrigerated centrifuge and spun at 2,500 rpm for 30 minutes. This resulted in the separation of several drops of blue-stained fluid which were collected in a capillary tube. No fluid was obtained from grossly normal (unstained) white matter. The

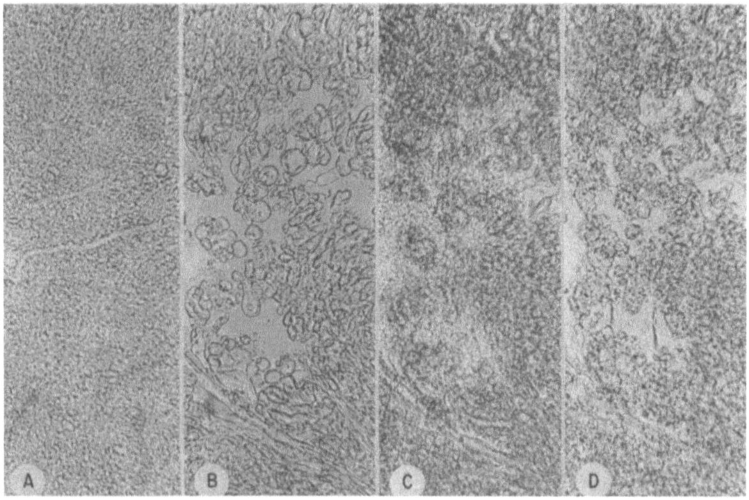

Fig. 3. Squash preparations of white matter; Normal white matter (a), edematous white matter (b), frozen edematous white matter (c), thawing edematous white matter (d).

remainder of this communication will deal with a chemical analysis of this fluid as compared with a sample of serum obtained in the case of the experimental material from the same animal at the time of sacrifice. The experimental material was obtained from dogs sacrificed four hours after injury. Some of the animals had also received about ten microcuries of radioactive (I^{131}) iodinated serum albumin prior to production of the lesion.

Electrolyte concentrations of serum and edema fluid were determined using standard micromethods, flame photometry for sodium and potassium and the Volhard method for chloride. The concentration of Evans blue was determined photometrically without prior separation of the dye-protein complex. Counts referable to the concentration of I^{131} were obtained in the routine manner. Total protein was determined by the Lowry technique (Lowry, et al., 1951). The material was subjected to electrophoresis on cellulose acetate strips using a barbitone buffer (Colab Laboratories, Chicago Heights, Illinois) at pH 8.6 and a current of one milliamp. The strips were removed after two hours, fixed in alcohol and stained by Ponceau S or the PAS technique. Quantitative studies were performed by dissolving portions of the strips in chloroform-ethanol 9:1 and determining the light absorption in a Coleman Spectrophotometer. Absorption at 520 mμ was used for the Ponceau S. It was found that at this wave length there was essentially no interference from the

Evan's blue on the strips. The PAS stained material was read at 680 mμ.

Immunoelectrophoretic studies were done in 0.8% Ionagar No. 2 (Colab Laboratories), dissolved in 0.027 M barbital buffer at pH 8.6 on 3 1/4" × 4" glass plates. Antiserum was produced by injecting rabbits intramuscularly with a mixture of equal parts of pooled dog serum and Freund's adjuvant. The animals were given 0.5 ml every three days for one week, no injections for three weeks, and one injection every week for three weeks. After this they were sacrificed by bleeding, the serum collected, and the antibody titer determined. It was not further purified. Antiserum directed against dog brain was also prepared. Several anesthetized dogs were perfused with normal saline injected into the internal carotid arteries. The internal jugular veins were severed. When the returning fluid was free of blood, the brains were removed and white matter collected by gross dissection. While the antigen consisted predominantly of white matter, it was not entirely free of gray matter. We have found that it is almost impossible to collect pure white matter in suitable quantity from the brains of experimental animals. The material was placed in a Waring blender and mixed with nine volumes of normal saline. Following centrifugation in the ultracentrifuge at 20,000 rpm for one hour, the clear supernatant was lyophilized. About 40 mg./ml of this material were redissolved in normal saline, mixed with an equal amount of Freund's adjuvant, and injected into rabbits as described above. The antiserum so obtained was designated "antibrain antibody." This antiserum was much weaker than that obtained from whole dog serum. Electrophoresis was performed at a current of 40 milliamps. The plate was cooled during this process by contact with heptane. After one hour, trenches were cut, the antibody added, and the plate was placed in an incubator at 37°C overnight. On the following morning the plate was washed with normal saline, the solution being changed every hour for 4 hours. After this, washing was continued for two more days, changing the solution twice a day. The plate was then dried and stained by Ponceau S with acetic acid differentiation. Some plates were photographed by indirect light prior to drying. It was found that all precipitin lines stained. Background staining was sometimes troublesome.

Results for electrolytes, dye and protein are given in the accompanying tables. The third column in each case is the mean of individual paired differences and not the difference of the means of the groups. Results were evaluated statistically by using Student's "t" test on paired comparisons. Five percent was chosen as the level of significance and the "two tailed" table of probabilities was used. The hypothesis tested is that the values are distinct from zero. Since all differences except for beta and gamma values were positive, the "ts" could justifiably be doubled testing the hypothesis that the values are greater than zero. Because of the small amount of edema fluid obtained in individual experiments, electrolytes and RISA concentrations were obtained in one set of experiments, dye and protein studies in a second set and immunoelectrophoretic studies in a third set. It should be borne in mind that the electrophoretic protein values were obtained in fluid which was stained in vivo by Evan's blue and the values may not be comparable to normal dog serum.

With respect to electrolytes, edema fluid contains significantly less sodium and chloride than serum (Table 1). It might, however, argued that the fluid is isotonic to serum with respect to these electrolytes and that in the method of isolation intracellular fluid is transferred to the edema fluid causing dilution. In keeping with this is the fact that the albumin of edema fluid is, on a percentage basis, as hypotonic to serum as is the sodium (Table 2). While this is a possibility, we are inclined to doubt it, since there is no good morphologic evidence of swelling of formed tissue elements at this time (Fig. 2) and no fluid is obtained when normal white matter is centrifuged. Direct analyses of edematous white matter associated with freezing lesions in cats 24 hours after injury have been reported (Pappius & Gulati, 1963). According to these authors the sodium content in this tissue is increased from 59 to 86 mEq/kilo of fresh tissue while the percent dry weight decreases from 31.2 to 22.1. Using their reported normal for serum sodium (154 mEq/L) and assuming that serum has a 10% dry weight, the former represents the addition of 397 ml of serum and the latter, 751 ml of serum to a kilogram of white matter. These mean figures also, therefore, represent the addition of a fluid to white matter which is hypotonic with respect to serum. However, because of the variance of the means, the fluid could also be isotonic or even hypertonic to serum. We are dealing here with a different species and time interval. What is needed to resolve this question is a direct analysis of edematous tissue in the dog four hours after injury.

On a percentage basis the decrease in chloride in edema fluid is greater than the sodium resulting in a higher molar ratio of sodium to chloride in edema fluid than in serum (Table 1). In the absence of selective binding in the process of preparation, a second artifact which must be considered, this would indicate that with respect to chloride, edema fluid contains disproportionately more sodium than serum. We have found this to be consistently the case for whole hemisphere analyses of monkey brains damaged by freezing at every time interval studied during the first 24 hours after injury.

TABLE 1

ELECTROLYTES IN SERUM AND EDEMA FLUID

	Sodium mEq/liter			Chloride mEq/liter			Sodium-Chloride molar ratio			Potassium mEq/liter
	E	S	S-E	E	S	S-E	E	S	E-S	E
n			11			12			7	15
$\bar{x}$	123.4	143.0	19.6	86.7	110.0	23.3	1.46	1.28	0.19	59.5
$s_{\bar{x}}$	2.4	2.0	3.4	1.5	1.2	2.2	0.01	0.01	0.02	2.2
t			5.7			10.6			9.5	
p <			0.001			0.001			0.001	
%	85.8	100		78.8	100					

TABLE 2

ALBUMIN AND EVAN'S BLUE IN SERUM AND EDEMA FLUID

	Albumin gms.%			Evan's Blue mg.%			Dye-Albumin molar ratio			RISA cts/min/mg		
	E	S	S-E	E	S	S-E	E	S	E-S	E	S	S-E
n			5			6			4			10
$\bar{x}$	1.87	2.14	0.25	16.4	31.8	15.4	0.52	0.95	0.43	7.51	9.02	1.51
$s_{\bar{x}}$	0.08	0.07	0.09	3.4	5.1	2.4	0.17	0.20	0.04	0.72	1.05	0.45
t			2.8			6.4			10.7			3.4
p <			0.05			0.01			0.01			0.01
%	87.4	100		58.0	100					83.5	100	

Edema fluid contains a quite high potassium concentration (Table 1). This may represent release of solid intracellular material into the fluid during the process of isolation. However, it is not unreasonable to assume that fluid adjacent to an area of cellular necrosis would have a high potassium content in the first few hours after injury and it has been reported that glia in tissue culture can survive a potassium concentration in this range (Friede, 1964). In the cat, four hours after injury there is an uptake of intravenous K^{42} in the edematous tissue adjacent to the lesion indicating the presence of an exchangeable potassium pool derived from serum (Bakay & Haque, 1964). This is decreased 24 hours after injury. Measurements of tissue potassium at 24 hours also show an increase in the concentration of potassium when the figures are recalculated on a dry weight basis (Pappius & Gulati, 1963) but the differences are not statistically significant. Analysis of edema fluid obtained in the monkey 48 hours after injury, within minutes of death and without prior centrifugation, showed a potassium concentration of 52.5 mEq/liter. Again, different time intervals and different species are involved.

In summary, because of the method of isolation, there is more than reasonable doubt that the electrolyte concentrations measured in this fluid represent in vivo values. They have validity only when they can be correlated with total tissue changes. At least the potassium change can be reproduced by mixing normal serum and white matter and collecting the fluid by centrifugation. The dye and protein changes to be discussed, however, cannot be so reproduced.

The concentration of Evan's blue in edema fluid is on a percentage basis even lower with respect to serum than the chloride (Table 2). Since this dye is known to form a complex with serum albumin (Allen & Orahorats, 1950) the values were recalculated on a molar ratio basis. The concentrations obtained in these animals are only about one-tenth the reported maximum binding capacity of albumin and the molar ratio in edema fluid is also less than that seen in serum (Table 2). Total hemisphere analyses in the monkey 12 hours after injury have shown serum equivalents from RISA studies of 3.20 ± 0.37 and from Evan's blue 4.47 ± 0.56 gm/100 gm. dry weight. This difference is significant on paired comparison testing (Clasen, et al., 1965). At 24 hours after injury the values are 4.59 ± 0.53 for RISA and 10.88 ± 2.23 for dye (Clasen, et al., 1966). The actual dye figures are 18.14 ± 1.51 at 12 hours and 16.64 ± 3.14 mgm/100 gm. dry weight of tissue at 24 hours. These figures show a retention of dye by tissue in the face of a falling serum level and suggest that the dye-albumin complex has been split with binding of dye by fixed tissue elements. The lower dye-albumin ratio in isolated edema fluid is probably a reflection of this same phenomenon occurring as early as four hours after injury.

Another factor which must be considered is the possibility of in vivo binding by fixed tissue elements. For instance, with respect to water and RISA, the changes in the whole monkey hemisphere 24 hours after injury are reasonably close (Clasen, et al., 1966). The fluid in the intercellular space (Fig. 2) could, however, be hypotonic to serum if a portion of the RISA were within glial cytoplasm. In the edema associated with freezing lesions in the cat 24 hours after injury, radio-autography (using I^{131}) revealed a diffuse distribution in edematous white matter when the RISA was given one hour before sacrifice (Bakay & Haque, 1964). On the other hand, in the edema associated with the implantation of extradural balloons in cats, uptake of RISA by glial cytoplasm was demonstrated six hours after injury (Cutler, et al., 1964). These authors used a different isotope (I^{125}) and injected the material during production of the lesion. Further data in this area are needed.

On cellulose acetate, human globulin is in most cases resolvable into five fractions (Fig. 4). These have been designated as two alpha and two beta subfractions plus a gamma fraction. In the dog there are only four fractions. By analogy with the human we have designated these as two alpha subfractions plus a single beta and gamma fraction. In the human the alpha fraction is more prominent than the beta; in the dog just the opposite is the case. As compared with the human, the level of gamma globulin in the dog is lower and the band is less distinct. In quantitative studies on the dog the origin was included with the gamma fraction and the two alpha fractions were combined.

The electrophoretic pattern of serum was modified by the presence of the dye (Fig. 5). More protein remained at the origin probably representing denatured material. As the proteins migrated to the anode, the albumin-dye complex was progressively split and the Evan's blue remained as a hemi-ellipsoid figure on the strip. The serum protein bands tended to form backward "C" figures around this area. On paper the dye remained at the origin. These facts are related to the high affinity of the dye for cellulose (Allen & Orahovats, 1950). In anion agar the dye migrated with the albumin.

In edema fluid the various bands were clearly recognized but appeared to be superimposed on a diffuse band in the globulin area. Quantitative studies showed a significant increase in the concentration of alpha globulin in edema fluid as compared to serum (Table 3). This excess globulin amounted to about 20% of the total protein of the edema fluid. It should be borne in mind that any protein from the end of the albumin band to the beginning of the beta band is, by definition, alpha protein. As with RISA, the concentration of electrophoretic albumin was less in edema fluid than in serum. Since the two determinations were not made on the same samples, direct ra-

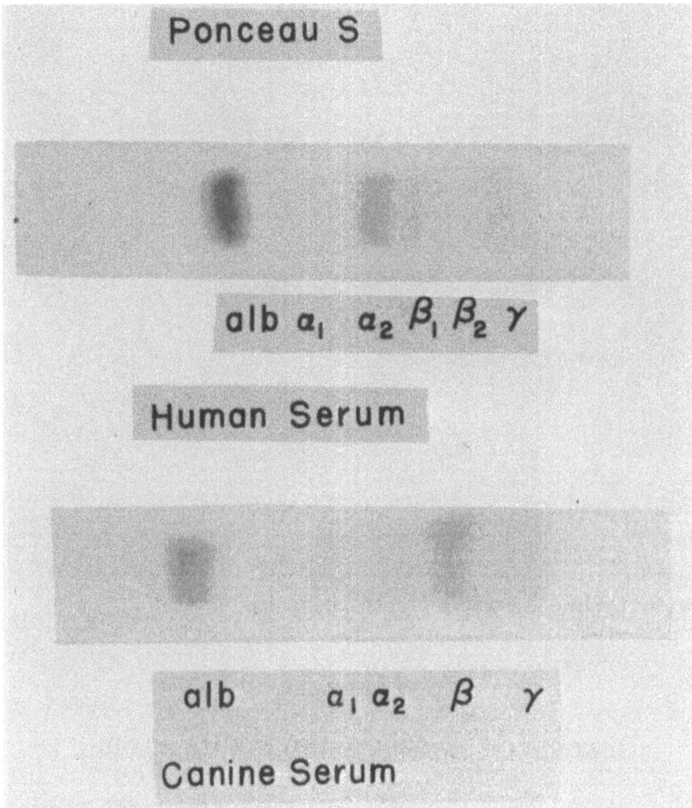

Fig. 4. Cellulose acetate electrophoresis.

tio comparisons cannot be made but the fact that the percent depression is essentially the same for both measurements suggests that the entity measured as electrophoretic albumin is in fact serum albumin.

In canine serum, PAS staining is essentially restricted to the globulins with the strongest staining in the alpha 2 and beta fraction (Fig. 6). In edema fluid distinct staining of the alpha 1 fraction is also seen. Quantitative studies (Table 4) showed an increase in the relative staining of the alpha fraction at the expense of the beta and gamma fractions. Using the same PAS technique (Colab Laboratory Manual) in Ionagar resulted in a staining of all fractions and a pattern indistinguishable from that seen with Ponceau S. The reasons for the difference in PAS staining with these two mediums are not clear.

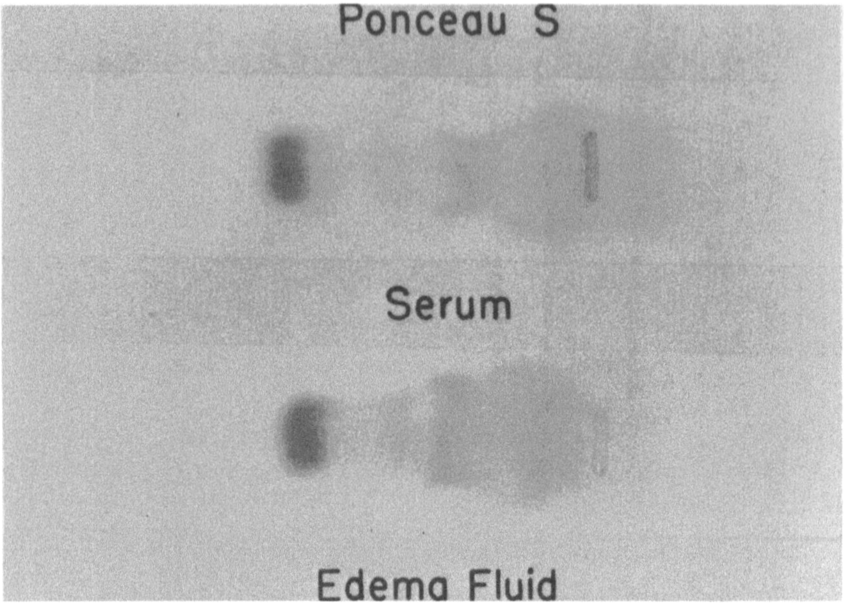

Fig. 5. Cellulose acetate electrophoresis.

TABLE 3

GLOBULINS IN SERUM AND EDEMA FLUID

	Alpha gms%			Beta gms%			Gamma gms%		
	E	S	E-S	E	S	E-S	E	S	E-S
n			5			5			6
$\bar{x}$	1.21	0.73	0.48	1.31	1.29	0.02	0.43	0.45	−0.01
$s_{\bar{x}}$	0.13	0.12	0.07	0.17	0.16	0.17	0.08	0.05	0.06
t			6.8			0.2			0.2
p <			0.01			ns			ns

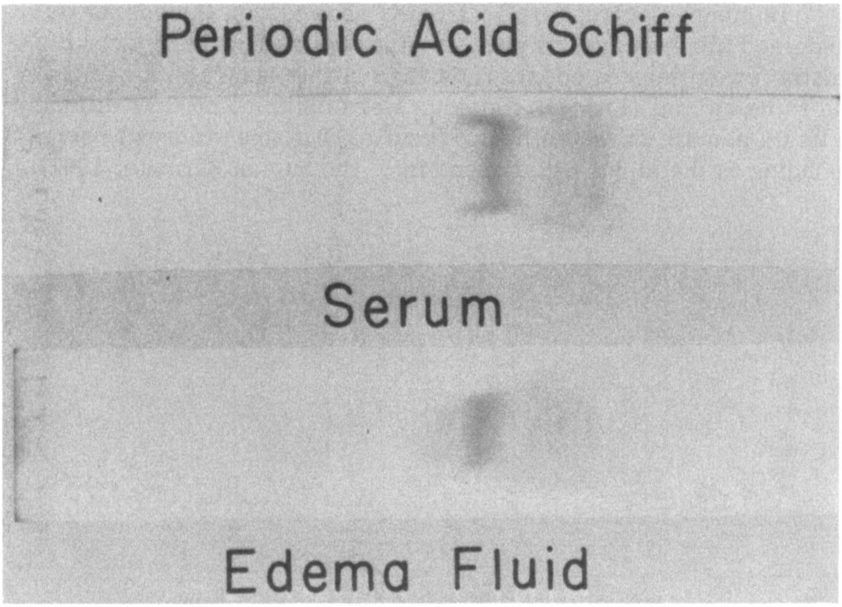

Fig. 6. Cellulose acetate electrophoresis.

TABLE 4

PERIODIC ACID-SCHIFF STAINING OF GLOBULINS IN SERUM AND EDEMA FLUID EXPRESSED AS PERCENT OF TOTAL

	Alpha			Beta			Gamma		
	E	S	E-S	E	S	S-E	E	S	S-E
n			7			7			7
$\bar{x}$	55.6	33.6	13.3	34.4	42.9	8.5	10.1	16.3	6.2
$s_{\bar{x}}$	4.3	5.3	3.5	4.0	1.9	3.1	1.7	2.2	2.5
t			3.8			2.7			2.5
p <			0.01			0.05			0.05

Immuno-electrophoretic studies showed that the edema fluid contained albumin and all classes of globulins but there were distinctly fewer lines in edema fluid than in the serum obtained from the same animal (Fig. 7). Patterns were obtained on four different animals and all showed similar results. The arch (arrow) corresponding to the alpha 1 glycoprotein of the human (Crowle, 1961)

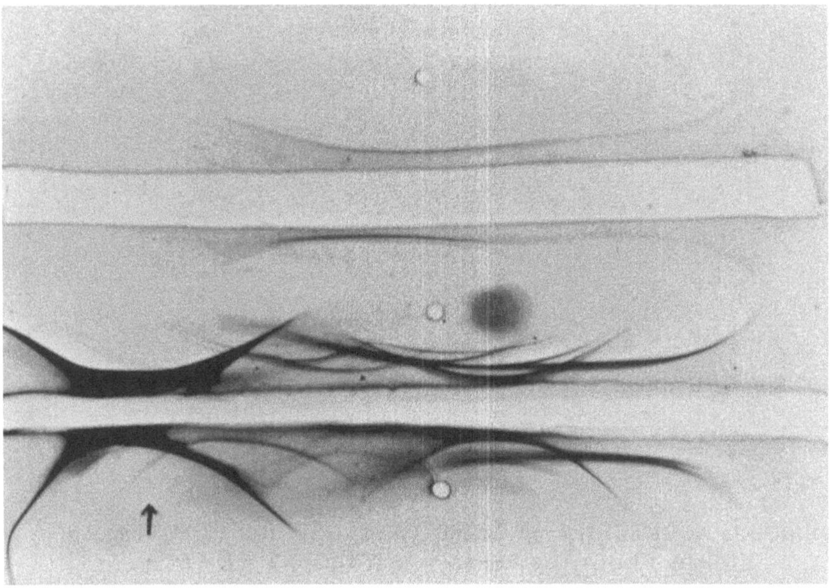

Fig. 7. Immuno-electrophoresis in Ionagar, dried and stained with Ponceau S. Outer holes: edema fluid. Center hole: serum. Upper trench: antibody directed against the saline soluble fraction of normal dog white matter. Lower trench: dog antiserum. Arrow: alpha 1 glycoprotein position in the human.

appears to be heavier in the edema fluid than in serum. This would suggest that the concentration of serum glycoprotein is increased in the edema fluid. The identification of this arch as a glycoprotein is based on analogy with the known human pattern. It may be that in the dog the pattern is different. We are currently studying this problem with purified canine glycoprotein fractions. The specificity of this arch depends upon the specificity assigned to the antigen-antibody reaction. The anti-serum was directed against serum factors. While tissue could contain a protein capable of cross reaction and with the same electrophoretic mobility as the serum protein, this seems to us unlikely. It is possible, however, that abnormal glia or perivascular cells could synthesize a protein antigenically and electrophoretically identical with serum glycoproteins. Again, this is unlikely.

The problem of artifacts involved in collection of edema fluid is of less importance in the interpretation of the protein findings than with the electrolytes. It might, however, be argued that, as with potassium, the excess globulin is released from the formed elements of the tissue during the process of centrifugation. Viewing only the protein patterns on cellulose acetate, this is not an unlikely explanation. This was the reason we attempted to prepare an antibrain antibody. As can be seen (Fig. 7), this antibody is directed principally against gamma globulin (7s and beta 2a) with a few faint lines probably both alpha and beta fractions (Crowle, 1961). That these proteins were not present in the brain extract because of incomplete saline washing, is suggested by the absence of the albumin line. Thus, if edema fluid contains a normal tissue protein, it is either washed out by saline perfusion or it is non-antigenic for the rabbit. Putting together the three facts that edema fluid contains more alpha globulin than serum, that this region shows increased PAS staining, and that there is a heavier line in the position of human alpha 1 glycoprotein, the most likely explanation for our findings is that edema fluid contains an increased concentration of glycoprotein relative to serum and that the source of this protein is the blood stream.

An analysis of the proteins in edematous white matter of the cat 24 hours after injury has been published (Klatzo, et al., 1958). The material was frozen, extracted with buffer, dialyzed and electrophoresed on paper. Normal white matter showd alpha, beta and gamma components and only a small amount of albumin, probably as a result of the blood content of tissue. Edematous tissue showed an increase in total protein and albumin. The percentage of albumin relative to the total protein was less in extracts from edematous tissue than in serum. Unfortunately, the globulin fractions were not resolvable by this technique. Extraction studies using sucrose preceded by in vivo perfusion have also been reported in dogs with brains made edematous by the implantation of psyllium seeds (Hauser, et al., 1963). Again, paper electrophoresis was used. Edematous brains showed an increase in extractable protein involving both gray and white matter. It should be noted that the authors studied samples containing varying amounts of gray and white matter. In no case was "pure" white matter studied. The authors report the presence of a "band 2" which they interpret as albumin in normal tissues. Edematous brains showed an increase in band 2 which accounted for one-half of the increase in total protein and is most probably due to serum albumin. The authors were unable to demonstrate an increase in the adjacent band 3. This leaves 50% of the protein increase unaccounted for. In a study of human material an increase in both the albumin and alpha fractions has been demonstrated using free boundary electrophoresis on extracts of edematous tissue (Kyota, 1959). In starch electrophoresis (Cumings, 1961), extracts of human edematous tissue have been reported as showing an increase in albumin, gamma globulin and band 5 (not further identified). What these studies all have in common is the demonstration of albumin plus other proteins in increased amounts in edematous cerebral tissue. The characterization of these other proteins varies with the electrophoretic medium. On the basis of our data we would say that various serum fractions are present. Whether this can account entirely for the protein increase must await the application of quantitative immunochemical techniques to this problem. It is of interest that in a form of edema not associated with positive PAS staining (triethyl tin edema), there is no increase in tissue nitrogen and on starch electrophoresis there is an increase in band 2, not in 1 (gamma globulin), 8 (albumin) or 5 (Kalsbeck & Cumings, 1962).

Of all the forms of experimental disease, the freezing lesion is probably the most unnatural. When the reaction to this injury is examined, however, a striking resemblance to many human diseases is seen. When it was found that edema fluid could be isolated by centrifugation of edematous tissue, an attempt was made to this with human autopsy material. It was found that fluid could be collected by this technique from white matter adjacent to abscesses, some tumors, and areas of hemorrhage, whether traumatic or vascular in origin. We have not been able to collect fluid from cases of anemic infarction with swelling, generalized anoxia or lead encephalopathy. This does not mean that the fluid from these cases is intracellular since we also have been unable to collect fluid from the experimental lesion itself where it is obviously extracellular in location. It is a question, we believe, of the relative proportions of fluid and solid elements. If this is high enough, fluid will be separated by centrifugation. We should like to close by presenting data from a single case.

The patient was a 33-year-old white female who had a radical mastectomy for adenocarcinoma five months prior to admission. Thre months later she developed focal seizures. For two weeks prior to admission she had been unable to feed herself. On physical examination she showed papilledema and a left hemiparesis. She was poorly oriented and expired on the second hospital day. At autopsy there was marked swelling of the right cerebral hemisphere which contained a 3 cm. in diameter metastatic nodule. On cut section of the fresh brain, the white matter adjacent to this nodule was swollen, wet and yellowish. Several grams of this tissue were collected by gross dissection, centrifuged as described above, and the separated fluid collected. On microscopic examination the edematous areas showed pools of PAS positive fluid interspersed between the fibers of the white matter. Clear areas with widely separated fibers but containing no such material were also seen.

The collected fluid was subjected to immuno-electrophoresis as described above. An attempt was made to use serum obtained from the patient at autopsy for purposes of comparison. This proved to be unsatisfactory; therefore, normal pooled serum was used. This was reacted against commercial human antiserum (Colorado Serum Company, Denver, Colorado) prepared in the horse. The results are shown in Figure 8. As with the experimental material, albumin and globulin are clearly present and an arch which may be a glycoprotein is heavier in edema fluid than in serum.

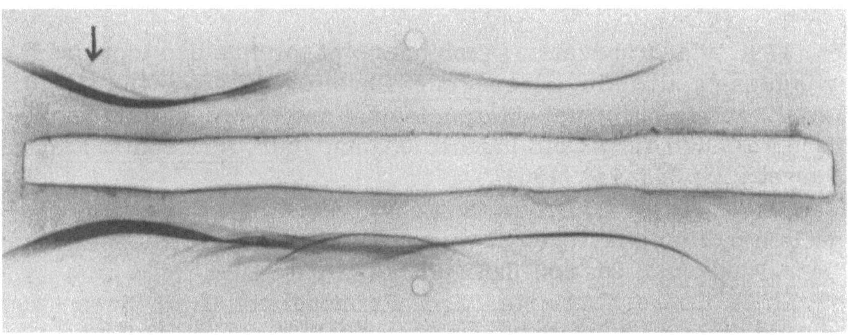

Fig. 8. Immuno-electrophoresis treated as above. Upper hole: human edema fluid. Lower hole: pooled normal human serum. Trench: human antiserum. Arrow: (?) alpha glycoprotein.

Our chemical findings with isolated edema fluid may be summarized by the statement that this fluid is qualitatively similar to but quantitatively distinct from blood serum. The alpha globulins are increased in edema fluid and this is believed to be the result of an increase in glycoproteins. It is our present hypothesis that the increased diffuse PAS staining observed with certain forms of human and experimental cerebral edema is a reflection of an increased glycoprotein content in edema fluid with respect to serum and that the PAS stain is, under these circumstances, a protein stain.

SUMMARY

Edema fluid was isolated from the brains of dogs with freezing lesions four hours after injury. This fluid was analyzed chemically and compared with serum. It showed a diminished concentration of sodium, chloride, Evan's blue and albumin, equal concentrations of beta and gamma globulins and an increased concentration of alpha globulins and potassium. The increased concentration of alpha globulin is attributed to an increased glycoprotein content. It is suggested that this is the cause of increased diffuse PAS staining in certain forms of cerebral edema.

REFERENCES

Allen, T. H. and Orahovats: Combination of tolidine dye isomers with plasma albumin, Amer. Jour. Physiol., 161; 473-482 (1950).

Bakay, L. and I. V. Haque: Morphological and chemical studies in cerebral edema. I. Cold induced edema, Jour. Neuropath. Exp. Neurol., 23; 393-418 (1964).

Clasen, R. A., D. V. L. Brown, S. Leavitt and G. M. Hass: The production by liquid nitrogen of acute closed cerebral lesions, Surg., Gyne., and Obs., 96; 605-616 (1953).

_____, P. M. Cooke, F. Martin, A. J. Raimondi and G. M. Hass: Use of vital staining in experimental cerebral edema, Fed. Proc., 16; 353 (1957).

_____, _____, S. Pandolfi, D. Boyd and A. J. Raimondi: Experimental cerebral edema produced by focal freezing. 1. An anatomic study utilizing vital dye techniques, Jour. Neuropath. Exp. Neurol., 21; 579-596 (1962).

_____, _____, _____, G. Carnecki and G. M. Hass: Steroid-antihistaminic therapy in experimental cerebral edema, Arch. Neurol. (in press, a)

_____, S. Pandolfi, D. Oelke and G. M. Hass: Reserpine in experimental cerebral edema, Neurol., 16; 1194-1204 (1966).

Crowle, A. J.: Immunodiffusion, first edition, New York and London: Academic Press (1961).

Cumings, J. N.: Soluble cerebral proteins in normal and edematous brain, Journ. Clin. Path., 14; 289-294 (1961).

Cutler, R. W. P., G. V. Watters and C. F. Barlow: I^{125}-Labeled protein in experimental brain edema, Arch. Neurol., 11; 225-238 (1964).

Friede, R. L.: The enzymatic response of astrocytes to various ions in vitro, Jour. Cell Biol., 20; 5-15 (1964).
Gregersen, M. I. and R. A. Rawson: The disappearance of T-1824 and structurally related dyes from the blood stream, Amer. Jour. Physiol., 138; 698-707 (1942).
Hauser, H. M., H. J. Svien, B. F. McKenzie, W. F. McGuckin and N. P. Goldstein: A study of cerebral protein and polysaccharide in the dog. III. Albumin changes in experimental cerebral edema, Neurol., 13; 945-952 (1963).
Kalsbeck, J. E. and J. N. Cumings: Experimental edema in the rat and cat brain. Jour. Neuropath, Exp. Neurol., 22; 237-247 (1962).
Kiyota, K.: Electrophoretic protein fractions and the hydrophilic property of brain tissue, Jour. Neurochem., 4; 202-216 (1959).
Klatzo, I., A. Piraux and E. J. Laskowski: The relationship between edema, blood-brain-barrier, and tissue elements in a local brain injury, Jour. Neuropath. Exp. Neurol., 17; 548-564 (1958).
Lowry, O. H., N. J. Rosebrough, A. L. Farr and R. J. Randall: Protein measurement with the Folin phenol reagent, Jour. Biol. Chem., 193; 265-275 (1951).
Pappius, H. M. and D. R. Gulati: Water and electrolyte content of cerebral tissues in experimentally induced edema, Acta. Neuropath., 2; 451-460 (1963).
Torack, R. M., R. D. Terry and H. M. Zimmerman: The fine structure of cerebral fluid accumulation. 1. Swelling secondary to cold injury, Amer. Jour. Path., 35; 1135-1147 (1959).

IGOR KLATZO
HENRYK WIŚNIEWSKI
OSKAR STEINWALL
EUGENE STREICHER

DYNAMICS OF COLD INJURY EDEMA

Cold injury edema may serve as an experimental model for ar edematous process in the brain tissue originating from an increase vascular permeability. Undoubtedly, this type of edema is of a para mount clinical importance as a dreaded complication of head injuri brain tumors, inflammatory processes, etc.

Since 1958 we have been using in our laboratory a standardize procedure consisting in a local application of a metal plate cooled t −50°C to the exposed cerebral cortex of the cat (Klatzo, et al., 195 Such application results in a sharply demarcated necrosis of the su perficial cortical layers and a progressive development of edema which shows a striking predilection to spreading through the white matter. By controlling the temperature of the metal plate and the time of application it was possible to achieve a degree of uniformit of the lesions which was adequate for observations related to dynar ics and effects of various experimental conditions.

The investigations presented below include a summarizing re view of our previous investigations, as well as some of the recent data pertaining to the factors which proved to exert an effect on the development and progression of cold injury edema.

OBSERVATIONS

Dynamics of a Standard Cold Injury Edema in Adult Cats.

The observations on the relationship between duration of the lesion, spreading of the edema and of the blood-brain barrier indicator were carried out in a large series of cats (Klatzo, et al., 1963) and revealed the following findings:

When one of the fluorescent indicators (fluorescein labeled albumin or sodium flourescein) was injected intravenously immediately preceding the cold injury, the area of edema, as ascertained by histological methods, always corresponded closely to that which was green fluorescent under the ultraviolet illumination. There was also a direct relationship between the extent of edema and the time elapsed since the production of the cold lesion (Table 1, A). Thus, e.g., after two hours the area of edema occupied only the white matter of the injured gyrus; at six hours it extended into the adjacent gyri and in cats sacrificed 24 hours following the operation it reached its maximal extension. It might be emphasized that edema always showed a striking predilection to the white matter, the cortex overlying the edematous white matter appearing conspicuously spared.

In another series of cats, the tracer was injected at various time intervals following the cold injury and the animals were sacrificed always one hour after tracer administration. In these cats the area of tracer penetration proved to be similar in each case, i.e., regardless of duration of the injury and of the extent of edema the area visualized by the green fluorescent indicators was confined to the small portion of the white matter underlying the site of cortical injury (Table 1, B).

Vascular Permeability in the Edematous White Matter

Although the observations presented above are themselves indicative that the vascular permeability is disturbed only in the regions immediately adjacent to the cold application, two types of experiments were designed to establish more conclusively this point.

In one of these experiments two albumin indicators labeled with contrasting in color fluorescent markers were used consecutively. The cats received immediately preceding the cold injury the red flourescent Rhodamine B labeled albumin (RLA) and several hours later the green fluorescein isothiocyanate labeled albumin (FLA). They were sacrificed a few hours after the second administration of an albumin indicator. The result of such experiments is exemplified in Fig. 1B. In this cat the FLA was given six hours after the cold injury and administration of the RLA. The animal was sacrificed two hours after the intravenous injection of the second tracer. It is apparent that the areas of green and red fluorescence are clearly separated. Also, microscopically, there was no evidence of any extravascular passage of the FLA into the edematous white matter invaded by the RLA.

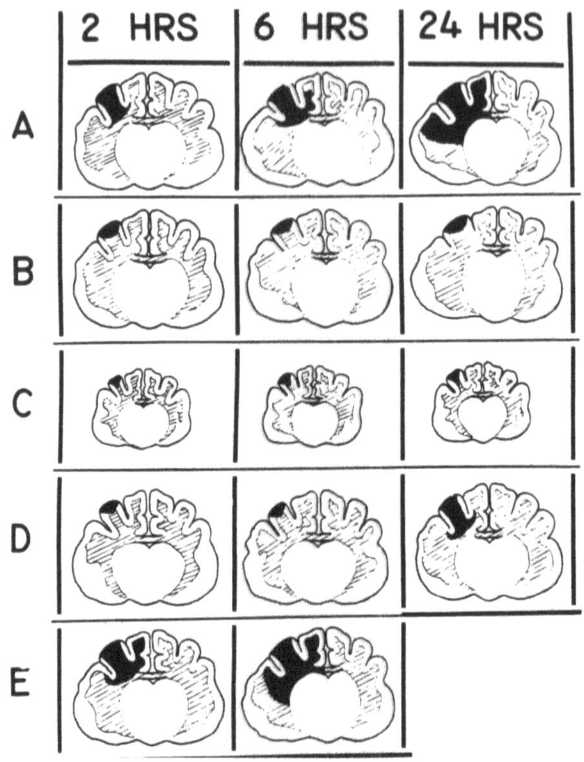

Table 1. Diagramatic representation of the tracer migration under various experimental conditions. (a) Adult cats in which a BBB indicator (FLA or sodium fluorescein) was injected intravenously at the time of production of the cold injury. (b) Adult cats in which an indicator was administered one hour before the sacrifice. (c) New-born kittens. (d) Adult cats in which the systolic blood pressure was maintained at 50 mm Hg. (e) Adult cats with 200 mm Hg systolic blood pressure.

In another experiment to test the vascular permeability in the area of edema radioautography using I^{125} labeled albumin was applied (Klatzo, et al., 1963). Cats injected with I^{125} albumin one hour before the sacrifice at 24 hours time interval following the cold injury showed no evidence of any extravascular passage of the tracer into the intensely edematous white matter with exception of a small region underlying the cold lesion (Fig. 1a).

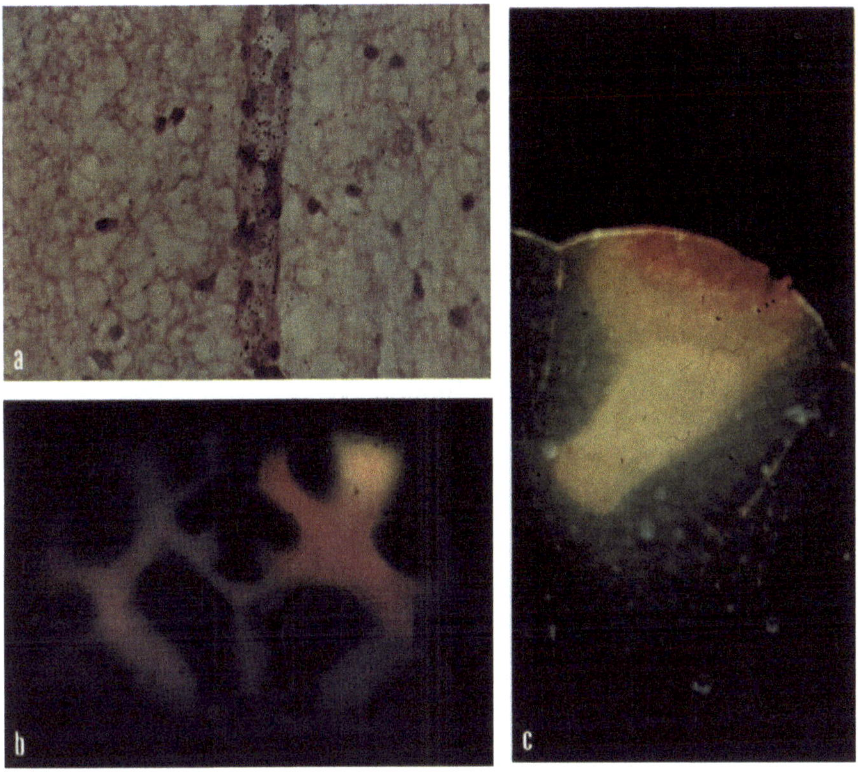

Fig. 1. (a) Edematous white matter in the cat with 24 hours cold lesion. I^{125}albumin was injected one hour before the sacrifice. There is no passage of the radioactive tracer outside of the blood vessel surrounded by intensely edematous tissue. Radioautograph, counterstained with hematoxylin and eosin, X320. (b) Cat injected with the RLA immediately before the cold injury. The FLA was administered at eight-hour time interval and the animal was sacrificed two hours later, i.e., ten hours following the operation. The area occupied by the red fluorescent RLA appears to be free of any FLA penetration. Photograph under the ultra violet illumination.
(c) Cat injected intravenously with the mixture of sodium fluorescein and Evans Blue-albumin complex at the time of cold injury and sacrificed two hours later. The area of edema is outlined uniformly by a yellow fluorescence, i.e., color of the mixture of both tracers, without any evidence of their separation at the periphery. A reddish color at the site of cortical injury is due to the affinity of red fluorescent Evans Blue-albumin to the necrotic tissue. A thin, cryostat-cut section under the oblique beam of ultraviolet light.

It appears that these two experiments demonstrate conclusively that the permeability of the blood vessels to serum proteins in the edematous white matter remains unaltered and that the extravascular migration represents the main route for spreading of the edema.

The Rate of Extravascular Migration

The purpose of the experiments described below was to ascertain whether the rate of extravascular migration through the white matter with regard to various substances may be to some extent dependent on their biophysical properties, such as molecular size or electrical charge. This was carried out by injecting at the time of cold injury a mixture of two tracers, either both fluorescent but of contrasting color, or one being fluorescent and another radioactive. In order to avoid artefacts with regard to easily diffusable substances the brain tissue after the sacrifice was rapidly frozen and the thin sections were prepared in the cryostat. The comparative distribution of two different tracers was assessed in the same section either by evaluation of the color of the fluorescence or by combined fluorescence-radioautography observations (Steinwall & Klatzo, 1965).

The double tracer application revealed that the rate of migration of various substances through the white matter was similar, which could be conjectured from the fact that the peripheral borders of tracers extension coincided in each combination used. (Figs. 1c, 2 and 3). This was evident comparing substances so different in molecular size as the FLA and C^{14} sucrose, or sodium fluorescein and Evans Blue-albumin complex. Also, the negatively charged FLA and the non-charged C^{14} inulin appeared to migrate through the white matter at similar rate.

Effect of the Systolic Blood Pressure

Considering the factors which could significantly influence the rate of extravascular migration of tracers from the site of injury the role of systolic blood pressure was evaluated. The level of the systolic blood pressure was affected by intravenous drip of 5% dextrose to which hyper- or hypotensive drugs were added and the con-

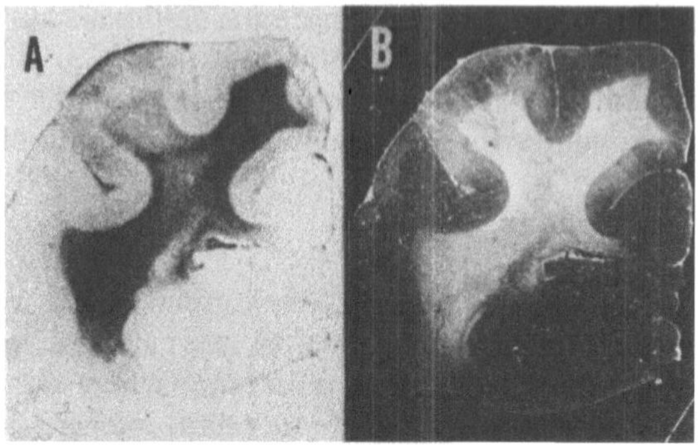

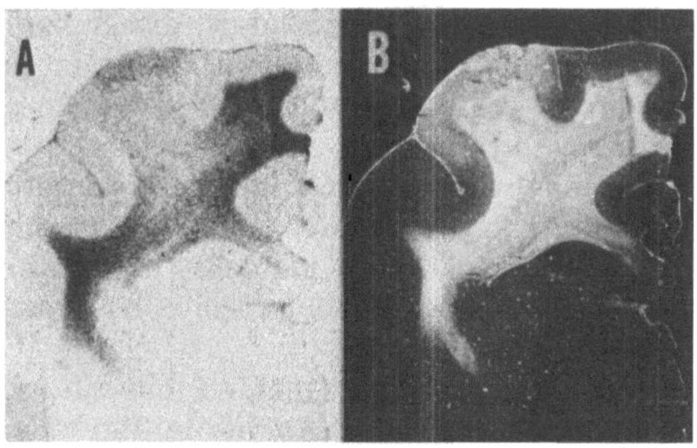

Fig. 2. (Top.) Cat injected with the FLA and C^{14} inulin preceding the cold injury and sacrificed after four hours. The area of the FLA (b) matche closely in its peripheral extension that of C^{14} inulin (a).

Fig. 3. (Bottom). Cat injected with the FLA and C^{14} sucrose, sacrificed seven hours after the operation. The respective distributions of the C^{14} sucrose (a) and FLA (b) indicate a similar extent of migration of both tracers.

tinuous blood pressure recording was obtained via the catheter introduced into the femoral artery and connected to the Gilson polygraph. By infusion of hyper- or hypotensive drugs the systolic bloc pressure was adjusted to a desired level. After administration of s dium fluorescein as a tracer the cold injury was performed and the cats were sacrificed at various time intervals. With each experimental animal, another cat having the cold lesion of the same duration but in which the blood pressure was not altered by the drugs, was sacrificed.

The results obtained from this investigation indicated a pronounced effect of systolic blood pressure on the dynamics of edem The elevation of the blood pressure produced a conspicuous accele ation in the spreading of the edema and the tracer. Thus, e.g., cats sacrificed two hours following cold injury in which the systolic blood pressure was maintained at 200 mm Hg by intravenous infusion of Levophed showed the area of edema and tracer penetration similar in extent to that seen in the normotensive animals after six hours (Table 1, E). Six hours of hypertension (200 mm Hg) resulted in almost maximal spreading of edema, the tracer extending into the white matter of the adjacent gyri (Table 1, E). Equally marked was also the effect of hypotension. Cats sacrificed two hours after cold lesion in which the systolic blood pressure was lowered to 50 mm Hg by intravenous infusion of Arfonad (0.05% in 5% dextrose) exhibited a remarkably small area of tracer penetration corresponding to that seen in the normotensive animals with cold lesion of 15 minutes' duration. The penetration of the tracer was only slightly deeper in hypotensive cats (50 mm Hg) sacrificed six hours following the cold injury. The area of edema in hypotensive cats with 24 hours lesion was comparable to that observed after four hours in animals which had no interference with regard to their blood pressure (Table 1, D).

Factors Related to the Brain Tissue Itself

The tendency of edema to involve preferentially the white matter indicates the presence of some factors in the brain tissue itself which influence the dynamics of edematous spreading. Investigating the effect of local brain injury in an experimental material other than adult cats we found two instances; namely, in sharks and in new-born kittens in which there was a striking resistance to the development of edema, although the inducing lesions were of comparable nature and intensity as in adult cats.

New-born Kittens

In spite of a prevailing clinical impression that the immature human brain is very susceptible to edema, our studies revealed a pronounced resistance of the kitten brains to the development of cold injury edema as compared with adult cats (Streicher, et al., 1965). Using both the FLA and the I^{125} albumin as the tracers it was apparent that in the new-born kittens even at 24 hours following the cold injury a tracer did not spread beyond the white matter of the injured gyrus (Table 1, C).

Sharks

Even more striking resistance of the brain tissue to edematous process following a traumatic injury was observed in sharks

(Klatzo & Steinwall, 1965). Investigating some aspects of the blood-brain barrier and the CSF pathways we discovered that even most drastic lesions, such as those produced by a direct application of dry ice or heated metal plate to the exposed cerebral cortex of the lemon or nurse sharks, failed to result in any recognizable edema or spreading of the tracers into the adjacent brain tissue (Fig. 4).

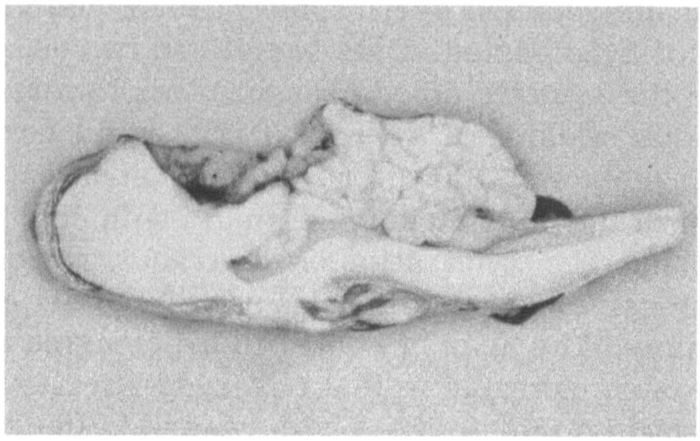

Fig. 4. Brain of a shark injected with Evans Blue-albumin and subjected to a severe heat lesion in the posterior part of the fore-brain. The animal was sacrificed three days after the operation. There are no signs of edema or extravasation of the indicator in the area surrounding the large tissue defect.

COMMENTS

The observations presented on the dynamics of edema following cold injury provide some insight into a so far obscure relationship between the brain edema and the blood-brain barrier (BBB). In numerous previous investigations on the BBB it was generally assumed that the staining of the brain tissue by a dye indicator invariably indicated a disturbed BBB function in such an area. Although this might have been the case in the studies on the BBB using an intravascular perfusion with chemical toxic agents followed almost directly by assessment of tracer distribution (Broman, 1949; Steinwall, 1961), our investigations demonstrated that in the BBB damage associated with cold injury edema the distribution of a tracer is mainly dependent on the extravascular migration, the extent of which is related to the time element. Whether this migration takes place primarily via extra- or intracellular compartments the techniques used in our investigations are inadequate to provide a definitive answer. On the basis of some previous observations, such as those pertaining to the distribution of fibrinogen, effects of supravital perfusion (Klatzo, et al., 1962), and to evaluation of thiocyanate and chloride spaces (Streicher, et al., 1964), we have been inclined to favor the possibility that edema spreads mainly via extracellular routes, the swelling of the tissue components, such as the astrocytes, being a secondary phenomenon. This assumption is now strongly supported by more recent electron microscopic observations which amply demonstrate the widening of extracellular spaces without rupture of the cell membranes in various types of experimental edema.

The indication that the substances of greatly diverse molecular sizes seem to migrate through the white matter at a similar rate is rather difficult to interpret. If the extravascular migration would depend only on a simple diffusion, one would expect perhaps some "lagging" of, e.g., serum proteins in comparison with relatively small molecular compounds such as sucrose or sodium fluorescein. Otherwise, it might be possible that mechanisms such as propelling of edema fluid by an undulating movement of glial membranes, which is characteristic for pinocytotic activity (Klatzo & Miguel, 1960), could provide an independent factor in spreading of edema.

The results concerning the effect of systolic blood pressure on the dynamics of cold injury edema appeared to be unequivocal. Undoubtedly, further experimental studies are required, particularly with regard to the relationship between duration and time of application of hypotension and its edema-reducing effect. Otherwise, it should be considered, that since the lowering of the blood pressure is a concommitant feature of hypothermia, it is possible that its beneficial effect on brain edema, so widely reported in experimental and clinical investigations, may be to a large extent related to hypotension.

The apparent resistance of shark and immature mammalian brains to the development of edema following a local cortical injury is presumably related to a variety of factors inherent in the structural and physiological features of the tissue. With regard to an immature mammalian brain, Dr. Tower's observations as presented at this workshop on difference in amount of swelling in vitro between immature and adult cat brains are most interesting and perhaps in some way related to our findings. Our knowledge concerning the properties of shark brain is very meager. Of some relevance to the dynamics of edema might be a strikingly different from mammalian arrangement of astrocytes in their relationship to blood vessels and pia (Klatzo & Steinwall, 1965), as well as the paucity of myelinated fibers in the fore-brain which was subjected to injury. Also, of some importance could be a remarkably low (30 mm Hg) systolic blood pressure in the sharks (Dr. E. Bering, personal communication).

SUMMARY

1. Observations on the dynamic aspects of the cortical cold injury indicate that the resulting edema spreads preferentially through the white matter via extravascular migration, the blood-brain barrier in the edematous white matter remaining undisturbed.

2. The rate of extravascular migration through the white matter appears to be similar for indicators of considerably different molecular size or electrical change.

3. The systolic blood pressure exerts a pronounced effect on the rate of edema progression.

4. An apparent resistance to the development of edema following a local brain injury was demonstrated in shark and new-born kitten brains.

REFERENCES

Broman, T.: The permeability of the cerebrospinal blood vessels in normal and pathological conditions, Copenhagen: Ejnar Munksgaard (1949).

Klatzo, I., A. Piraux and E. J. Laskowski: The relationship between edema, blood-brain barrier and tissue elements in a local brain injury, J. Neuropath. Exp. Neurol., 17, 548-564 (1958).

_____ and J. Miquel: Observations on pinocytosis in nervous tissue, Ibid., 19, 475-487 (1960).

_____, _____ and R. Otenasek: The application of fluorescein labeled serum proteins (FLSP) to the study of vascular permeability in the brain, Acta Neuropath., 2, 144-160 (1962).

_____, H. Wisniewski and D. E. Smith: Observations on penetration of serum proteins into the central nervous system, proceedings of the symposium on the biology of neuroglia (Buenos Aires, October 1963), Progress in Brain Research, Elsevier, Vol. 15, 73-88 (1965).

_____ and O. Steinwall: Observations on cerebrospinal fluid pathways and behaviour of the blood-brain barrier in sharks, Acta Neuropath 5, 161-175 (1965).

Steinwall, O.: Transport mechanisms in certain blood-brain barrier phenomena: a hypothesis, Acta Psychiatr. Neurol. Scand., 36, Suppl. 150, 314-318 (1961).

_____ and I. Klatzo: Double tracer methods in studies on blood-brain barrier dysfunction and brain edema, Proceedings of the 17th Congress of Scandinavian Neurologists (Goteborg 1964), Acta Neurol. Scand., 41, Suppl. 14, R31/1-R31/5 (1965).

Streicher, E., P. J. Ferris, J. D. Prokop and I. Klatzo: Brain volume and thiocyanate space in local cold injury, Arch. Neurol., 11, 444-448 (1964).

_____, H. Wisniewski and I. Klatzo: Resistance of immature brain to experimental cerebral edema, Neurology, 15, 833-836 (1965).

J. W. F. BEKS
C. A. ter WEEME
E. J. EBELS

ALTERATIONS IN THE INTRAVENTRICULAR PRESSURE IN CATS AFTER COLD INDUCED EDEMA

The experiments were set up in order to register the alterations in the intraventricular pressure in cats during the development of brain edema resulting from a cortical lesion cold-induced by Klatzo's method. With the aid of a cooling thermoprobe which was put on the intact dura of the left frontal lobe, a decrease of temperature to −30°C was achieved. In contrast with other investigators we left the cooling thermoprobe in its place during the entire course of the experiment so as not to influence the intracranial pressure relations by decompression. The pressure was measured in the cella media of the right lateral ventricle, in which a needle was introduced by stereotactic means (Fig. 1).

The average initial pressure in the ventricle amounted to 80 mm water. The first symptoms of compression of the brain stem occurred about two hours after the cooling at an average intraventricular pressure of 1500 mm water. These symptoms were changes of respiration (Cheyne- Stokes breathing) and increase of the arterial blood pressure. About 20 minutes after the appearance of the firs symptoms, apnea occurred, whereafter the intraventricular pressure increased to a maximum level of about 2500 mm water. At this moment we noticed pilomotor action and decerebrate rigidity. Immediately hereafter the intraventricular pressure decreased to a level beneath the initial value and the animal would die if no further measures were taken. The arterial blood pressure reached its highest value (3000 mm water) simultaneously with the maximal value of the intraventricular pressure. The venous pressure hardly showed any change (Fig. 2).

Light microscopic observations showed hyperemia and degeneration of the brain parenchyma, with vacuolisation and spongiosis of the "neuropil" and degeneration of neurons. In the white matter the changes were of two kinds: directly under the cortex and probably as a direct result of the application of cold we saw desintegration and destruction of the myelin sheaths with pyknosis of the oligodendroglia nuclei. In the deeper white matter the well-known picture of edema was seen, with separation of otherwise undamaged myelin sheaths and normal oligoglial cells (Fig. 3). Leakage of P. A. S. positive fluid through the wall of the vessels was observed, especially in the damaged cortex and white matter and also to a lesser degree in the edematous white matter (Fig. 4). The fluid seems to collect at the lower border of the lesion and hence to spread through the white matter, sparing the corpus callosum, optic radiation and internal capsule to a large extent.

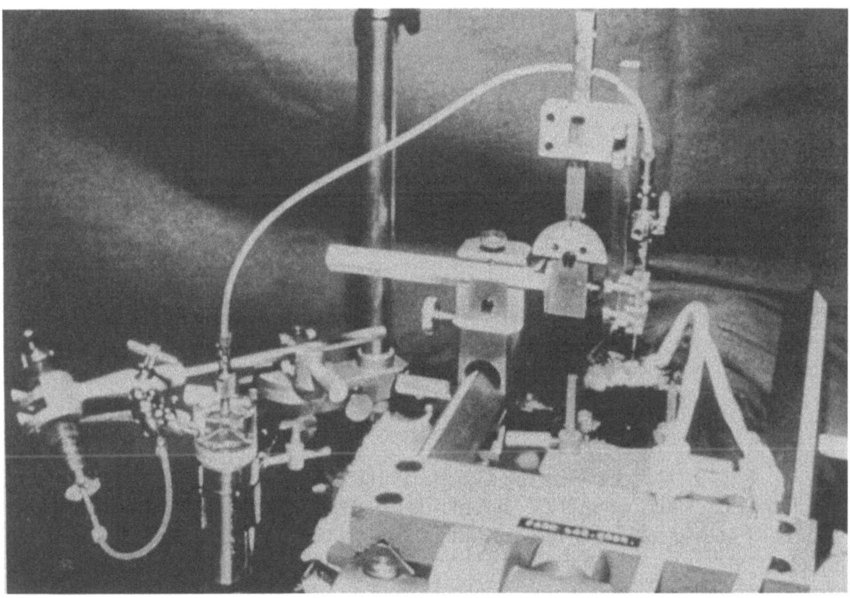

Fig. 1. Position of the cat in the stereotactical apparatus, with the thermoprobe on the left hemisphere and the needle in the right lateral ventricle.

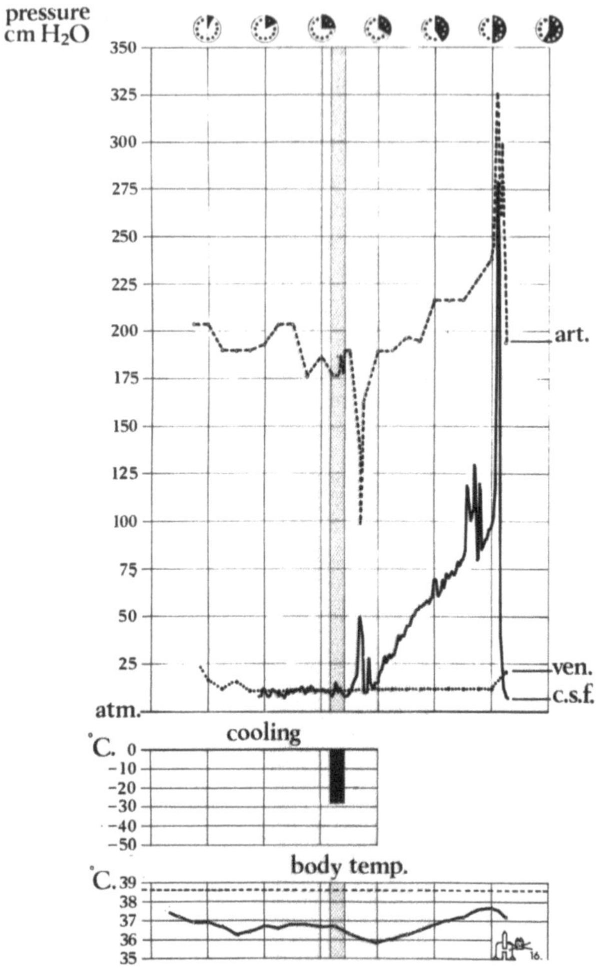

Fig. 2. Curves showing C.S.F. (right lateral ventricle) and arterial (A. femoralis) and venous (V. femoralis) pressures during an experiment. The body temperature of the animal is registered throughout the experiment.

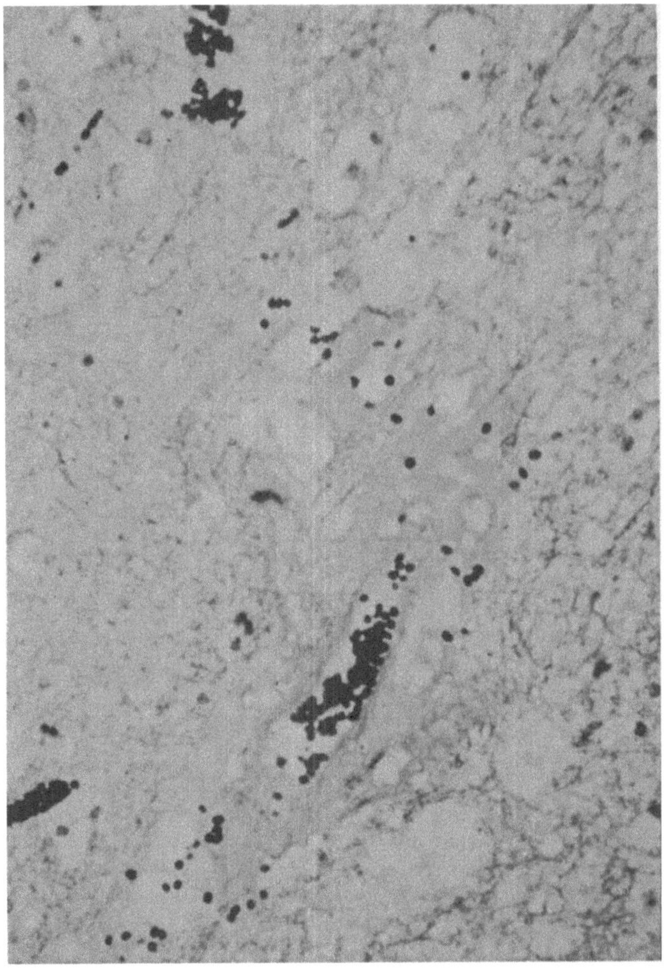

Fig. 3. Leakage of fluid through vessel walls in the damaged cortex.

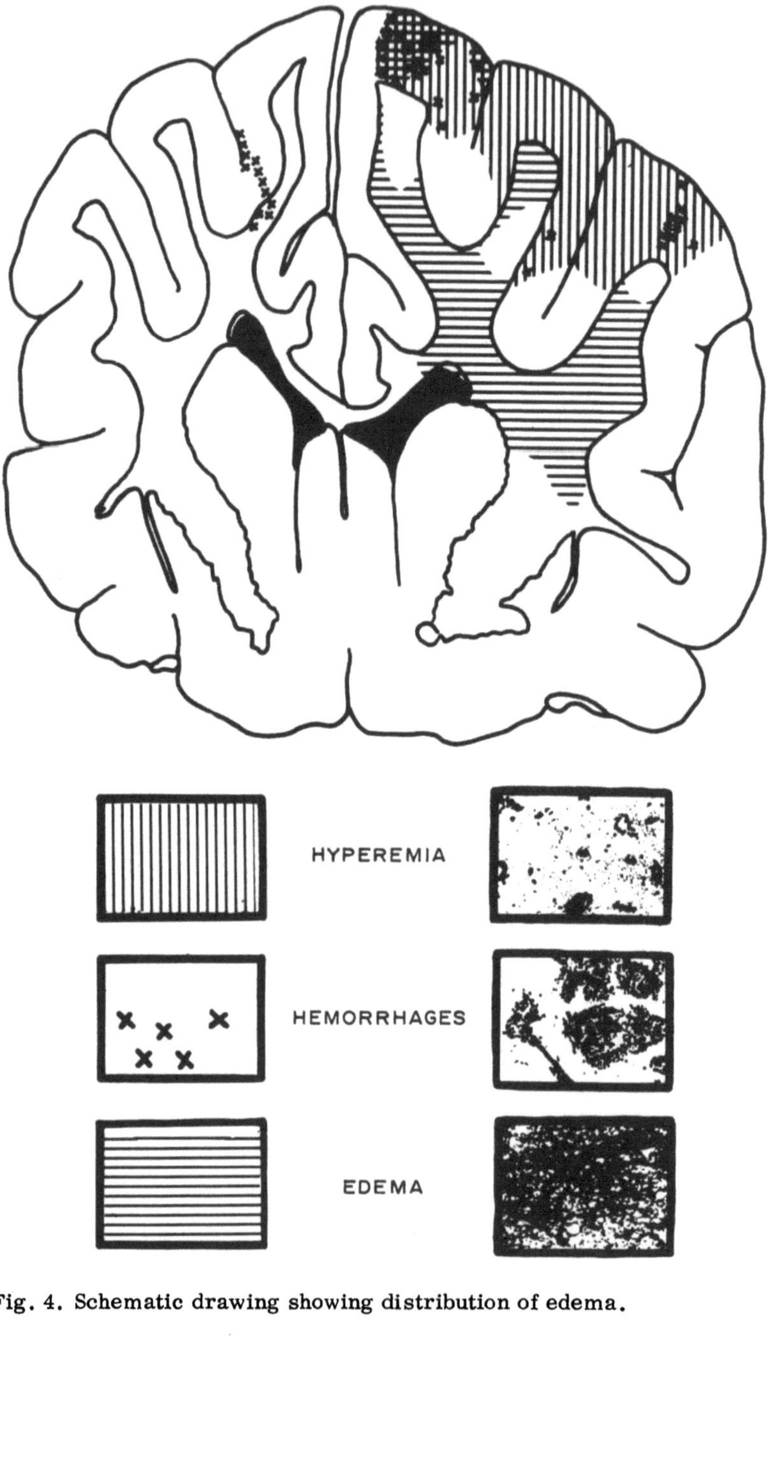

Fig. 4. Schematic drawing showing distribution of edema.

ASAO HIRANO
H. M. ZIMMERMAN
SEYMOUR LEVINE

FINE STRUCTURE OF CEREBRAL FLUID ACCUMULATION*

X. A REVIEW OF EXPERIMENTAL EDEMA IN WHITE MATTER

INTRODUCTION

Although cerebral edema has been studied for many years, conclusive evidence as to the precise origin, location and morphological nature of the edema fluid had to await both the advent of the electron microscope and improved techniques of preservation. The development of better techniques has permitted us to carry out a series of studies which, we feel, provide some information clarifying the edema process. Edema is a condition which affects primarily white matter. Therefore, in our experiments we studied several different types of white matter injury. One type of injury followed implantation into the brain of the relatively bland polysaccharide isolated from Cryptococcus neoformans. Another type of injury followed implantation of the powerfully necrotizing chemical agent, silver nitrate. A third type of injury was of systemic, auto-immune origin, that is, experimental allergic encephalomyelitis (EAE).

*This investigation was supported by the United States Public Health Service Research Grant No. B-3533 from the National Institute of Neurological Diseases and Blindness, National Institutes of Health, and Grant No. 317-2 of the National Multiple Sclerosis Society.

MATERIALS AND METHODS

Cryptococcal Capsular Polysaccharide

Pellets of a mixture of equal parts by weight of cryptococcal polysaccharide mixed with inert graphite were implanted unilaterally in the anterior end of the hemispheric white matter in a total of 28 adult female rats. These rats were divided into two groups. The first group consisted of two rats sacrificed 24 hours and two rats sacrificed 48 hours after implantation. Celloidin and paraffin-embedded sections were prepared after the conventional immersion fixation with 10 per cent neutral formalin. Sections were stained with hematoxylin and eosin (H & E), cresyl violet, periodic acid-Schiff (PAS)-luxol fast blue (LFB) and Woelcke stains, as well as by silver impregnation techniques. The second group consisted of 24 rats. These were sacrificed at six, 12, 24, 36 and 48 hours and at three, four, seven, 14, 21, 28, 35 and 100 days after implantation. Their brains were fixed by perfusion via the heart with a solution of 4% formaldehyde and 6% sucrose at pH 7.4 followed immediately by Dalton's fixative. Seven different sites were sampled after slicing each brain in a horizontal plane: the implant region, three portions of white matter in the callosal radiation (proximal, middle and distal portions) on the side of the implant, the corpus callosum on both the side of the implant and the opposite side, and finally the callosal radiation of the opposite side. The blocks of tissue were dehydrated after brief post-fixation in Dalton's fixative and were embedded in Vestopal-W. In order to study the morphologic features of the implanted chemicals under similar conditions, but without interference from tissue reaction, pellets of cryptococcal polysaccharide alone, graphite alone, or a mixture of equal parts of polysaccharide and graphite were implanted into the brains of three additional freshly killed rats that had been pretreated intraperitoneally with 1,000 units of heparin. The dead rats were cooled on ice, and the region of the implant was removed for electron microscopic study within four hours. Sectioning of the blocks from all animals was performed with a Porter-Blum ultramicrotome. Thick sections prepared from each Vestopal block were stained with toluidine blue, cresyl violet and silver impregnation techniques for light microscopy. Guided by the findings, thin sections were cut from the appropriate region in the same blocks. The specimens were stained with lead hydroxide or with 2% uranyl acetate and examined with the RCA EMU 3F electron microscope. Further details concerning implantation, and other technical matters have been presented previously (Levine, et al., 1963; Hirano, et al., 1964a).

Silver Nitrate

Pellets of a mixture of equal parts by weight of silver nitrate and graphite were implanted unilaterally in the forebrain of ten adult female rats (Levine, 1963; Levine, 1965). These animals were divided into three groups. The first group consisted of two rats sacrificed 24 and 48 hours after implantation. Paraffin-embedded sections were prepared after the conventional immersion fixation with 5% glutaraldehyde, phosphate buffered at pH 7.4. Sections were stained with H & E, and PAS-LFB stains. The second group consisted of six rats which were sacrificed at 24, 48 and 72 hours after implantation. Their brains were fixed by perfusion with 5% glutaraldehyde in phosphate buffer at pH 7.4, followed by immersion in Dalton's solution, dehydration and embedding in Epon. The third group consisted of two rats which were killed one and two days after implantation. They were fixed by immersion in 5% glutaraldehyde, followed by immersion in Dalton's fixative, dehydration, and embedding in Epon. Sectioning, staining and electron microscopic examination were carried out in a manner similar to that employed in the polysaccharide experiment (Hirano, et al., 1965c).

Hyperacute Allergic Encephalomyelitis

Female Lewis rats (Microbiological Associates) were maintained on Purina Laboratory Chow and tap water. Hyperacute EAE was produced by injecting a mixture of 200 mg. (wet weight) guinea pig spinal cord homogenate and 0.6 ml. pertussis vaccine made up to a final volume of 3.0 ml. with saline, into the peritoneal cavity. In one experiment, five rats with no clinical signs, two with weakness of tail only, and one with hind limb weakness were selected from a large group, early on the eighth day after sensitization. At this time, most of the rats had clinical evidence of EAE, and we could be certain that even the asymptomatic animals had early histologic lesions. In another experiment, six rats with clinical signs varying in severity from loss of tail tonus to quadriplegia were selected. The rats were perfused with 5% glutaraldehyde solution in phosphate buffer at pH 7.4. The lower spinal cord (site of predilection of hyperacute EAE) was dissected out of the vertebral column. Blocks were sectioned from lumbar and sacral cord, conus medullaris, nerve roots and cauda equina. The blocks were post-osmicated in Dalton's fixative, dehydrated and embedded in Epon. After sectioning and staining, specimens were examined with the electron microscope. Further details concerning technical matters have been reported previously (Levine & Wenk, 1964, 1965; Levine, et al., 1965).

RESULTS

Cryptococcal Capsular Polysaccharide

Light Microscopy

The celloidin or paraffin-embedded preparations of the rat brain, made by conventional immersion fixation in formalin, showed selective morphological alterations in the white matter. The site of implantation was marked by a well-localized black mass of implanted graphite. The graphite was chemically inert and merely served as excipient, binder, lubricant and marker for the implanted material. A wide, optically empty zone was evident in the callosal radiation on the side of the implant during the acute phase (up to 48 hours after implantation). This pale band extended a remarkably long distance along the white matter. The involvement often extended into the corpus callosum, but the white matter on the opposite side usually remained intact (Levine, et al., 1963).

By contrast, the Vestopal embedded thick sections which were fixed by perfusion with formalin and osmium, demonstrated no optically empty spaces except for the lumens of blood vessels distended by the perfusion. Instead, darkly stained material was clearly seen (Fig. 1). This material originated from the implant and extended into the distal part of the involved white matter during the acute stage. The optical density of the material gradually decreased with time as well as with distance from the implant (Hirano, et al., 1964a).

By the third and fourth days after implantation (the subacute phase) the fluid flow decreased. One week after implantation (the chronic phase) isolated chains of fluid material were seen in the interfascicular glial cells (Levine, et al., 1963; Hirano, et al., 1965a, 1965b).

Electron Microscopy

In the involved white matter during the acute stage, the arrangement of myelinated nerve fibers was obviously disturbed by the presence of a diffusely distributed electron-dense substance which had separated individual fibers and groups of fibers. At higher magnification, this substance revealed a highly electron-dense reticulated texture without discrete morphological units. In order to determine the exact nature of this material, electron microscopic examination was carried out on a variety of substances which were implanted into the forebrain of dead animals. We found that the material in question was indeed morphologically identical with the cryptococcal polysaccharide that had been implanted, and not some endogenous material produced in response to the implantation (Hirano, et al., 1964b). This polysaccharide had exactly the same appearance, when examined in situ, as part of the capsule of cryptococcal yeast cells (Levine, et al., 1964). The cytoplasm and cell wall of the Cryptococcus neoformans were surrounded by the polysaccharide material which made up the capsule. It had the same reticulated, electron-dense structure as the purified polysaccharide. Visualization and identification of this material was greatly facilitated after staining with heavy metals like uranyl acetate or lead hydroxide (Hirano, et al., 1964b).

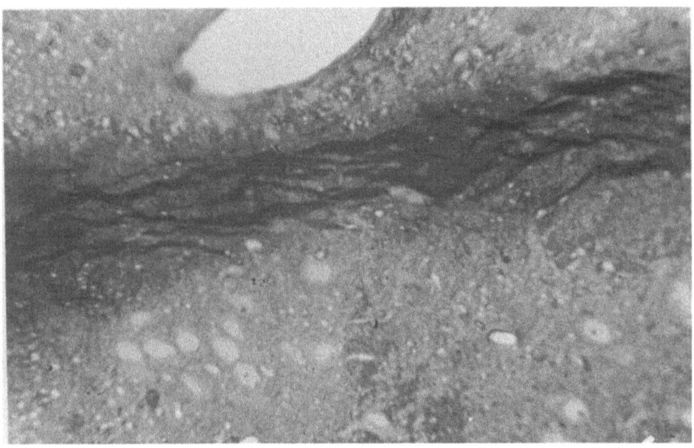

Fig. 1. Involved callosal radiation 12 hours after polysaccharide implantation. The lumen of a vessel is clear and empty as a result of perfusion. There is no optically empty space in the cerebral tissue proper. There is a flow of darkly stained fluid in the white matter. Vestopal-W embedding, cresyl violet stain (reduced).

In our experiments, the white matter on the opposite side of the implant served as a control. In the normal white matter, both myelinated and non-myelinated fibers were compactly arranged, and there were no empty spaces except for vascular lumens which were empty and distended due to perfusion. No electron-dense fluid was observed, and the anatomical arrangement between myelinated nerve fibers was normal. The outermost major dense line of the myelin sheath was surrounded by a less dense line similar in appearance to the intraperiod line. There were intraperiod lines between adjoining myelin sheaths (Fig. 2). There were triangular areas formed by juxtaposition of three adjacent myelin sheaths. The extracellular space in normal white matter was largely restricted to these very small triangular areas.

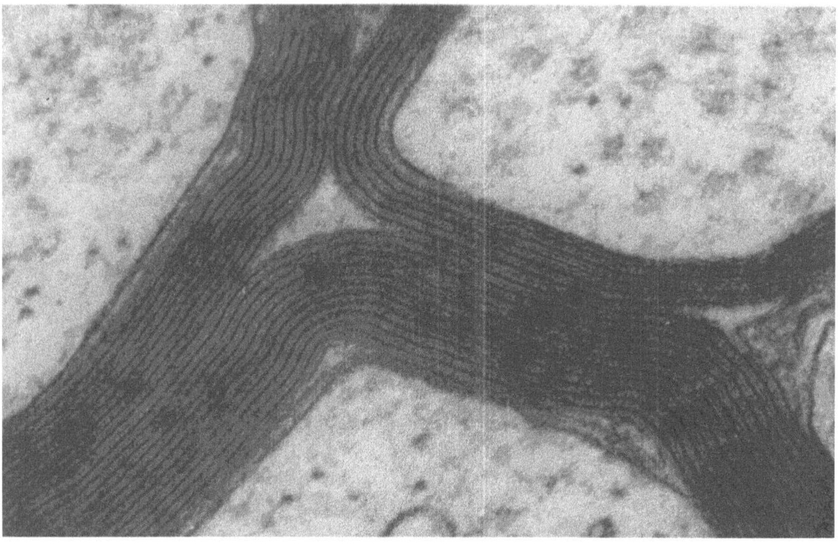

Fig. 2. High magnification of intact contralateral callosal radiation 48 hours after polysaccharide implantation. The extracellular space is not noticeable except for a triangular area formed by three separate myelin sheaths. This is surrounded by a low density line similar in appearance to the intra-period line. There is an intra-period line between two adjacent myelin sheaths. X136,000 (reduced).

At high magnification of the involved white matter, this extracellular space had been broadened by the intrusion of polysaccharide-rich fluid (Fig. 3). The presence of an intraperiod line between two adjacent myelin sheaths was often still visible. One could see that the outermost major dense line was still surrounded by a less dense line similar to the intraperiod line. Therefore, the location of the polysaccharide-rich fluid material was in the greatly distended extracellular compartment of the white matter. There was no splitting of the myelin lamellae or separation of the outer loop.

The polysaccharide-rich fluid was also in contact with the plasma membranes of the glial and neuronal cell bodies and their processes. However, the vast majority of neuroglial cells in the distal white matter revealed no intracytoplasmic accumulation of the fluid during the acute stage despite proximity of the extracellular fluid (Hirano, et al., 1964a).

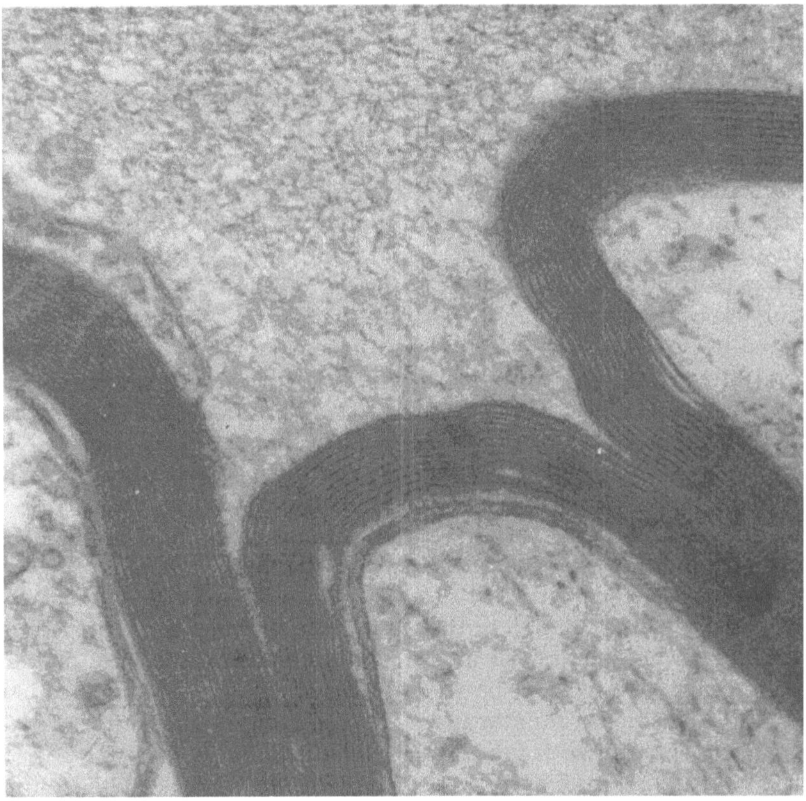

Fig. 3. High magnification of involved callosal radiation 48 hours after polysaccharide implantation. There are three adjacent myelin sheaths. The fluid, filled with electron-dense reticulated material, occupies the greatly distended extracellular space. X108,500 (reduced).

Thus myelinated and non-myelinated nerve fibers as well as individual glial cells in the white matter were often widely separated from each other by large areas of fluid. However, there was remarkable preservation of the perivascular glial processes in the distal portion of an affected white matter. The astrocytic foot processes kept their normal anatomic relation to the basement membrane and to the adjacent feet. Separation of the perivascular astrocytes from the basement membrane or from each other was not observed, and there was a continuous band of glial perivascular feet. However, glycogen granules in the swollen cytoplasm of the vascular feet were frequently increased in number. Preservation of astrocytic foot processes and basement membranes was observed at large as well as small vessels. Similarly, the pia-glial membrane formed a continuous anatomical demarcation between Virchow-Robin spaces and the pool of extracellular fluid in the cerebral parenchyma (Fig. 4).

In the early phase of fluid spread, and only in areas close to the implant, the extracellular space contained a second type of fluid. This second type of fluid had a fine granular texture without reticular substance or discrete morphological units (Hirano, et al., 1964b). The texture and density of this fluid resembled blood plasma. The two types of fluid had different staining reactions to heavy metals. The polysaccharide-rich fluid was light and almost transparent in unstained sections, while the finer textured second type of fluid was darker. After staining, however, the relative densities were completely reversed. The affinity for heavy metals of the polysaccharide-rich fluid gave it a greater relative density than the fine-textured fluid in stained sections. This second type of fluid was always located between the polysaccharide-rich fluid and tissue, especially between fluid and blood vessels near the implant (Fig. 5). The basement membranes of vessels at the site of implant were often infiltrated with the second type of fluid, which also filled the distended perivascular spaces. A gap in the perivascular ring of astrocytic vascular feet was seen occasionally. As a result of this gap, direct communication was evident between this second type of extracellular fluid and the basement membrane. The second type of fluid was occasionally connected with the basement membrane in an area between ruptured edges of a vascular foot (Hirano, et al., 1964b).

Although the major portion of the fluid was confined to the extracellular space, a small amount of fluid entered the intracellular compartment in the acute phase (Hirano, et al., 1964c). Near the implant, some fluid entered glial and neuronal cytoplasm through ruptured plasma membranes. Near the implant, as well as in the distant white matter, some of the fluid material was engulfed by phagocytosis into macrophages. However, these phagocytes were few in number.

It is important to emphasize that the location of the fluid changes considerably as the lesion ages. By the third and fourth days after implantation, the bulk of the fluid had left the extracellular space and many interfascicular glial cells with intracellular fluid accumulations could be found. This change was virtually complete by one week. The cells involved were primarily the interfascicular oligodendroglia (Levine, et al., 1963; Hirano, et al., 1965a). They were identified in both light and electron microscopy by their appearance, arrangement in rows, and their location and frequency

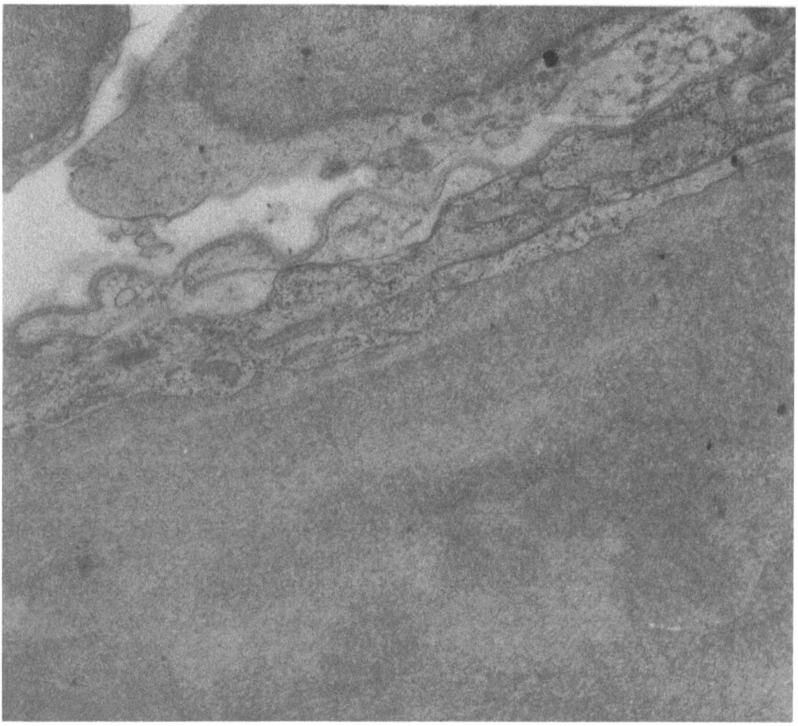

Fig. 4. Callosal radiation 24 hours after polysaccharide implantation. Virchow-Robin space (above), which appears empty due to dehydration preceding embedding, contains two mononuclear cells. Cerebral parenchyma contains a pool of electron-dense polysaccharide-rich fluid. Pia-glial membrane separates perivascular space from intracerebral fluid. There is no separation or disruption of pial membrane or subpial astrocytic glial processes. X15,600 (reduced).

in white matter. They became distended by large grape-like clusters of vacuoles filled with polysaccharide-rich fluid. The astrocytes, too, took up polysaccharide material, which appeared as diffuse infiltration of the cytoplasm, or large lakes of fluid, or multiple small focal cystic collections near the Golgi apparatus (Hirano, et al., 1965b). A similar reaction was observed even in the ependymal cells (Hirano, et al, 1966). In these glial cells, the intracellular ma-

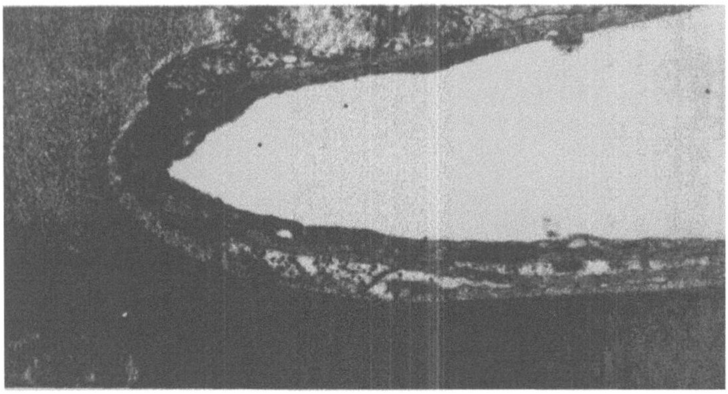

Fig. 5. Callosal radiation 24 hours after polysaccharide implantation. Electron-dense polysaccharide-rich fluid fills much of the field (left and bottom). Lumen of vessel is empty. A narrow band of astrocytic perivascular foot processes maintains its normal continuity, although gaps were seen occasionally in other fields. Between the perivascular foot processes and the polysaccharide-rich fluid, there is a narrow band of less-dense (hematogenous) fluid. X18,000 (reduced).

terial persisted for at least 100 days with no evidence of toxic effect, inflamatory reaction, digestion or degradation.

Silver Nitrate

Light Microscopy

The position of the implanted pellet was seen as a black mass of graphite which was surrounded by a well demarcated cylindrical zone of silver impregnated brain tissue. Most vessels in the zone were heavily impregnated with silver (Levine, 1965). In contrast to the relative preservation of structure in the impregnated zone, surrounding brain tissue showed severe necrosis, hemorrhage and edema. In additon to the perifocal edema, there was also severe edema in the callosal radiation and corpus callosum, mostly on the side of implant (Levine, et al., 1963). Pools of eosinophilic and PAS-positive amorphous fluid resembling plasma surrounded vessels and extended among the white matter bundles.

Electron Microscopy

Edema fluid was identified as an homogenous, granular, fine-textured substance which appeared indistinguishable from blood plasma. Although direct comparison between edema fluid and blood plasma was unattainable in perfused brains, they appeared identical in specimens fixed by immersion (Fig. 6).

The fluid was most often observed in proximity to vessels. The basement membranes were infiltrated by the plasma-like fluid which often extended into the distended extracellular space through gaps between disrupted perivascular feet. The separation and disruption of the perivascular ring of astrocytic foot processes was often extensive, and completely naked endothelial rings floated not infrequently in pools of fluid in the severely involved white matter (Fig. 6). The endothelial cells often became very thin and irregularly folded, as observed in immersion fixed specimens. However, direct communication between plasma in the vessel lumen and perivascular fluid was not observed in electron micrographs. Foci of the vascular basement membranes were often indistinct in these vessels. The fluid spread into the extracellular spaces between myelinated nerve fibers in a manner similar to that described in the previous polysaccharide experiment (Fig. 7). However, in contrast to the polysaccharide experiment, regular separations of the outer loop and the outer myelin lamellae were observed in some of the myelinated fibers in severely edematous areas (Hirano, et al., 1965c). The plasma-like fluid extended into the widened space between the major dense lines.

Hyperacute Experimental Allergic Encephalomyelitis

The early lesions of hyperacute EAE were characterized by exudation of plasma into the subarachnoid spaces and the extracellular spaces of spinal cord and roots, and by diapedesis of mononuclear and polymorphonuclear inflammatory cells and erythrocytes (Levine, et al., 1965). The subarachnoid space was filled with plas-

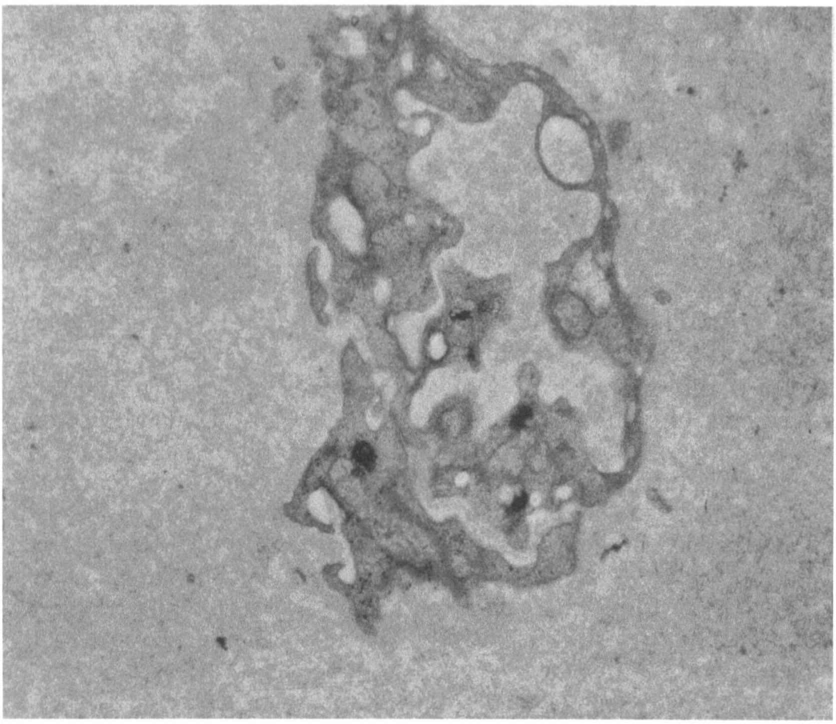

Fig. 6. A blood vessel floats in edema fluid in white matter 48 hours after silver nitrate implantation. Immersion fixation. Edema fluid appears identical with the plasma within the lumen of the vessel. X20,000 (reduced).

ma-like fluid. The pia and the subpial layer of astrocytic processes were preserved without obvious separation. The extracellular spaces of the spinal cord were distended and filled with plasma-like fluid (Fig. 8). Extracellular fluid in the cord parenchyma was most abundant around vessels and in the subpial areas. Findings in basement membranes and perivascular astrocytic foot processes around involved small vessels were essentially similar to those observed in the silver experiment previously described. In addition, however, leukocytes often migrated from vessels through gaps between adjacent endothelial cells. Passage of plasma through these gaps was seen at the site of leukocyte migration. Passage of plasma through endothelial gaps unaccompanied by inflammatory cells was not observed.

In rats with a more advanced disease, the edema fluid con-

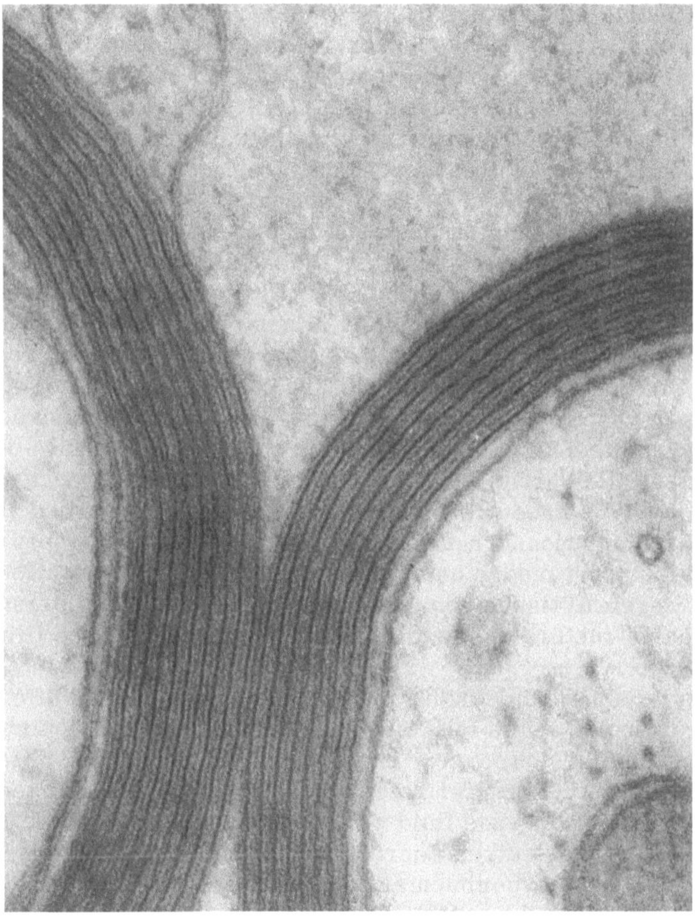

Fig. 7. Callosal radiation 48 hours after implantation. Plasma-like fluid fills the distended extracellular space between myelinated nerve fibers. X174,000.

tained large amounts of fibrin, especially around vessels. Various cellular reactions and alteration of myelin and other tissue elements became progressively more evident. Similar changes have been illustrated in other studies of EAE (Luse & McDougal, 1960; Bubis & Luse, 1964a, b; Lampert & Carpenter, 1965).

DISCUSSION

Since the advent of electron microscopic investigation in the field of neuropathology, cerebral edema and swelling have been actively investigated in order to locate the accumulated fluid precisely (Torack, et al., 1959, 1960; Gerschenfeld, et al., Luse & Harris, 1960, 1961; Evans, et al.; Raimondi, et al.; De Robertis; Ishii & Tani; Aleu, et al., 1964, 1965; Gonatas, et al., 1963, 1964; Koizumi). These electron microscopic reports vary considerably from one experimental condition to another, as recently reviewed by Zimmerman in 1964.

The site of accumulation of fluid has been reported to be in the glial cells of the cortex exclusively (Torack, et al., 1959, 1960; Gerschenfeld, et al.; Luse & Harris, 1960, 1961; De Robertis; Ishii & Tani; Koizumi), almost exclusively in large clefts within the myelin sheath (Aleu, et al., 1963), or in great part in the extracellular space in the white matter (Gonatas, et al., 1963, 1964). In spite of such differences in respect to the site of involvement at the ultrastructural level, a common feature can be pointed out: the appearance of pale, clear and swollen areas in certain specific structures. Such enlarged spaces which displace pre-existing structures are regarded as sites of fluid accumulation. That is, accumulation of fluid has been interpreted by indirect means as evidenced by structural alteration of the adjacent cerebral tissue components. Accumulated fluid presumably has a clear structureless texture in electron micrographs (Hirano, et al., 1964b).

Our experimental findings presented in this report differ from the above reports in the following ways. First, our fixation was perfusion, not immersion, except in a few special instances. Second, we studied mainly white matter rather than cortex. Third, we demonstrated an electron-dense fluid which was subject to positive identification under the electron microscope, rather than clear empty spaces. The three experimental conditions selected for our study were not investigated by others.

Our first experiment with cryptococcal polysaccharide provide a clue as to the location of fluid material in the white matter. Flow of polysaccharide in the white matter was seen only as optically empty zones in the paraffin or celloidin embedded preparations prepared by conventional immersion fixation in formalin (Levine, et al., 1963). Later, application of fluorescent antibody methods revealed that specific fluorescence, representing polysaccharide, was selectively distributed in the white matter and was co-extensive with a vascular lesion (Levine, 1963). Actual visualization of stained polysaccharide and its further precise localization was then investigated by light and elec-

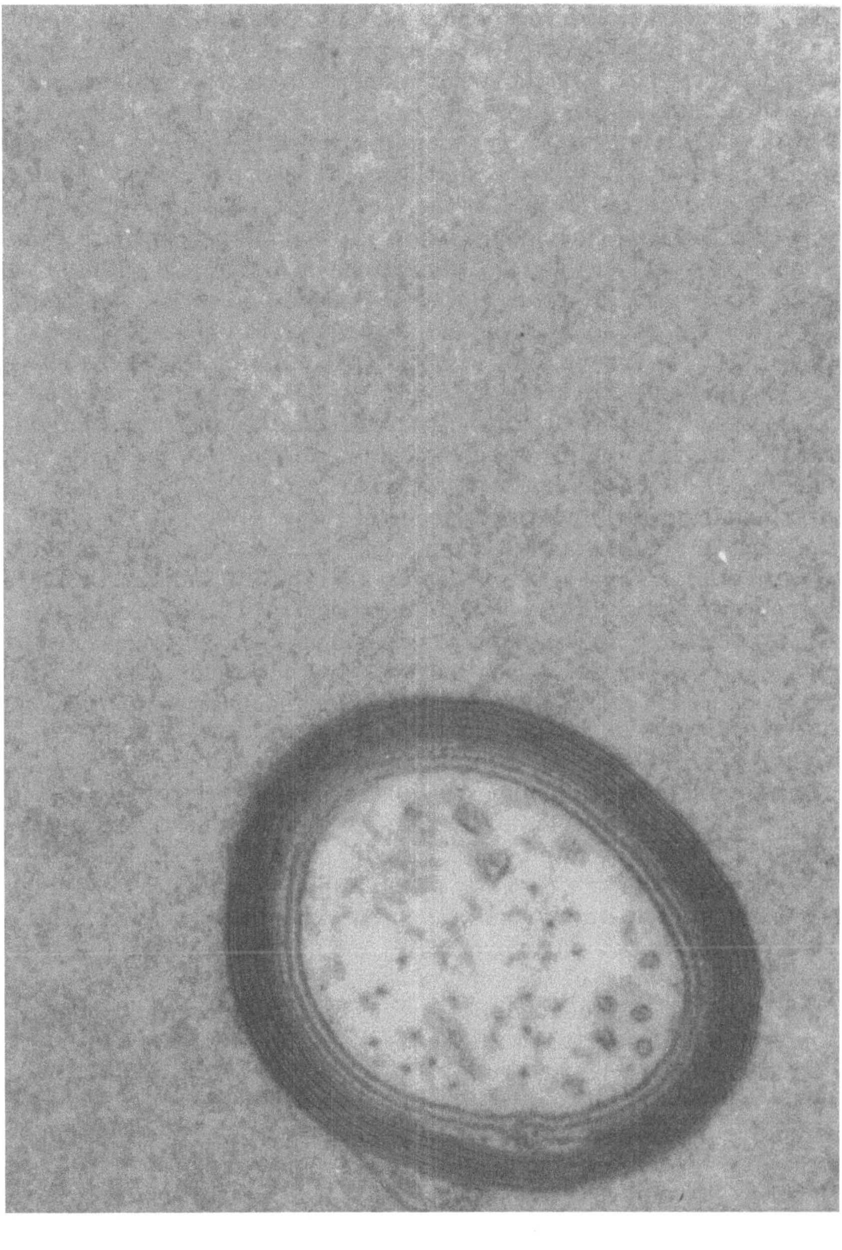

Fig. 8. White matter in the spinal cord of an animal with experimental allergic encephalomyelitis. A myelinated nerve fiber is surrounded by a pool of plasma-like fluid in the extracellular space. X99,200 (reduced).

tron microscopy using brains fixed in toto by perfusion. By this method, colored or electron-dense fluid material was identified in the greatly expanded extracellular compartment of the white matter during the acute phase of the experiment. With the electron microscope, this material was characterized by a reticular appearance and by strong staining with heavy metals, a feature not present in any normal central nervous system constituent in the adult or infant rat. Since we were not aware of the electron microscopic appearance of cryptococcal polysaccharide, identification and recognition of this substance was needed. This material appeared identical with the purified cryptococcal capsular polysaccharide placed in a dead animal's brain, and had exactly the same appearance when examined in situ, as part of the capsule of cryptococcal yeast cells. These observations indicate that the electron-dense fluid contained cryptococcal polysaccharide, that it originated from the region of the implant, and that it had moved a considerable distance in the white matter by way of distended extracellular spaces.

Furthermore, in the early phase of fluid spread, and only in areas close to the implant, a second type of fluid was identified in the extracellular spaces. This plasma-like fluid was thought to be of hematogenous origin because of its structural features, staining reaction, proximity of vessels and occasional relation to gaps in the perivascular ring of astrocytic foot processes. It should be emphasized that throughout the experiments on polysaccharide implantation, interruptions of astrocytic vascular feet were rare and confined solely to the site of the implantation during the acute stage, where they were presumably caused by mechanical injury. Also, it has been shown that the blood-brain barrier was intact except for mild disruption at the site of implantaion, presumably due to the same mechanical injury (Levine, et al., 1963). More information on this subject was obtained from other experiments, in which silver nitrate was implanted intracerebrally, and plasma-like fluid formed the exclusive element of the edema.

Silver nitrate produced local necrosis and widespread edema of white matter associated with markedly increased permeability of the blood-brain barrier. Pools of PAS-positive amorphous fluid surrounded vessels and extended among the white matter bundles. The texture of this fluid appeared identical with blood plasma and also with the second hematogenous type of fluid observed in the polysaccharide experiment. In contrast to the well preserved astrocytic vascular foot processes seen in the polysaccharide experiment, the rings of astrocytic feet were often disrupted. Plasma-like fluid infiltrated the basement membranes and communicated freely with the distended extracellular spaces.

This plasma-like edema following implantation of silver nitrate can also be produced by intracerebral implantation of other inorganic and organic compounds (Levine, et al., 1963). Furthermore, it is similar to the edema in human brains caused by a variety of pathological conditions (Feigin & Popoff) and to the edema in animal brains caused by experimental cold injuries (Clasen, et al.; Klatzo, et al.; Bakay & Haque). The plasma-like edema fluid was also observed with electron microscopy, following intracerebral implantation of living cryptococcal cells as well as killed, lyophilized cryptococcal yeast cells, as part of the inflammatory reaction (Levine, et al., 1964). This fluid was also found by us, under electron microscopy, in human biopsy specimens of cerebral neoplasms. In an electron microscopic study of cold-induced edema, Bakay and Lee recently reported that the extracellular space of the white matter is enlarged and filled with seemingly proteinaceous exudate. Finally, it should be emphasized that a pool of this plasma-like fluid may be caused not only by direct injury but also by a systemic immunological mechanism, experimental allergic encephalomyelitis.

In conclusion, polysaccharide implantation experiments provided a clue as to the location of the edema fluid. Because of the innocuous nature of the polysaccharide, tissue preservation was excellent and the edema fluid was clearly localized for the most part in the extracellular space.

The next step was the recognition of the second, finer textured type of edema fluid. This fluid was found in a variety of experimentally induced edemas: silver nitrate, cryptococcus, or bacterial endotoxin implants and experimental allergic encephalomyelitis. Furthermore, this type of fluid accumulation was always associated with a change in the blood-brain barrier and often also with a disruption of astrocytic vascular feet. In addition, the electron microscope has revealed a remarkable morphological similarity between intravascular plasma and the edema fluid. As a result of all these findings we conclude that this type of edema fluid, commonly formed in a number of pathological conditions, is derived from blood plasma.

SUMMARY

Cryptococcal polysaccharide was implanted into the rat brain and its selective spread in the white matter was studied with light and electron microscopy, after the whole brain was fixed in situ by perfusion.

The cryptococcal polysaccharide in fluid was observed as an

electron-dense reticular substance with uranyl acetate or lead hydroxide stains. It originated from the region of the implant and moved a considerable distance in the white matter by way of the extracellular space during the acute stage. The location of fluid change considerably as the lesion aged. The fluid flow was reduced in three to four days, and the fluid exclusively localized within the glial cells after one week.

In the early phase of fluid spread, in areas close to the implant the extracellular space contained a second type of fluid. The latter was thought to be of hematogenous origin because of its structural features, staining reaction, proximity to vessels and relation to gaps in the perivascular ring of astrocytic foot processes. Fluid of this type was the essential element of the pool of fluid produced in response to the intracerebral implantation of silver nitrate. This plasma-like fluid was caused not only by direct injury, but also by a systemic immunological mechanism, experimental allergic encephalomyelitis.

REFERENCES

Aleu, F. P., R. Katzman and R. D. Terry: Fine structure and electrolyte analyses of cerebral edema induced by alkyl tin intoxication, J. Neuropath. exp. Neurol., 22, 403-413 (1963).

_____, F. L. Edelman, R. Katzman and L. C. Scheinberg: Ultrastructural and biochemical analysis in cerebral edema associated with experimental mouse gliomas, Ibid., 23, 253-263 (1964).

Bakay, L. and I. U. Haque: Morphological and chemical studies in cerebral edema. 1. Cold induced edema, Ibid., 23, 393-418 (1964

_____ and J. C. Lee: Ultrastructural changes in the edematous central nervous system. Program of the American Academy of Neurology, Seventeenth annual meeting, April 30, 1965, Neurology, 15, 292 (1965).

Bubis, J. J. and S. A. Luse: An electron microscopic study of experimental allergic encephalomyelitis in the rat, Amer. J. Path., 44, 299-317 (1964a).

_____ and _____: Ultrastructure of the leptomeninges in experimen tal allergic encephalomyelitis, Neurology (Minneapolis), 14, 616-622 (1964b).

Clasen, R. A., P. M. Cooke, S. Pandolfi, D. Boyd and A. J. Raimond Experimental cerebral edema produced by local freezing. 1. An anatomic study utilizing vital dye techniques, J. Neuropath. exp.

Neurol., 21, 579-596 (1962).
De Robertis, E.: Some old and new concepts of brain structure, Wld. Neurol., 3, 98-111 (1962).
Evans, J. P., E. Tani and A. J. Raimondi: Electron microscopic study of brain swelling, Trans. Amer. Neurol. Assn., 28-29 (1961).
Feigin, I. and N. Popoff: Neuropathological observations on cerebral edema. The acute phase, Arch. Neurol., 6, 151-160 (1962).
Gerschenfeld, H. M., F. Wald, J. A. Zadunaisky and E. De Robertis: Function of astroglia in the water-ion metabolism of the central nervous system, Neurology (Minneapolis), 9, 412-425 (1959).
Gonatas, N. K., H. M. Zimmerman and S. Levine: Ultrastructure of inflammation with edema in the rat brain, Amer. J. Path., 42, 455-469 (1963).
_____, S. Levine and R. Shoulson: Phagocytosis and regneration of myelin in an experimental leukoencephalopathy, Ibid., 44, 565-583 (1964).
Hirano, A., H. M. Zimmerman and S. Levine: The fine structure of cerebral fluid accumulation. III. Extracellular spread of cryptococcal polysaccharides in the acute stage, Ibid., 45, 1-19 (1964a).
_____, _____ and _____: The fine structure of cerebral fluid accumulation. IV. On the nature and origin of extracellular fluids following cryptococcal polysaccharide implantation, Ibid., 45, 195-207 (1964b).
_____, _____ and _____: Fine structure of cerebral fluid accumulation. V. Transfer of fluid from extracellular to intracellular compartments in acute phase of cryptococcal polysaccharide lesions, Arch. Neurol., 11, 632-641 (1964c).
_____, _____ and _____: Fine structure of cerebral fluid accumulation. VI. Intracellular accumulation of fluid and cryptococcal polysaccharide in oligodendroglia, Ibid., 12, 189-196 (1965a).
_____, _____ and _____: The fine structure of cerebral fluid accumulation. VII. Reaction of astrocytes to cryptococcal polysaccharide implantation, J. Neuropath. exp. Neurol., 24, 386-397 (1965b).
_____, _____ and _____: The fine structure of cerebral fluid accumulation. IX. Edema following silver nitrate implantation, Amer. J. Path., 47, 537-548 (1965c).
_____, _____ and _____: The fine structure of cerebral fluid accumulation. VIII. Reaction of ependyma to cryptococcal polysaccharide implantation, J. Path. & Bact. 91, 149-156 (1966).
Ishii, S. and E. Tani: Electron microscopic study of the blood-brain barrier in brain swelling, Acta Neuropath. (Berlin), 1, 474-488 (1962).
Klatzo, I., A. Piraux and E. J. Laskowski: The relationship between

edema, blood-brain-barrier and tissue elements in a local brain injury, J. Neuropath. exp. Neurol., 17, 548-564 (1958).
Koizumi, J.: Electron microscopic studies on the cerebral cortex in the so-called experimental edema and dehydration, Psychiat. Neurol. Jap., 66, 763-779 (1964).
Lampert, P. and S. Carpenter: Electronmicroscopic studies on the vascular permeability and the meçhanism of demyelination in experimental allergic encephalomyelitis, J. Neuropath. exp. Neurol., 24, 11-24 (1965).
Levine, S.: Cerebral white matter: Selective spread of pneumococcal polysaccharides, Science, 139, 605-606 (1963).
_____: Silver impregnation of blood vessels in vivo, I: Introduction of silver behind the blood-brain barrier, II: Chemocautery with silver nitrate, Exper. Med. & Surg., 23, 70-81 (1965).
_____, A. Hirano and H. M. Zimmerman: The reaction of the nervous system to cryptococcal infection: An experimental study with light and electron microscopy, The 44th Annual Meeting of the Association for Research in Nervous and Mental Disease, New York, December 5 (1964).
_____, _____ and _____: Hyperacute allergic encephalomyelitis, Electron microscopic observations, Amer. J. Path., 47, 209-221 (1965).
_____ and E. J. Wenk: Allergic encephalomyelitis: A hyperacute form, Science, 146, 1681-1682 (1964).
_____ and _____: A hyperacute form of allergic encephalomyelitis, Amer. J. Path., 47, 61-88 (1965).
_____, H. M. Zimmerman, E. J. Wenk and N. K. Gonatas: Experimental leukoencephalopathies due to implantation of foreign substances, Ibid., 42, 97-117 (1963).
Luse, S. A. and B. Harris: Electron microscopy of the brain in experimental edema, J. Neurosurg., 17, 439-446 (1960).
_____ and _____: Brain ultrastructure in hydration and dehydration, Arch Neurol., 4, 139-152 (1961).
_____ and D. B. McDougal, Jr.: Electron microscopic observations on allergic encephalomyelitis in the rabbit, J. exp. Med., 112, 735-742 (1960).
Torack, R. M., R. D. Terry and H. M. Zimmerman: The fine structure of cerebral fluid accumulation, I: Swelling secondary to cold injury, Amer. J. Path., 35, 1135-1147 (1959).
_____, _____ and _____: The fine structure of cerebral fluid accumulation, II: Swelling produced by triethyl tin poisoning and its comparison with that in the human brain, Ibid., 36, 273-287 (1960).
Raimondi, A. J., J. P. Evans and S. Mullan: Studies of cerebral edema, III: Alteration in white matter: electron microscopic study

using ferritin as labeling compound, Acta Neuropathologica, 2, 177-197 (1962).
Zimmerman, H. M.: Some contributions of electron microscopy to problems in pathology, Bulletin of the New York Academy of Medicine, 40, 831-862 (1964).

JOSEPH C. LEE
LOUIS BAKAY

ELECTRON MICROSCOPIC STUDIES ON EXPERIMENTAL BRAIN EDEMA

Experimental brain edema was produced in rats by triethyltin hydroxide feeding, and in cats by focal extradural freezing and by inducing hypercapnic hypoxia. The animals were killed by perfusion with buffered 4% glutaraldehyde; normal and edematous brain tissues were post-fixed with 1% osmium tetroxide. The Maraglas-embedded material was cut on a Porter-Blum Ultramicrotome, and the sections were stained with lead citrate.

In triethyltin edema, the ultrastructural change was characterized by the accumulation of excess fluid between the myelin lamellae, rendering a split of the myelin (Fig. 1). This split started in the white matter of the spinal cord on the third day of feeding before the appearance of neurologic signs and ascended to involve the white matter of cerebellum and cerebrum, a sequence comparable with the observed order of paraplegia, quadriplegia and apathy. The change persisted after clinical recovery following resumption of a normal diet for 25 to 45 days. The myelin split was always at the less dense lamellae (Fig. 2), and the resulting vacuoles were clear but became electron dense when demyelination began. Demyelination and phagocytosis were observed in the late and recovery stages.

In cold-induced edema, the changes, seen only in the ipsilateral hemisphere of the lesion, reached a peak at 24 to 48 hours after freezing. The astrocytes and their processes, particularly the perivascular processes, were dilated in both the gray and white matter (Fig. 3). Enlargement of the intercellular space occurred only in the white matter, and the enlarged space contained electron dense material of seemingly proteinaceous nature (Fig. 4). The blood capillaries in the vicinity of the freezing lesion showed numerical increase of large and small pinocytotic vesicles (Fig. 3). These changes were similar to those produced by heat and electric coagulation (unpublished data). By using ferritin as a tracer, we found that the uptake of ferritin particles was greater in the edematous than in the control brain tissue. The particles were present in the pinocytotic vesicles, situated freely in the cytoplasm and basement membrane, associated with granular bodies, and lodged in the intercellular space (Fig. 5). The ultrastructural changes and the uptake of ferritin were greatest in the region adjacent to the lesion and decreased with increasing distances therefrom. Our findings suggest that the permeability of the blood-brain barrier is increased in the neighborhood of the freezing lesion and that the extravasated fluid and solutes spread through intra- and extracellular routes to more distant areas.

In hypercapnic hypoxia induced by hypoventilation and CO_2 retention, the CSF pressure of the cat rose from 50 to 170 mm. H_2O at the end of a three hour period. The arterial blood pH was reduced to about 6.9, with pO_2 around 30 and pCO_2 above 110. The brain was swollen. The astrocytic processes in the gray and white matter were moderately dilated. The intercellular space was enlarged slightly but only in the white matter (Fig. 6). The internal membranes (cristae) of the mitochondria in the neurons were occasionally disrupted or dissolved, while the endoplasmic reticulum of the neuronal and glial elements was moderately distended (Fig. 7). These changes were comparable to those of ischemic edema produced by ligation of the internal carotid artery (unpublished data).

In conclusion, electron microscopy shows that edematous changes depend on the causative agents and the duration of damage. Intracellular and extracellular edema may exist concomitantly, but the latter occurs only in the white matter under the experimental conditions reported here.

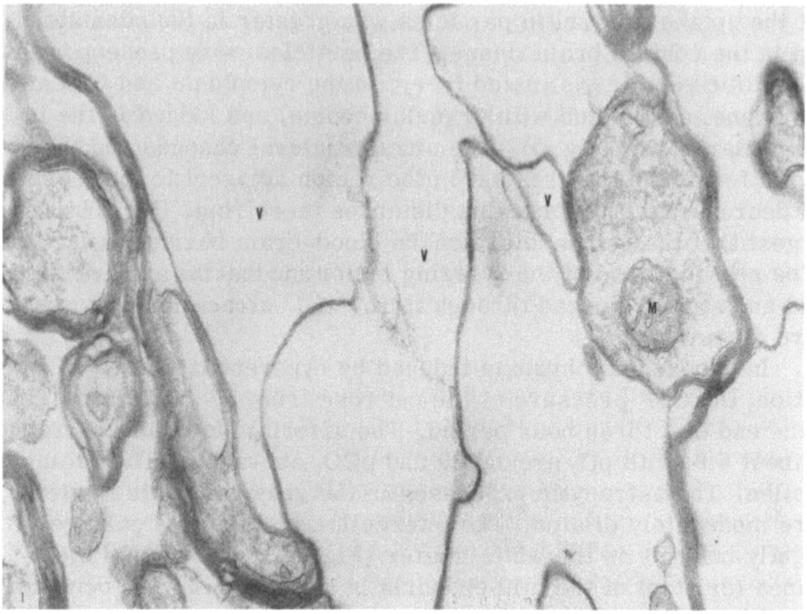

Fig. 1. Cerebral white matter of a rat fed with triethyltin for 11 days. Note the repeated splits of myelin sheaths to form electron clear vacuoles (V) of various sizes. The mitochondria (M) and other organelles of the axon appear intact. X13,000 (reduced).

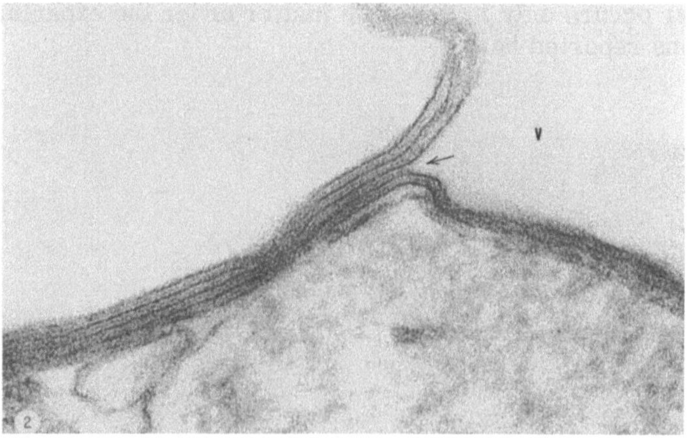

Fig. 2. Cerebellar white matter of a rat fed with triethyltin for seven days. The arrow indicates the myelin split at the less dense lamella. V = part of a vacuole. X50,000 (reduced).

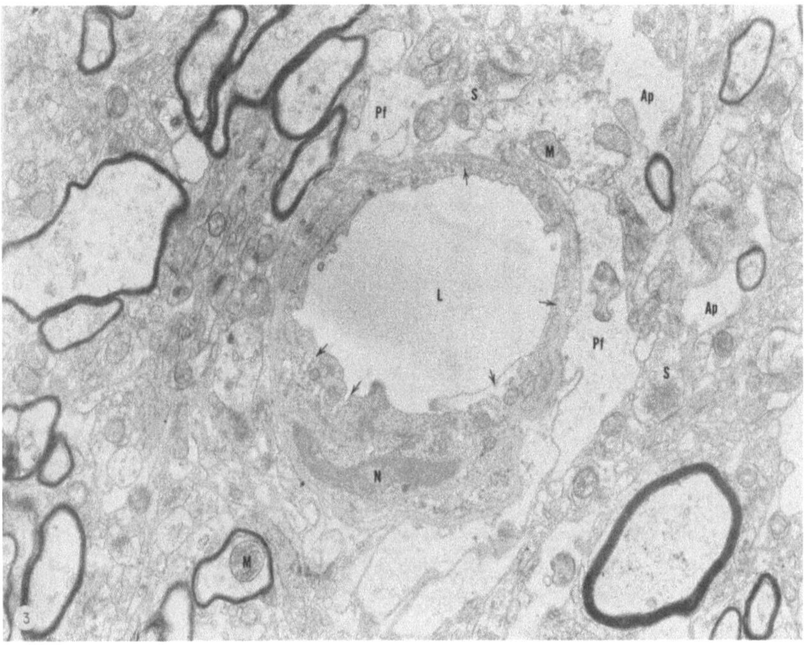

Fig. 3. Deep layers of cerebral cortex of a cat in the vicinity of the freezing lesion produced 24 hours before. The perivascular feet (Pf) and astrocytic processes (Ap) are dilated, but the intercellular space is not enlarged. The myelin sheaths, mitochondria (M), and synapses (S) show no change. Note the increase in the number of pinocytotic vesicles (arrows). L = lumen of a capillary; N = nucleus of endothelial cell. X6,000 (reduced).

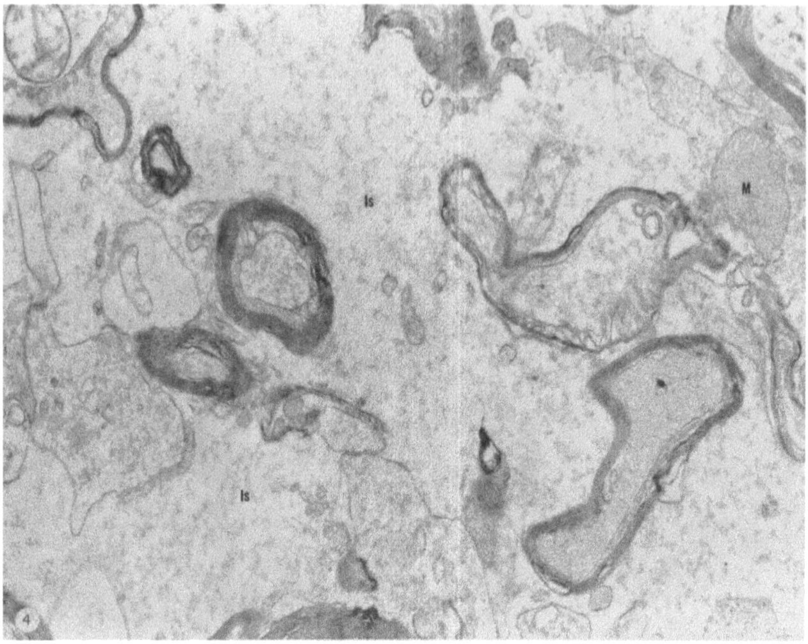

Fig. 4. Cerebral white matter of a cat adjacent to a six-hour lesion. The intercellular space (Is) is enlarged, but the mitochondria (M) and other organelles of the axons are normal. There is electron-dense material in the enlarged intercellular space. X12,500 (reduced).

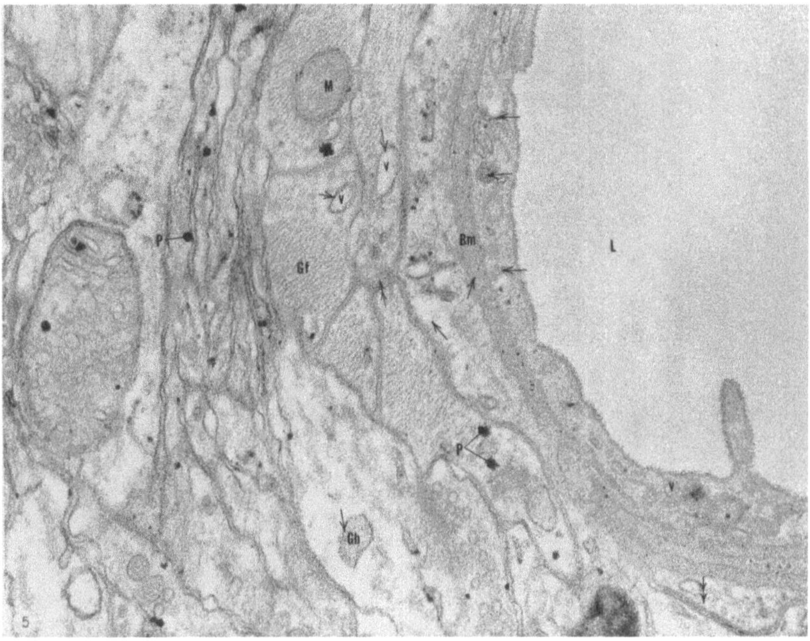

Fig. 5. Cerebral cortex of a cat in the neighborhood of a 24-hour lesion. Ferritin was injected 30 minutes before death. Ferritin particles (arrows) are present in the vesicles (v), free in the cytoplasm and basement membrane (Bm), associated with granular bodies (Gb) and lodged in the intercellular space (double arrows). L = lumen of a capillary; Gf = astrocytic glial filaments; M = mitochondria; P = lead precipate. X20,000 (reduced).

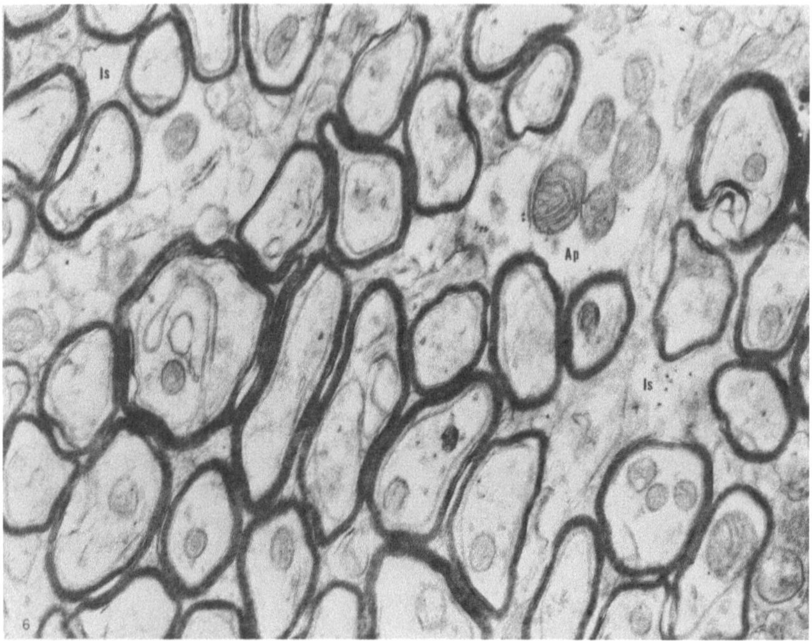

Fig. 6. Cerebral white matter of a cat under hypercapnic hypoxia. The enlargement of the intercellular space (Is) is minimal. Note a moderately dilated astrocytic process (Ap) containing normal mitochondria (M). X13,000 (reduced).

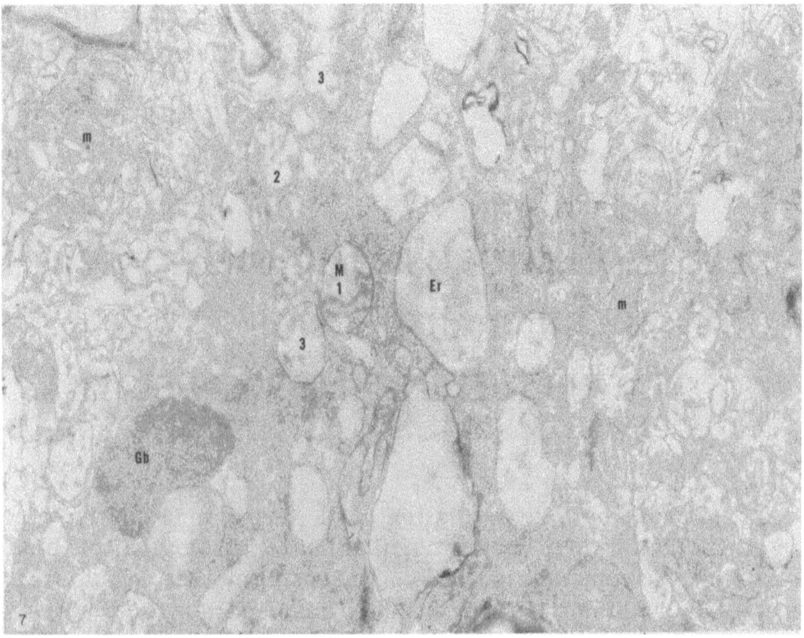

Fig. 7. Cerebral cortex of a cat under hypercapnic hypoxia. Part of the cytoplasm of a nerve cell is shown in the center. The mitochondria (M) reveal various stages of dissolution (1, 2, 3). The endoplasmic reticulum (Er) is distended. Mitochondria (m) of the axonal terminals and glial processes are, however, intact. Gb = granular body. X14,000 (reduced).

W. WECHSLER
E. RIVERSON
J. M. SCHRÖDER
P. KLEIHUES
J. F. PALMEIRO
K. A. HOSSMANN

ELECTRON MICROSCOPIC OBSERVATIONS ON DIFFERENT MODELS OF ACUTE EXPERIMENTAL BRAIN EDEMA

The morphologic investigation of the phenomena involved in brain edema has been a very intriguing neuropathological problem. Electron microscopy has become an essential method in this field, because it facilitates the recognition of abnormal extracellular and/or intracellular fluid accumulation. Cerebral edema produced under various experimental conditions has been investigated by this technique in order to achieve a more precise localization of the pathologically accumulated fluid in the brain tissue.

Thanks to improved techniques (perfusion fixation and embedding in polyester) it is possible to obtain satisfactory preservation of the brain tissue not only in the cortex but also in the deep white matter. This is of special importance since in many types of brain edema the white matter is the more vulnerable part. Our own endeavor has been to study experimental models related as closely as possible to human pathology. The following experiments have been employed in the production of cerebral edema: traumatisation of the brain in adult mice (Schröder, & Wechsler, 1965a), localized injection of diphtheria toxin into the cat brain (Kleihues, Wechsler & Zülch, 1965), epidural cerebral compression with laminaria according to a method by Riverson, et al. (1966), and sinus obstruction and/or ligation of the jugular veins (experimental procedures carried out by Palmeiro and Hossman).

METHODS

The brains were fixed by perfusion with buffered 6.25% glutaraldehyde, post-fixation in a 1% osmium-tetroxyde-mixture buffered to a pH of 7.2 according to the method of Wohlfarth-Bottermann (1957) for two to four hours; embedded in Vestopal W; electron micrographs Zeiss EM 9.

RESULTS

In the first two experiments the pathological changes observed ranged from necrosis to uncomplicated brain edema. In the latter, associated with brain compression and venous congestion, the dominant alterations were serous and plasmatic edema especially in the white matter of the cat's hemisphere (see Zülch).

The present report summarizes some aspects of our observations in the acute stage of brain edema with special regard to the following problems: (1) the different reaction patterns of the gray and white matter; (2) the ultrastructural details of serous (protein-poor) and plasmatic (protein-rich) edema, as well as the so-called acute "Ödemnekrose" (Jacob, 1940) and the "plasmatische Infiltrationsnekrose" (Scholz, 1949), special forms of necrotizing edema; (3) the correlation of the extent of the enlargement of the extracellular spaces to the varying severity of the tissue lesions; and finally (4) the problem of the structural background of the blood brain barrier (BBB) in the edematous gray and white substance.

OBSERVATIONS IN THE GRAY SUBSTANCE

In all the experimental models we have carried out extensive light microscopy to determine the nature, the topographical distribution, and the chronology of the lesions. Electron microscopy has been only applied to study special problems, e.g., the alteration in early stages or the precise localization of the abnormal fluid accumulation. All the findings reported demonstrate tissue alterations of short duration, whereby only the series of brain trauma in mice have been completed and published (Schröder and Wechsler, 1965). The results of the other experimental models will be published in detail later.

The ultrastructural substrate of the microspongy state in the region of cortical edema, e.g., in brain trauma, brain compression and brain intoxication is due to a generalized swelling of astroglial elements in the perivascular and perineuronal regions, and all over the neuropil, without any necrotic changes of these cells (Fig. 1b). During the early stages of edema, proliferation of the endoplasmic

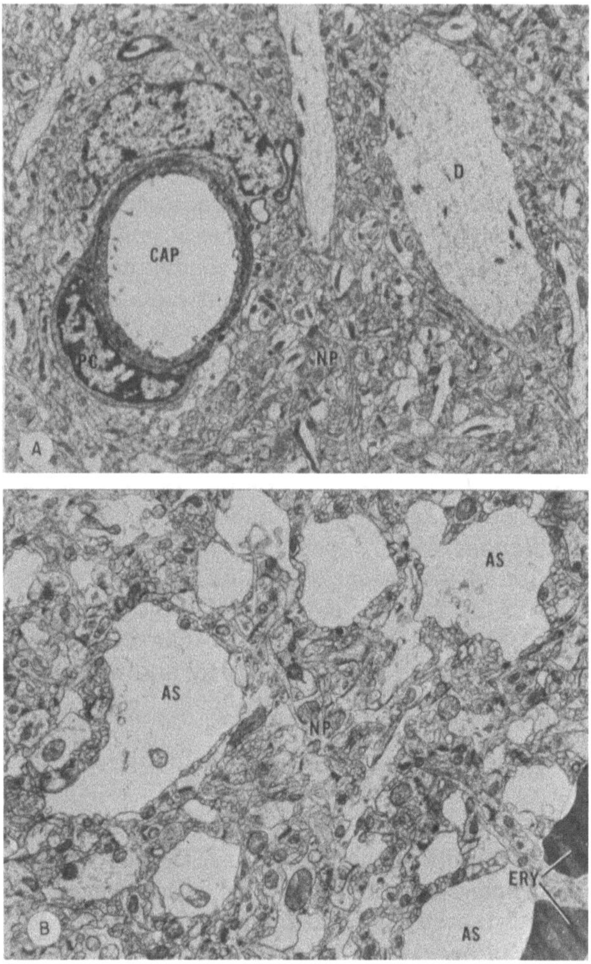

Fig. 1. Fine structure of the gray substance (cerebral cortex of the cat and the mouse): a) normal adult cat cortex of the hemisphere with the fine processes of the neuropil (NP). CAP — capillary, D — 2 apical dendrites, n.b. the lack of a wide extracellular space (No. 10713, X5,500, reduced;) b) perifocal edematous region, 12 hours after traumatization of the mouse brain. Generalized swelling of the astrocytic processes (AS), without changes of the neuropil (NP) and the extracellular volume. ERY — erythrocytes, lying within the locally widened extracellular space (No. 7174, X8,000, reduced).

reticulum, the mitochondria, the glycogen particles and the glial filaments are not prominent features. Such reactive protoplasmic astrocytes have been observed by means of electron microscopy in later stages of edema, e.g., in cortical brain trauma (Hager, 1964; Schröder & Wechsler, 1965), and as reported by Hirano, Zimmermann & Levine (1965a) after cryptococcal polysaccharide implantation in the chronically edematous white matter. Changes of the nerve cells, the nerve fibers and the oligodendrocytes are not conspicuous. No increased interstitial (extracellular) space was present in the zone of cortical edema (Fig. 1b), confirming the original observations reported by Gerschenfeld, et al. (1959), Torack, Terry and Zimmermann (1959), Luse and Harris (1960, 1961), Niessing and Vogell (1960), Ule (1962). The most prominent feature of the changes in cortical cerebral edema is the fact that the astroglia practically bears the whole burden of abnormal fluid accumulation. That means cortical edema represents not a primary structural but a primary pathophysiological disturbance.

New aspects regarding the expansibility of the extracellular space in the gray matter have been elucidated by studying diphtheric intoxication and brain traumatization. These models offer the opportunity for a comparative study of edema and necrosis. Of course, there is no sharp demarcation between the necrotic and the edematous zones. Therefore, we would like to distinguish three topographically defined regions on the basis of their histopathology: (1) next to the traumatic injury or the central focus of diptheria injection a zone of necrosis; (2) a so-called "Zwischenzone;" and (3) a perifocal edematous region. In the so-called "Zwischenzone," edematous changes and partial tissue necrosis intermingle with one another, thus representing the stage of an acute "Ödemnekrose." Figure 2 represents the alterations in such a zone. Generalized astrocytic swelling occurs. Apart from this, we find disseminated lesions of the neurones, while the nerve fibers are less involved. In contrast to uncomplicated or "pure" edema, there is a slight irregular distension of the extracellular space, sometimes with protein-rich exsudation (Fig. 2). The slight widening of the extracellular space, as well as various degrees of reversible and irreversible changes of the nerve and glial cells, indicate a more severe lesion of the tissue. It is difficult to determine if this enlargement of the interstitial space represents a primary phenomenon, or a secondary effect of partial tissue necrosis.

The changes in the necrotic zone can be more easily understood. In the initial stages of necrosis, nearly all the dying neuronal and glial cells become watery; some of them are shrunken. In contrast to the pure edema, however, this is followed by the destruction of the cell membranes and irreversible liquefaction (Fig. 3).

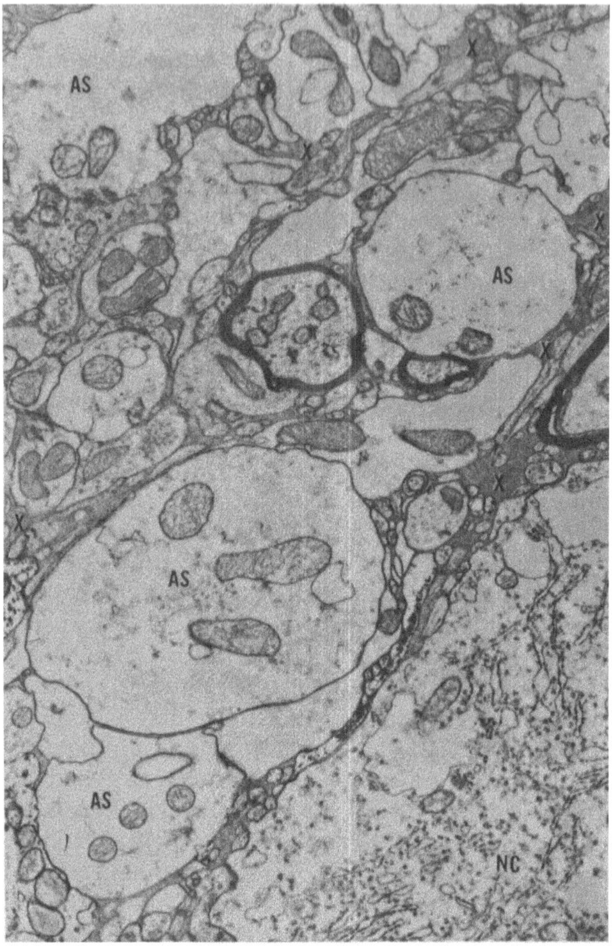

Fig. 2. The so-called "Zwischenzone" between necrosis and edema in the gray substance (acute "Ödemnekrose"), basal ganglia of the cat, 40 hours after local diphtheric intoxication. More severe lesions, with swelling of the astroglia (AS), disseminated minor swelling of the nerve cells (NC), and moderate distension of the extracellular space (x), with plasma-like interstitial exudation (No. 12876, X13,500, reduced).

This means that an increase in interstitial volume in the necrotic area is a result of a primary structural damage.

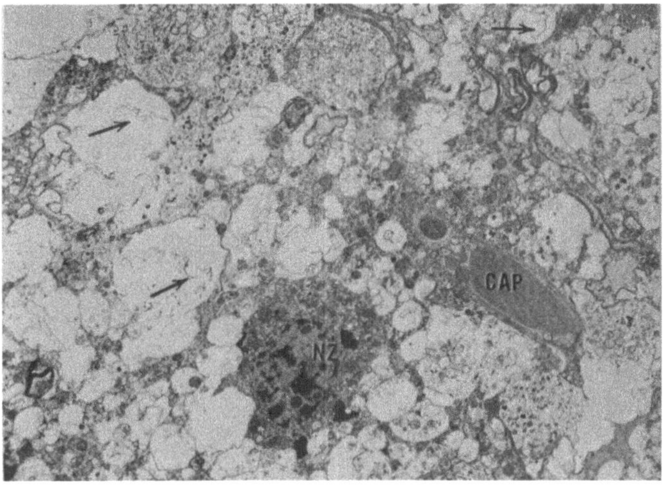

Fig. 3. Necrotic zone of the mouse cortex, 11 hours after trauma. Generalized swelling of neuronal and glial processes with beginning destruction of cell membranes NC — pyknotic nerve cell, CAP — capillary (No. 6895, X4,500, reduced).

OBSERVATIONS IN THE WHITE MATTER

In all our experiments we have found that serous (protein-poor) edema of the white matter is regularly accompanied by an extreme enlargement of the extracellular space and a dissociation of the myelinated fibers (Fig. 4b). A generalized swelling of the astrocytes is visible. The oligodendroglia are not involved in the same manner as the astroglia during the acute phase of edema. Pronounced alterations of the oligodendroctyes, representing possibly acute swelling and mucoid degeneration, have been described by Hirano, et al. (1965b), in later stages of edema after cryptococcal polysaccharide implantation. It is difficult to evaluate in the initial stages of edema of the white matter the time relationships underlying the cellular and the interstitial changes. In general, we can adopt the idea that swelling of astrocytes and widening of the extracellular space may develop side by side.

The plasmatic (protein-rich) form of edema is acidophilic in nature, and can be demonstrated easily in Masson-preparations. In our experiments with brain compression, venous congestion and diphtheric intoxication, we found both serous and plasmatic edema. The electron microscopic study of such a plasmatic form of edema revealed

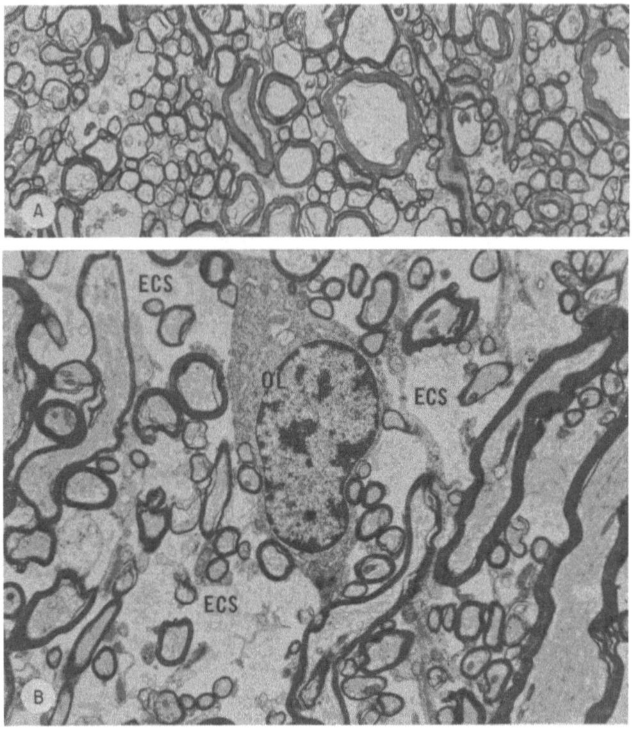

Fig. 4. Normal and edematous white matter in the hemisphere of the cat: a) Normal white matter: close contact of the nerve fibers, relatively small amount of intervening glial processes (No. 11072, X4,500); b) edema of the white matter, one day after epidural implantation of laminaria (brain compression). Dissociation and enlargement of the extracellular space (ECS) due to a serous (protein-poor) interstitial fluid accumulation. No significant regressive changes in the oligodendrocytes (OL) and the nerve fibers (No. 13995, X6,000).

an electron-dense material of homogeneous or fine granular appearance, spreading within an extremely enlarged extracellular space (Fig.5). Similar observations on plasma-like exsudative phenomena have been made by Hirano, et al. (1964), and Levine, et al. (1965). In such regions of protein-rich edema, the swollen astrocytes appear definitely more pale than the interstitial fluid, indicating that the extracellular protein-rich fluid is not exuded by the astrocytes. On the other hand, it seems that the astrocytes do not absorb an appreciable amount of this fluid despite the intimate contact with this extracellular liquid. Where nerve fibers are surrounded by plasma-like fluid, there is no limiting membrane to demarcate the fluid

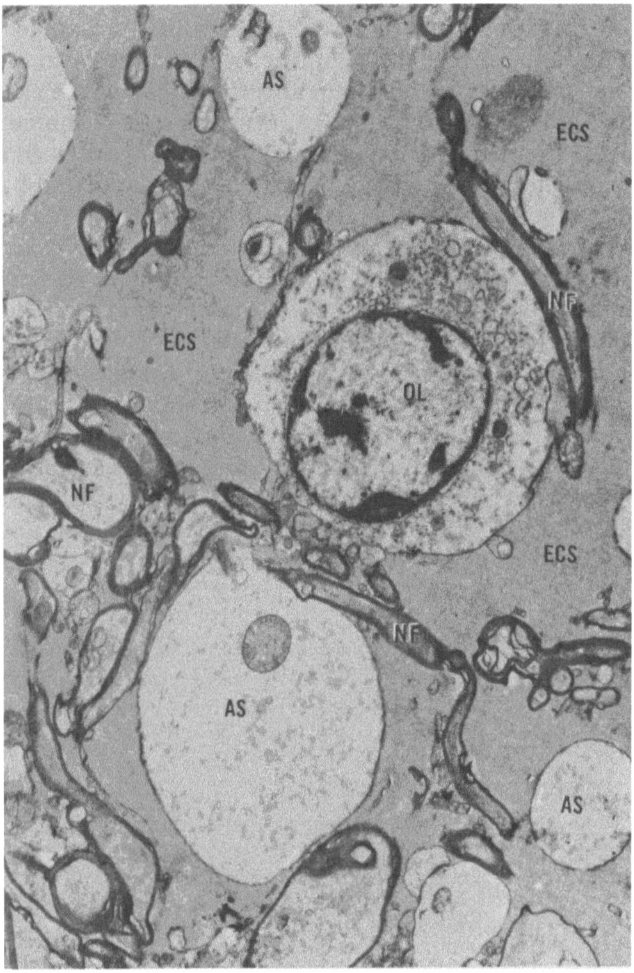

Fig. 5. The fine structural details of a plasmatic (protein-rich) form of edema of the white matter; venous congestion, two days after experimental obstruction of the sinus and ligation of the jugular veins. Separation of the nerve fibers within a pool of electron-dense interstitial fluid (ECS), marked swelling of the astrocytic cells, while the oligodendrocyte (OL) presents a minor degree of swelling (No. 13148, X8,000).

from the outermost myelin lamellae. According to Scholz (1949), the secondary hypoxic effect of protein-rich interstitial fluid is of importance for alterations of the nerve fibers of a primary and a secondary nature. But we do not want to go into detail, because this problem is still under investigation.

Summarizing our preliminary findings in serous and plasmatic forms of edema of the white matter, we would like to emphasize that there are no essential structural differences with regard to distention of the extracellular space, dissociation of the nerve fibers, and generalized swelling of the astrocytes. Differences in chemical composition of the interstitial fluid have to be elucidated by histochemical and biochemical techniques. If we adopt the idea of Scholz, that the protein-rich edema can induce a secondary hypoxia, we must consider that the sequelae of serous and plasmatic edema in the white substance may be different from one another. This leads to the problem of acute "Ödemnekrose" and necrotizing edema.

In the zones of necrosis (brain trauma, toxic lesions) there is a total destruction of the cellular elements. In the so-called "Zwischenzone," more pronounced regressive changes of the glial cells and the nerve fibers may occur. Summarizing our findings in the white matter, we would like to emphasize that in all three of the above-mentioned topographically defined zones, the extracellular space shows a primary significant enlargement.

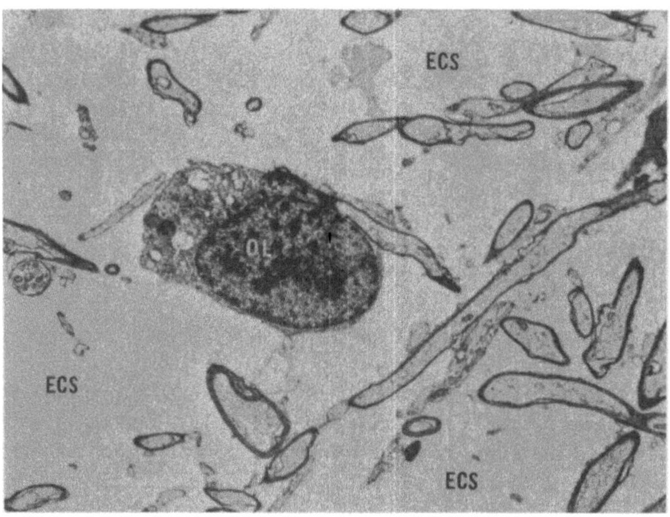

Fig. 6. The so-called "Zwischenzone" of the white matter, in which edema and partial tissue necrosis are intermingled (acute Ödemnekrose"), 30 hours after diphtheric intoxication of the cat brain. More severe lesions with extreme enlargement of the extracellular space (ECS) and dissociation of the nerve fibers; OL — pyknotic oligodendrocyte (No. 12813, X5,500, reduced).

VASCULAR CHANGES

Brain edema defined as a pathological increase of fluid within the brain tissue is accompanied by changes of the vascular permeability. Edematous changes occur in connection with varying degrees of disturbances of the blood brain barrier (BBB) function. Electron microscopy of normal (see, e.g., Hager, 1961) and developing (see, e.g., Wechsler, 1965) central nervous system has convincingly demonstrated that the peculiar morphological characteristics of the BBB are determined by (1) the very continuous extracellular space which has a distance between the cell membranes of 200 Å approximately, (2) the lack of a true pericapillary space, and (3) a complete pericapillary sheath composed of astrocytic foot processes closely attached to the basement of the capillary wall. The functional view of BBB effects is analogous to events in cell membranes and special cell transport. In spite of the above-mentioned anatomical peculiarities, the role of the endothelial layer of the cerebral capillaries in the regulation of the permeability or the transfer properties cannot be overlooked.

For the study of BBB disturbances in brain edema, among the most appropriate methods so far employed have been fluorescence microscopy and autoradiography. Electron microscopy gives us, however, the opportunity to study the structural background of the glial-vasal relationships under normal and pathological conditions (Hossmann, Schröder & Wechsler, 1965). Even in zones with a severe breakdown of the BBB function, demonstrable, e.g., by Evans-blue, it can still be difficult to find ultrastructural changes which can be interpreted as a structural basis of the microscopically demonstrated pathological alteration of permeability. In this connection, it is necessary to bear in mind that blood vessels chosen for electron microscopic investigations represent only a very small part of an extensive vascular system affected by such disturbances of the BBB. We find it necessary, however, to demonstrate some representative observations in the gray and white matter.

In the gray matter (cortex, basal ganglia), the normal relationship between the capillary and its surrounding glial processes is preserved, in spite of the swelling of the perivascular astrocytes. Also, there is no enlargement of the extracellular space and the pericapillary space (Fig. 7a). In the region of the plasmatic exsudation, on the other hand, a widening of the extracellular space can occur. Figure 7b shows a small vein of the cortex with plasma-like exsudation. There is no fenestration of the wall of the vessel. The adventitial cell shows some signs of activation. Within the true perivascular space of this small vein, limited by the vascular basement membrane and the glial basement membrane, one can see elec-

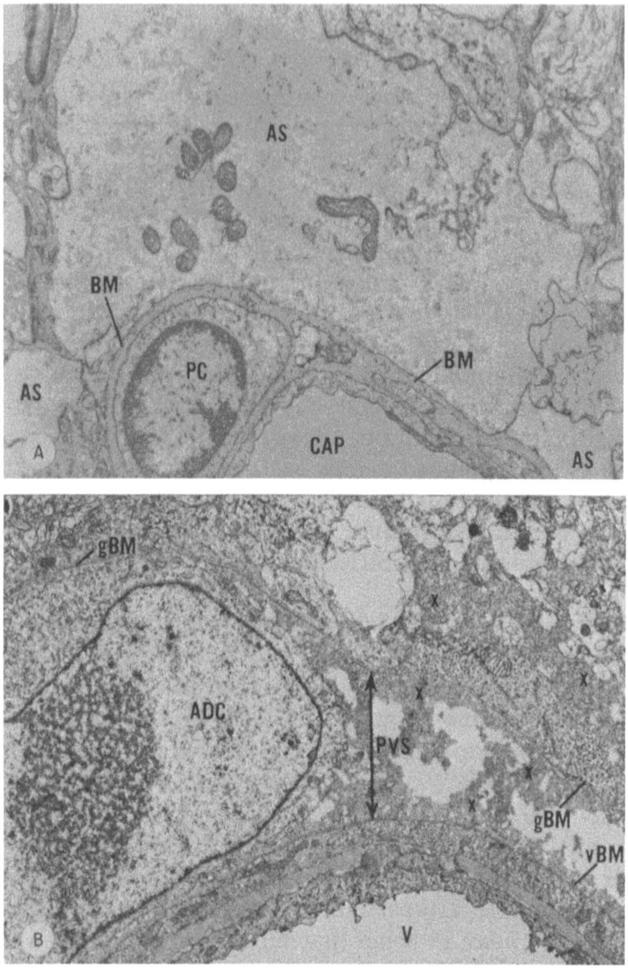

Fig. 7. Capillary and small vein in the edematous cortex of the cat: a) capillary (CAP), no separation of the swollen astrocytic foot processes (AS) from the vascular basement membrane (BM), 24 hours after brain compression. PC — pericyte (No. 13745, X13,000; b) small vein (V) with electron-dense plasma-like fluid (x) in the free perivascular space (PVS), limited by the vascular (vBM) and the glial basement membrane (gBM). Electron-dense fluid of the same appearance (x) fills the locally distended extracellular space of the damaged perivascular nervous tissue. ADC — activated adventital cell. Brain compression three days after implantation of laminaria (No. 12770, X9,000).

tron-dense plasma-like fluid. It is interesting to note that a substance of the same nature is also visible outside the glial shealth border and within the neuropil spreading throughout irregularly enlarged extracellular space (Fig. 7b).

In the edematous white matter the astrocytic foot processes also maintain their normal anatomical relationship to the vascular basement membran e (Fig. 8a). Sometimes rarely occurring slight separation of a part of perivascular astrocytes from the basement membrane may be observed (Fig. 8b). In any case, the tendency to preserve the intimate contact between astroglial processes and the small vessels is a very striking feature observed in our experiments, even when the extracellular space has been extremely enlarged.

All these observations indicate that in brain edema the morphological substrate of BBB does not necessarily show changes which can be detected by electron microscopy. It may be that such disturbances of the BBB are probably related more with functional than with structural changes of the vascular bed. Further studies are necessary to clarify these problems.

DISCUSSION AND SUMMARY

(1) In summarizing our findings, we would like to stress the essential differences in the reaction patterns of the gray and white matter under the conditions of edema (i.e., a primary pathological accumulation of fluid within the brain tissue). In the gray matter, this accumulation of fluid manifests itself mainly in intracellular compartments. In the white matter, the extracellular space, on the contrary, serves as the main channel for collection and spread of edema fluid. The essential peculiarities in the reaction patterns can be attributed to a relatively higher degree of expansibility of the extracellular space in the white matter, with a resultant dissociation of the nerve fibers, whereas in the gray matter the adhesion forces between adjacent cell membranes remain effective (Schröder & Wechsler, 1956b; Fig. 9). The ease with which the edema fluid spreads through the white matter could be explained by the fact that this fluid is localized mainly in a distended continuous extracellular space. In the white matter there is, independent of irreversible primary structural changes, a remarkable tendency for generalization of the primary regional edematous focus. The development of edema in the gray substance (e.g., cortex or basal ganglia) on the other hand, is of a more localized nature, which was well explained by Luse and Harris (1960): "Accumulation of the fluid within a cellular space is con-

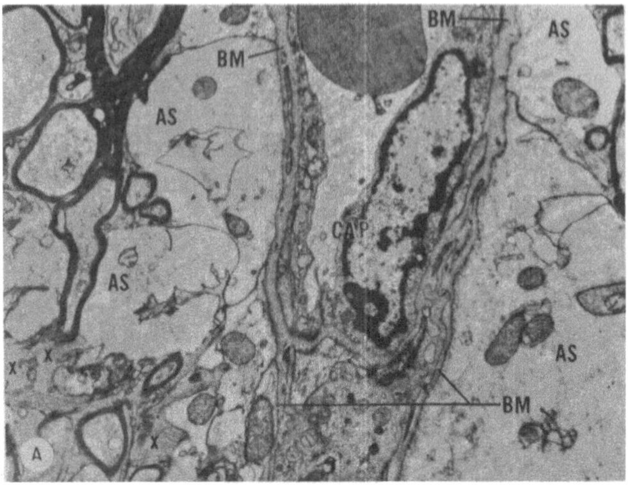

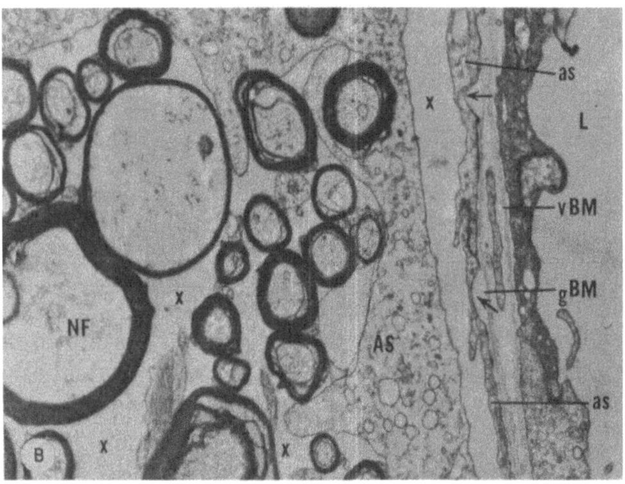

Fig. 8. Capillary and small vein in the edematous white matter of the cat: a) no prominent changes of the capillary; preservation of the normal anatomical relationship of the vessel wall and the swollen astrocytic processes (AS). BM — vascular basement membrane of the capillary (CAP) x — electron-dense edema fluid in the distended extracellular space. Two days after venous congestion (No. 13035, X7,500); b) portion of the vessel wall of a small vein (V) with the vascular (vBM) and the glial (gBM) basement membrane. Minimal retraction of the astrocytic foot processes (as) from the glial basement membrane indicated by an arrow; no gap between the two processes (as), but separation of the next perivascular astrocytic sheath cell (AS). x — enlargement of the extracellular space, NF — nerve fiber, L — lumen. 3 days after brain compression (No. 12925, X14,500).

sonant with the localized edematous response (of the cortex) to a focal zone of damage. If the accumulation of fluid were within the extracellular space localization of the fluid would be impossible, since this space is continuous throughtout the cerebrum." This latter idea of the authors can be taken as a basis for the explanation of the more generalized nature and spreading tendency of the edema fluid in the white matter.

Since the spread of edema in the white matter does not occur to the same extent in all regions, it would be of interest in future investigations to probe into the possible reaction of topographically different regions, e.g., the usually most severely affected centrum semi-ovale of the cerebral hemispheres, and on the contrary, the relatively spared long fiber tracts such as the internal capsules, the corpus callosum, the optic radiations, and finally the subcortical arcuate fibers. Similar topographical investigations could also be carried out in the gray substance, e.g., in cytoarchitectonically different regions of the cortex and the basal ganglia. Lastly, interest could also be directed to the changes in the various ependymal zones, and the regions which normally lack a BBB.

(2) The study of the fine structural equivalents of serous (protein-poor) and plasmatic (protein-rich) edema in the white matter leads to the conclusion that there are no basic primary structural differences. In each case the main features are dissociation of the nerve fibers, enlargement of the extracellular spaces, and swelling of the astrocytes. Serous and plasmatic forms of edema may represent only different stages or different severities of BBB disturbances. The interpretation of the alterations of other tissue elements can present difficulties, since one has to consider and differentiate between primary and possible secondary changes (sequelae of edema).

(3) We may add a few words about the expansibility of the extracellular space in relation to various severities of tissue lesions. We would like to refer again to the findings in brain trauma and diphtheric intoxication which allowed the classification of the lesions into three zones: (1) zone of necrosis, (2) the so-called "Zwischenzone" (intermediate zone with edema and partial necrosis), and (3) the perifocal edematous region. Figure 9 is a schematic presentation of the different degrees of expansibility in the above-mentioned zones. It would be of benefit to study the underlying causes of the stability or instability of cellular contacts in the brain. With respect to our findings in brain traumatization (Schröder & Wechsler, 1965a), we have published a hypothesis in another paper (Schröder & Wechsler, 1965b).

(4) Finally, we would like to define brain edema as an abnor-

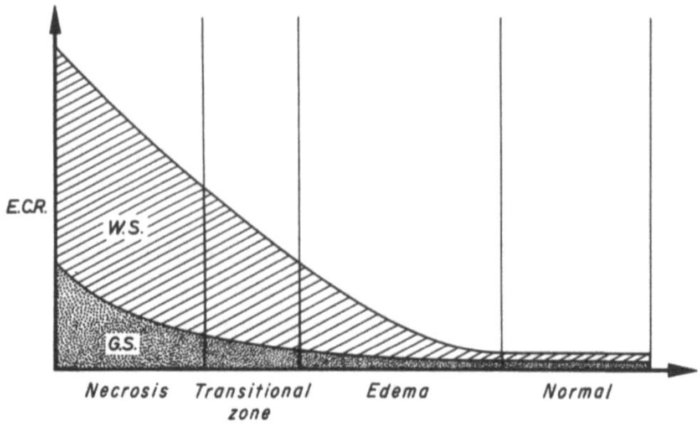

Fig. 9. Expansibility of the extracellular space (ECR) in the gray substance (GS) and the white matter (WS) in relation to differences in the severity of the tissue lesions (generalized schematic representation; see discussion).

mal intra- and/or extracellular fluid accumulation with unique primary and different secondary tissue effects (sequelae).

REFERENCES

Gerschenfeld, H. M., F. Wald, J. A. Zadunaisky and E. D. P. De Robertis: Function of astroglia in water-ion metabolism of the central nervous system, Neurology, 9, 412-425 (1959).

Hager, H.: Elektronenmikroskopische Befunde zur Feinstruktur der Hirngefässe und der perivasculären Räume im Säugetiergehirn. – Ein Beitrag zur Kenntnis des morphologischen Substrates der sogenannten Bluthirnschranke, Acta Neuropath., (Berlin), 1, 9-33 (1961).

_____: Die feinere Cytologie und Cytopathologie des Nervensystems, in: Veröffentl. morphol. Pathol. Heft, 67, Stuttgart: G. Fischer-Verlag (1964).

Hirano, A., H. M. Zimmermann and S. Levine: The fine structure of cerebral fluid accumulation. – III. Extracellular spread of cryptococcal polysaccharides in the acute stage, Am. J. Pathol., 45, 1-19 (1964).

_____, _____ and _____: The fine structure of cerebral fluid accumulation. – VII. Reactions of astrocytes to cryptococcal polysaccharide implantation, J. Neuropath. exp. Neurol., 24, 386-397 (1965).

____, ____, and ____: Fine structure of cerebral fluid accumulation. — VI. Intracellular accumulation of fluid and cryptococcal polysaccharide in oligodendroglia, Arch. Neurol., 12, 189-196 (1965).

Hossmann, K. A., J. M. Schröder and W. Wechsler: Das morphologische Substrat der Bluthirnschranke unter physiologischen und pathologischen Bedingungen, Verh. Dtsch. Ges. Path., 49th Meeting, 350-357 (1965).

Jacob, H.: Über die diffuse Markdestruktion im Gefolge eines Hirnödems (Diffuse Ödemnekrose des Hemisphärenmarkes), Z. ges. Neurol. Psychiat., 168, 382-395 (1940).

Kleihues, P., W. Wechsler and K. J. Zülch: Elektronenmikroskopische Befunde aus den perifokalen Ödemzonen des Katzengehirns nach lokaler Diphtherie-Intoxikation, Naturwissenschaften 53, 202 (1966).

Luse, S. A. and B. Harris: Electron microscopy of the brain in experimental edema, J. Neurosurg., 17, 439-446 (1960).

____ and ____: Brain ultrastructure in hydration and dehydration, Arch. Neurol., 4, 139-153 (1961).

Niessing, K. and W. Vogell: Elektronenmikroskopische Untersuchungen über Strukturveränderungen in der Hirnrinde beim Ödem und ihre Bedeutung für das Problem der Grundsubstanz, Z. Zellforsch., 52, 216-237 (1960).

Riverson, E., P. Kleihues, B. Schultze and W. Wechsler: Experimentelles Hirnödem nach epiduraler Kompression, Verh. Dtsch. Ges. Path., 50 Tg, 441-446 (1966).

Scholz, W.: Histologische und topische Veränderungen und Vulnerabilitätsverhältnisse im menschlichen Gehirn bei Sauerstoffmangel, Ödem und plasmatischen Infiltrationen, Arch. Psychiat. Z. Neurol., 181, 621-665 (1949)

Schröder, J. M. and W. Wechsler: Ödem und Nekrose in der grauen und weissen Substanz beim experimentellen Hirntrauma (Licht- und elekronenmikroskopische Untersuchungen), Acta Neuropath., 5, 82-111 (1965a).

____ and ____: Zur Frage unterschiedlicher Adhäsionskräfte zwischen den Zellmembranen in der grauen und weissen Substanz des Gehirns, Naturwissenschaften, 52, 86-87 (1965b).

Torack, R. M., R. D. Terry and H. M. Zimmermann: The fine structure of cerebral fluid accumulation. — I. Swelling secondary to cold injury, Am. J. Path., 35, 1135-1147 (1959).

Ule, G.: Elektronenmikroskopische Studien zum experimentellen Hirnödem. Proc. 4. Int. Kongr. Neuropathol., München, Vol. 2, 118-124 (1961): Stuttgart, G. Thieme-Verlag (1962).

Wechsler, W.: Die Entwicklung der Gefässe und perivasculären Gewebsräume im Zentralnervensystem von Hühnern (Elektronenmikroskopischer Beitrag zur Kenntnis der morphologischen Grundlagen der Bluthirnschranke während der Ontogenese), Z. Anat. Entwickl. Gesch., 124, 367-395 (1965).

Wohlfarth-Bottermann, K. E.: Die Kontrastierung tierischer Zellen und Gewebe im Rahmen ihrer elektronenmikroskopischen Untersuchung an ultradünnen Schnitten, Naturwissenschaften, 44, 287-288 (1957).

JAIME MIQUEL
WEBB HAYMAKER

BRAIN EDEMA INDUCED BY PARTICLE AND ULTRAVIOLET RADIATION

Interest in the study of experimental brain edema has stimulated the development of a variety of edema-producing techniques. Among others, extradurally inflated balloons (Ishii, et al.), and freezing of the cortex (Bakay & Haque; Clasen, et al., 1957, 1962; Klatzo, et al., 1958; Pappius & Gulatti), have been used in an effort to elucidate the pathogenesis of traumatic brain edema. Although, since Rachmanov's observations in 1926 radiation has been known to produce brain permeability disturbances, and although an edematous process following irradiation has been demonstrated, there has been no study directed at utilizing radiation-induced injury as a "model" for the study of pathogenesis of brain edema or of the effectiveness of therapy. This is rather surprising since radiation offers unsurpassed versatility in the production of brain lesions in any area or depth desired. Brain edema reproducible with great uniformity should be easily achieved by the simple expedient of exposing the brain of a series of animals to identical radiation dosage. These considerations prompted us to undertake the present study on rat and cat brain edema induced by particle and ultraviolet (UV) radiation.

MATERIAL AND METHODS

A total of 25 female Sprague-Dawley rats, three weeks of age at the time of irradiation, and 92 adult cats of both sexes, were used in this study. For the rats, the radiation source was the heavy ion linear accelerator (HILAC) at the University of California in Berkeley, which delivered 41.6-Mev alpha particles at 24,000 rad/min. For the cats, the 88-inch cyclotron in Berkeley was used. Some of the cats received 31-Mev protons at 40,000 rad/min, and others, 120-Mev alpha particles, at 40,000 rad/min. For UV irradiation, the Osram HBO 200 high pressure mercury lamp was used.

Methods of irradiation of rat brain with alpha particles have been described in detail elsewhere (Miquel & Haymaker). With the rats under sodium pentobarbital anesthesia, the scalp was incised in the midline and reflected, and the animals were mounted in special holders. The aperture through which the particles passed was 10 mm in diameter, sufficient to irradiate most of the dorsal surface of the cerebrum. Doses and sacrifice times are shown in Table 1. In the experiments on the proton-irradiated cat brain, the animals were first anesthetized with sodium pentobarbital. The proton beam was directed to the dorsal aspect of the head through an aperture 4 cm in diameter. Exposure of cats to the 120-Mev alpha particles was performed as indicated for proton irradiation, but in the alpha-particle irradiated cats the skin and muscle over the

TABLE 1

IRRADIATION OF RAT BRAIN WITH 41.6-MEV ALPHA PARTICLES FROM THE BERKELEY HILAC: RADIATION DOSES AND TIME OF SACRIFICE

Number of Brains Studied	Radiation Dose (rad)	Time of Sacrifice
3	12,000*	24 hrs.
3		48 hrs.
3		72 hrs.
3		14 days
2		30 days
2	24,000*	24 hrs.
2		48 hrs.
2		72 hrs.
3		14 days
2		30 days

*These values represent surface doses.

cranium were reflected prior to exposure. In the cat the surface dose for both the alpha particles and the protons was 40,000 rad, and the depth of penetration in the brain, approximately 4 mm. At this depth, the (peak) dose for the alpha particles was 6.7 times the surface dose, and, for the protons, 3.6 times. After irradiation the animals were sacrificed at the time intervals indicated in Table 2.

TABLE 2

PARTICLE IRRADIATION OF CAT BRAIN WITH 40,000 RAD*: RADIATION ENERGY AND TIME OF SACRIFICE

Radiation Energy	Source	Time of Sacrifice
120-Mev alpha particles	88-inch cyclotron	24 hrs. (2)**
31-Mev protons	88-inch cyclotron	24 hrs. (3)
		4 days (2)

*This value represents the surface dose.
**Number of brains studied.

Prior to UV-irradiation, the cats were anesthetized by intraperitoneal injection of sodium pentobarbital, and parietal craniotomy performed. The dura was incised and reflected over the cranium. The exposed area of leptomeninges in the right inframarginal area (Fig. 1a) was approximately 20 × 10 mm. Pieces of gauze were placed around the opening to shield the skin, muscle and bone during UV-exposure. For irradiation, the HBO Osram lamp was used without filters. After a warm-up period of approximately five minutes, the lamp was placed above the head of the cat in the position shown in Fig. 1b. In order to obtain a reproducible lesion, it was essential that the light beam be placed exactly on the exposed meningeal surface. This was easily accomplished by closing almost completely the diaphragm in the lamp housing, thus dimming the light. After directing the light beam to the exposed brain the diaphragm was completely opened and exposure of the cerebral surface was carried out for the periods indicated in Table 3. After completion of the exposure, the scalp wound was sutured. The same procedure was used for cerebellar UV-irradiation.

For studies of blood-brain barrier (BBB) permeability, most of the animals were injected with sodium fluorescein or Evans blue. The technical procedures have been previously described (Miquel & Haymaker). At the various time intervals shown in Tables 1, 2

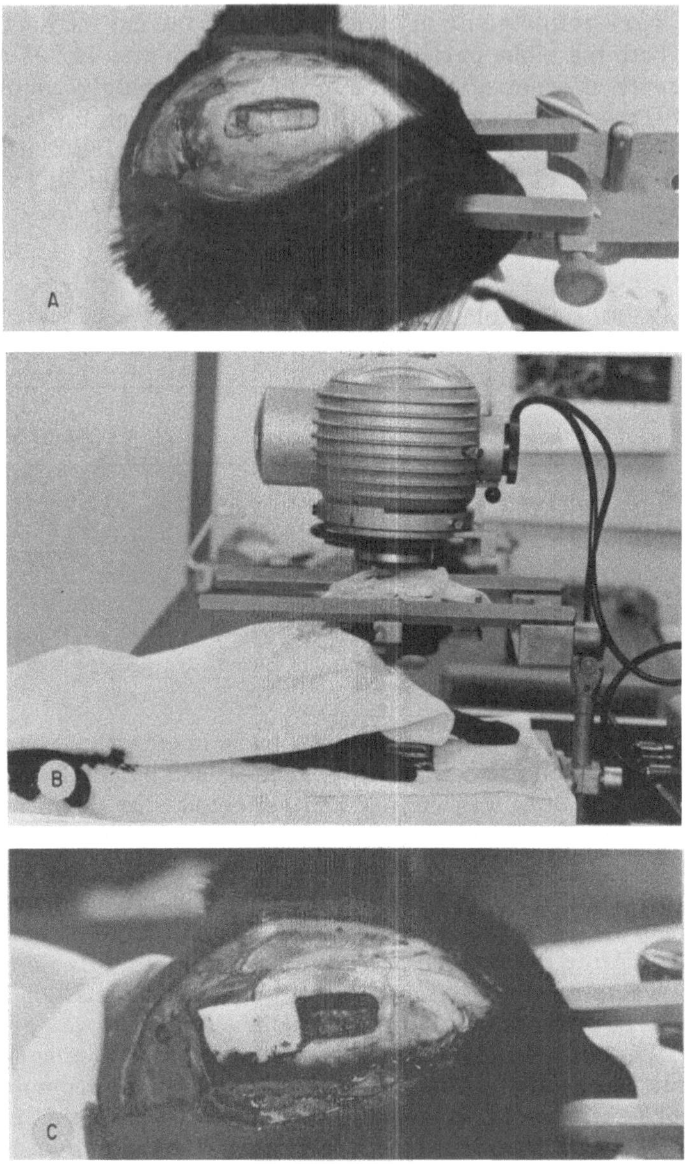

Fig. 1. Technique for the induction of cerebral edema in the cat by ultraviolet radiation: a) Craniotomy at the level of the inframarginal gyrus; b) Set-up for brain irradiation with use of the Osram HBO 200 Lamp; c) Demonstration of BBB damage induced by UV radiation. Penetration of Evans blue in the cortex is evident immediately after exposure.

TABLE 3
UV IRRADIATION OF CAT BRAIN:
DURATION OF EXPOSURE AND SACRIFICE TIME

Number of Brains Studied	Exposure Time	Time of Sacrifice
2	15 min.	6 hrs.
6		24 hrs.
2	30 min.	1 hr.
6		3 hrs.
2		4 hrs.
19		6 hrs.
21		24 hrs.
5		2 days
2		3 days
3		4 days
5		7 days
3		15 days
2		30 days
Total 78		

and 3, the rats were sacrificed by decapitation, and the cats, by severing the major blood vessels in the thorax. The brains were removed and sectioned coronally into blocks 3-4 mm in thickness. After fixation, the following histological and histochemical technique: were used: gold chloride method of Cajal for astrocytes, Holzer for astroglial status, Penfield's modification of Río Hortega for oligodendroglia and microglia, PAS-luxol fast blue-gallocyanin, PAS-hematoxylin following amylase digestion, and dimedone-PAS-gallocyanin. In addition, water content was determined in samples of white matter from four control and seven UV-irradiated brains. This was accomplished by weighing the tissue samples on tared coverslips in a torsion balance before and after drying overnight at 100°C.

RESULTS

Rat Brain Irradiation

BBB disturbance and the histological features of the cortical injury induced by alpha particles have been described in detail elsewhere (Janssen, et al.; Klatzo, et al., 1961; Miquel & Haymaker, 1965). In the present experiments, the white matter of the brains showing abnormal permeability to sodium fluorescein had the histological appearance of an edematous process (Fig. 2a). Widening of perivascular spaces and general loosening of the tissue was observed. Glycogen accumulation was present in the cortex in the vicinity of the necrotic zone and also in glial cells in the edematous white matter (Fig. 2b). Cajal's gold chloride technique revealed marked enlargement of the astrocytes as compared with those of the white matter elsewhere in the same brains.

Cat Brain Irradiation

The particle-irradiated cats showed intense sodium fluorescein or Evans-blue penetration in the necrotic zone at 24 hours and four days postexposure (Fig. 3). The indicators had also widely penetrated the underlying white matter. The histological appearance was that commonly associated with an edematous condition. PAS-positive material was observed in interstitial spaces, particularly in the vicinity of capillaries. Also, the perikaryon and processes of astroglia were clearly demonstrated due to the intensity of their PAS-positive coloration. In the edematous area, the astrocytes were markedly enlarged. In the cortical area, irradiation resulted in coagulation necrosis in 24 hours. The necrotic tissue was infiltrated by glycogen-laden leucocytes, while the parenchyma was free from glycogen. On the other hand, abundant glycogen granules were found in the cortical tissue situated at the border of the necrotic zone (Fig. 4a, b, d). The glycogen deposits were located predominantly in the gray matter, with few, if any, glycogen granules in the subcortical white matter (Fig. 4a, c).

When Evans-blue was injected immediately preceding UV-irradiation, staining of the brain cortex was already evident on completion of the exposure (Fig. 1c). It was also shown that when Evans blue was injected one hour before sacrifice, at 24 hours after irradiation, only the injured cortex stained although the white matter of the whole irradiated hemisphere was edematous. By contrast, when the injection was given immediately after UV exposure, the coloration was a faithful indicator of the spread of edema, an observation made also by Bakay and Haque, who used trypan blue as an indicator of edema in brains in which the cortex was frozen. The cats used in our experiments for standarization of the UV-irradiation technique were, therefore, injected with Evans-blue at the completion of the exposure time. Following UV-irradiation for 30 minutes, the animals sacrificed one hour after completion of the exposure showed Evans-blue staining limited to the injured cortex. At three hours, the edema had spread to the white matter but was usually limited to the injured gyrus (Fig. 5a). In the animals sacrificed from three to six hours after exposure, the extension of

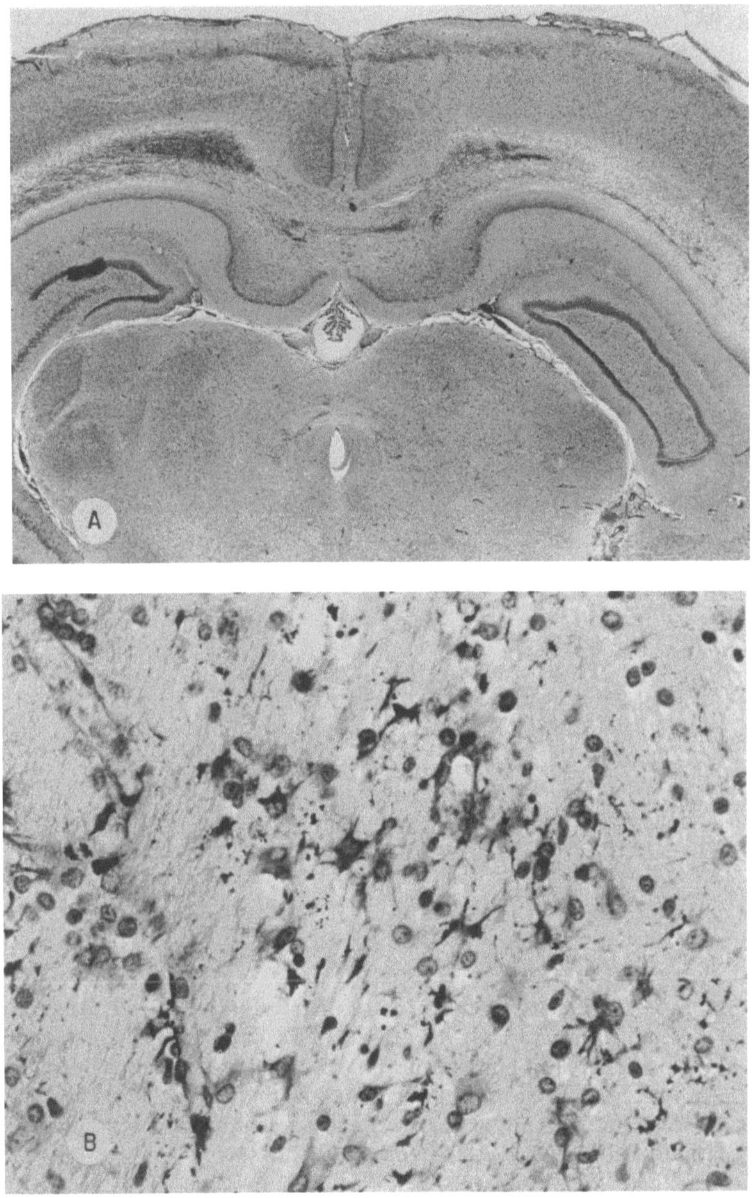

Fig. 2. Rat cerebrum at three days after exposure to 24,000 rad proton radiation: a) Necrosis at the level of the Bragg peak band and edema of the corpus callosum. PAS-luxol fast blue-gallocyanin. X12.4; b) Glycogen-containing astrocytes in the edematous area. Dimedone-PAS-gallocyanin. X375.

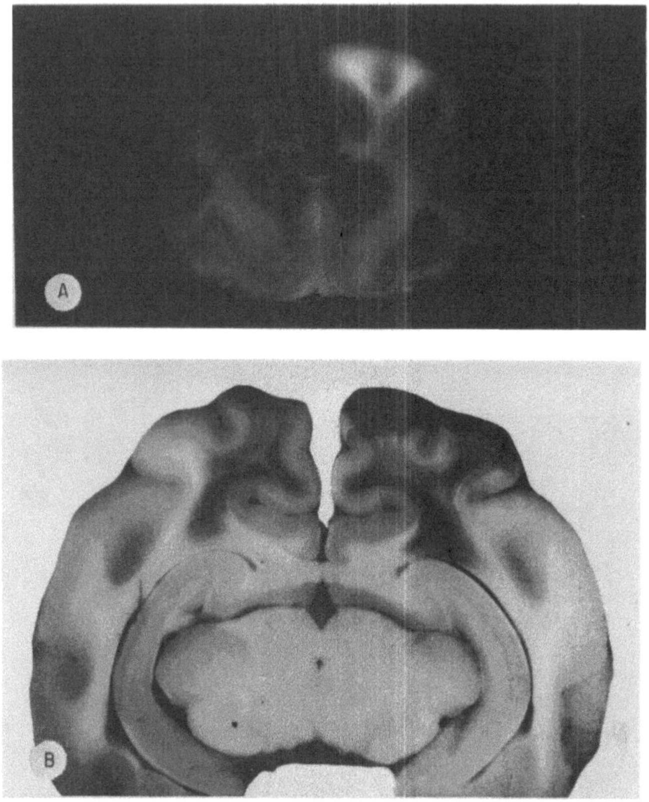

Fig. 3. Permeability disturbances in particle-irradiated cat cerebrum: a) Sodium fluorescein penetration at four days following exposure to 40,000 rad protons. The photograph, made in UV light, shows permeation of sodium fluorescein in the irradiated area and underlying white matter. X1.9; b) Evans-blue staining of necrotic and edematous areas 24 hours after irradiation with 40,000 rad alpha particles. X2.5.

edema was somewhat variable from animal to animal. It was only at the 24-hour interval that the edema was uniform. At this time the edematous condition had spread to almost the entire hemisphere in all the animals receiving 30-minute UV-radiation (Fig. 5b). When the exposure time was only 15 minutes, the animals sacrificed at 24-hour postexposure showed dye penetration and edema half way

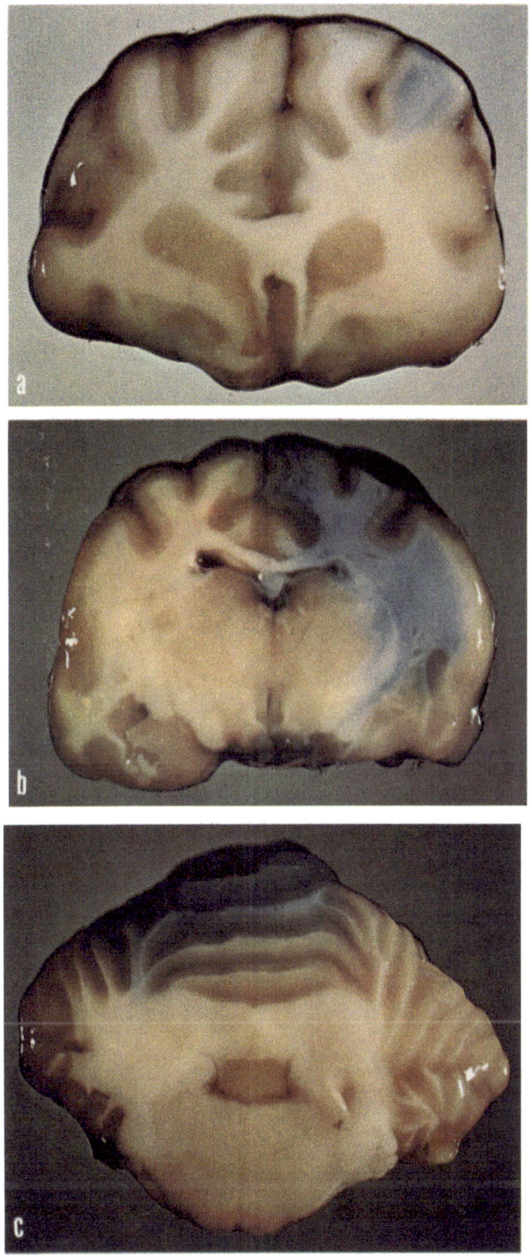

Fig. 5. BBB Penetration by Evans blue in UV-irradiated cat brain; a) Cross section of cat cerebrum at three hours after irradiation. X1.75 (reduced); b) Cross section at 24-hour postexposure. The dye penetration reaches to almost all the subcortical white matter of the irradiated hemisphere. X2.1 (reduced); c) Cerebellum at 24-hour postirradiation. The dye penetration is much more limited than in the cerebrum at the same time interval.

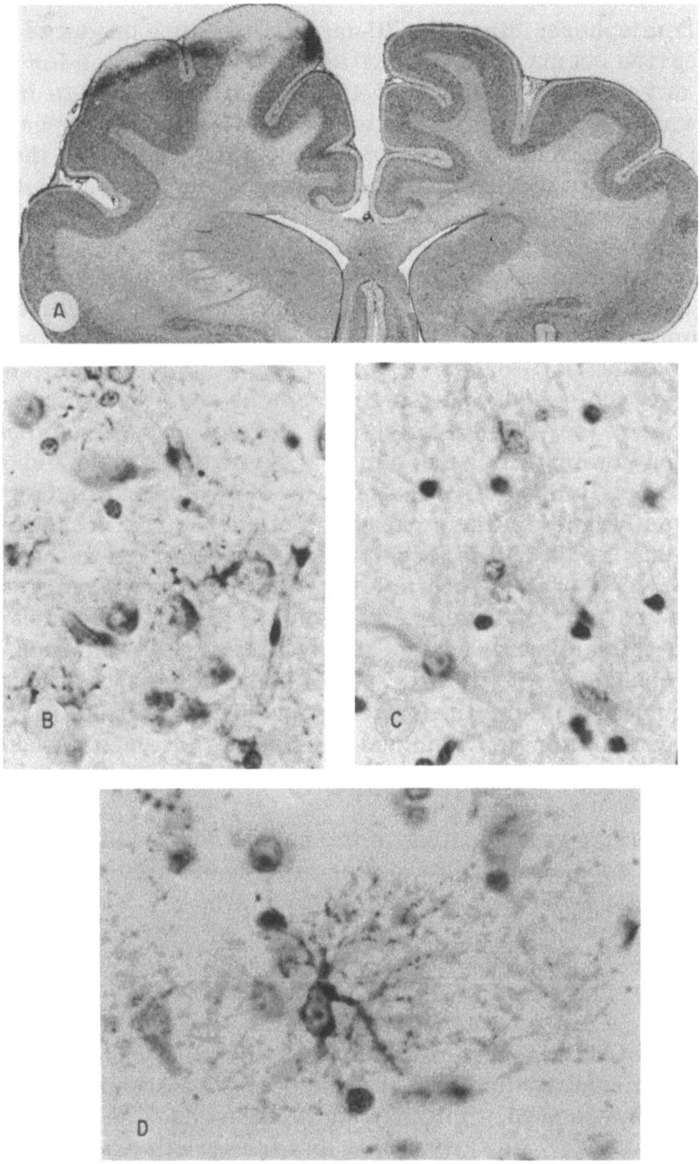

Fig. 4. Sections from the same brain as shown in Fig. 3a: a) Cortical necrosis in the irradiated zone and adjacent glycogen deposits in the gray matter. Very little glycogen is present in the white matter. Dimedone-PAS-gallocyanin. X3.9, reduced; b) Glycogen-containing astrocytes in the cortical area next to proton-induced injury. PAS-gallocyanin. X685, reduced; c) Swollen PAS-positive astrocytes (no histochemically demonstrable glycogen) in the adjacent edematous white matter. PAS-gallocyanin. X685, reduced; d) Heavy staining of the perikaryon and processes of a protoplasmic astrocyte due to their high glycogen content. Dimedone-PAS-gallocyanin. X220 (reduced).

down the hemisphere. Since the 30-minute exposure produced a more extensive edema, this irradiation time was selected for the induction of "standard edema." At 48 hours after 30-minute irradiation, the widening of the white matter of the affected hemisphere was still very evident. An hemorrhagic infarct was observed in the zone of maximal damage in the cortex. At three to four days after exposure, the widening of the white matter was definitely reduced. At seven days, although Evans blue was still present in the affected hemisphere when injected at irradiation time, the white matter had reverted to its normal width. At the 30-day interval, the cortex still showed some penetration of Evans blue, but none was observed in the white matter.

The morphological changes occurring in the necrotic and edematous zones of the UV-irradiated cats were observed from one hour to 30 days after exposure. Shallow cortical necrosis and an accumulation of PAS-positive material in the white matter (Fig. 6a) were constantly noted in the acute stage of edema. As in the particle-irradiated brains, glycogen accumulation was observed in the cortex in the vicinity of the necrotic zone (Fig. 6b), but was very sparse in the white matter. Glycogen deposits in the cortex were still noticed in the animals sacrificed at 30 days after UV-irradiation. The astrocytic changes were striking. At 24 hours, they showed marked hypertrophy (Fig. 7), and, thereafter, suggestive hyperplasia (Fig. 8). In general, the histological findings paralleled those described by Klatzo, et al., and by Bakay and Haque in cat brain edema induced by freezing.

The average water content of the normal white matter was 69.2%. In the edematous white matter at 24 hours following UV irradiation the water content was raised to 80.2%.

DISCUSSION

The fact that exposure of the brain to ionizing radiation may result in permeability disturbances and edema has been recognized since Rachmanov and Mogilnitzsky and Podljaschuck showed in mice and rabbits injected with trypan blue that the irradiated part of the brain became blue. More recently, Clemente and Holst (1953, 1954) observed alterations in the permeability of cerebral vessels of the monkey following irradiation. Trypan blue injected intraperitoneally revealed a marked impairment of the BBB of the hypothalamus and medulla oblongata. Following exposure of the mouse to X-radiation, cerebellar edema was observed by Schümmelfeder, et al. The cerebellum had the characteristics of an extracellular edematous process with the widened intercellular spaces containing sparse hemor-

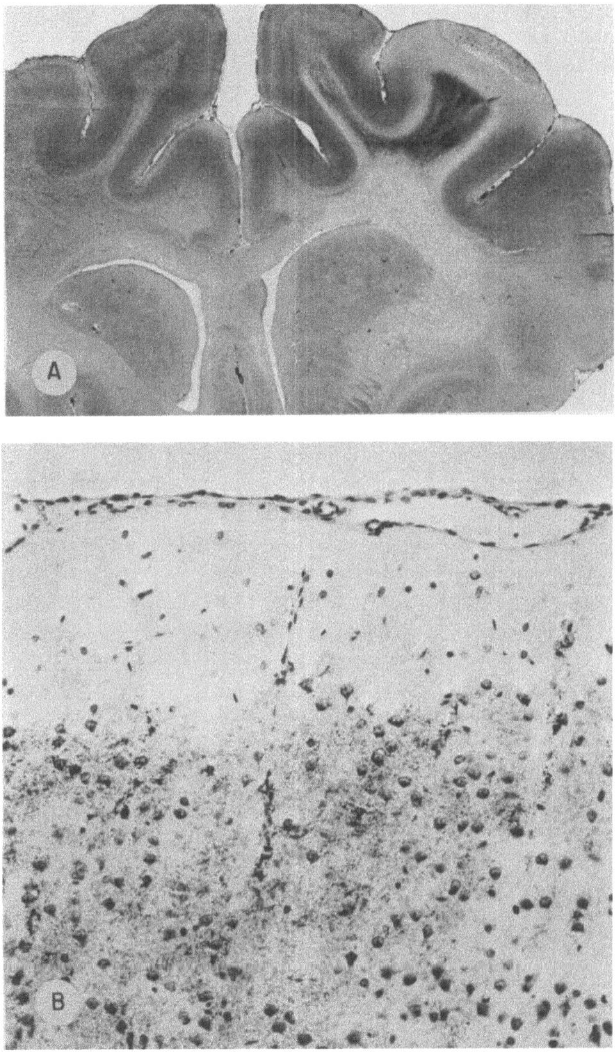

Fig. 6. Sections of cat cerebrum exposed to UV radiation. X2.1: a) Shallow cortical necrosis and PAS-positive material in the white matter at 4 hours after exposure. PAS-luxol fast blue-gallocyanin. X3.5; b) Glycogen accumulation in the cerebral cortex at 24 hour postirradiation. X140.

rhages. Electron microscopic studies of the irradiated cortex were carried out by Hager, et al. In the irradiated area of the cerebral cortex, all the astroglial processes were considerably enlarged.

Increased permeability of brain structures has also been dem-

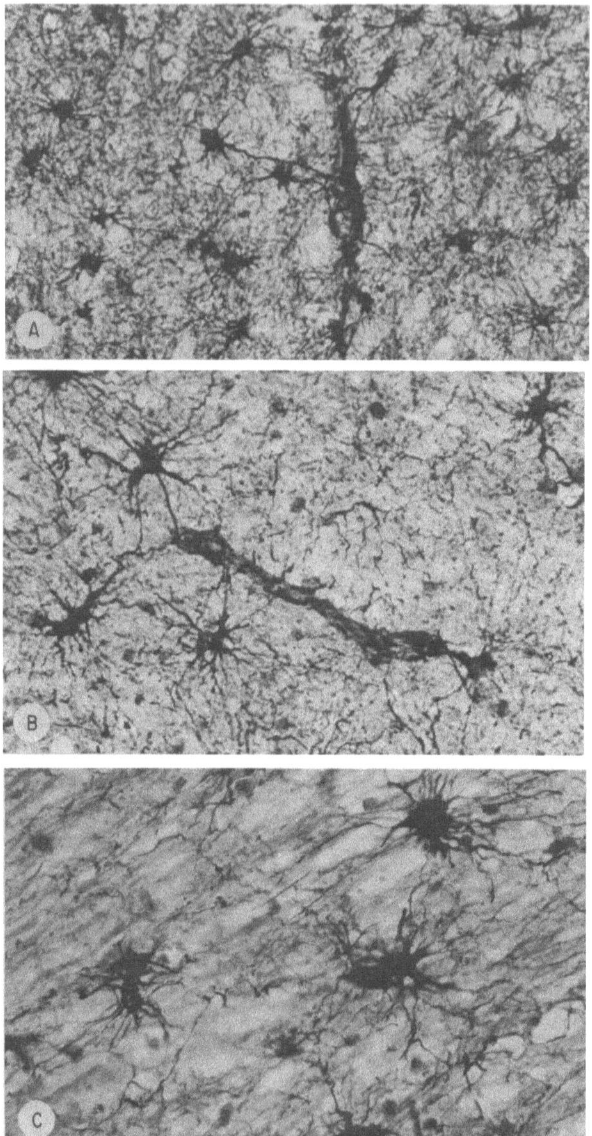

Fig. 7. Acute astroglial changes in edematous white matter. Cajal's gold chloride impregnation at 24 hours after UV-irradiation: a) Astrocytes in the white matter of the non-edematous hemisphere; b) Astrocytes in the edematous white matter; c) Astrocytes in another area of the edematous hemisphere.

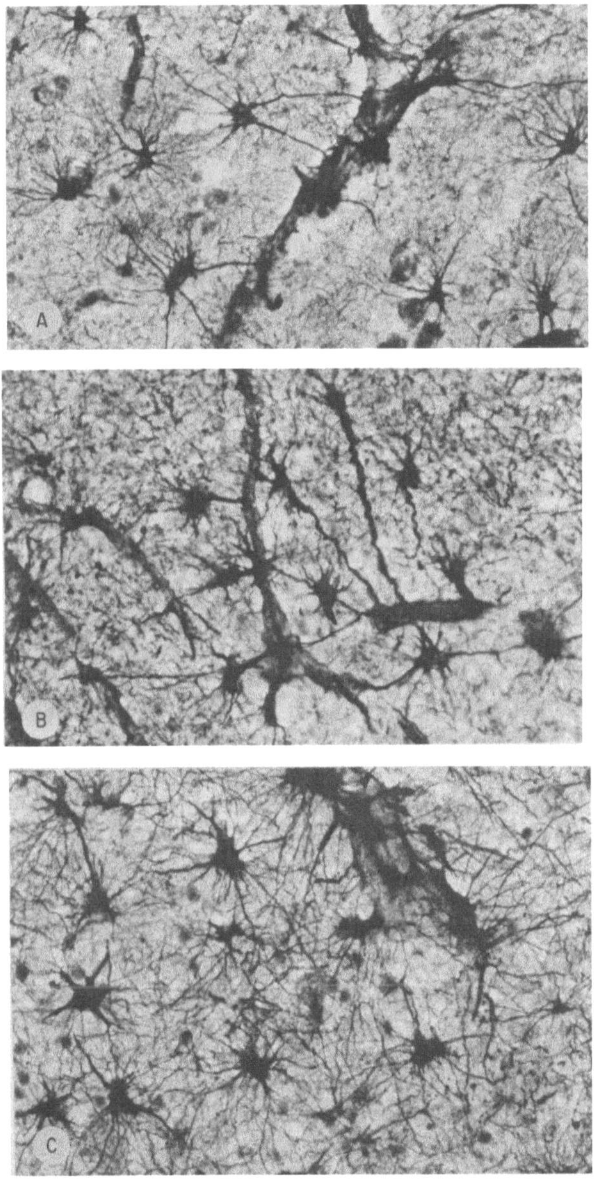

Fig. 8. Chronic changes in the astrocytes of UV-irradiated cat brain. Cajal's gold chloride impregnation. X375: a) Normal astrocytes in the non-edematous white matter of an animal sacrificed at seven days postexposure; b) Hypertrophy of fibrous astrocytes in the white matter of the edematous hemisphere seven days after irradiation; c) Astrogliosis in the irradiated hemisphere at 15 days' postexposure.

onstrated following exposure to particle radiation. As reported by Larsson, proton irradiation of the rat brain resulted in vascular engorgement and penetration of trypan blue into the brain parenchyma. Furthermore, sodium fluorescein was observed by Van Dyke, et al., to penetrate in the brain tissue of rats, monkeys and rabbits following exposure of the brain to alpha particles. Also, Janssen, et al., observed typical white matter edema following alpha-particle irradiation of the rat brain. Klatzo, et al., (1961) noted that penetration of fluorescein-conjugated serum proteins proceeded from the injured cortex to the underlying white matter, in the absence of hemorrhage or necrosis in the white matter. It seems that permeability disturbances and edema are common sequelae of exposure of the mammalian brain to electromagnetic and particle radiation. Our experiments show the usefulness of radiation as an injurious agent in inducing edema in the rat and cat brain. Although the cold-lesion technique has produced a wealth of information on monkey and cat brain, our attempts to use it in the rat were not successful. By contrast, particle radiation appears to be a rapid and reliable technique for producing brain edema. An advantage is that the irradiation can be done through the intact skull.

Our studies showed that UV-irradiation is an effective means of producing cerebral and cerebellar edema in the cat. The severity of the lesion and ensuing edema were proportional to the irradiation time. A 30-minute exposure of the cerebral surface resulted in edema which spread through the white matter of almost the entire hemisphere. At this time the cortical zone of necrosis was shallow, and ample tissue was therefore available for chemical studies of the edematous process. The edematous process was uniform throughout the hemisphere at 24 hours. UV-induced edema thus constitutes a satisfactory model for the study of the pathogenesis of the edema and of the efficacy of therapy.

The experimentally-induced edema observed in the present study may be considered similar to that produced clinically by infarctions, abscesses, tumors, and surgical intervention. In clinical and radiation-induced experimental edema, the histological changes are practically identical, both being characterized by exudation of fluid with separation of the neuroglial meshwork and progressive astroglial reactions. In clinical conditions, certain tissues of the brain have a special tendency to become edematous, whereas others are less affected. The white matter of the cerebral hemispheres is particularly vulnerable, but not the corpus callosum or the internal and external capsules or the anterior and posterior commissures. Gray matter, in general, is less affected. In UV-induced edema the relative resistance of the corpus callosum to edema is clearly demonstrated by the observation that the edema never spread to the contralateral hemisphere. A similar observation was made by Clasen, et al. (1962), in monkey brain edema produced by freezing. In our experiments the cerebellum also showed a remarkable resistance. As illustrated by Fig. 5C, the Evans blue at 24 hours after exposure was much less widespread than in the cerebral tissue at the same time interval. The astroglial swelling and subsequent astrogliosis observed in our experimental material also have a counterpart in the changes described by Greenfield in edema around tumors.

Glycogen accumulation has been observed in epidermal basal cells exposed to UV-radiation (Daniels, et al.), but to our knowledge the present report is the first on glycogen accumulation following UV-irradiation of the cerebrum and cerebellum. It seems that glycogen increase is a general response of the astroglial cells to radiation, and indeed to any injurious agent. Glycogen accumulation has been observed around stab wounds of the brain (Friede), in brain tissue exposed to particle radiation (Klatzo, et al., 1961) and X-radiation (Miquel, et al.), and in lesions induced by freezing of the cortex (Miquel).

SUMMARY

Particle-irradiation of the rat and cat brain is a satisfactory means of inducing brain edema. The radiation is effective when delivered through the intact skull.

In the cat, ultraviolet irradiation of the cortex resulted in uniform cerebral and cerebellar edema. At 24 hours after exposure, although the necrotic zone produced by the UV was very superficial, the edema spread through the affected hemisphere.

Radiation-induced edema is a useful model for histological, histochemical and biochemical observations. This model may also be useful for studies dealing with the therapy of brain edema.

ACKNOWLEDGMENTS

We are indebted to Dr. Igor Klatzo for his suggestions during the pursuit of this work. We acknowledge the technical assistance of Mrs. Frances Hobbisiefken and Mr. P. Lundgren and the assistance in photomicrography rendered by Miss Ella L. Craig. We also wish to express appreciation to Dr. Graeme Welch and his staff of the Lawrence Radiation Laboratory for the cyclotron operation.

REFERENCES

Bakay, L. and I. U. Haque: Morphological and chemical studies in cerebral edema. I. Cold induced edema, J. Neuropath. exp. Neurol., 23, 393-418 (1964).

Clasen, R. A., P. M. Cooke, S. Pandolfi, D. Boyd and A. J. Raimondi: Experimental cerebral edema produced by focal freezing. I. An anatomic study utilizing vital dye techniques, Ibid., 21, 579-596 (1962).

_____, R. R. Prouty, W. G. Gingham, F. A. Martin, and G. M. Hass: Treatment of experimental cerebral edema with intravenous hypertonic glucose, albumin and dextran, Surg. Gyn. Obst., 104, 591-606 (1957).

Clemente, C. D. and E. A. Holst: Pathological changes in the blood brain barrier, neuroglia and EEG induced by X-irradiation of the heads of monkeys, Proc. 19th Internat. Physiol. Congr. Montreal, pp. 273-274 (1953).

_____ and _____: Pathological changes in neurons, neuroglia, and blood-brain barrier induced by X-irradiation of heads of monkeys, A.M.A. Arch. Neurol. & Psychiat., 71, 66-79 (1954).

Daniels, F., D. Brophy and W. C. Lobitz: Histochemical responses of human skin following ultraviolet irradiation, J. Invest. Dermatol., 37, 351-357 (1961).

Friede, R.: Die Bedeutung der Glia für den zentralen Kohlenhydratstoffwechsel, Zbl. allg. path. Anat., 92, 65-74 (1954).

Greenfield, J. G.: The histology of cerebral edema associated with intracranial tumours (with special reference to changes in the nerve fibers of the centrum ovale), Brain, 62, 129-151 (1939).

Hager, H., W. Hirschberger and A. Breit: Electron microscope observations on the X-irradiated central nervous system in the Syrian hamster. In: Response of the Nervous System to Ionizing Radiation (ed. by T. J. Haley and R. S. Snider), New York: Academic Press, 261-275 (1962).

Ishii, S., R. Hayner, W. A. Kelly, and J. P. Evans: Studies of cerebral swelling. II. Experimental cerebral swelling produced by supratentorial extradural compression, J. Neurosurg., 16, 152-166 (1959).

Janssen, P., I. Klatzo, J. Miquel, T. Brustad, A. Behar, W. Haymaker J. Lyman, J. Henry and C. Tobias: Pathologic changes in the brain from exposure to alpha particles from a 60-inch cyclotron. In: Response of the Nervous System to Ionizing Radiation (ed. by T. J. Haley and R. S. Snider), New York: Academic Press, 383-409 (1962).

Klatzo, I., J. Miquel, C. Tobias, and W. Haymaker: Effects of alpha particle radiation on the rat brain including vascular permeability and glycogen studies, J. Neuropath. exp. Neurol., 20, 459-483 (1961).

_____, A. Piraux and E. J. Laskowsky: The relationship between edema, blood-brain barrier and tissue elements in a local brain injury, Ibid., 17, 548-564 (1958).

Larsson, B.: Blood vessel changes following local irradiation of the brain with high-energy protons, Acta Soc. med. upsal., 65, 61-71 (1960).

Miquel, J.: Unpublished observation.

_____ and W. Haymaker: Astroglial reactions to ionizing radiation, Progr. in Brain Res. 15, 87-114 (1965).

_____, I. Klatzo, D. B. Menzel, and W. Haymaker: Glycogen changes in X-irradiated brain, Acta neuropath., 2, 482-490 (1963).

Mogilnitzsky, B. and L. D. Podljalschuk: Röntgenstrahlen und sogen. "hämatoenzephalische Barrière," Fortschr. Röntgenstr., 41, 66-75 (1930).

Pappius, H. M. and D. R. Gulati: Water and electrolyte content of cerebral tissues in experimentally induced edema, Acta neuropath., 2, 451-460 (1963).

Rachmanov, A.: Zur Frage über die Wirkung der Röntgenstrahlen auf des Zentralnervensystem, Strahlentherapie, 23, 318-329 (1926).

Schümmelfeder, N., K. J. Ebschner, H. D. Bergeder, and E. Krogh: Strahlennekrose am Kleinhirn nach einzeitiger, hochdosierter Röntgenbestrahlung, Virchows Arch. path. Anat., 334, 32-55 (1961).

Van Dyke, D. C., P. Janssen, and C. A. Tobias: Fluorescein as a sensitive, semiquantitative indicator of injury following alpha particle irradiation of the brain. In: Response of the Nervous System to Ionizing Radiation. (ed. by T. J. Haley and R. S. Snider) New York: Academic Press, 369-382 (1962).

J. CERVOS-NAVARRO

BRAIN EDEMA DUE TO IONIZING RADIATION*

For this investigation we used twenty macaca mulatta, all abou one year old. The heads were X-irradiated under Nembutal anesthesia. The dose was 2.700 r and the voltage 145 Kv at 19 mA. The brain was removed between one hour and six days after irradiation. Small fragments of white matter from the parietal lobe were submitted to OsO_4 fixation, either directly or after prefixation with glutaraldehyde. These fragments were then embedded in Vestopal and observed in the electron microscope.

Apart from the neuropathological findings, the presence of edema was determined in two ways. The cerebrospinal fluid pressure was measured, and the free water content determined. In monkeys, at the employed dose the edema is moderate. The first indication of brain edema appeared a few hours after irradiation and was manifested by an increase of 5% in free water content.

Variations in the treatment of the material caused differences in the histological pattern of the white matter. Edematous tissue fixed directly in osmium exhibited a marked distension of extracellular spaces (Fig. 1). Occasional splitting of myelin lamellae was found, but not more than in normal tissue fixed directly in osmium.

The prefixation with glutaraldehyde gave rise to a better conservation of the membranes and better preservation of cell content, especially of the filaments and the structureless coagulated protein. Nevertheless, it could be observed that the extracellular space is increased, too (Fig. 2). The cell membranes of the glial processes

*Supported by a grant from Bundesministerium für Wissenschaftliche Forschung (St. Sch. 205/66).

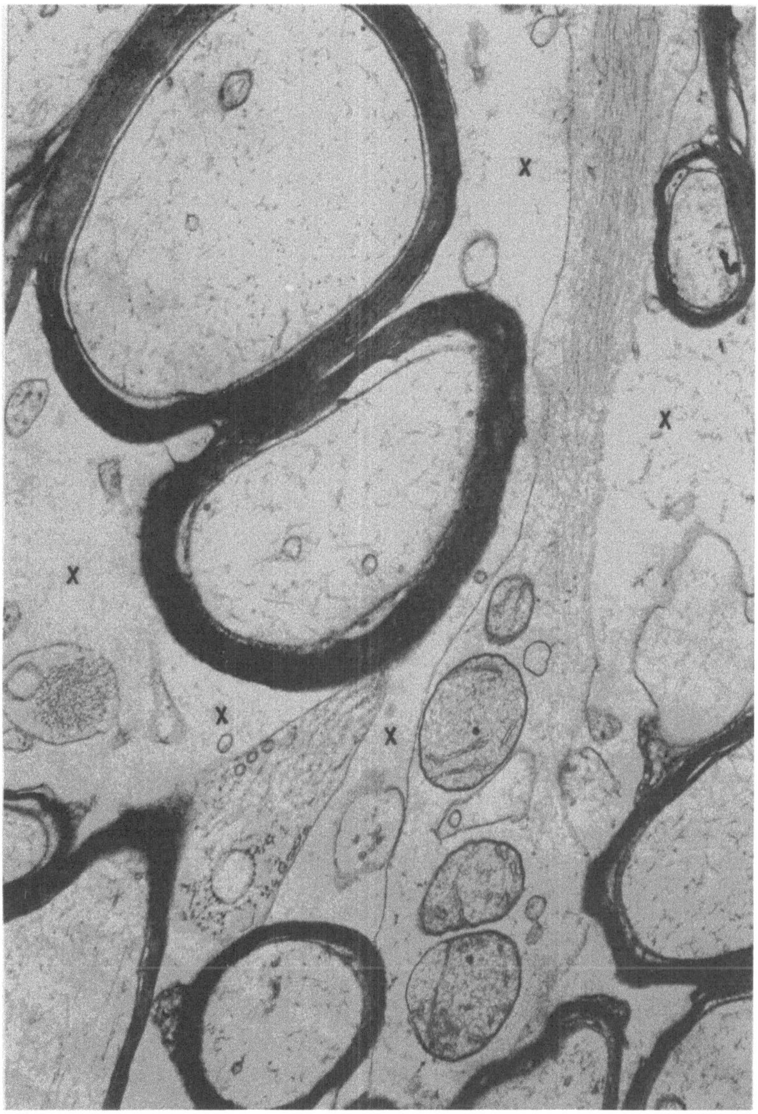

Fig. 1. White matter of monkey cerebrum six hours after irradiation; fixation directly in osmium. Extracellular space (x) is clearly enlarged. X27,000.

in the edematous zone are always intact, both with prefixation in glutaraldehyde and without.

Beside the spaces formed by separation of neighboring cellular structures there are some of the latter that rested together

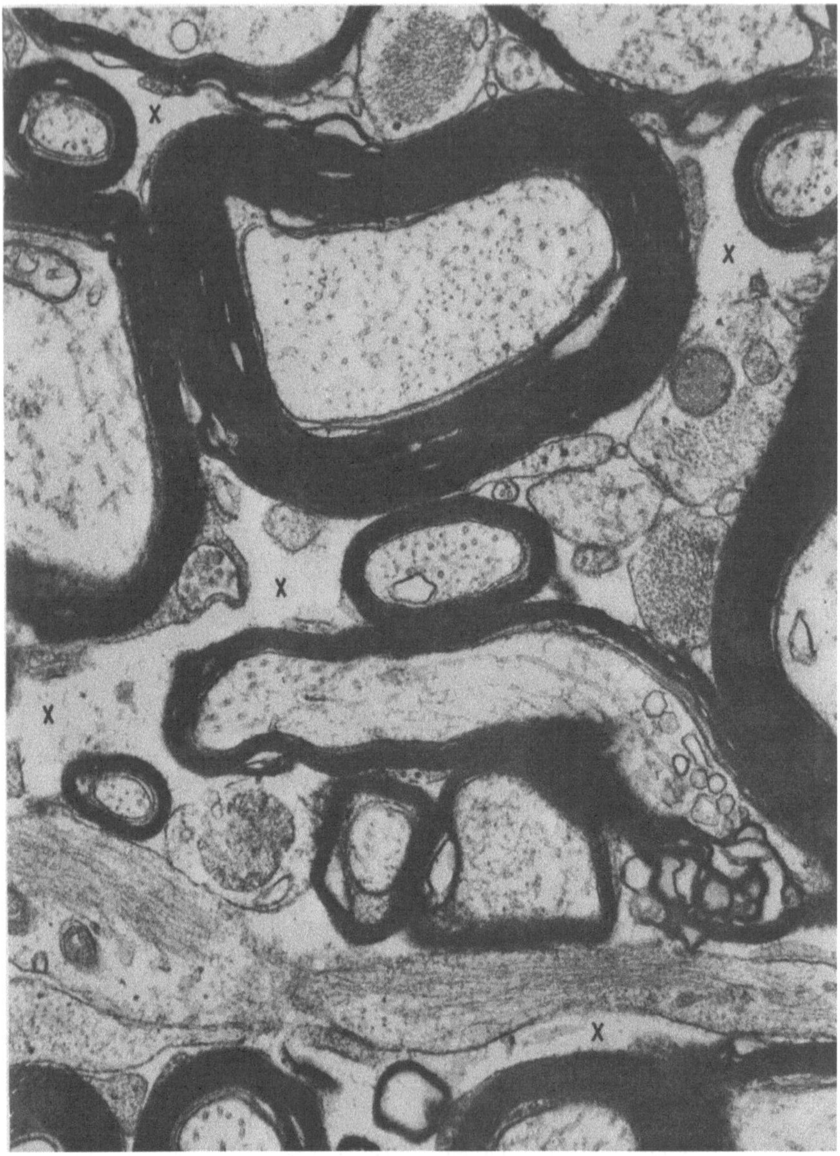

Fig. 2. White matter of monkey cerebrum six hours after irradiation; prefixation for three hours in glutaraldehyde; better preservation of cell content. Extracellular space (x) is moderately increased. X30,000 (reduced).

separated only by intercellular clefts of about 200 Å. The size of the increased spaces was found to be directly related to the degree of edema, but this applies only to the early stage of edema as seen during the first 30 hours after irradiation. After this time, cellular swelling becomes frequent. Intracellular swelling appeared as enlargement of the spaces in the endoplasmic reticulum. This enlargement can be found in glial cells as well as in nerve cells, but mainly in the former.

Variations in the site of edematous alterations occurred not only in different animals receiving the same doses and sacrificed at the same time, but they occurred also in different blocks of the same specimen. It was thought that perhaps the variations could be explained by different depth of the examined area from the cortex, but this supposition was not confirmed. Now we intend to search for a possible relation between the state of the capillaries in an area and the intensity of the edematous alterations in the same area.

One can see different alterations of the capillaries in the same brain and in capillaries which are very close to each other: 1) an increase of number and size of the pinocytotic vesicles (Fig. 3); that in capillaries of non-irradiated animals was rarer; 2) a swelling of endothelial cells (Fig. 4); and 3) in limited stretches, enlargement of the perivascular space (Fig. 4) with separation of the glial and endothelial basement membranes one from another.

Capillaries without morphological changes can be found in irradiated brains as well as capillaries with endothelial swelling or enlargement of the perivascular spaces in normal brains. Of course, we cannot relate all the ultrastructural alterations in our material to edema, because this is just one reaction of the nervous tissue to irradiation.

Glycogen accumulation in glial cells (Fig. 5) and reactive changes in myelinated and unmyelinated nerve fibers were present in about 50% of irradiated monkeys. These alterations have been described by others in irradiated brain. Further studies may elucidate if these changes are usually present in edematous tissue. Regarding the glycogen content of edema, a number of conflicting observations have been presented at this symposium. Therefore, in our opinion, the discussion of this subject may be worthwhile.

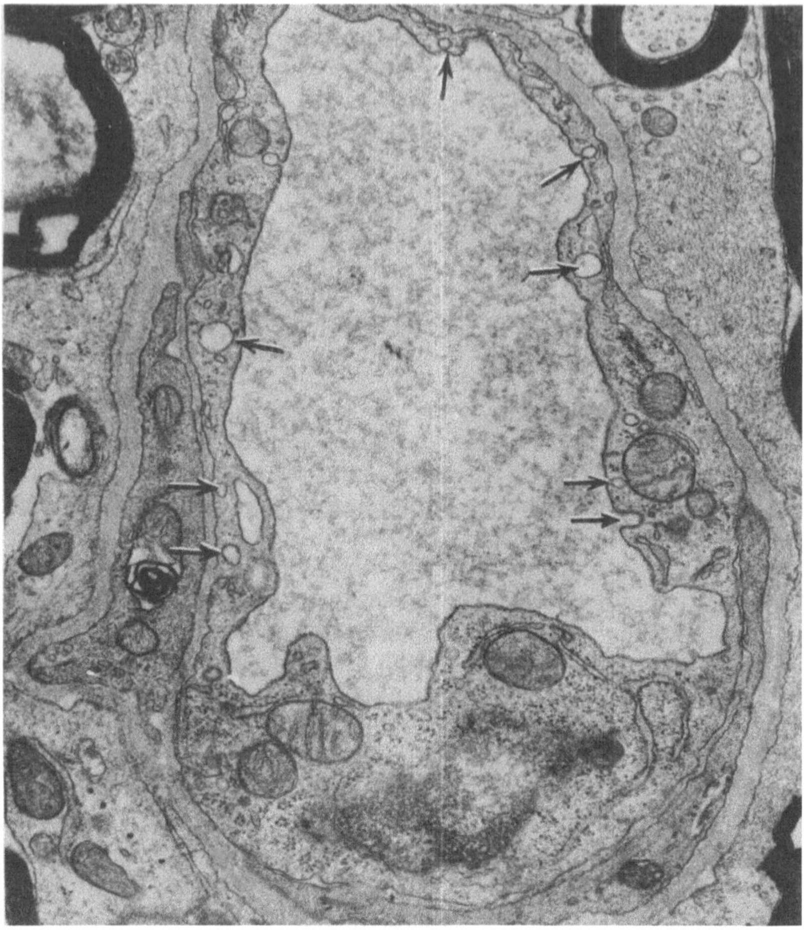

Fig. 3. Capillaries in the white matter of monkey cerebrum three hours after irradiation; increase of number and size of pinocytotic vesicles (arrows). X25,000 (reduced).

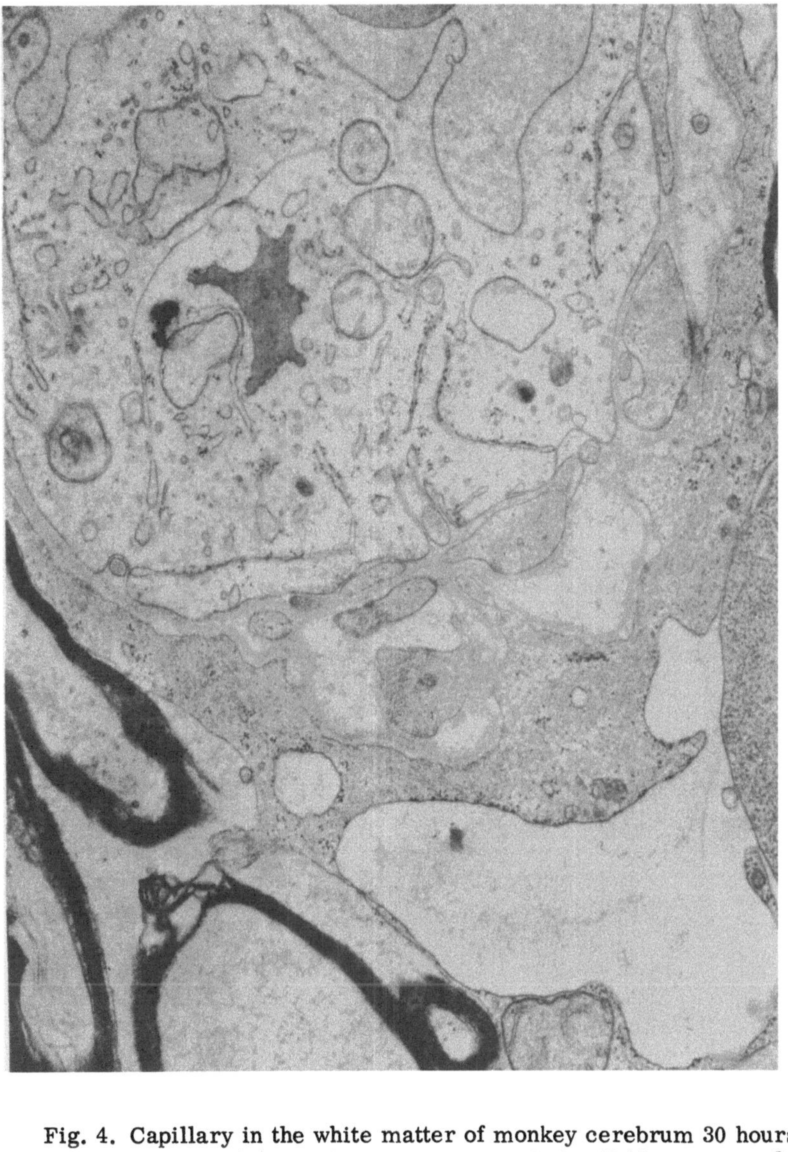

Fig. 4. Capillary in the white matter of monkey cerebrum 30 hours after irradiation; lumen (L); Swelling of the endothelial cell (e); perivascular spaces (x). X25,000 (reduced).

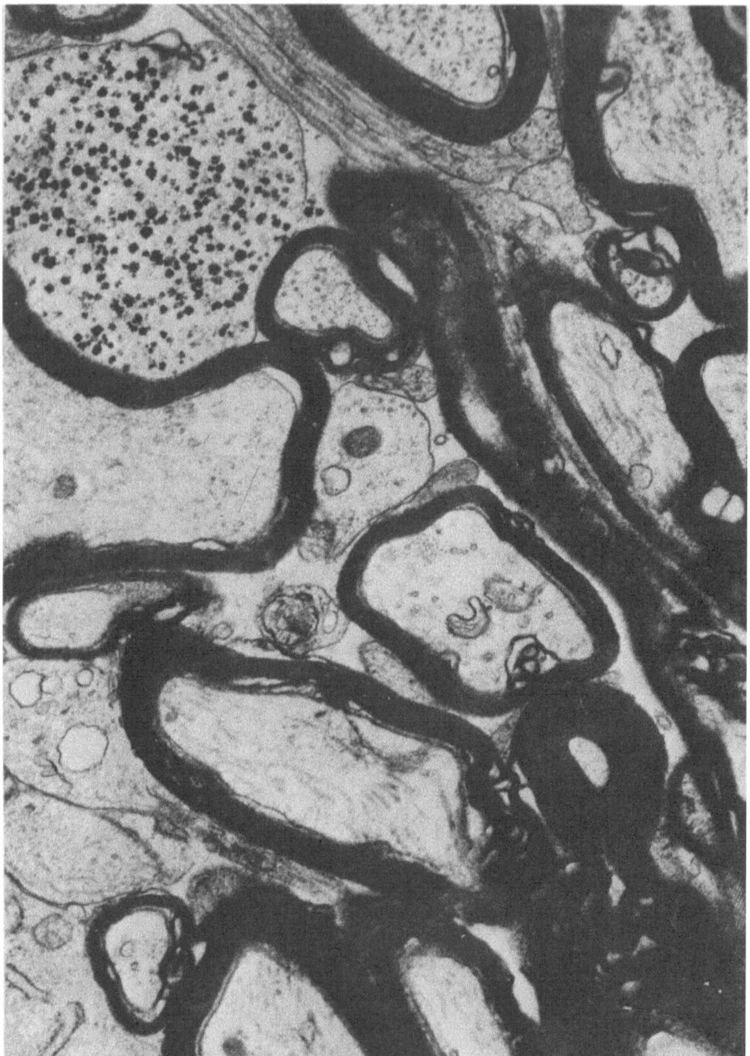

Fig. 5. White matter of monkey cerebrum 24 hours after irradiation; glycogen granules in a glial cell in the upper left. X27,000.

WERNER LIERSE
HERBERT D. FRANKE

EFFECTS OF X-IRRADIATION ON GUINEA PIG BRAIN

AN ELECTRONMICROSCOPICAL AND HISTOCHEMICAL STUDY

Our previous studies have shown that X-irradiation of guinea pig brain results in an initial increase of pinocytosis in capillary endothelium and brain edema during the first hours and days (Franke & Lierse, 1965). The purpose of this study was to ascertain whether this edema persists and/or other changes develop in the capillaries in the next six months. Klatzo, et al. (1961, 1962), Miquel, et al. (1963), have demonstrated that the permeability of the rat brain capillaries increases and that at the same time the metabolism of carbohydrates is disturbed. We found accumulations of glycogen as well as mucopolysaccharides in the brain of guinea pigs.

MATERIALS AND METHODS

The heads of 98 adult female and male guinea pigs were subjected to X-irradiation while the rest of the body was shielded by lead. The unanesthetized animals were immobilized for irradiation in a special animal holder of plastic material. The region of the brain was exposed. The mean weight of the animals was 400 g. Technical data: Siemens-Stabilipan, 200 kV, Filter 0.5 mm Cu, HVL 1.1 mm Cu, 20mA, FSD nearly 40 cm. The roentgen beam was focused over the right and left side of the brain. Therefore the dose distribution inside the brain was homogeneous. The X-rays were delivered at a rate of 100 R/min, measured with the normal cham-

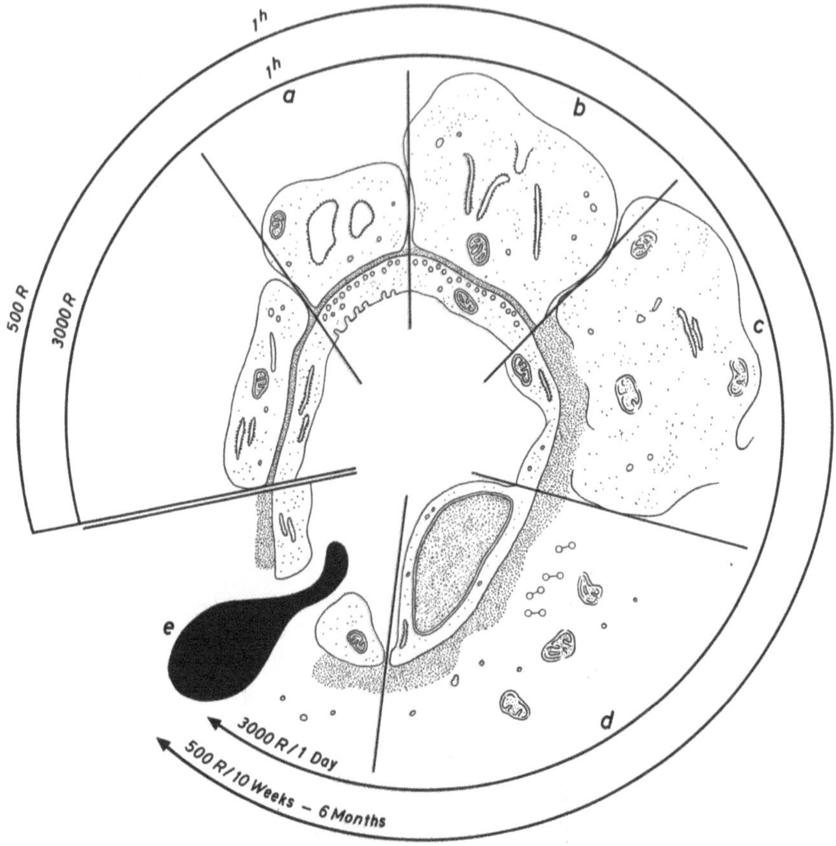

Fig. 1. The alterations following x-irradiation in guinea pig's brain: a) Increase of pinocytosis in the endothelium; b) Swelling of pericapillary astrocytes; c) Rupture of the glial cell membranes; d) Swelling of endothelium and disintegration of the basement membrane.

ber of the Simplex-Dosimeter (Physik.-Techn. Werkstätten, Freibur in the "brain-midline" of a phantom. The skull-skeleton of an adult guinea pig was filled with plastic material (Plastoid (R), Röhm and Haas; specific density 1.15) and was shaped like the head of a guinea pig. This phantom was fixed in the same position beside the guinea pig's head. Each animal was exposed together with the phantom, and for each exposure the dose was measured and recorded. The unfractionated dose levels were 100 R, 500 R, 1000 R, 2000 R, 2500 R, 3000 R and 4000 R. Postradiation sacrifice time was one and 24 hou six, nine and 14 days, ten weeks and six months.

In all animals which were used for electronmicroscopy small pieces of cortex and cerebellum were removed immediately after decapitation. The tissue was placed in osmium tetroxide buffered according to the method described by Dalton. After dehydration the material was embedded in Vestopal or Epon and stained with the lead hydroxide and uranyl acetate. All photographs were prepared with the Elmiskop I (Siemens) or the EM 9 (Zeiss). A second series of animals was anesthetized and perfused via the ascending aorta with Gendre's fluid. After dehydration the specimens were embedded in paraffin and sections of the cerebrum at the level of the frontal lobe, of the thalamus, of the occipital lobe and of the cerebellum were stained with periodic acid Schiff reagent, Astra blue, Ruthenium red and Kongo red. Some sections were incubated with amylase prior to staining.

RESULTS

The results concerning the pathogenesis of brain edema following X-irradiation are summarized in Figure 1. The lowest radiation dose at which an increase of pinocytosis in capillary endothelium was observed was 100 R and one hour following exposure. At this time an enlargement of the pericapillary feet of astrocytes was not seen. Subsequently only the pinocytosis of the endothelium increases and the endoplasmic reticulum of the pericytes enlarges. After 500 R the brains showed a still further increase of pinocytosis and the enlargement of the endoplasmic reticulum of the pericytes is seen after one hour following exposure. Nine days later we see a swelling of the pericapillary astrocytes. However, before this swelling the endoplasmic reticulum of these cells is enlarged. Similarly, swelling of the astrocytic processes is visible at one hour following the exposure to 1000 R. Following a higher dose, such as 2000 R or 3000 R, this swelling of astrocytes may be seen also at one hour, but hemorrhages are evident at the same time. Perhaps an important factor causing the hemorrhage is a swelling of the nuclei of the capillary endothelium because the capillaries may become blocked. We have seen such swelling of the endothelium nuclei a short time following 3000 R or at six months following 500 R. The lumen of these capillaries is nearly blocked. The endothelium and the pericytes are not damaged. Other authors have commented upon the durability of the capillary walls following irradiation (Maxwell & Kruger, 1965). In general we find the vessels intact, but not the adjacent elements of swollen endothelial nuclei. Before a disruption of capillaries is visible the cell membrane of the pericapillary astrocytes rupture and an enlarged extracellular

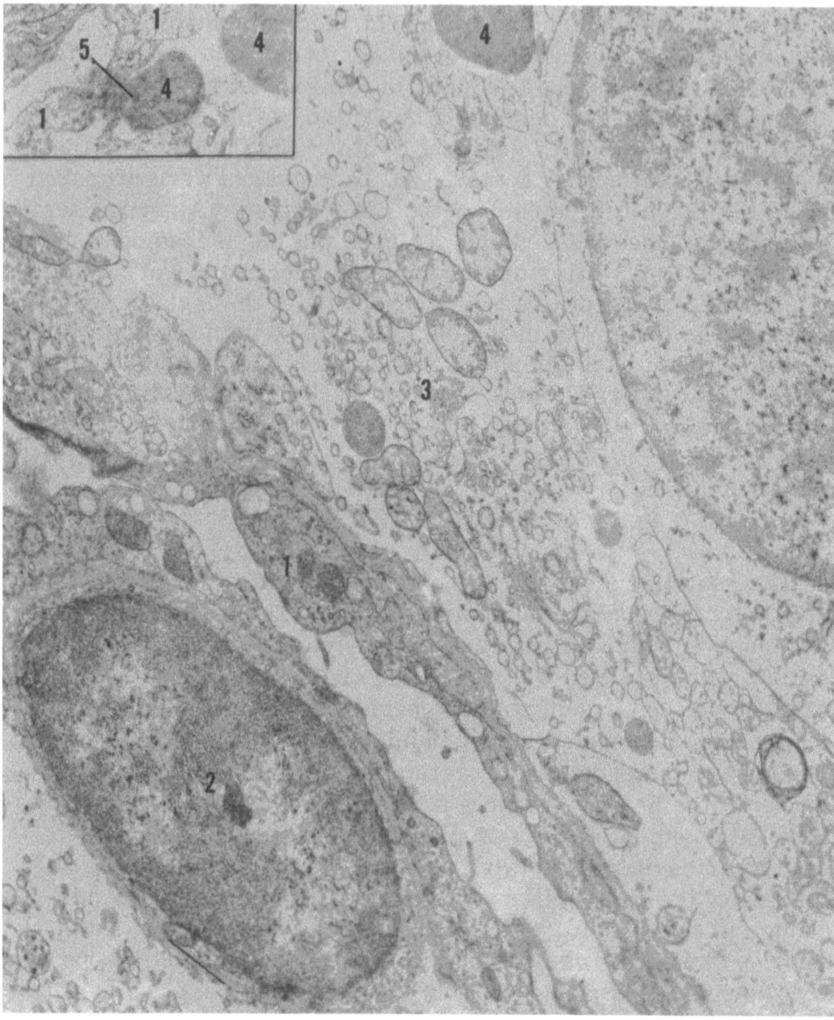

Fig. 2. Disintegration of the pericapillary astrocytes in the white matter of the guinea pig's cerebellum 24 hours after exposure to 3000 R: 1) Capillary endothelium with pinocytotic vesicles; 2) Pericyte which is surrounded by the basement membrane; 3) The astrocytic cell membrane is damaged and the enlarged extracellular space is filled with microsomes, mitochondria and a red cell (4); 5) The hemorrhage and the penetration of the red cell. X18,000 (reduced).

space develops which is filled with Golgi profiles, vesicles of endoplasmic reticulum and swollen mitochondria (Fig. 2). If the capillary is ruptured, the junctions between and adjacent endothelial cells disappear and the red cells lie between the endothelium. The endothelium itself is not damaged. Following the same dose of 500 to 3000 R, we find histochemical alterations in glial as well as neuronal elements. The intensity and distribution of PAS positive material is dependent on the dose and on the time following the irradiation. In comparison with the findings in the rat brain (Klatzo, et al.; Miquel, et al.; Brownson, et al.), the brain of guinea pigs appears more sensitive to X-irradiation. The PAS positive material in our preparations is not completely negative after the incubation with amylase prior to staining. For that reason, the Astra blue fluid has been used for identification of mucopolysaccharides. Such accumulations, i.e., glycogen, acid groups of mucopolysaccharides and glycoproteides, were observed in both the neurons and the glial elements. 500 R. The granules were conspicuous in the cerebral cortex and in the frontal lobe (Fig. 3). Twenty-four hours after exposure to 1000 R, the granules were seen in the whole cortex of the cerebrum and the hippocampus, but not in the white matter. Both the gray and white matter of the cerebrum and cerebellum contained accumulations following exposure to 3000 R (Fig. 4). Six months after 3000 R glycogen and mucopolysaccharides were demonstrated in the frontal lobe only. Glycogen granules and mucopolysaccharides were absent in all centrally located structures, i.e., thalamus and corpus striatum.

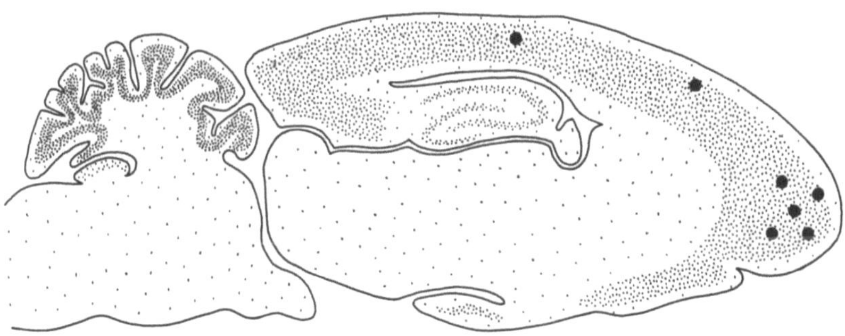

Fig. 3. The distribution of glycogen and mucopolysaccharides (O) in the guinea pig's brain 24 hours after 500 R or six months after 3000 R.

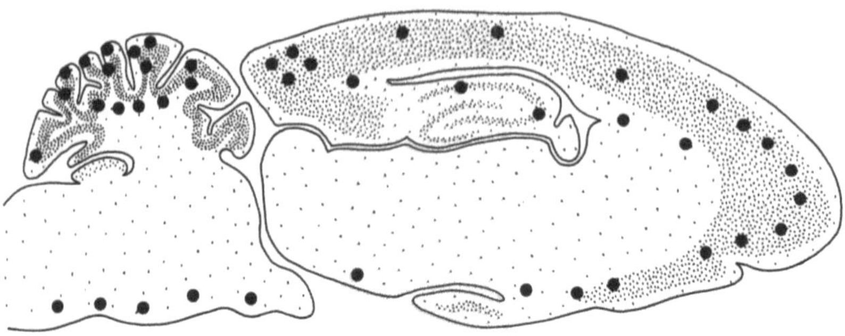

Fig. 4. The distribution of glycogen and mucopolysaccharides (O) in the guinea pig's brain 24 hours after 3000 R.

REFERENCES

Brownson, R. H., D. B. Suter, J. L. Oliver and D. A. Diller: Acute brain damage induced by x-irradiation with special reference to rate and recovery rates, Neurology (Minneapolis), 13, 1011-1020 (1963).

Franke, H. and W. Lierse: Elekronenmikroskopische Untersuchungen über Hirnveränderungen des Meerschweinchens nach Röntgenbestrahlung, Fortschr. Röntgenstr., 102, 78-87 (1965).

Klatzo, I., J. Miquel, W. Haymaker, C. Tobias and L. S. Wolfe: Observations on appearance of histochemically-demonstrable glycogen in the rat brain as effect of alpha-particle irradiation, Proc. Sympos. Effects Ioniz. Rad. on the Nerv. Syst., Vienna: Internat. Atomic Energy Agency, 285-296 (1962).

_____, _____, C. Tobias and W. Haymaker: Effects of alpha particle radiation on the rat brain, including vascular permeability and glycogen studies, J. Neuropath. exper. Neurol., 20, 459-483 (1961).

Maxwell, D. S. and L. Kruger: The fine structure of astrocytes in the cerebral cortex and their response to focal injury produced by heavy ionizing radiation, J. cell Biol., 25, (May), 141-157 (1965).

Miquel, J., I. Klatzo, D. B. Menzel and W. Haymaker: Glycogen changes in x-irradiated rat brain, Acta neuropath., 2, 482-490 (1963).

Wolfe, L. S., I. Klatzo, J. Miquel, C. Tobias and W. Haymaker: Effect of alpha-particle irradiation on brain glycogen in the rat, J. Neurochem., 9, 213-218 (1962).

C. L. CAZZULLO
P. L. GIORDANO
G. INVERNIZZI

HISTOLOGICAL AND HISTOCHEMICAL ASPECTS OF THE EARLY EFFECTS OF ROENTGEN IRRADIATION ON THE NERVOUS SYSTEM OF RABBITS

In our clinic we have been studying for some time various aspects of experimental brain edema produced by different methods (acute phlogosis, water intoxication, etc.). In this area of investigation we included also observations on early effects of roentgen irradiation in the nervous system.

According to the literature, the early lesions are observed following at least a 1000 R dose; the changes appear in the first few hours after radiation as damage in the gliovascular system with formation of a diffuse perivascular and microglial edema, whereas the swelling of neuronal elements is variable (Greco, et al.; Gerstner, et al.; Scholz, et al.; Halier, et al.; Giordano & Invernizzi).

The contribution of histochemical observations with regard to effects of roentgen radiation on the nervous system has been rather limited. Many investigations were specially concerned with variations of both RNA and DNA following irradiation. A remarkable reduction in nucleic acids was described, particularly in granular and Purkinje cell layers of the cerebellum (Tognacca, et al.; Rabassini, et al.; Brownson; Pisani, et al.; Schummelfeder).

It has been pointed out by several investigators that histological and histochemical changes due to a dose of approximately 1000 R are fully reversible (Davidoff, et al.; Brown, et al.; Lebedinskij, et al.). This applies also to associated type of cerebral edema.

The purpose of our studies was to elucidate the morphological changes in the central nervous system following the roentgen irradiation, as well as to analyze the composition of extracellular edema by histological and histochemical methods.

MATERIALS AND METHODS

Our experiments were carried out on 30 male adult rabbits of 3000 g. average weight divided into three groups of ten animals in each. Every group received 1000 R to an area of 4 cm^2 on the vertex. The radiation was performed at 40 cm distance, using a 0.5 mm. primary copper filter and a 3 mm. secondary aluminum filter (the same filtration as for deep therapy). The hardness of radiation corresponded to 180 kv tension and 10 mA intensity. The rabbits were sacrificed by exsanguination from carotid arteries at two and six hours after irradiation. The animals belonging to the third group were killed five months later. After formalin fixation the brains were embedded in paraffin and the histological and histochemical procedures applied were as follows: (A) hematoxylineosin, Nissl, gallocyanine, Spielmeyer; (B) Periodic Acid Schiff (PAS) according to McManus; Alcian Blue, according to Lison. (A) and (B) methods were also applied following 30, 60 and 120 min. digestion by hyaluronidase and sialidase.

RESULTS

From a histological point of view, our observations can be summarized as follows: (1) most affected was the vascular system revealing enlargement of Virchow-Robin spaces and a remarkable edema spreading into the surrounding parenchyma (Fig. 1); (2) there were three different types of edema localization: (a) perivascular, limited strictly to Virchow-Robin spaces, (b) perivascular but with infiltration of the surrounding parenchyma, and (c) perivascular as in (a) but showing in addition discrete edema foci near the vessels; (3) the myelin sheaths, even those in immediate proximity of the affected blood vessels, were not particularly affected; (4) the oligodendroglia showed a remarkable swelling.

The histochemical observations on composition of perivascular and interstitial edema revealed the following.

By application of McManus reaction we demonstrated neutral polysaccharides, glycoproteins, mucoproteins and lipoproteins. Lison reaction revealed acid mucopolysaccharides. PAS proved to be slightly positive in the perivascular space only. These observations were in accordance with those on phlogistic cerebral edema

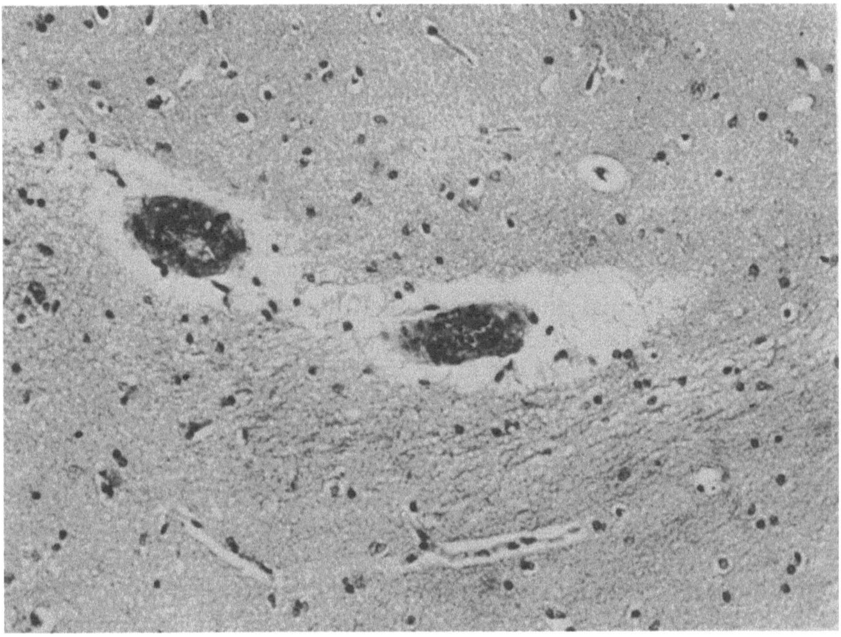

Fig. 1. Ammon cortex, hematoxylin-eosin stain; X450; perivascular edema infiltrating the surrounding parenchyma.

(Cazzulo; Cazzulo & Ravasini). Conversely, Alcian Blue staining was consistently positive both in the perivascular space and diffusely in the surrounding parenchyma (Fig. 2).

This method demonstrates different acid mucopolysaccharide fractions and particularly: (a) hyaluronic acid, (b) sialic acids, (c) A, B, and C chondroitin sulphates, and (d) heparin and heparin-like compounds. Although these substances are usually present in the normal nervous tissue, our experiments revealed the acid mucopolysaccharides to constitute a most relevant component in areas of perivascular and interstitial edema. For further histochemical differentiation of these substances, we applied testicular hyaluronidase and sialidase digestions. The former digests primarily hyaluronic acid and A and C chondroitin sulphates, whereas B chondroitin sulphate, sialic acids and heparin-like compounds remain unaffected.

In our experiments testicular hyaluronidase digestion did not affect at all Alcian Blue positive foci of edema. Similar results were obtained with sialidase digestion which acts specifically on sialic acids. These results indicate that the Alcian Blue positive staining in areas of edema depends primarily on the presence of B chondroitin sulphate and heparin-like substances. Currently we are trying to elucidate further the nature of these substances.

Our histological and histochemical observations revealed no essential differences with regard to animals sacrificed two to six hours as well as five months after irradiation. This is in agreement with other investigators applying small doses of X-rays (Davidoff, et al.; Brown, et al.).

To complete our studies we carried out experiments on animals affected by cerebral phlogosis. Our previous observations on this condition stressed the perivascular edema, localized primarily in the white matter around small veins and even arteries, as the main pathogenic feature. Initially transudative features prevail; later the edema is characterized by serous exudation. In the early stages of edema, transudates are difficult to demonstrate histologically due to the small content of proteins. Hematoxylin-eosin stain reveals merely a conspicuous widening of pericellular and Virchow-Robin spaces. In the stage of serous exudation, the blood vessels reveal irregular outlines due to compression by the edema. The lumina are engorged with blood due to stasis; the surrounding parenchyma shows serous imbibition. Contents of Virchow-Robin spaces stain in acidophilic fashion and reveal a slight PAS-positive reaction (Cazzullo; Giordano & Invernizzi). These observations were also confirmed by studies carried out on animals in deep hypothermia where the development of the disease could be followed en ralenti (Cazzullo & Ravasini; Giordano, Invernizzi & Ravasini).

The application of histochemical procedures to brains of rabbits sacrificed 10 days after induction of experimental phlogosis showed the following. In this phase of the process, the histological observations revealed the presence of copious perivascular cuffings and edema infiltrating the surrounding tissue. The histochemical reactions in these areas revealed slight PAS-positive and strong Alcian Blue-positive staining, which remained unchanged following testicular hyaluronidase and sialidase digestions, i.e., indicating the presence of B chondroitin sulphate or heparin-like substances.

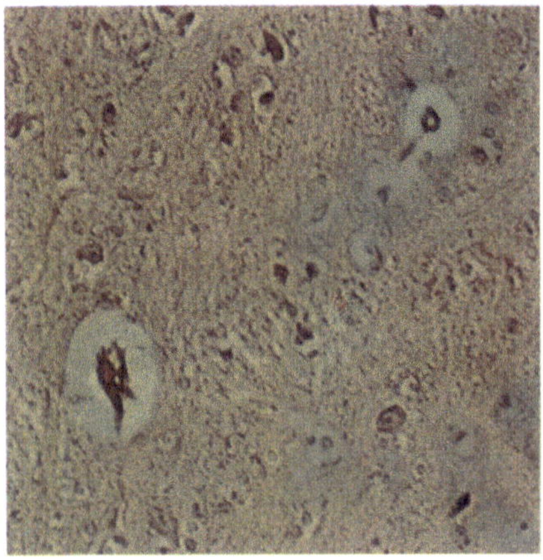

Fig. 2. Brain stem, Alcian Blue stain; X180; the Lison's method shows strongly positive staining of the perivascular edema.

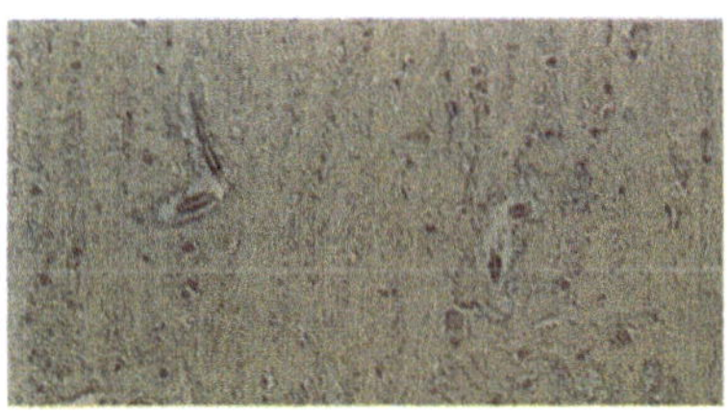

Fig. 3. Brain stem, Alcian Blue stain; X180; perivascular and interstitial edema infiltrating the surrounding parenchyma are strongly Alcian Blue-positive.

REFERENCES

Aleksandrovskaya, M.: The effect of different doses of ionizing radiation on the morphology of the brain and internal organs of animals under physiological and pathological conditions, Radiobiology – Transact. All. Union Conf. Use Isotopes Nucl. Radiat. in Russian Science and Economy, Izd. Akad. Nauck SSSR, Moscow, 168 (1958).

_____: Some data on the effects of ionizing radiation on the central nervous system of animals, Transact. Inst. Higher Nerv. Act. Pathophysiol. Series, Ibid, Moscow, 211 (1958).

Brown, D. G., D. P. Sasmore and L. P. Jones: In: Response of the Nervous System to Ionizing Radiation, (ed. by R. S. Snider), Internat. Symp. Chicago, 1960, New York: Academic Press (1961).

Brownson, R. H.: Changes induced in the rat central nervous system following cumulative exposure to X-irradiation, J. Neuropath. Exp. Neurol., 20, 206 (1961).

Cazzullo, C. L.: Le encefalomieliti demielinizzanti. Clinica, anatomia patologica, eziopatogenesi, Relaz. XII Cong. Naz. Neurol., Abano 4-7 (April 1956).

_____: Allergia e sistema nervoso, in: Melli G. Allergia, malattie allergiche e allergosimili (ed. by Vallardi), Milano vol. II, 1743,

_____: Antigens of experimental allergic encephalomyelitis, Sist. Nerv., 15, 353 (1963).

_____ and A. Ferraro: Studi sulla encefalomielite sperimentale allergica acuta e cronica nella scimmia, Atti X Cong. Ital. Neurol., 130 (1949).

_____ and _____: Ricerche ed osservazioni semeiologiche sulla encefalomielite sperimentale allergica acuta e cronica nella scimmia, Riv. Pat. Nerv. Ment., 71, 533 (1950).

_____ and C. Ravasini: Histochemical studies on unspecific phlogosis of nervous system, IV Intern. Cong. of Neuropath. 4-8 München, vol. I, 187 (September 1961).

Davidoff, L. M., C. G. Dyke, C. A. Elsberg and I. M. Tarlov: Effect of radiation applied directly to brain and spinal cord. I. – Experimental investigations on Macacus Rhesus monkeys. Radiol., 31, 451 (1938).

Gerstner, H. S. and S. P. Kent: Early effects of head X-irradiation in rabbits, Radiat. Res., 6, 626 (1957).

Giordano, P. L. and G. Invernizzi: L' edema cerebrale infiammatorio sperimentale. Studio elettroencefalografico, semeiologice e morfologico nel gatto, Biol. Lat., 17, 773 (1964).

_____ and _____: Studio sperimentale sull'effetto di piccole dosi di radiazioni roentgen sul sistema nervoso centrale, e tentativi di protezione con farmaci antireazionali, XV Cong. Ital. Neurol. Salice Terme (Pavia) 26-28 (April 1965).

_____, _____ and C. Ravasini: Studi sulla prevenzione dell'edema cerebrale da flogosi sperimentale: azione dell'ipotermia profonda, Ibid.

Greco, S., A. Pasqualino and G. Pisani: La radiosensibilità del neurone, VI Cong. Naz. Radiol. Med. Atti, vol. I, 1 (1962).

Hager, H., W. Hischberger and A. Breit: In: Response of the Nervou System to Ionizing Radiation, (ed. by R. S. Snider), Internat. Symp. Chicago, 1960, New York: Academic Press (1961).

Haymaker, W. W., J. H. Nauta, J. C. Sloper, G. Laquer, F. Vogel and J. E. Pickering: The effect of barium-140, lanthanum-140 (gamma) radiation on the central nervous system and pituitary gland of macaques, J. Neuropath. Exper. Neurol., 17, 12 (1958).

Lebedinskiy, A. V. and Z. N. Nakhinitskaya: Effects of ionizing radiation on the central nervous system, Amsterdam: Elsevier (1963).

Hotchkiss, R. D.: A microglial reaction resulting in the staining of polysaccharides structures in fixed tissue preparations, Arch. Biochem., 16, 131 (1948).

Lison, L.: Alcian Blue 8 G with Chlorantine fast red 5 B. A technic for selective staining of mucopolysaccharides, Stain Technol., 29, 131 (1954).

McManus, J. F. A.: Histological and histochemical uses of periodic acid, Ibid., 23, 99 (1948).

Pisani, G. and P. Fumagalli: Pathologica Diencephalica, Symposium Internat. (Milano) 606 (1956).

Rabassini, A., C. S. Rossi and C. Gregolin: Variazioni del contenuto di ATP, ADP e AMP nel cervello di ratti sottoposti ad irradiazio con raggi W X, Giorn. Biochim., 9, 217 (1960).

Scholtz, W.: Histologische und topische Veränderungen und Vulnerabilitätsverhältnisse in menschlichen Gehirn bei Sauerstoffmangel Odem und plasmatischen Infiltrattionen, Z. ges. Neurol. Psychiat

_____ and Y. K. Hsu: Late damage from roentgen irradiation of the human brain, Arch. Neurol. Psychiat., 40, 926 (1938).

Schummelfeder, N.: In: Response of the Nervous System to Ionizing Radiation, (ed. by R. S. Snider), Internat. Symp., Chicago (1960), New York: Academic Press (1961).

Tognacca, M. L. and G. Savino: Studio istofotometrico delle prime alterazioni del DNA dopo irradiazione, nelle cellule gangliari del ganglio di Gasser di ratti irradiati, con 50-60 r., Boll. Soc. Ital. Biol. Sperim., 42, 125 (1962).

DISCUSSION

ZIMMERMAN: May I ask Dr. Clasen a question purely for clarification? When you talk about experimental edema fluid, are you referring to all types of experimentally produced edema or only to the cold injury type? I ask this because there is some morphological evidence and some other evidence as well, indicating that the fluid is in different locations and possibly of a different composition. Therefore, the question is are you, in your experiments, dealing purely with the cold injury or have you also worked with triethyl edema?

CLASEN: We have only worked with cold injury; however, you have reported on edema fluid which showed increased periodic acid-Schiff (PAS) staining following the implantation of certain substance into the cortex of rats (Amer. J. Path. 42: 97-110). I would think that these findings are comparable to that. They are not comparable to systemic triethyl tin edema because in this situation the edematous tissue is not PAS positive. In many human conditions, the edematous tissue is also PAS positive. This includes the cerebral edema associated with some tumors, hemorrhages (traumatic or spontaneous), abscesses, and lead encephalopathy. In other words, I would say that what I have shown has some relevance to those edematous conditions in which the tissue shows increased PAS staining.

ZEMAN: I would like to ask Dr. Bakay what the rationale was to use C_{14} glycine as a tracer in edema studies. This amino acid is probably one of the amino acids most easily equilibrated between various fluid compartments, as we have found in unrelated studies.

BAKAY: I can answer that easily. There was no particular rationale to use this tracer except that we were gearing ourselves for electron microscopic radioautography at this time, and as a preliminary step we took some regular histological autographs. It is true that glycine equilibrated rapidly; it is the simplest aminoacid, and it is, to a greater extent, an indicator of metabolic activities than it is of membrane permeability. However, we found that there was a very significant difference in various conditions, due to permeability or metabolic factors, because in traumatic edema we found a much more complete equilibration in a much shorter time than we did in triethyl tin edema, which did not differ from the normal. In traumatic edema the concentration of glycine was identical to that of the choroid plexus under normal circumstances, indicating a break-down in the barrier as far as this tracer is concerned. So we utilized this with some reservation as far as its exact rationale is concerned. I could not show you radioactive albumin radioautographs, and that is the reason we actually settled on radioactive aminoacid. You cannot demonstrate the depostion of radioactive albumin in triethyl tin edema because it never gets into the edema fluid.

BRENNER: Some questions to Dr. Bakay, Dr. Clasen and Dr. Klatzo. What do you think about opening of the dura during the cold application? We came back to the closed method because incarcerations of cortical veins and venous infarctions could not be inhibited in the open method and changed our artificial lesions.

We think that neurosurgical problems of brain edema, its prevention and treatment, can be examined by investigations of this cold injury edema as a basic method. The main advantage is its constant reproductibility, so it looks like the prototype of artificial edema. Our own experiments were carried out on more than 130 cats and rabbits. Under general anesthesia an unilateral trepanation was performed and a cold was applied at the temporal region for 30 seconds by the method of Klatzo. A heating unit inside the cold metal block could stop the cooling rapidly so that the freezing time was always constant. 5 minutes afterwards, 50 μC of a Radioiodinated Serum Albumin Solution were administered intravenously. The animals were sacrificed 24 hours later by an aortic perfusion of the upper half of the body. After 5 minutes, the blood has been washed out completely. The brain was taken out and also the sharp marked necrotic area excided. The amount of I 131 was estimated in the normal and edematous hemisphere as in the blood. The increase of albumin in the involved brain was nearly 600 - 700%.

On this basic method we tried to get experimental answers about the antiedematous effect of some drugs: concentrated albumin, Diamox, vitamins, calcium, etc. These experiments showed some interesting details.

If we want to establish a basic method of experimental edema simulating those conditions occurring in human pathology, we must expect that the disturbances in blood–brain barrier and turnover of albumin take place shortly after injury and, therefore, the tracer or radioactive material must be applied also shortly after the experimental injury and not prior to sacrifice.

A last question to Dr. Klatzo: You demonstrated a slide showing the increase of edematous area after raising and a decrease after lowering systolic blood pressure. Did you expect those results in contrast to general clinical experience, and can you explain them?

BAKAY: We can dispose of the first three questions since we did not open the dura, and consequently there was no direct damage to the brain; there was no herniation of the brain, no venous thrombosis. The method was essentially that of Klatzo, but it was simplified. We made a hole in the bone, did not touch the dura and covered it with a layer of Saran plastic wrap, and applied a CO_2 cylinder, 9mm in diameter, directly to the plastic wrap. At the end of 3 minutes, which we chose for no particular reason, but I don't think it makes too much difference, you get more of an edema than you do after a shorter time. After we removed the CO_2 cylinder (it was easily removed since it did not adhere to anything), we waited for a few seconds and then the Saran wrap could be easily removed. Now we applied vital dyes, but I cannot elaborate on this since time is so short. Trypan blue showed the same spatial and temporal distribution as the radioactive iodinated serum albumin, from which we concluded (which has been mentioned already many times) that practically all, or at least most vital dyes in the brain are protein bound, and it hardly makes much difference whether one studies the protein or the trypan blue. Only very little of this dye remains diffusible. The essence of these experiments which I did not have too much time to point out, was that this is a very protein-rich serum exudate and derives directly by rupture from the capillaries or from the venules at the site of the cortical freezing lesion and then seeps fairly slowly into the underlying edematous white matter, which, in itself, as Dr. Klatzo and others pointed out, is not particularly permeable for proteins, so that here is a locus minoris resistentiae from which the whole edema fluid derives and seeps into the white matter.

PAPPIUS: Since my own efforts to produce edema by hypoxia and hypercapnia have been singularly unsuccessful, I would like to ask Dr. Bakay what criteria he used to establish that edema was present in his experiments on hypercapnia and hypoxia.

BAKAY: These were last-minute slides and they looked that way. Actually this only indicates one point which I think is pertinent, and the same holds true for P^{32}, but I thought that perhaps sodium would be the most appropriate label here to show that if we do animal experiments under various circumstances where we separate four major components involved in asphyxia, namely, hypoxia itself, hypercapnia, which always associates with asphyxia under clinical conditions, increased venous pressure, and the effect of CO_2 alone, then we end up with these kinds of figures. If the oxygen saturation is lowered very considerably and if the CO_2 retention is high with a low pH, then, and only under such circumstances, do we get a truly significant increase in cerebrospinal fluid pressure. The increase of cerebrospinal fluid pressure, however, and I would like to emphasize that very much, is definitely not a direct indication of an increase in brain volume, because it can also be caused by other factors. I think it is a mistake to assume that intraspinal fluid pressure equals an equal increase in brain volume, because in this case much of this increased pressure is due to an increased volume of cerebrospinal fluid. But the fact remains that under such circumstances increased pressure could be correlated to an increase in brain volume which was noticeable on inspection and also an increase in the water content which I cannot show you in tabular form; this amounted only to about 2% as far as the percentage of fluid in the unit of wet brain is concerned, but when calculated to dry brain it came up to about 10%. This is not a great deal of edema, because most other edemas, when calculated to dry weight, indicate an increase of 25, 35, 50%, so this 10% is a modest but still significant degree of edema. We also found in these hypercapnic hypoxic brains a moderate but definite enlargment of both glial cells and intercellular clefts under the electron microscope. I cannot comment on this any better yet, since as yet we do not have any data.

ZÜLCH: Dr. Bakay, is there any detailed morphological evidence for your concept, if I rightly understood your words a few minutes ago, of the edema being formed in the cortex and seeping from there 2 or 3 cm wide into the white matter? That would be, according to what we have seen in our experiments, a very difficult idea to assume. Is there morphological evidence available, or is it only evidence from the tracer findings?

BAKAY: I based this opinion on radioactive isotopic studies on brain edema, and this concept derives basically not only from radioactive isotopic but also from straight chemical analysis. Now, e.g., this seepage which autographically seems to originate at the lesion and with the passage of time goes deeper and deeper into the white matter, also correlated to a chemical concentration gradient. Again, if you take simple things, which are perhaps less misleading than others, such as sodium, there is a very interesting relationship in the chemical sodium content, completely irrespective of the radioactive sodium determinations. In the lesion itself, which is essentially a hemorrhagic necrosis, which is mainly clotted blood with very little of the original brain tissue remaining, we got sodium values that were almost up to the sodium values of plasma. And indeed, what we see there is mainly plasma. Now, when we get to the edema itself, which is nearest to the white matter, we have very high sodium values, twice normal almost, 85 or 90 m Eq per liter, and if one goes deeper, this gets lower, and at the margin of the edema, which is perhaps already outside the edema, we go down to the normal 45 or 50 m Eq liter values, so there is a concentration gradient. Morphological data will be given by Dr. Lee in a subsequent paper which will involve this very same experiment.

SIESJÖ: Did I understand you right that an increase in CSF pressure means an increase in CSF volume?

BAKAY: No. An increase in CSF pressure can mean such a variety of things that it is hard to go into it. Increased CSF pressure can mean increased brain volume, increase of cerebrospinal fluid volume, most usually the combination of both, and it can reflect, as it does in tetralogy of Fallot, just venous engorgement. The same thing happens if you give 20% CO_2 inhalation to the animal. You might get a somewhat increased pressure which, in this case, is due to an increase in the vascular bed of the intracranial cavity; so in any given case it is extremely difficult to differentiate these factors from each other.

SIESJÖ: I thought you said that in your hypercapnic-hypoxic cats the increase in CSF pressure was due to an increase in CSF volume.

BAKAY: No. I believe that part of the increase in hypercapnic hypoxia was due to an increase in brain volume, but that, in itself, would not have explained its high rise. I think that in addition to increased brain volume there is also an increased production of cerebrospinal fluid. The same thing happened in a moiety of edema, which I don't want to go into at all, but which we carried out; namely, edema due to water intoxication. If you studied the CSF pressure under water intoxication, you get very high cisternal pressures and this is certainly to a great extent due to cerebrospinal fluid production, which is increased when the blood is hypotonic. It is very hard in these cases to distinguish which compartment of the three in the intracranial cavity is mainly responsible for the increased pressure.

SIESJÖ: But you would propose that there might be a mechanism producing more CSF?

BAKAY: Yes, I think so.

BRIGHTMAN: Dr. Bakay, I cannot share your disappointment that Ferritin was confined to membrane-bounded structures in your swollen glial processes. The pinocytotic uptake of Ferritin is one thing, the passage of water and electrolytes through a membrane by direct diffusion, quite another. I would be concerned, however, about finding freely dispersed Ferritin in a swollen process. Such a deposition is probably artifactual.

BAKAY: Again I want to refer to Dr. Lee's paper who will present our data at a somewhat later time from the electron microscopic point of view. I did not want to give the impression that these experiments with Ferritin are either conclusive or terribly significant in one view or another. The point I want to make is that in light microscopic radioautography, even if you use a magnification of 2000 or so, which is about the limit, you still cannot definitely say whether the I^{131} albumin granules, and we assumed that they are undissociated, are intracellular or extracellular, because with light microscopic resolution you cannot make this distinction. We are working on radioautography on the electron microscopic level, and maybe this will be the answer. In the meantime, Ferritin is a useful tool, and since we found such a variety of the deposition of Ferritin, this is a warning for us not to assume that the radioactive albumin is all intracellular because of active pinocytosis, or all extracellular because there could be a variety of factors involved.

EVANS: Professor Zülch has already expressed some concern over the experimental model that has been used. I would not for a moment decry the means that are employed in various experimental techniques in the effort to understand more fully the nature of edema. However, I do believe that it is important, for those of us who must think in clinical terms, to employ models which simulate more closely the clinical problems with which we are dealing. Again, this is not an objection to the approach used by Dr. Klatzo. On the other hand, I would submit that the method which Dr. Ishii has been using, and on which I had hoped he would speak today, is a closer approximation of the clinical conditions with which we deal. I know that Dr. Bakay has used this method also, and he may have something further to say to this.

BAKAY: I very much agree with what you said. All these experimental edemas are, of course, except perhaps for the toxic ones, not quite the prototype of human edema, and this has to be understood from the beginning. At the same time, a great number of the experimental tools that we are now applying, radioactive isotopes or even electron microscopy, requires a quick death with immediate recovery of the brain, preferably after immediate perfusion at the preagonal stage. These are things that relegate us to animal work. When one tries to apply the results to humans, then the strangest things occur. For instance, it is well known that in peritumoral edema there is an increased uptake of almost any isotope that you might apply. This, incidentally, injects another interesting point: Is brain scanning, which we clinically use for tumor detection, truly indicative of the size of the tumor or does it occasionally misleadingly show a bigger tumor than there really is, on account of the perifocal edema which also gives a positive scan. Dr. Planiol and I worried about that for some time. Nevertheless, in edema, whether peritumoral or other, there is usually an increased isotope uptake. However, when one examines human material, as I said, the strangest things happen. This is a post-mortem human brain, about 4 days after the injection of P^{32} for diagnostic purposes. The patient died and I made a gross autograph from the brain. This is the area of the operation with some tumor remaining alone, and as you see, there is a considerable edema in this hemisphere. Now here is the P^{32} autograph, this being the normal hemisphere showing the good pattern of mostly cortical and periventricular P^{32} distribution. Here is quite a bit in the tumor and in the contused exposed parts of the brain. There is nothing in the edema, so this is exactly the opposite of what we might expect, and this is where human pathology usually differs from experimental findings.

ZÜLCH: Could I add one morphological observation? Since 1940 I have been staining a great number of brains with brain tumors with Massons trichrome and trying to find by the different stainability a change which consisted of an increase in volume in the white matter and a loss of stainability of the myelin sheaths. I was particularly interested in the stainability with Masson's blue. There is a definite difference between peritumoral edema and other edemas of the white matter because peritumoral edema is not stainable with Masson's at all. We found only one exception to this rule. If there was a very recent necrosis or fresh hemorrhage into the tumor, as it occurs often in glioblastomas, the edema was heavily stained with Masson's blue, which means to me an edema which is probably very rich in proteins. There are quite different forms of peritumoral edema, according to Masson' stain; it may be serous, it may be plasmatic, i.e., high in proteins. The very nature can only be classified biochemically or by tracer studies.

BAKAY: As a matter of fact, there is some chemical proof to that. Kyota wrote a paper a few years ago in the Journal of Neurochemistry, in which he separated mostly peritumoral edemas in 2 groups: a simple group and a complicated one. The point was that in the simple group there was fluid but not very much in the way of increased protein concentration. In the so-called complicated groups there was an increase of a number of protein compounds, both albumin and some globulin. Obviously there is quite a variety of peritumoral edemas as far as their proteinaceous or non-proteinaceous nature is concerned.

ZIMMERMAN: I was getting concerned about a combination of Professor Zülch and the neurosurgeons in this discussion, but now that Dr. Tower wants to join us we shall continue.

TOWER: As a first approximation, this problem might be clarified, if we recall what we have seen in these last couple of days. If there is necrosis and hemorrhage, as Professor Zülch has pointed out, then we are probably dealing with disturbances of vascular permeability to a rather gross degree. This situation would correspond to the observations which Dr. Klatzo and Dr. Bakay have been showing us this morning. On the other hand, in the absence of such changes, there may still be impairment of circulation to tissue surrounding a tumor, and certainly in cerebral cortex, as Rall, et al. (Life Sci. 1 (2): 43, 1962, Van Harreveld, et al. (J. Cell Biol. 25: 117, 1965), and we have found, associated with intracellular swelling in cells, the identity of which we need not specify at this time. These distinctions may help to resolve the problems developing in this discussion.

TERRY: With regard to the problem that Dr. Bakay brought up related to the scanning of brain tumors, we have used an experimental model involving the Brown-Pearce carcinoma implanted into the rabbit brain. In association with Drs. Scheinberg, Herzog, Schecter and Zingesser, we have studied the location of tritium-labelled mercuhydrin in these animals by scintillation counting, light and electron microscopic radioautography. We did not use the isotopic mercury because it has too long a path-length for high resolution. In the hemorrhagic center of these tumors there is obviously extracellular label at a very early stage. This material diffuses outward, or at least there is a concentration gradient outwards beyond histologically definable neoplasm into the adjacent white matter. I cannot yet say as to whether this is intracellular or intercellular.

LOWENTHAL: I would add something to the discussion of necrosis. I think that in human brains far away from the tumoral lesion, in edematous tissue, we can find abnormal proteins and in increase in water content and sodium content, e.g., in periventricular white matter there is at a distance from the lesion a distinct, important increase in water content and sodium content in edematous brains. Therefore, two questions to Dr. Clasen: If I understood you correctly, you are working on an edematous kind of liquid at the level of the lesion but not on extracts of brain proteins. This will explain, I think, some differences between your results and ours, but I would also like to know if you obtain that liquid at levels other than at the level of the lesion.

Can you characterize a protein fraction only by its mobility rate on cellulose acetate or on agar? I think that at the same level different protein fractions could move, and as you have no pure fractions, it could be difficult to give an exact definition of these fractions. Also with immunoelectrophoresis you do not work on isolated material.

CLASEN: The answer to the first question is that the necrotic lesion and the immediately surrounding area was avoided in the collection of edematous white matter, and therefore this fluid comes from tissue which shows no morphologic evidence of necrosis by light or electron microscopy at this time interval. In answer to the second question, the supposition I made was based upon the correlation of three findings, the third one of which was the reaction with antibodies directed against serum proteins.

Dr. Brenner raised a few points which he also directed to me. The answer to his first question is our lesions were produced through the intact skull and therefore the dura was never opened. In this technique, absolutely perfect contact between the instrument and the skull is necessary. Under these conditions, it takes from 5-10 minutes in the dog and from 3-5 in the monkey to produce a rather massive lesion. With respect to the Evans blue data, in order to measure this in tissue, the dye must first be removed. This is done by homogenating the tissue with the detergent "teepol" and then extracting the dye on a cellulose column. The dye is eluted by alkaline acetone solution. This technique was originally described by Campbell, et al., for serum (J. Lab. Clin Med., 52: 768-777, 1958). We adapted it to tissue and a 95% recovery (both as a dye solution and as a dye-serum protein complex) was obtained from homogenized brain. It is, however, necessary to extract the dye shortly after the tissue is removed. If this is delayed for a period of several weeks, the extraction of the dye becomes extremely difficult. The relationships between experimental and human disease is almost a philosophic question. I should like to point out that most of us who work in experimental pathology also study human material and apply to it the insights gained from experimental animals. When one does this, it is clear that the reaction to injury which occurs around freezing lesions is very similar to that seen in many human conditions, especially around hemorrhages or some tumors and certainly around abscesses. I should also like to point out to Dr. Evans that the last slide I showed was of human material.

EVANS: I would like to ask Dr. Clasen if he does not agree, as I am reasonably sure he does, that differences in age, in species, and in experimental approach play a significant role in the experimental results. I think we understand one another clearly on these points, do we not?

ZIMMERMAN: Any further questions? If not, I would like to go back to the paper by Drs. Kolkmann and Ule on tin poisoning. Are there any questions?

SEITELBERGER: From my experience I would like to contradict the suggestions of Dr. Kolkmann about the basis of different types of spongy state in white matter. As I tried to outline in my paper, the spongy state of white matter in spongy necrosis of the Canavan type, as well as the spongy state of the gray matter type (van Bogaert and Bertand), is due to dystrophic astroglial changes. In these conditions I could not find primary changes of the myelin sheaths. As far as combined degeneration of the spinal cord is concerned, we find that the primary change is localized in the axons in the form of a swelling of the axons and that the myelin sheaths degenerate secondarily. This lesion produces the "Lückenherde" of combined degeneration. So far in our experience with spongy state in human neuropathology, a correlate to the experimental tin edema changes of the myelin sheaths does not exist.

TOWER: Dr. Kolkmann stated quite definitely that the swelling within myelin lamellae in alkyl tin edema is in the potential extracellular spaces between these lamellae. Is this view generally accepted by electron microscopists, or is there some argument on this point? I think it would be worth knowing whether anyone localizes the swelling within the cytoplasm of the oligoglial cell as it wraps around to form the myelin lamellae, or is it actually within this potential extracellular space between the various lamellae as they form the sheath?

ZIMMERMAN: Dr. Tower, do you want a vote of the electron microscopists present here this morning, or will one of them volunteer to supply the information? Dr. Lee?

LEE: I would like to substantiate Dr. Kolkmann's finding of the myelin split in triethyltin edema. However, there are two points which we cannot confirm. One is about the survival time of animals after tin intoxication. In our hands, the rats could survive up to 45 days or longer if we let them, after discontinuation of feeding with TET. Another point concerns the dilatation of the intercellular space shown in Dr. Kolkmann's electron micrographs. We were unable to find in our material such dilatation either in the gray or white matter. With regard to Dr. Tower's question whether the intra- or inter-period line of the myelin represents the potential extracellular space during myelinogenesis in the embryo, it is, in my opinion, still not yet settled. Up to the present time, not all the electron microscopists in the field of nervous system agree that the mechanism of myelinogenesis in the central nervous system is the same as that established in the peripheral nervous system.

ZIMMERMAN: Dr. Terry, you were one of the first people to describe the intramyelin splitting. Will you answer Dr. Tower's question?

TERRY: I think, Dr. Tower, that very few electron microscopists have much doubt that this space is analogous to the original extracellular space in the central nervous system as it would be in the periphery. As to whether it represents a potential extracellular space is perhaps another question. But at least in the periphery, Robertson showed in the experiments in which he soaked peripheral nerve in hypotonic and hypertonic solutions that he could again evoke a split there in the intraperiod line. Our original experiments, essentially duplicated by Dr. Lee, did not reveal this widened intercellular space between intact sheaths as demonstrated here by Dr. Kolkmann.

KOLKMANN: First the question of Dr. Terry. The widening of the extracellular space between intact myelin sheaths in cases of diethyl tin dichloride poisoning was not a very conspicuous finding, but we have seen it.

And our answer to Professor Seitelberger: Our special attention was directed to the lesion of the myelin sheaths, which in this form certainly is not only limited to the TET intoxication but also represents quite a distinct form of myelin damage, which can be found also in other cases of spongy degeneration of the white matter.

JELLINGER: I would like to stress Professor Seitelberger's disagreement with your statements, and I would like to ask you whether you have ever seen progressive lesions of astroglia in TET-induced edema.

KOLKMANN: No.

JELLINGER: But we all know that we can observe them in pseudospongy and spongy states of various genesis, as was demonstrated by you. Whereas the type of pseudospongy state in TET-induced edema is known to be a fully reversible lesion, this is not the case in other pseudospongy conditions known in general neuropathology, e.g., in funicular myelosis or in degenerative diseases. I would like to emphasize that we are not allowed to deduce from experimental lesions final states and end results seen in human neuropathology, e.g., in combined tract degeneration or in infantile spongy states. Though they may have some similarities, they seem to be of quite different pathogenesis, as we can infer from light microscopic findings. Though I am no electron microscopist, I would like to warn about comparative deductions from light microscopically defined stages of certain processes and experimental electron microscopical data.

KOLKMANN: The funicular myelosis and the infantile spongy degenerations are certainly not identical with the TET alterations. We never have said that. But the partial phenomenon of splitting of the myelin lamellae occurs, maybe as a transitory phenomenon. Naturally this appearance doesn't exclude glia reactions.

We are not the first to notice the histological similarity of TET alterations and spongy degeneration. I think that Dr. Cumings, together with Dr. Kalsbeck, in 1963 in the Journal of Neuropathology and Experimental Neu-

rology, Volume 23, page 245, has mentioned this histological similarity, working with triethyl tin hydroxide.

WECHSLER: May I ask Dr. Kolkmann a question? We have heard several contributions on the subject of *spongy state*. Referring back to classical neuropathology, we can find the spongy state, *e.g.*, in Pick's disease or in funicular myelosis of the spinal cord. Nowadays there is quite a lot of discussion about the spongy state. Considering brain edema and other pathological lesions in the CNS, we can also detect morphological equivalents of a spongy state. Therefore, *the spongy state is a syndrome*, and it would be a good thing to have a discussion of terminology about the spongy state, otherwise this term becomes a confusing one.

TERRY: Drs. Torack, Zimmerman and I reported on tin poisoning of neuropil of rats. Some years ago we showed quite clearly, I think, swelling of astrocytic processes. Drs. Aleu, Katzman and I studied tin poisoning in rabbits and again we showed mild but definite swelling of astrocytic processes in that material.

CUMINGS: I would like to make two comments. First of all, as far as I understood it correctly, you introduced Canavan's disease as one form of spongy degeneration comparable, if that is not too strong a word, to the effects of organic tin. I think we should keep Canavan's disease out of our discussion, in that biochemical studies have shown it to be a totally different type of disorder. From all the lipid studies I have done I am quite confident that you will find the other spongy states are not the same as those that you find in Canavan's disease. The other comment I would like to make is that it is only the triethyl tin, as in fact it is the triethyl lead, that will give rise to any pathological condition, because if you use tetraethyl lead, it is converted to triethyl lead before the pathological reactions take place.

KLATZO: To elevate the systolic blood pressure we used Levophed (Roche Laboratories), and Arfonad (Winthrop Laboratories) was employed to induce the hypotension. Both drugs were given with 5% dextrose by intravenous infusion.

EBELS: Our facilities and the number of animals we can use for our experiments are limited. One of the disturbing things in our experiments which Dr. Wechsler referred to in the discussion was the great variation between the reactions on the application of cold in different animals, even with a fairly well-standarized set-up. Now you in your paper, Dr. Klatzo, as well as Dr. Clasen in his, confidently compare the results in the different animals at different times (2, 4, 6 hours, etc., after the application). Is this a "statistical" confidence, or is the variation between the different animals in your experiments less than in ours, possibly due to technical reasons?

KLATZO: The main factors which can affect the intensity and dynamics of resulting edema due to cold lesion are: (1) the duration of cooling, (2) the temperature of the metal plate, and (3) the amount of pressure exerted on the exposed cerebral cortex by the applicator. There is no problem in being exact with regard to the cooling time. In our laboratory the temperature of the applicator (-50°C.) is checked each time by the thermocouples embedded in the metal plate. The most difficult thing to control is the pressure of the applicator which depends on the person performing the procedure. We try to minimize the variability of this factor by having a large experimental series of cats performed by the same investigator who tries to be as "uniform" as possible in touching the exposed cortex. It is rather surprising how very reproducible the lesions are under these circumstances. Of course, individual variations occasionally occur, but using a large series of animals the effect of various factors influencing the dynamics of edema can be demonstrated unequivocally.

CLASEN: I believe part of that question was directed at me. In my opinion, quantitative figures can only be compared by applying statistical techniques, and means published without standard deviations have little meaning. One weakness in any statistical analysis is that real differences between groups may not be demonstrable because of the variances of the factors measured. This is unavoidable and must simply be faced in interpreting negative results. I can only say that I believe that our own experimental design is a sound one.

BRENNER: A question to Dr. Klatzo. How do you explain the difference between your results and the clinical experience as a relation between general blood circulation pressure and staining of edematous areas by fluorescein-labelled albumin? Did you expect these results or the contrary?

KLATZO: My experience is limited to experimental data and I am hesitant to make any comparative evaluations with complex clinical conditions.

BRENNER: In the introductory speech we heard that improvement of general blood circulation is able to prevent edema, and your results showed just the contrary.

KLATZO: I assume that clinical cases of brain edema are usually associated with a variety of factors which are difficult to assess and which may be basically different from those operative in our experimental conditions. Thus, in a patient with a severe head injury, brain edema may be of anoxic origin due to shock or more local interference with the cerebral circulation and it seems likely that in such a case the elevation of blood pressure improving oxygen supply to the brain may improve edematous condition.

BRENNER: But the blood pressure of 50 is less than 40% of the original pressure of 130.

KLATZO: Again, I would like to emphasize that it is difficult to compare clinical conditions such as those complicated, e.g., by circulatory insufficiency, anoxia, thrombosis, etc., with our experimental model. We are inclined to interpret the dynamics of cold lesion edema in rather simple terms. We have demonstrated that spreading of edema depends primarily on the extravascular migration of serum contents through the white matter. We assume that the propelling force for this migration is related to the hydrostatic pressure of the blood and our experiments on the effect of the systolic blood pressure support this assumption. To make a comparison, one can imagine the bursting of an irrigation pipe in the desert. How far the water will spread in the ground will be, to a great extent, dependent on the water pressure in the pipe.

BROMAN: I should like to comment on Dr. Klatzo's report, because I think it is a very important paper. His experiments serve as a model for the development of edema in many different kinds of lesions with bearing also on diseases and lesions of the human brain. I think that previously most of us had misunderstood this spreading of the edema and thought of it as caused by a mysterious propagation of a barrier damage. Instead, the barrier damage is local and the increasing edema is the result of other dynamic factors. This has elucidated a very important problem.

WECHSLER: Dr. Klatzo, do you have any explanation why there are such remarkable differences in the vulnerability of the white matter, if you compare your findings on neonatal cats with adult cats?

KLATZO: The difference between immature and adult cat brain, with regard to cold injury edema, is a very interesting problem, but I cannot offer any explanation. How much this difference may be related to ultrastructural or biochemical aspects would be difficult even to speculate at this moment. Also, I am uncertain how significant a role can be attributed to a remarkably low systolic blood pressure in the new-born kittens. Perhaps some clues will be obtained from Dr. Tower's studies demonstrating the differential swelling of immature and adult cat brain tissue in vitro.

WECHSLER: We have done some light and electron microscopic investigation on the development of the brain and the spinal cord, and I want to add something on this particular point. During the development of the white substance (in the hemispheres and the spinal cord of chicken embryos), it is interesting to see that in both, at various stages of development, there is a constant narrow continuous extracellular space about 200 Å in width. During the early stages of myelination, the already formed thin myelin sheaths come into closer and closer contact with one another, and at the site of direct contact there is an obliteration of the extracellular space with the resultant establishment of an intraperiod line. In a paper published some months ago by Dr. Schröder and me, we put forward the hypothesis that exactly these special contacts which are only found in the white matter show a higher degree of ability for separation compared with the relatively more stable cellular contacts in the gray substance. With respect to your findings, I would, therefore, say that the completely immature and the partially myelinated white substance in fetal animals resemble the adult gray substance as far as the extracellular space is concerned. That means that the less pronounced tendency for spreading of edema in the immature white substance can have something to do with these structural interstitial peculiarities.

TOWER: Dr. Wechsler has brought up an important point, and I would like to comment on possible differences between chicken and kitten, since the developmental period in the kitten is quite long. After birth, the maturation of neurons in cerebral cortex takes about a month, and myelination of cortical axons does not begin until about 2 weeks of post-natal age and continues until about 3 months of age. The studies of kitten brain maturation by Drs. Purpura and Pappas at Columbia are still in progress, so that we cannot say too much until a full series of sections is available. But certainly for the neonatal kitten, I agree with Dr. Wechsler that from a rather over-simplified point of view, the white matter and gray matter are similar and certainly quite different from what is observed in mature brain. Clearly, Dr. Klatzo is wise to be cautious about drawing conclusions about the meaning of these findings.

KATZMAN: Just one question to Dr. Lee in reference to the hypercapnic anoxia. I wonder if the disruption of the endoplasmic reticulum and mitochondrial cristae that you see in this condition might also occur in the sever hypercapnia, if you produced it just alone, or the anoxia alone. The reason I ask this is that it might be supposed that the reduction in pH produced by CO_2 would decrease binding of calcium to phospholipids and that this might, by itself, reduce membrane integrity.

LEE: Thank you for your comment, Dr. Katzman. Unfortunately, we did not carry out any electron microscopic study on animals under hypercapnic or hypoxic condition alone. This is because our electron microscopic work was an extension of the histologic, chemical and autoradiographic studies by Dr. Bakay who found cerebral edema produced only by hypercapnic hypoxia. Therefore, I cannot answer your question, but it may be of considerable interest, as you pointed out, to study and compare the ultrastructural changes, if any, induced by hypoxia and hypercapnia separately.

FONCIN: I want to confirm Dr. Lee's observation about edema or, rather, hypoxic brain swelling, associated with aneurysms. Both with the optical microscope and with the electron microscope, my findings are quite comparable: ischemic manifestations and especially their acute form, as well as hypoxic brain swelling, are a prominent feature in brains of patients dying with supratentorial aneurysms.

ZIMMERMAN: I am a little concerned about the discussion of the various types of edema which Dr. Wechsler described. When I felt that we were dealing with a serous or plasmatic type of edema and asked whether this was so on the basis of the chemical findings which were reported earlier this morning, namely the changes in globulin and albumin, I was assured that there was essentially no difference. Then we come to third type of edema which Dr. Wechsler proposes, namely necrotizing edema, and for the sake of uniformity I wonder if Dr. Wechsler would be willing to agree that what he really is describing is edema with necrosis, not a necrotizing edema. In other words, is it the edema that is producing the necrosis of the tissue, or is it purely that edema accompanies a tissue-response to injury in which necrosis is also present? If you concede that, then we have no argument; if you don't concede it, I would like to propose that we talk about edema associated with necrosis as necrotizing edema, and edema associated with hemorrhage as hemorrhagic edema, etc.

KLATZO: I think it becomes quite apparent from this symposium that brain edema can be related to distinctly different pathophysiological mechanisms. Unquestionably, elucidation of these mechanisms is very important and it should enable us to arrive at comprehensive classification of edemas. Such classification, however, must be based on essential, qualitative characteristics derived from morphological as well as physiological criteria. Thus, I wonder whether classification of edemas by Dr. Wechsler into serous, plasmatic and necrotic types is justifiable, since it reflects merely the differences in morphological appearance of the same basic phenomenon, namely, the vascular injury. Personally, I believe we now have sufficient data to divide edemas into two major types. The first, vasogenic, originates primarily from vascular injury and is associated with extravascular migration of serum contents, enlargement of extracellular spaces, disruption of the blood-brain barrier as assessed by conventional tracers, and increase in sodium, chloride and proteins as measured by biochemical methods. The second type, which may be called cytotoxic, depends primarily on cellular swelling of individual component elements of nervous parenchyma due to cytotoxic effect of various noxic agents such as, e.g., anoxia or triethyl tin. In this type of edema, there is no extravasation of serum, no enlargement of extracellular spaces, no visible disturbance of the blood-brain barrier, and the biochemical characteristics are quite different.

WECHSLER: We started from two different points of view. The first concept was offered to you by Professor Zülch, defining different forms of brain edema according to pathogenesis and localization. In our electron microscopic paper, we started from common morphological findings in brain edema I do not want to stress the differences between serous and plasmatic edema too much, but nevertheless we can see these forms in our experiments. We found both, serous and plasmatic edema in our experimental animals, e.g., under the conditions of compression of the hemispheres or in venous congestion. In brain compression, it was interesting to notice that during the first and second day, there was more plasmatic edema than later, so that on the third day one could only detect diffusely spreading serous edema. I absolutely agree with Dr. Klatzo's concept that these differences must be explained on the basis of different degrees in the intensity of permeability changes of the blood brain barrier (BBB). Now to the somewhat confusing term of "necrotizing edema." I am sure all of you know the famous paper of Prof. Jacob on "Ödemnekrose," and of Prof. Scholz, my former teacher in neuropathology, on "plasmatische Infiltrationsnekrose." I think it is difficult to answer Dr. Zimmerman's question as to whether there exists a true form of necrotizing edema, or whether such observations represent only a combination of necrosis and edema. I think that both possibilities may occur.

ZÜLCH: I would like to add to Dr. Wechsler's statements going back to clinical observations. We have heard a paper by Dr. Glowacki who spoke of the edema as a space occupying factor in supratentorial lesion in which, as we now know, the brain is full of fluid. Now, this fluid cannot only be deduced from our experiments if we make venous blockages at the level of the sinuses but it is well-known from our observations in human pathology that we actually have a heavy accumulation of edema fluid in the brain. I now go back to the case of a young man who had a ligature of the right transverse sinus. For some reason, probably due to anatomical variations, this often leads to brain edema by venous blockage. He had a papilledema of 3 diopers for 3 months and no neurological findings apart from the palsy of an eye abductor muscle. He had never had any EEG findings, and he came out of this without any damage to his mental or other functions of the brain, as far as one can deduce from clinical investigations. And he went into the academic field with good success In this case we assume that the white matter was not badly damaged, although there must have been edema for months. This is in contrast to another case pertaining to an infected brain lesion, such as we saw in war wounds. There we saw a complete myelin sheath destruction after 4 days. In these cases we have a protein-rich edema, which is definitely strongly stained with Masson's blue. The myelin sheaths in this case actually disappeared after 4 days, although the cortex was, as far as I remember, quite well preserved. So I think there must be different forms of edema or different effects of edema on the human brain tissue, particularly on the myelin sheaths. And this is what Jakob wanted to call "necrotizing edema." There must be different forms of edema, at least in human pathology. I wonder if these do not also exist in experimental pathology.

ZIMMERMAN: I can't refrain from answering Dr. Zülch regarding the experimental differences in edema. For some years now, Dr. Hirano and I, and Dr. Levine, have been attempting to analyze the tissue response to injury with and without the production of edema by using various chemical substances. We found that if we use a cryptococcus and implanted it in the brain in the same manner that Dr. Hirano described this morning, we got an inflammatory response in which polymorphonuclear leukocytes, necrosis, hemorrhage and edema were all present. But if we used the purified polysaccharide we could eliminate the necrosis essentially, and we could eliminate the hemorrhage, and then we got only edema. The edema was protein-rich and, I think, intercellular in the white matter primarily, and was not different from the edema that has been described in many other experiments using different modalities. If we conceivably would use different injurious agents, we could produce what you would call, and what in human pathology is, "necrotizing edema" in the sense that there is both necrosis and edema present. But I think that these are two separate factors in a response of tissue and that the edema is not the primary and most important element in the response.

ZÜLCH: What is the primary factor which destroys the myelin sheath? In the case to which I was referring, there were no hemorrhages and certainly no inflammation in the neighborhood, since this was a case where the actual abscess was at least 5-6 cm distant. There had been edema seeping through the white matter of the whole hemisphere.

ZIMMERMAN: I think that in many inflammatory processes the edema precedes some of the other elements of the inflammatory reaction. An edema is an early manifestation, and later on, within a matter of hours or days the other elements of the inflammatory process also follow. Now, in some reactions there may never be any other element of inflammation, like a leukocytic response or even an hemorrhagic response, whereas in other instances some inflammatory response is also added to the process.

ZÜLCH: I think this is definitely true. We see all this in pathology, but if we go farther into this matter, we will have our traditional discussion on "inflammation," which is now thirty or forty years old and which we will probably never settle. There may be serous inflammation, if you call my form of necrotizing edema a serous inflammation, then I quite agree.

FEIGIN: I would like to support the contention of Dr. Zülch and Dr. Wechsler that edema can cause necrosis of the white matter and result in cavitation of these tissues. I differ from them, however, in thinking that the edema which causes such changes is not of a special type but differs from the others only in severity and possibly duration.

SHIRAKI: I would like to put a question to Dr. A. Hirano concerning the experimental "allergic" enephalomyelitis. In this type of experimentation as well as in neuromyelitis optica which represents a type of demyelinating encephalomyelitis and preferentially occurs in the Japanese, severe plasmatic transudations, as a rule, occur in the periadventitial parenchyma. Plasmatic fluids, however, consist of two types: one is represented by fibrinous networks of a high-molecular nature; another is serous fluid of a low-molecular nature. How far could you differentiate those two types of plasmatic transudations under an electron microscope?

HIRANO: Recently we have studied a hyperacute form of experimental allergic encephalomyelitis. This work was presented in detail by Dr. Levine in Atlantic City, New Jersey, during the 1965 meeting of the American Association of Neuropathologists and was published in the American Journal of Pathology, 47; 61-88, and 47; 209-221 (1965).

In the early phase of the experiment, electron dense plasma was found around the blood vessels, as I have just illustrated. Later, fibrin appeared within these pools of extravascular plasma. The fibrin was easily identified and the fine structure corresponded to that described by Kisch in Experimental Medicine and Surgery, 22; 237-245 (1964). In our experiment, I was not aware of any significant difference in the plasma before and after the appearance of the fibrin.

It should be pointed out that our experimental model is significantly different from the condition referred to by Dr. Shiraki. In our experiment, which was always acute, the plasma evidently accumulated continously in the parenchyma, and the animal finally died of this condition.

TORACK: I wonder if Dr. Lee has examined the blood vessels of the shark and has found any reason for the lack of hemorrhage and exudation in this necrotic lesion. He has also mentioned some differences between cerebral and cerebellar swelling in a rat due to triethyltin. Is there any other difference except in the degree of dilatation and myelin splits?

LEE: To answer Dr. Torack's first question, we did examine the blood vessels of the shark's brain after electric coagulation. The main changes were the increase in the formation of pinocytotic vesicles of different sizes and a certain amount of hydration of the basement membrane of the blood capillaries. We also observed hemorrhage, as evidenced by the presence of blood cells, in and nearby the lesion. However, this hemorrhage did not give rise to enlargement of the intercellular space in the gray matter. The electron dense material, representing possibly the exudates, was found in the moderately enlarged intercellular space where myelinated nerve fibers were concentrated. As to the second question about the difference in the reaction of the white matter of the spinal cord, cerebellum and cerebrum to triethyltin, we found that the difference was quantitative rather than qualitative. In other words, the same type of changes occurred at various levels of the central nervous system, but the degrees of severity were different in the early stages of intoxication.

BAKEY: There is one point I would like to mention as far as the sharks are concerned. Their plasma is very considerably different from the plasma of mammals, not only in salinity but also in protein profile. These shark brains were perfused with shark saline (which we have been told is the appropriate saline for shark), and its constitution compares to the normal shark plasma. We are still a little bit worried whether there might be some perfusion artifact in the shark brains which we have not encountered in mammalian brains.

KLATZO: With regard to the lemon shark brain I would like to mention a remarkable arrangement of astrocytes which is basically different from that seen in mammals. The astrocytic cells, stained by Cajal's gold chloride, appear to lie applied with their main cell bodies directly to the blood vessels and to the pial surface sending their processes away from blood vessels and pia without any formation of vascular foot plates.

ZIMMERMAN: I think we now understand the reason why we love sharks.

BROMAN: I would like to point out from a clinical point of view that there are a lot of vicious-circle mechanisms involved in the brain edema. One of the most well-known deals with secondary necrosis as a result of an edematous condition, e.g., by the compression of the blood vessels supplying herniated brain regions. There is another question I would like to ask Dr. Zülch pertaining to a case with reversible cerebral symptoms and normal EEG. What is the proof that there was a brain edema in this case?

ZIMMERMAN: I suggest that we leave the next five minutes for discussion of the other papers dealing with ionizing radiation. Are there any questions or remakrs about edema due to ionizing radiation?

TERRY: I am very much interested in Dr. Miquel's findings that glycogen is not quantitatively increased in these altered astrocytes. We see what looks much like increased glycogen in astrocytes in many diseases and experimental conditions. Does this indicate a change in its form such as an abnormal aggregation? Or is there some other disparity between the electron microscopic and the quantitative study?

MIQUEL: We have been talking about astrocytes in the edematous white matter. That is where we find little increase in glycogen, but we certainly find striking glycogen increase in the gray matter in the areas adjacent to a lesion. We have seen a glycogen increase in injuries induced by alpha-particle irradiation in cats and rats, by proton radiation in cats and monkeys, and near the cortical lesions induced by freezing and by UV-radiation. According to our experience, glycogen accumulation is largely a response of the gray matter to injury. In certain instances we have seen also glycogen granules in the injured white matter but in lesser amounts than in cortex. The glycogen deposits are not produced by a redistribution of the normal glycogen content of the brain but indicate a real glycogen increase, as ascertained by chemical analysis.

SHIRAKI: I would like to ask Dr. Lierse the following two points. What was the condition of exposure? I mean the brain only was exposed or the whole body was exposed? The reason for this question is that in certain cases of hepatocerebral diseases a conspicuously large number of glycogen granules deposits not only in the cytoplasmic processes of astrocytes but also in their nuclei, and, as far as I saw in your slides, glycogen granules deposit in the astrocytic nuclei. I would like to know about the condition of exposure and the existence of liver damages.

LIERSE: Only the heads were irradiated, not the whole body. And to the second question: we see at first glycogen and mucopolysaccharides in the pericarya of astrocytes, but not in all regions. The first glycogen granules appear in the frontal lobe above the basal gray matter in the commisura anterior. Following a higher dosage, all regions, gray and white matter, are affected. In the later stages we also find glycogen granules in the nuclei of astrocytes, neurons, and oligodendroglia.

WOLMAN: I want to ask Dr. Invernizzi whether the changes he has shown could correspond to the grape-like formations which have been extensively discussed in the Italian literature about thirty years ago and in the German literature, too. Couldn't it be the same thing which some people consider to be an artifact, others a non-specific change: Buscaino-bodies?

INVERNIZZI: No, I don't think so.

ROUND TABLE DISCUSSION

Moderator: R. D. ADAMS

ADAMS: Ladies and gentlemen, may the afternoon session be convened. First of all, I would like to make two general remarks: to thank Dr. and Mrs. Seitelberger for preparing what I consider to be an excellent meeting and for gracing the social events they have so kindly prepared. Next, I think I express the gratitude of all English-speaking members of this audience for the kindness of our German confreres in forcing all of their thoughts and expressions into the English language. We realize that this is a trial to them, but it has been extremely important and helpful to us.

It is more or less axiomatic, I believe, that all acute and many subacute and chronic diseases of the human nervous system cause disorders of function that cannot be easily explained by the pathological anatomy of the disease itself, the main features of the lesion. And further, from the pathological side, there are always changes in and around the lesions, reflected at times by swelling of tissues, that may relate more directly to the clinical phenomena of the disease than do the overt lesions themselves. This swelling of tissue varies in degree, appearing to depend to some extent on the size and on the locale of the lesions, and on their nature. Even the most casual neuropathological study of different types of lesions suggest that the swelling of the tissue in and around the lesion may relate to any one or a combination of several elements, such as vascular congestion, hemorrhage, infarct necrosis, extravasation of serum or other elements of plasma, or swelling of nerve cells and medullated fibres. Since most of the acute or subacute lesions are focal, therefore brain swelling is usually focal.

The study of a series of cases in which different stages of a given lesion are visualized in biopsy or autopsy specimens, informs us that the tissue swelling may occur at particular phases in the evolution of the lesion, bearing certain relationships to other elements of the tissue change. In each disease, probably, there is a specific sequence of alteration; and, if swelling of the tissue occurs, it is but one aspect of complexity of pathological processes. In infarct necrosis, for example, the destroyed tissue invariably becomes congested and swollen within a few minutes, depending upon the adequacy of circulation through the damaged vessels, but the surrounding brain is rarely swollen to a significant degree. In contrast, in pyogenic inflammatory foci swelling, exudation, and congestion exceed necrosis, and the surrounding brain undergoes much swelling, especially the white matter, and this may extend throughout the cerebral hemisphere, as you know. In gliogenic tumors and in secondary carcinomatous deposits, the neoplastic tissue frequently swells on its own accord due to vascular occlusion and hemorrhage. Again there is widespread pallor and volumetric increase of the surrounding tissue, particularly in white matter, with only slight alteration of medullated fibres, as seen under the light microscope, and some change in the astrocytic glia. In hypoxia, which is usually associated with circulatory failure, gray matter and sometimes white matter become necrotic in a certain anatomic pattern, and there is variable, but usually not prominent swelling in necrotic nerve and glial cells and medullated fibres. Compression of the brain by tumors and hematomas, when relieved by surgery permits swelling of both gray and white matter, with proliferation of only astrocytes to mark later the disturbance. In hyponatremia and water intoxication, and in certain obscure toxic states in infancy, the entire brain, gray and white matter, swells without significant alterations in nerve and glial cells, at least for the first hours or a day or two.

One could extend a discussion of this kind to include practically every known disease in pathology. Therefore, if we take the broadest view of our subject, it encompasses all of neuropathology. But this would be, I think, a rather pointless exercise and one which would not at all lead us to the heart of the problem which we are here to discuss. The principal idea to be imparted, I think, is that in each disease or its lesion—if there is to be swelling, it represents but one aspect of the pathological process. And we have to keep in mind always that taking the element of edema out of the context of disease is highly artificial; in fact, it may result in a rather misleading way of thinking, certainly a way of thinking that is extremely disorienting to the average neuropathologist. Nevertheless, I think there is some benefit to come from at least studying the subject that we have been pondering these last two or three days.

Perhaps the first question that we should address ourselves to this afternoon must have been posed originally by those who planned this colloquium: whether or not there are certain disease states in which the swelling of the lesion and the brain tissue surrounding it reaches such proportions as to contribute significantly to the hazard of the disease, producing a serious, though at times evanescent, functional derangement. The metastatic tumor, gliomatous tumors, cerebral abscess at once come to mind as standard examples of widespread edema that goes way beyond the limits of the lesion. If one looks at the leading articles on the subject of cerebral edema, written by Greenfield, Kernohan, Zimmerman and many others, the importance of localized edema is clearly set forth. (Cerebral trauma offers a far less clear illustration because hemorrhage and necrosis figure most prominently in the common forms of this condition.) The answer to this question as to whether it is profitable to study edema as a separate entity is obviously in the affirmative. Similarly it seems clear that diffuse swelling of the brain without other visible change represents another entity of great significance. Both clinicians and pathologists appreciate this fact, especially that the functional disorder, i.e. the symptomatology, may depend upon brain swelling; and further that the difficulty in understanding the nature of the basic pathology and in delimiting the edematous zone accounts in part for the inexactitude of many clinical-pathological and clinical-anatomical correlations.

The second problem, and one which deserves more extended consideration, concerns a proper terminology for some of the conditions that we have been discussing. This is not a matter of idle quibbling over terms. The right choice of words will reflect our mode of thinking about these conditions. You have already heard in the first day reference to the work of Reichardt, who attempted to distinguish brain edema from brain swelling. Throughout this colloquium the term "edema" has been employed. But this term seems to lack precision in that it has more than one meaning in medicine. For example, it is most widely applied to states in which fluid accumulates in tissues, as in cardiac failure where there is high venous pressure, or in nutritional edema, or renal failure where there is hypo-albuminemia. Here, unfortunately, the function of the swollen tissue, which is usually connective or adipose tissue, is almost impossible to evaluate. It is curious that the brain and most visceral organs do not participate in such edematous states. Again the term "edema" has been used to designate any condition in which there is an accumulation of water within or around a lesion, whether the fluid be between or in cells, and without reference to the mechanism of such swelling. Little attention usually has been given to the components of the swollen tissue, whether they be blood, protein, white cells, or water. Hence it is not clear whether edema properly designates the abnormality or is merely a convenient term to indicate one obvious aspect of many different pathological processes. Obviously there is no point in referring to ischemic necrosis or hemorrhage by the term edema. Brain swelling, on the other hand, has sometimes been used to describe volumetric increase in tissue from whatever cause, due to an increase in any one of the aforementioned substances. This does not commit us to an assumption that only the water content is increased. However, Reichardt had already used the term "brain swelling" for a diffuse edema which he thought was intracellular. It is of interest that up to this point in our discussions there has not been a complete delineation of purely intracellular edema, at least in human beings. This is an ideal to be striven towards, but one which we have not by any means achieved.

Concerning terminology, my own recommendation would be that we actually use the term "brain swelling" for all these states, specifying it as regional or focal when it is restricted to an area in or near a lesion. Modifying adjectives could be employed to indicate whether this volumetric increase is due mainly to blood, serum or other fluid. We could use the term "edema", i.e. edematous regional swellin to refer to those states where fluid seems to be the main element of the p hological process. This is a descriptive term and commits us in no way to anything more than what we can see. I feel we are not prepared to speak of edema as a separate entity in most human pathological states. Similarly, we could refer to diffuse volumetric increase as a diffuse or generalized brain swelling and specify that it is due to edema or ischemic necrosis or hypoxia, etc. Always the term should be used in relation to the disease which has led to it. In other words, we should speak of brain abscess with regional brain swelling of edematous type. I would like to hear comments on this matter of nomenclature, because I think they would be useful in the monograph which is to ensue. Dr. McMenemey, what is your opinion about terminology?

McMENEMEY: I do not think I can improve upon what you have said, Dr. Adams. I did not bring my Greek lexicon with me(!) but someone has kindly looked up the word edema in the dictionaries. According to Saunders it is "the presence of abnormally large amounts of fluid in the intercellular tissue spaces of the body." Dorland gives the same. Webster defines it as "an abnormal accumulation of serous fluid"—Dr. Wechler will be interested to note that: "in the interfibrillar spaces of connective tissue or in the fibrous cavities", which means, I suppose, that according to Webster, the brain has to be excluded. According to MacNalty, 1961, edema is "the presence of excessive amounts of fluid in the intercellular spaces of the body due to increased transudation of fluid from the capillaries." This more precise definition necessitates a specific mechanism for edema formation which we may not feel able to accept in its entirety.

I believe that from the practical point of view of the clinician we should use the word swelling; it gives the right concept of a continuous process dangerous for the patient and therefore it is the term I should favour. A brain swelling, of course, may be local as well as diffuse and spreading. There are alternative terms that one could use: Dr. Zimmerman speaks of fluid accumulation and that is very precise: we could only make it more precise by saying "liquid accumulation", thereby excluding an accumulation of gas! "Tumor cerebri" is another obvious term that we should like to use: it is absolutely correct, except for the fact that we regularly employ the word "tumor" to cover neoplasms and granulomas. "Hydrocephalus" again is strictly correct but it has come to have an entirely different meaning. If we follow Saunders then we should only use the word edema when we have certain knowledge that the liquid is lying extra-cellularly in the brain. Except by implication, it is impossible to know if in any particular case liquid is lying outside cells or if it has already been absorbed by avid processes of astrocytes. Nevertheless, a histological preparation which shows the separation of myelin fibres and the presence of plasma outside vessels provides reasonable assumption that a state of edema existed within the brain at the time of death. When we are prepared to use the word edema in respect to the brain it should be hyphenated— "brain-edema" or perhaps we should coin a word like "encephaledema." Although I do not like it, it would have the advantage that its two components are derived from the same language.

BAKEY: I looked up the etymology of edema some time ago. Edema is a very old Greek word, it is a common word and it has no medical connotation, as far as original Greek is concerned. The medical connotation came fairly late; it was assumed that edema is a predominantly interstitial or intracavitary exudate. Originally, however, edema which was used about the time of Aristoteles, means nothing more than increase in volume or tumescence or turgor.

FONCIN: I welcome Dr. Adams's suggestion to use the term "swelling" on a morphological basis and I would like to warn of the dangers involved in too many a priori classifications which are semantic traps rather than research guidelines.

ADAMS: All we can do is suggest a terminology whereby we can discuss these several pathological states. Are there any further comments on this topic? Perhaps we should not pursue it too far.

A similar terminological difficulty arises in connection with this "spongy state" (status spongiosus). Our colleague, Dr. Seitelberger, has struggled with this condition and has reached the conclusion that there probably is nothing similar in such diverse states as B_{12}-deficiency with status spongiosus of the white matter of the spinal cord, Pick's disease and Jakob-Creutzfeld's disease with status spongiosus of the cerebral cortex or Canavan's disease with its peculiar status spongiosus of cerebral cortex and white matter. Here again imprecise terminology has resulted in the formulation of inapposite concepts of disease. Dr. Seitelberger recommends that we eliminate further discussion of status spongiosus from this colloquium.

Before the neuropathologists take the floor, I would ask them their views on other states in which the tissues and their water content seems to be increased or in which the cerebrospinal fluid is increased. For example, what is known about meningial hydrops or pseudotumor cerebri? Obviously, there should be some reference to this condition in a symposium of this kind. There have been a number of experimental studies using radioactive isotopes, such as those of Dr. William Sweet and Dr. Bertram Selverstone. And what about the uremic brain? It has been said by a number of people that in uremia there is swelling of the brain. Yet in our experience very few of the uremic brains are actually swollen and those that are usually turn out to have malignant hypertension, and are really examples of hypertensive encephalopathy. This form of brain swelling is due, as Byrom has shown, to multiple foci of ischemic necrosis resulting from arterial spasm. And what should be said of the condition of the cerebral tissues beneath the chronic subdural hematoma after the clot is removed? And should some kind of a statement be made, perhaps by Dr. Cummings, about Canavan's disease in which there is an obvious increase in water? No reference has yet been made of a whole group of conditions loosely called "toxic encephalopathies." Most of these cases are infants and children in whom brain swelling occurs at a prodigious rate over a period of hours or days often with fatal outcome. As a rule, the pathologist finds nothing in microscopic sections of the brain except a series of minor alterations largely of artefactural nature; light microscopy has not really thrown much light on the whole subject. These latter conditions call attention to a point that was made by a number of workers, that diffuse cerebral swelling of edematous type occurs more rapidly in children than adults. It might be suggested that Professor Seitelberger call upon some of the participants of this symposium to make a statement about some of these conditions.

We come now to one of the first sections in this symposium, that of the clinical manifestations of cerebral edema. The lecture by our colleague, Dr. Hoff, called attention to the fact that cerebral swelling may express itself by signs of focal derangement of brain function, increased intracranial pressure, and/or temporal lobe and cerebellar herniation. While this is true, it must be obvious to all who reflect upon these matters that such statements could apply as well to brain tumor, abscess, subdural hematoma, and any of many other diseases. To list these as the clinical expressions of cerebral edema is not particularly helpful. One fact so far ignored is the temporal aspect of the functional disorder in regional brain swelling. For example, in glioma of the brain it is the rapidly advancing, transitory (if operation relieves the situation or corticosteroids are used) symptomatology that appears to be most clearly related to the regional brain swelling of edematous type. Moreover, these symptoms may fluctuate over hours, and may vary with the level of the intracranial pressure in certain general ways for reasons that are not clear. With reference to the increased intracranial pressure of hyponatremia and water intoxication, the cerebrospinal fluid pressure is increased and, as a rule, the patient convulses and rapidly lapses into coma. But his coma is certainly not due merely to the raised intracranial pressure, for the pressure may be higher in meningial hydrops where the state of consciousness is perfectly preserved. Here the functional cerebral disorder manifestly depends upon an altered state of the parenchymal elements, caused probably by a shift in blood electrolytes and probably by impairment of some intracellular energy mechanism that paralyzes the cells. It seems entirely impossible at the present time to designate a clinical picture of diffuse cerebral swelling. One can only indicate those parts of particular syndromes in specific disease states which appear to depend upon brain swelling. Probably in each of these states brain swelling in relation to the lesion will have a time course all its own. This is not meant to repudiate the idea that it would ever be possible to delineate a particular syndrome of brain swelling. Could some of the neurosurgeons and neurologists in the audience comment upon this point and correct my views if they are exaggerated?

CAVENESS: I think Dr. Adams is stating the case too strongly. Anything that involves the nervous system has to express itself externally in accordance with that part which is involved. Now, is there a clinical picture of edema in trauma? I made a point of stating how complex the effects of trauma are. But if one singles out those cases of closed head injury in which swelling is the principal feature, one observes a meaningful constellation of symptoms and signs. These include, progressively, a decrease in alertness, restlessness, followed by the signs and symptoms of increasing intracranial pressure and those related to tentorial or foramen magnum herniations. One can find this without evidence of extra- or sub-dural hematomas.

The regional involvement from local injury, similarly, is dependent upon the function of the area that is involved. The time-course that you referred to is an important part in the clinical picture. It should be mentioned that in closed head injuries signs and symptoms can develop within 2 hours or be delayed for 72 hours.

ADAMS: Do you believe it possible at the present time to separate out the parts of the syndrome that are due to hemorrhage, traumatic necrosis, and herniation in such a way as to be left with a syndrome of brain edema?

CAVENESS: One cannot, without specific examinations. A swollen brain may be mainly edematous, or edematous plus hemorrhage, or edematous plus hemorrhage plus necrosis.

Might I make two other comments? I would like to accentuate again the clinical impression that a damaged brain is much more sensitive to anoxia than a nondamaged brain in regard to swelling. And, finally, may I reiterate our conviction that future advances in the management of head injury are going to depend a great deal on the better understanding and correction of the processes involved in brain swelling?

ZÜLCH: Our present task is to define a syndrome which could be the consequence of a pure accumulation of fluid in the brain. At this point I should like to point out that the French and also the German schools of neurosurgery speak of the "posttraumatic edema" on the third, fourth and fifth day after trauma. At this time, the primary sequelae of trauma have disappeared, but very often you have a secondary deterioration and then these symptoms will disappear again. They may consist of focal signs, for example a Babinski reflex, a difference in the width of the pupils, some slight paresis of brain nerves or of one extremity, or of symptoms like aphasia. Naturally, the neurosurgeons have been trying to find causes other than this hypothetical edema, yet they have not found them up to now. I have also to cite some experiments of Scholz which, unfortunately, have never been repeated. He examined the cortex of animals where he had produced concussion and found a disruption of the circulation in the cortical capillaries, so that one could hypothetically (because it has yet to be proved by a series of experiments) speak or think of a disregulation of circulation with an ensuing diffuse edema of the brain.

ADAMS: I think there can be no doubt that when the tissue swells it produces symptoms. It would be most unwise to reject that notion. The only point is whether it is possible at this time to make a definitive statement about there being a particular syndrome that relates to the swelling per se.

BROMAN: As a clinical neurologist I know quite well that there is no such sign. We must rely on indicative symptoms. As a convincing, though not 100%, proof, we may use a series of pneumoencephalographams showing changes in volume consistent with the diagnosis. Thus, we may need more than one pneumoencephalogram to make the existence of a brain edema probable.

ADAMS: Yes, further serial electroencephalography and serial arteriography could be used to delineate a volumetric increase in the damaged part of the tissue.

BAKAY: I almost hate to say that, because I am sure it will be a misleading statement in many ways, but it was mentioned by other authors a number of times. Could this not be specific for edema in a person whose intracranial pressure is increased, who has no local neurological symptoms indicating a tumor, a hematoma or something like that, who shows no evidence of herniation, either clinically or by radiological methods, and who becomes somnolent and develops stupor, with all the other factors bring ruled out? Dr. Evans and his group, and Bronson Ray and other investigators showed that simply increasing intracranial pressure to unprecedented heights does not cause real change in the state of consciousness. I do not want to comment on the vital signs, for that is another matter. It is equally true that people with pseudotumor cerebri can have a very high pressure, papilledema, and be perfectly clear and alert. And yet, if such a tumor develops with the elimination of all the other factors, it might be explained by cerebral hypoxia due to edema, the edema enlarging the diameter of the Krogh cylinders. In other words, in the brain as in any other organ, capillaries supply or support a certain area, which is the Krogh cyliner. The oxygen pressure falls from the capillary to the outermost edge of this cylinder. If such a tissue is blown up by edema and the distance from the capillary to the remote part of the Krogh cylinder increases, the patient becomes hypoxic and, hence, stuporous.

ADAMS: Dr. Evans, would you like to comment on whether you find there to be a specific, identifiable syndrome, apart from any given disease, which may be identified clinically? Do you recognize edema syndrome?

EVANS: I believe, Dr. Adams, that one should emphasize that the calvarium is occupied by brain tissue, by the circulating blood volume, by the cerebrospinal fluid, and, when present, by a lesion. We know from the studies carried out by Ryder in our Cincinnati laboratories a good many years ago, that one can, by the addition of normal saline to the lumbar space, safely raise the intracranial pressure to the range of 1200 to 1400 mm. of water. In most instances, conscious patients were not even aware that something was going on. There is no question that high ranges of pressure can be tolerated for brief periods of time. On the other hand, lower ranges of pressure, if productive of shift of a portion of the intracranial contents, may cause serious trouble. Let me cite an example. I had occasion to perform a hemispherectomy upon a child and I deliberately left the choroid plexus intact, hoping that it would fill the hemicalvarium with fluid which would be in contact through the foramen of Monro with the normal cerebrospinal fluid pathways. Unfortunately, however, the foramen of Monro obstructed. Following discharge from the hospital, the child was brought back by his mother because of increasing dullness. The pressure in the hemicalvarium was found to be approximately 400 mm. of water. Shortly thereafter, the child became comatose and the pupil dilated upon the operated side. It was then clear that the cerebrospinal fluid, which was being formed by the intact choroid plexus and whic was unable to communicate with the normal pathways was, in fact, acting as a lesion and was causing a herniation of the brain stem through the tentorial ring. Such mechanical shifts are of extreme importance. Another example of the interrelationship of these factors is that of lead encephalopathy. Here the tremendously high pressures are a reflection of the involvement of brain tissue itself. In considering the whole spectrum of these four elements, one must always bear in mind the parameter of time. A final clinical point is the rapid deterioration that may be seen following a seizure, as pointed out by Dr. Caveness. The sudden increase in the circulating blood volume associated with hypoxia and accummulation of CO_2 may often tip the balance in a most adverse fashion. We see this most strikingly in the seizures that occur in lead encephalopathy, following which a child's condition may deteriorate dramatically.

ADAMS: We all seem to feel that there are certain symptoms produced by swelling of the brain tissue and brain edema, but they will always have to be considered in terms of the lesion with which they are connected. It seems doubtful if there is a specific syndrome of cerebral swelling or edema as a separable entity.

LOWENTHAL: Can EEG give some information on the cerebral edema?

ADAMS: I am sure there are very definite instances where a given lesion and the local swelling which it engenders has seemed to cause both a progressive symptomatology and a progressive change in EEG. The answer, I would think, would be yes, but that you could not look at the EEG and say that it reflected edema rather than hemorrhage or some other change. This, like serial arteriography, might be the same in hemorrhage as in progressive edema.

LOWENTHAL: I have the impression that without focal lesion you can have EEG alteration purely due to edema.

ADAMS: You mean a diffuse EEG abnormality?

LOWENTHAL: Yes, more or less.

ADAMS: Perhaps so, but one immediately encounters problems of herniation and displacement of central structures which might be responsible.

ZEMAN: Inasmuch as there seems to be some difficulty in distinctly diagnosing edema, and considering the fact that the edema might become a cerebral lesion, the question arises whether we should not consider the introduction of some other methods by which edema could be more positively diagnosed. One possibility which comes to mind would be the determination of the impedance (both electrical and acoustic). Electrical impedance of the nervous tissue has already been successfully employed to determine the water content of tissues by using the Faraday principle.

FONCIN: I have done some work with Professor Gougerot (2nd Int. Cong.

Med. Electr. 1959) on the impedance of intracranial contents, but we have never seen any relation to edema, the only factor appearing to be the blood flow.

CUMINGS: I can only answer this in regard to animals. In the monkey you can distinguish cortex from white matter, and you can distinguish the presence of edema spreading in both white matter and cortex. I have only had experience with that, of course.

ADAMS: Perhaps we might leave this topic for the moment and turn to the question of the human diseases in which either focal, regional or diffuse edema figure most prominently. It must be admitted that because of limitations of time none of our neuropathology colleagues has been able to give a complete description of any one of these diseases. You heard an account of peritumoral plasmatic edema and serous edema and necrotizing edema, as presented by Dr. Wechsler and Dr. Zülch. However, in human neuropathology, just to take an example, peritumoral brain swelling cannot clearly be ascribed to congestion of vessels, extravasation of blood, exudation of plasma, nor is it possible to indicate the full extent of the edema in the surrounding tissues. Nonetheless, in the summary of the final deliberations of the group, it would be useful to have statements on the pathological changes in these cerebral diseases that we have been mentioning. Perhaps Dr. Zülch could undertake to do this for us.

ZÜLCH: I don't think there is time to give any more details of the histology of various forms of edema, but it is really very interesting to see what happens in them. We have, for instance, seen in these acute edemas mitotic proliferation in the oligodendroglia, and there was no doubt that it must have been the oligodendroglia because it was interfascicular. We have seen various other changes in the oligodendroglia which are very near to what Alzheimer described as amoeboid glia. Most of the cells described by Alzheimer in his original work were astrocytes, whereas these were oligodendroglia which were particularly acidophilic, being very red in H. and E. and blue in Masson's stain. I think we have even been able to reproduce the electron microscopical pictures of this change. I think we know very well from light microscopy all the tissue elements in our five models and could find the analogous changes in electron microscopy.

WECHSLER: I think there is still some confusion about the serous and plasmatic forms of edema. I would like to emphasize once more that we were able to demonstrate the ultrastructural equivalents and details of such edema changes. Serous and plasmatic forms of edema do not necessarily represent two separate entities of edema, because the obligatory primary changes (distention of the extracellular space, dissociation of the nerve fibers, swelling of the astrocytes) in the white matter are identical. The essential difference seems to be of a more biochemical nature, since the content of protein and possibly other component of the edema fluid are different.

It was interesting for me to hear from different American colleagues that the term "necrotizing edema" is not the right translation for "Ödemnekrose" in the sense of Jacob. They suggested that the proper interpretation would be "edematous necrosis." Maybe this was also the reason for some confusion. (To avoid misunderstandings we have, therefore, applied the original German terms in our final manuscript.)

Finally, I want to say something about primary and secondary lesions. The primary lesions in brain edema are the generalized swelling of the astroglia, which occurs in the gray and the white matter; in the white matter there is also a primary widening of the extracellular space. With respect to the nerve fiber changes in the edematous white matter in early stages, we have to distinguish between primary lesions and the sequalae of the edema. What happens to the nerve fibers in the white matter? In our electron microscopic findings we can recognize three forms of alterations: (1) primary lesions of the myelin sheath, (2) degeneration of the myelin complex as a result of a primary axonal lesion, and (3) under the conditions of "Ödemnekrose" myelin alterations due to a primary damage of the supporting oligodendroglia.

TOWER: I wish to raise a small objection to Dr. Wechsler's categorical statement that the primary process in edema is the swelling of astrocytes. This may or may not be so, but I do not think we have the final story here. It is a characteristic of the astrocyte to swell under almost any insult you give it, and one of the worst insults you can give is when you fix for electron microscopy. If this is not done properly, the astrocytes will swell and yet there may not have been any swelling of astrocytes before you started to process the tissue. Although I think you may be right in certain circumstances, we are not in a position to so state categorically at this time. I can conceive of just the opposite, namely, that the influx of fluid could be primarily extracellular and then as a result of some change in the characteristics of the astrocyte and its membrane, the fluid suddenly shifts within the astrocyte where you then visualize it. Until we have agreements on techniques and valid sequential analyses, we ought to be very careful about such conclusions.

CLASEN: I am quite convinced that the early stage of the edema associated with freezing lesions is exclusively an accumulation of fluid in the extracellular compartment.

WECHSLER: It is, of course, necessary to talk about this problem. The technical procedures are important. We are working with adult cats. Under general anesthesia, we do tracheotomy and intubate the animals, then we start with artificial respiration after pneumothorax. After opening the thorax, exposing the heart and clipping the aorta descendens, we perform initial fixation by perfusion (via aorta ascendens) with buffered glutaraldehyde of 6.25% for 15-30 minutes. The brain is removed and immediately bathed in cold buffered 1%-osmium-textroxide-postassium-dichromate-mixture. There are, of course, minor changes due to these procedures and the embedding techniques, but we have achieved regularly satisfactory results in our experimental animals. I would like to know what happens to the brain tissue at the ultrstructural level during your biochemical preparation procedures.

ADAMS: The whole question of tissue sequelae to brain edema was discussed this morning and there was some disagreement about it. I think part of the trouble lies in the fact that it is probably impossible with the microscopic methods in current use to separate the lesion from the regional swelling. Therefore, once the lesion has been permitted to resolve any persistent deficits in the tissue might just as well have been due to whatever caused the primary disease as to the edema itself. Surely in the laboratory animal a diffuse edema produced by the injection of hypotonic, hypo-osmolar solution may disappear leaving absolutely no change or functional deficit. Dr. Zimmerman, would you care to comment on this subject?

TORACK: I think at this time it would be appropriate since we have heard on several occasions about the artifact inherent in electron microscopy, also to point out and bring to the foreground the artifact that I refer to the incubation of tissue slices, either fixed or unfixed, in a physiological medium. We have already had some indication that across the cut surfaces of all these cells there is an early and significant infiltration of large particles. I have also done this in relationship to Thorotrast. I have seen Thorotrast enter these cells, and I might add not only in glial cells, but also in neurons, in a significant quantity.

ADAMS: We have, of course, devoted a large part of this meeting to the experimental induction of various types of brain edema, and, in the final analyses, I suppose, one of the most useful results would be a clear description of the methods of producing the different models of cerebral swelling in animals, and the interpretation of the mechanisms of these different forms of edema. Dr. Zimmerman, would you consent to summarize the very sizeable literature on experimental brain swelling, discussing types, causes and mechanisms and then endeavouring to relate the types to some of the human diseases in which cerebral swelling is prominent.

ZIMMERMAN: Were I to carry out the dictate of our chairman, we would be here until tomorrow at this hour without any interruption for sleep and food, and so I will attempt merely in general terms to summarize what has been accomplished to date in various forms of experiemental endeavors to produce edema in animals in the nervous system and to try very briefly to compare these findings with those few states in man with which we are familiar. These happen to be relatively few for reasons which will become apparent as I go along.

Some ten years ago when the light microscope was found wanting in the solution of the problem of cerebral swelling versus cerebral edema, a group of investigators began working with an experimental model, using the electron microscope, in hope of determining whether swelling is an intracellular or intercellular condition, or perhaps both. A few of us who began work at that time were cautious enough to try to avoid the use of the terms "edema" and "swelling," and this is the reason, Dr. McMenemey, that my group selected the term "fluid accumulation." Now you may prefer the word liquid to fluid, and you may prefer some other word for accumulation, but the fact is that we attempted to avoid any preconceived notion, simply because light microscopists had already reasoned that there was either an inter- or an intra-cellular (or both) accumulation of fluid in the brain. So we and others began working with models that would create fluid accumulation in the nervous system without any other form of injury.

One of the things that disturb me in this meeting so far is the use of terms such as anoxia as the equivalent of cerebral edema. I do not believe that these two terms are necessarily equivalent. One may get edema as the result of anoxia, and one may get edema as part of the response to trauma. Or one may get edema as part of the response to a bacterial infection with the creation of an abscess in the nervous system, but these reactions are not the equivalent of edema.

It was found quite by chance that triethyl tin poisoning tends to produce an accumulation of fluid in the nervous system without any other demonstrable lesion. This happened to be a good model except for the fact that the early workers, including my group, hit by chance upon cortical gray matter for study. So we published a paper stating that there is no intercellular fluid ac-accumulation and that the edema of the nervous system, the fluid accumulation, if you will, in the nervous system in triethyl tin poisoning, is due to a swelling of clear cells within gray matter. This was accepted for a time, because others also happened to work with gray matter. It was not long, however, before those who went a little deeper into the subcortical white matter found that the fluid actually is an intercellular accumulation. And so a third group, who worked with gray and white matter in the same model, the rat, soon found that in white matter the fluid is an intercellular accumulation primarily, and in the gray matter it is primarily an intracellular glial, probably astrocytic, accumulation.

On a number of occasions Dr. Tower has repeated the fact that we are looking, essentially, at artifacts, when we look at the electron microscopic view of animal brains in which fluid has accumulated. I happen to feel that both the light microscopists and the electron microscopists do create artifacts when they examine tissue. The only hope is, of course, that these artifacts are reproducible, and because they are reproducible one ultimately comes to interpolate these changes in such a way as to come to some valid conclusions. It so happens that the intercellular space in gray matter in these experimental animals remains constant, at about 150 to 200 Å units. The astrocytes, despite the fact that we dehydrate the tissue and shift fluid from cells to extracellular spaces or conversely, remain fairly constant. But the white matter still maintains large spaces which are not shifting, and for these reasons, I believe, the electron microscope does give you a fairly valid view of what goes on both in gray and white matter.

It is important to remember that following the experimental edema production with triethyl tin almost simultaneously other types of injury to the nervous system were created and studied. I believe that perhaps even Dr.

Klatzo's experiments with freezing the cerebral tissue antedated the work with triethyl tin by some years, at a time, however, when electron microscopy was still not well enough developed or was not used. Soon, of course, many people repeated the experiments of Dr. Klatzo and discovered that the triethyl tin lesion is slightly different from the one with freezing. Primarily the lesion with freezing is in the white matter and there is an excessive accumulation of fluid in intercellular spaces. This fluid is protein-rich, and so forth.

Other modalities have since been used; we, in our laboratory, have used cryptococcus polysaccharide in the production of edema. We soon discovered that we were not studying edema alone but a massive inflammatory response when we employed the live organisms. Dr. Levine supplied us with an extract of the cryptococcus capsule which we found produces edema alone, and is an excellent material for the study of fluid accumulation. Dr. Hirano this morning described some of the changes that occur with cryptococcus polysaccharide implantation. Dr. Levine and others have been using purified tuberculoprotein in experimental models, one produces edema almost exclusively, but when one uses the purified lipid fraction of the tubercle bacillus, one produces massive necrosis of myelin plus edema. Which comes first, is the problem that is unanswerable in such an experimental model. People have used, and we also have used, silver nitrate. Silver nitrate produces necrosis plus edema, and even some hemorrhage. Others have used hypoxia and I believe that in hypoxia edema develops, but I do not believe that the hypoxia creates the edema primarily. It produces also ganglion and glial cell injury, and blood vessel damage, and a lot of other things in which edema is only part of a generalized extensive process. We ourselves have used hypoglycemia. We have found the same kind of injury to ganglion cells in the brain with hypoglycemia that you see with hypoxia, except that the brain is shrunken and not swollen, just the reverse process occurs under these circumstances.

There are, in addition to this simple accumulation of fluid in the nervous system, other changes that occur that produce secondary effects. You can't produce swelling of the brain from fluid accumulation without compressing blood vessels, without interfering with nutrition, without interfering with oxygen uptake and perhaps even with the CO_2 absorptive mechanism. It is important to realize that it is the type of injury that one has to consider when one talks about experimental cerebral fluid accumulation. And one undoubtedly also has to think in terms of the animal that is used. Dr. Tower and others have indicated that the cat behaves somewhat differently from the ape, and certainly the mouse behaves differently from the rat, electron-microscopically and otherwise, in the accumulation of fluid. But the general principles, the ones that I have tried to enumerate, namely that by and large in the gray matter the cellular accumulation of fluid is the predominating element, and in the white matter by and large the accumulation of intercellular fluid is the predominating element, apparently remains true for all species. One has to keep a further thing in mind, namely the time after injury at which you examine the specimen. This holds true for the biochemical as well as for the electron microscopic analysis of the tissue.

We have shown, and Dr. Hirano has tried to emphasize, that the mere implantation in the corpus callosum of the rat's brain of a small pellet of cryptococcal polysaccharide is followed in a matter of a very few minutes by the accumulation of fluid along the myelinated sheaths. This raises another problem: many of us have been talking today about the light microscopic appearance of oligodendroglial swelling, and I think a word of caution is necessary here. What, with the light microscope, looks like the swelling of the oligodendroglia may not, under the electron microscope, actually be that. One may find that the oligos are not swollen at all in these circumstances, that the fluid merely occupies the interoligodendroglial tissue spaces, lining up the oligodendroglia in long columns. With the light microscope it is just not possible to resolve the site of the lesion. This, by the way, is also true for the so-called spongy state which we have been discussing. Dr. Gonatas, and, I believe, Dr. Terry also has found that in certain types of spongy state, like the Jakob-Creutzfeldt condition, the vacuolization isn't in the interstitial tissue at all, it is not even in glial cells, it is apparently swelling of the dendritic processes of the neurons.

If one considers species and time, one must also consider the site of injury as I have indicated, whether it be gray matter or white matter that is injured, or whether it is gray or white matter that you examine following the injury. I have already stressed the fact that the type of injury is important, whether it be freezing, whether it be anoxia, whether it be triethyl tin poisoning, or a host of other types. Cyanide has been used as well as a variety of purified chemical substances in producing the lesion.

As to the source of the fluid, I had hoped that Dr. Clasen would indicate that, at least in triethyl tin poisoning, the type of fluid that we find is relatively protein-poor and consists of a transudate, and that, as a contrast, the fluid one sees in freezing, in cold injury, is protein-rich as he has indicated, and probably also represents a transudate from the blood vessel lumen. He did not like to say that there was much of a difference in the two conditions, if I understood him correctly, and I do not believe that this necessarily disproves the notion that in both instances the fluid accumulation is derived from the vessel lumen. I think both of us would agree as to that. There is no shift, I believe, of fluid from cells of the brain or free-existing fluid to the extracellular space, or vice-versa from the extracellular space into cells in cerebral edema without the participation of blood plasma, the plasma from blood vessels in these various injurious states. We have fairly good evidence to indicate that the fluid accumulation in excess, whether it be intracellular or intercellular, is derived from the lumen of the blood vessels, probably capillaries, perhaps also arterioles and venules.

I have already mentioned that there are at least two places where fluid accumulation occurs. We have seen (I believe Dr. Torack when he was in my laboratory demonstrated this fact) that under certain circumstances the intracellular fluid in gray matter can reach such proportions that the cell membranes actually rupture. Even under these circumstances, Dr. Tower, we haven't seen an increase in the intercellular tissue spaces in gray matter, even with the rupture of the cell membranes of the glial cells, from massive intracellular fluid accumulation.

What of the human counterparts? It has been easy, of course, to work with the experimental animal model, and it has not been as easy to work with man. There have, however, been attempts in recent years to study fluid accumulation, especially in biopsy specimens obtained by neurosurgeons during operative procedures for brain tumors. So far as I can judge from the findings in man that others have described, and from those in our own laboratory, the fluid in the white matter is predominantly intercellular. We have much less data from specimens of gray matter. But in gray matter, there appears to be cellular swelling of the kind that we have seen in the experimental animal, and, I think, in that regard the animal model and man seem to be comparable. We have not seen and at least I am not aware of biopsy specimens of primary brain swelling in man, other than perhaps in two or three instances of pseudotumor cerebri. Here again, when the white matter was examined, there seemed to be an intercellular fluid accumulation. These studies are, by a long way, not so extensive as those in the experimental animal, and therefore, Dr. Adams, I do not think that I can summarize in any fuller detail what the state of affairs is in human swelling. No one, so far as I know, has yet tried to look at biopsy specimens of white matter of uremic patients. There is evidence, from light microscopy, however, that there is an accumulation of fluid, even to such an extent as to produce spreading apart of the myelin sheaths to produce what some people have called demyelination, which I think, as I believe you do, is merely a seepage of fluid out of damaged blood vessels into the surrounding perivascular zones with separation of myelin.

ADAMS: Have you examined any children's or animal's brains that are caused to swell very markedly by hyponatremia or hypo-osmolarity?

ZIMMERMAN: I have not, but I wonder if Dr. Terry has. He has examined so many biopsies.

ZÜLCH: At the end of this meeting one has to ask how the concept of brain edema, formulated in the period of light microscopy and presented to you here in this symposium, to be modified according to the new data from the literature of recent years and the findings summarized in this meeting.

1) What we called the "equivalent" of cortical edema can be explained now as an hydropic swelling of the astrocytes and their processes.

The question, whether this is a primary change of the glia or a secondary uptake of fluid from the extracellular spaces, as suggested earlier in the period of light microscopy, seems not yet finally decided, particularly since Lampert showed a transient enlargement of the extracellular spaces of the cortex in the triethyl tin edema, which disappeared very soon, when an intracellular enlargement of the astrocytes began to appear and since Tower as a biochemist formulated the concept that the astrocytes may not swell primarily but may take up extracellular water by a special change in the membrane.

I have to stress here the fact, that in some occasions, for instance in our experiments on venous obstruction, we have definitely seen an accumulation of the "blue" fluid "in" the pericellular and pericapillary spaces of the cortex with the light microscope (Masson's trichrome-stain).

2) The earlier light microscopic observations on an extracellular edema in the white matter are now elucidated further by the electron microscopical findings. The fluid accumulation is either rich in proteins, "plasmatic" as we call it and Masson-positive,—or "serous" and "watery" and Masson-negative. We have not sufficient evidence yet to state that the formation of this edema is entirely perivenous, as proven in the case of microembolism, or whether it may be partly pericapillary as we have seen in the light microscopic observations in venous obstruction. Our electron microscopic data do not suffice to clarify this question. Here we would like to suggest a more adequate correlation between the light microscopic findings and electron microscopy and, furthermore, with the data obtained by permeability studies with "tracers." For instance, in the cold-induced necrosis of the cortex with edema in the white matter only one light microscopic picture was given in this symposium by Beks and this showed a perivenous edema in the white matter. Perhaps the actual site of formation of the gross edema in these cases could be better clarified by serial observations with the light microscope. This site may be the veins in the white matter.

I was happy to hear Dr. Sluga's observations on a topographical correlation between the swelling of the myelin sheaths and the neighboring oligodendroglia, which corresponded to our early description of the grapelike swellings of the myelin sheaths (1940) which now are so beautifully portrayed ultrastructurally.

One question is left open to me at the end of this symposium. Neither our own findings in electron microscopy nor those shown here suffice to decide whether the "paling" and enlargement of the white matter around malignant gliomas results from a swelling of the myelin sheaths alone, i.e., from an intracellular accumulation of fluid, or from an intercellular serous edema in the white substance. This can probably only be decided on the base of experimental malignant brain tumors.

The model of TET seems to me to be particularly interesting because it may come out that it corresponds exactly to the primary brain swelling in the definition of Reichardt and our own earlier findings.

In summarizing, I want to emphasize once more my opinion that all our discussions ought to begin with the clinical state and the morphological and biochemical findings on brain edema in man. We have to utilize our results for the bedside in the form of suggestions for therapy. All theoretical investigations ought to consider this in choosing models.

ADAMS: Dr. Klatzo very properly calls attention to the fact that in the experimental models there are at least two identifiable forms, one in which there is a vascular injury, altered vascular permeability, seepage of protein, increased sodium, chloride, water and changes in the white and gray matter that Dr. Zimmerman has described, and with blood brain barrier abnormality being very conspicuous, and another one in which there seems to be no vascular component at all, or barrier effect. I believe in our discussion there has been given little attention to this latter form and it is one of the great deficiencies in the experimental studies, since these might be some of the most easily induced forms of relatively pure edema without very general injury to tissue.

TERRY: Dr. Luse at Washington University studied neuropil in rabbits, I believe, made hyponatremic by arterial infusions of water. The neuropil showed, as in all other neuropil studies, swelling of clear cells which she identified, at that time, as oligodendroglia.

ADAMS: We have several other subjects to discuss, having to do with the study of experimental models, the chemical analyses, and the electron microscopy, but there will first be an intermission.

ADAMS: We come now to the last parts of our discussion. Dr. Broman, in view of the fact that one of the major forms of experimental and human brain swelling seems to depend upon alteration of the blood-brain barrier, and in view of the fact that various dyes are regularly used to demonstrate this change, would you care to comment upon the correct use of these dyes? It has been pointed out to me by a number of workers, including you, that there is great importance in using the appropriate dye at the right time, i.e., when the injection is made, in relation to death.

BROMAN: When we want to make detailed studies of dysfunctional states of the blood-brain barrier system, i.e., the various mechanisms responsible for the restriction of blood-brain passage, it may be important to use different tracers corresponding to the material handled by the particular mechanisms involved. In geral, however, we restrict our concept of a blood-brain barrier damage to the lesions which give rise to extravasation of plasma solutes such as acid dyes or other organic ions, which normally are unable to pass from blood to brain and, furthermore, are more or less prone to protein binding. This type of BBB damage, which is most commonly referred to in experimental work in general, implies primarily a disturbance of the vascular (endothelial) permeability, the last term used in its biological sense. Earlier as well as recent observations, now also supported by electronmicroscopical findings, demonstrate the unique permeability properties of the endothelium of the cerebral vessels and characterize also those arteries and veins in the brain and in the pia which have no glial membrane apposed to the endothelium.

In the demonstration of BBB damage with such indicators, we must be aware of the possibility that various artifacts may distort the picture. Slight mechanical pressure may impair the BBB, something which certainly may occur in neurosurgical operations, even by cautious manipulation of the brain. Under experimental conditions the tracer might, after some time, migrate outside the area of BBB damage, as we have seen exemplified today.

By passing out in the cerebrospinal fluid through a damaged choroid plexus epithelium, the tracer dye may stain the ventricular walls as well as the outer brain surface "secondarily" without underlying barrier damage in these areas. These and other artifacts may be particularly difficult to control when using nonvisible tracers such as most radioactive indicators, which are very convenient for quantitative assay. Therefore, it may sometimes be advantageous in such studies of BBB damage to use concurrently an easily visualized tracer for the outlining of the injured area, and as an aid in the detection of artifacts.

Under certain circumstances EEG has been found usable for the testing of BBB dysfunction. The barrier defect is revealed by intravenous administration of normally barred EEG-activating drugs. In studies in our laboratory this method has been used for studies on the course of reversible and irreversible chemotoxic impairment of the BBB (Flodmark and Steinwall). Although an irreversible injury could exist for a short period without detectable influence per se on the neuronal activity, as seen in EEG, it gradually gave rise to increasing EEG deterioration and also to the development of a brain edema.

ADAMS: Dr. Tower, would you assume responsibility for coordinating the principal ideas that have emerged from the biochemical studies of fluid compartments?

TOWER: Let me preface my remarks by saying that I am delighted to be serving as a sort of devil's advocate here, because I think that one of the important features of this workshop is the stimulation of discussion and thought and open expressions of opinion. Dr. Torack is welcomed as a latecomer to the club of in vitro artifacts in incubated brain slices. We have all been aware of this problem for many years, much longer than I have been in the field. Certainly the incubated brain slice is a very poor substitute for the intact, functioning brain in vivo. In such slices, the neurons no longer display spontaneous electrical activity, there is no capillary circulation, and there is swelling under virtually all in vitro conditions. Surely, these are artifacts formidable enough for anyone. However, quite remarkably, despite all this, one can measure really respectable potential differences across cell membranes (Gibson and McIlwain: J. Physiol. [London] 176: 261, 1965). One can demonstrate the ability of these cells still to transport Na^+ out and K^+ in against significant concentration gradients. One can show that such slices maintain good P/O ratios, and so on, so that such incubated slices are not dead or so terribly abnormal as some might wish to suppose.

Now to the topic of my discussion. The problems of fluid compartmentation in the central nervous system are quite evident from the presentations that we have heard. If I could summarize all of this in a single idea, it would be the complexity of the situation. I had the feeling, at least in the early part of our proceedings, that some were trying to make things too simple. I am heartily in favor of simplification as long as there is a good basis for it, but to insist upon a simple two-compartment model composed of an extracellular and an intracellular space is, I think, incorrect and does not take account of what we know about the complexity of the central nervous system.

In this regard, Professor Heinrich Waelsch recently reintroduced and emphasized the concept of compartmentation in the central nervous system (Page 313 in Structure and Function of the Cerebral Cortex, edited by Tower and Schadé, Elsevier, 1960). There are morphological compartments which are familiar to all of you: the three which Dr. Evans has discussed, namely, the vascular, the cerebrospinal fluid-interstitial, and the cellular or tissue compartments. The tissue compartment is further subdivided into gray matter and white matter, and each of these is not necessarily similar in all brain areas. In white matter there are at least 4 cell types and in gray matter there are 5. All these cells are further subdivided into perikaryon and processes, which do not necessarily exhibit the same metabolic and functional attributes. And within the cell there are many particulate subdivisions, such as mitochondria, nuclei, etc.

If we regard all this from a biochemical and fluid distribution point of view, it obviously must be complex, whether we can measure the complexity or not. There is a vascular fluid compartment. And there is a cerebrospinal fluid compartment, which most investigators agree is coextensive with the interstitial fluid of the tissue. With regard to interstitial fluid, there is a question whether this may be coextensive with fluid within the lumen of the endoplasmic reticulum of cells. Siekevitz (page 17 in Ciba Symposium on Regulation of Cell Metabolism, 1959) thinks this is a likely possibility. In another tissue, the thymus, Mirsky and colleagues (Proc. Nat. Acad. Sci. (U.S.) 47: 907, 1961) strongly suggest that the cell nuclei are invested by extensions of the endoplasmic reticulum and are thus, in fact, surrounded by extracellular fluid. I find this a little difficult to conceptualize, but they report experimental data which would be consistent with their suggestion. Within the cytoplasm of the cell there are other fluid compartments, the mitochondria, the endoplasmic reticulum or microsomes (if not part of the extracellular fluid system) and the nucleus. Thus, I do not think we should leave this meeting with the idea that the distribution and compartmentation of fluid in the central nervous system is a simple matter or that we necessarily have adequate means of evaluating what is occuring with respect to the fluids in these various compartments.

As biochemists we have presumed upon the electron microscopists and argued with them and perhaps invaded their territory more than we should have, because we have been and are anxious to be able to correlate what we measure with the morphology of the tissue in question. This is why we worry about artifacts. Dr. Zimmerman, I certainly don't object to your point of view. I agree with you. But there are artifacts, and the reason we appear to harp on the point is that for so long most electron microscopists insisted that there were no extracellular spaces in the central nervous system. It is a pleasure to attend a meeting on the nervous system where extracellular space is not a dirty word. Here it is perhaps worth reiterating a point I made earlier. When attempting to quantitate extracellular space in an electron micrograph, one must realize what is involved. We are looking at what was originally a three-dimensional structure. If one considers the 150 Å space between two cells as a cylinder and calculates how much wider this space would have to be to take up 30% extra fluid, it would have to widen to only 170 Å. This difference would be rather difficult to appreciate visually. Similarly, if for the sake of illustration, one assumes an astrocyte to be a sphere of diameter 10μ and that it swells 30%, the diameter need only increase to 10.9μ. Finally, if one assumes a 150 Å wide intracellular space to represent only a 10% space, how much wider would such a cylinder of fluid have to be to provide a 30% extracellular space? The width would have to be only 260 Å. I see Dr. Katzman is disturbed, but I think you will find that when considered from a volumetric point of view this is how it works out. My point here is that the changes are relatively small, so that we tend to be arguing about minutiae. I suspect many of us have not appreciated how little the dimensions on electron micrographs need to change to correspond to rather sizable volume changes.

On the other hand the indicators, like inulin, sucrose, thiocyanate, sulfate, etc., are not without problems either. We have generally assumed that some of them, like inulin, are extracellular. Very likely they are under most condtions, but they are not necessarily always so, as some investigators have shown (Ames, et al., J. Physiol. (London) 177: 246, 1965). Inulin may pose special problems, as Chen, et al., (Proc. Soc. Exp. Biol. Med. 113: 584, 1963) and Phelps (Biochem. J. 95: 41, 1965) have reported. On the other hand, some investigators have tended to bandy about results with certain indicators without realizing the problems inherent in their use. I want to make this point especially with reference to sulfate and thiocyanate, as they are used in vivo. Like iodide, certain organic acids, etc., these two indicators are transported actively out of the central nervous system, i.e., from CNS→blood (Pollay and Davson, Brain, 86: 137, 1963; Streicher, et al, Am. J. Physiol. 206: 251, 1964; Richmond and Hastings, Ibid, 199: 814, 1960). Thus, if one uses sulfate, for example, as a measure of space in the central nervous system, the reference of these tissue measurements to plasma sulfate levels will give an erroneously small sulfate space for brain tissue; whereas reference to CSF sulfate levels will yield tissue sulfate spaces of the same order of magnitude as found for inulin, chloride, etc. Now, the neurophysiologists should have something to say here because they require at least a functional extracellular or extraneuronal space. Impedance studies and microelectrode studies would insist that there is an appreciable space which must be at least functionally extracellular. In the case of the leech nervous system, Kuffler and colleagues (J. Neurophysiol. 27: 645, 1964) have shown that this must in fact, as well as function, be extracellular. I would hesitate to equate the leech with mammals, but here, at least, is well-documented evidence that the relatively narrow interstitial spaces between glial cells and neurons actually do serve for the transport of nutrients and electrolytes to support activity of the neurons. Interpretations of biochemical data have been questioned here, because my figures do not agree with someone else's, and theirs do not agree with another set of figures. This is clearly mostly a technical problem which should be of less concern to us at this time than the fact that we do measure such spaces. Regardless of the fact that one set might be only 50% of someone else's values, the spaces are there.

The real questions are: where are they morphologically and, even more important (as Dr. Pappius indicated at the close of her paper), how can we utilize any of our space measurements to calculate the distribution of electrolytes? These, to me, are the really vital questions, because until we are able to calculate such distributions, the full understanding of problems like edema will elude us. Unless we can properly conduct studies, e.g., with ^{24}Na and ^{42}K, to see how and at what rate such cations enter or leave swollen astrocytes for example, I don't think we will appreciate all the problems involved nor be able to fully evaluate therapeutic measures. Unfortunately, as Dr. Pappius has pointed out, we are not at the stage where we can calculate the cation composition within an astrocyte or within a neuron. To be sure, McIlwain and his colleagues have developed some good approximations (J. Physiol. (London) 176: 261, 1965; Biochem. J. 95: 289, 1965), but they are still working essentially with a two-compartment model. Their intracellular compartment comprises 5 different cell types, and one may not, a priori, say that all have the same electrolyte composition within them. Furthermore, other factors are involved when one considers pathological situations affecting distribution of fluids and solutes. We know relatively little about these. In situations in which either oxygenation or circulation or both in the brain are abnormal, we must also consider what happens to parameters like lactic acid, ammonia, pH, CO_2, etc. and how changes thereof may affect the way in which water and the inorganic ions we commonly measure are shifted from one compartment to another. Calcium has been mentioned and is also important. We know very little about it in neural tissues and are not yet able to distinguish how much is free and how much bound or where it is bound. In addition the changes in conformation of membranes with swelling must be taken into account because of the fixed charges in membranes. If the size of a cell increases or decreases, with stretching or shrinking of its membranes, the number of exposed or hidden charges may be altered and this will have a bearing on how much water and what sort of ions can be held on either side of the membrane.

I do not mean to make all this too complicated, but I want you to realize that these are not easy problems and that the reasons why we may not be completely in agreement or why we may be unable to give you some of the answers here because of the very complexity. Let me recall two studies in this regard which I consider quite important. First, what happens following circulatory arrest? I will not review the numerical data we presented but merely emphasize that this becomes an important problem when dealing with clinical material. It is seldom that even in a biopsy one can obtain a brain tissue sample under ideal experimental conditions. If the surgeon encounters a bleeder, that biopsy specimen may have to sit with no blood supply for many minutes before you can get your hands on it, and thus changes may ensue which no longer represent the state of the tissue at the time you wanted to biopsy it. And if you study post-mortem material, there can be changes related to the post-mortem state of no circulation, no oxygen, etc. rather than to the state of the person when he died or when you studied his disease on the ward. Secondly, I want to recall for you the study of Birks (Canad. J. Biochem. Physiol. 40: 303, 1962), who perfused sympathetic ganglia with perfusates containing sufficient cardiac glycoside to inhibit specifically cation transport (pump) systems in ganglion cells. Regardless of any artifacts which might be present, the electron micrographs of such ganglia clearly showed massive swelling of endoplasmic reticulum lumina; dark and shrunken mitochondria; pale, watery cytoplasm of neurons; and swollen axon terminals and synaptic vesicles. Under the same conditions but with a low sodium perfusate or a chloride-free perfusate, Birks observed that most of these changes could be prevented. The point of this example is that a great many changes can be produced simply as a result of interfering with normal matabolism or function of certain specific components of the tissue. The final result viewed by electron microscopy might be extremely difficult to interpret unless one knew exactly what had occurred and could experimentally vary one condition at a time in order to assess all possible contributory factors.

There are obviously many problems from our point of view still to be solved. I think we should congratulate Dr. Pappius for showing us in subcortical white matter an edema which can be understood, at least initially, from a biochemical point of view, since so little has been done in this area subsequent to the observations of Stewart-Wallace (Brain 62: 426, 1939) some 25 years ago. I regret that we could not have had the opportunity to hear from some others who have contributed to these problems, notably Drs. McIlwain, Lajtha, Van Harrevald, Woodbury and De Robertis. Despite the fact that they were not able to be present, their contributions to and influence on our discussions must be obvious to many of you. By way of summary, I do feel that we have finally arrived at the point where we can agree that there is considerable interstitial or extracellular fluid in the brain, and this conclusion is perhaps one of the major achievements of this Workshop. I had hoped that Dr. Davson would be able to continue the discussion by telling us something about comparisons between edematous situations in other tissues and the brain, but in his absence I will pass on to ask Dr. Katzman to give us a better correlation than I can between the biochemistry and electron microscopy of edema.

ADAMS: May I now call on Dr. Katzman?

KATZMAN: The assignment that Dr. Tower has given me is a relatively easy one compared to other matters that have been discussed here today, since there is really a remarkable agreement between the various groups who worked on experimental cerebral edema as far as the biochemical and some of the electron microscopic changes observed are concerned. In this regard, I might just address one word to Dr. Adams, that those of us working in experimental edemas are really ultimately interested in diseases of humans. But studies in humans had progressed very, very slowly before the experimental cerebral edemas were tackled directly, and I do not think this workshop would have been possible without the various experimental models that many of us had been working on. The kind of experimental cerebral edema that most resembles that observed in human disease processes is the kind of edema which I have called focal edema, in which there is a lesion, a cold injury, an implanted tumor, or a polysaccharide that is implanted in the brain, and around this area there is a breakdown of the blood-brain barrier and swelling of the tissue. All of the various workers in these circumstances have found an increase in water and sodium and an increase in proteins. Both Dr. Clasen's group and Dr. Lowenthal's group have found that these proteins to the largest extent resemble the proteins present in the serum, but that there are certain minor but perhaps very significant changes in the nature of the albumin that is present in the edemas and in the relative amount of glycoprotein present in the edemas. Dr. Klatzo has suggested that in these focal edemas the fluid accumulates via the leak in the injured capillaries, and in the white matter where the edema is extracellular, this is probably true. However, there does seem also to be a breakdown of the blood-brain barrier in these cases in the cortex, where this extracellular fluid has not obviously penetrated. The second form of edema, that many of us have studied, is that of triethyl tin edema. This, in fact, did produce human disease, when it was present in a preparation sold in France in the mid-1950's for the treatment of furunculosis, and there was an epidemic of increased intracranial pressure due to this disease. It was the autopsies in a few of these patients showing swollen brains that led to the experimental studies which have shown an increase in water and salt, without an increase, according to most laboratories, in the albumin or other serum proteins in the fluid. And here the fluid is confined in the gray matter within the astrocytic processes, and in the white matter within myelinic blebs or myelin splits. A third form of edema that is very important in children is that of water intoxication. Dr. Pappius has presented data on this form of edema during this conference. She noted that it differs from the other forms of edema in that there is only accumulation of water without any change in the relative sodium or potassium concentration. Whereas in other edemas one has an increase in sodium and water, in the water intoxication there is simply water intoxication of the brain. The fourth kind of edema has been the most controversial. This is the anoxic-hypercapnic edema that Dr. Lee and Dr. Bakay have talked about and which several laboratories have had some difficulty in producing.

With a considerable amount of agreement about these findings in experimental edemas, there is, on the contrary, considerable disagreement concerning the issues that Dr. Tower raised. I must agree with Dr. Tower that the brain is very complex, and that there is certainly probably more than one compartment. And Ranck (Experimental Neurology, 7:153, 1963), in a very elegant study of the electrical impedance of the brain, found it most useful to explain the electrical impedance by assuming that there were a least three compartments: that of the extracellular space, that of the glia cells, and that of the neurons. Nicholls and Kuffler, as Dr. Tower has pointed out, have shown that a small extracellular space between cells of a 150 to 200 Å is sufficient to take care of the fluid needs of the leech ganglia in terms of its electrical activities. We do not need to have more than that in order for the nerve tissue to function. The question then arises: what, in fact, is the true extracellular space of the brain? Is it the 2 to 5% that most electron microscopists believe to be present? Or is the 10 to 15% that Dr. Oppelt and Dr. Rall have presented? Or is it the 30 to 50% that Dr. Tower has presented? I do not agree with Dr. Tower that this is an unimportant argument. I think that this is of great significance, that it is very difficult to resolve, but I do not think that all of the artifacts present are those due to fixation in electron micrographs. There are as many artifacts and as many complexities in the physiological experiments as in the experiments carried out by morphologists in studying the ultrastructure. I should just like to point out a few of these.

There are somewhat different artifacts or assumptions in the experiments of Dr. Tower and the experiments of Dr. Oppelt and Dr. Rall. In Dr. Tower's experiments in vivo in animals he injected a tracer into the cisterna magna and then followed what happened over the cortex several hours later. He operated upon the animal, removed spinal fluid, cut out the underlying piece of brain and measured the content of his tracer in the brain and in the spinal fluid, and compared this ratio. But this is essentially a kinetic experiment in which there is a constantly changing level in the spinal fluid. And yet this is used in these experiments to measure what really ought to be a steady-state measurement, i.e., the extracellular fluid of the brain. One can see that in a given area of the cortex the fluid that passed over that area a few minutes earlier might have had a higher concentration of the tracer than the fluid at the time of the biopsy. This has already been pointed out by Dr. Oppelt. There is a second artifact, but I think it is inherent in this experiment and cannot be avoided. That is the question of what tissue are you measuring. When you remove a piece of cortex and then blot it gently on tissue paper, as Dr. Tower has done, and then measure the amount of tracer in this tissue, you undoubtedly have, first of all, adhering to the outer surface of this tissue, a small amount of the spinal fluid that was originally present, because in Dr. Tower's experiment he did not wash this out. If, on the other hand, you do wash out the spinal fluid, you might wash away some of your tracer. You are really caught in this kind of experiment. Secondly, you have pia and arachnoid which are actually extracellular tissue present in this piece of tissue that you removed. You also have the pial investure around the blood vessels as they enter this tissue. One would expect, under these circumstances, that if you got into higher and higher species where you have thicker and more blood vessels, more pia and more convexities in the tissue, you might have a greater apparent "extracellular space." If you had some way, and I do not know of any way, of getting into the tissue proper itself, without these artifacts, the space measured might be somewhat lower.

The very excellent experiments of Dr. Oppelt and Dr. Rall used a technique which I personally happen to use regularly, and I ought not to say there is any artifact associated with it, namely the steady state ventricular cisternal perfusion. Here, with this kind of perfusion you do have a constant level of your tracer in the adjoining fluid. When you do this experiment, there are a number of assumptions that one must make in order to make any calculations. Dr. Oppelt has listed many of these assumptions. I would like to add some more assumptions and emphasize some he has specified. One assumption that he makes is that the kind of diffusion kinetics that applies to a plane can also be applied to what essentially is a sphere. When you have tissue around a ventricle, this is acting as one sphere outside another sphere. This will give a somewhat different diffusion curve than the one that is used mathematically by Dr. Oppelt, and this curve will be even sharper in its fall-off. Secondly, as Dr. Oppelt has stated, if you have any diffusion of your tracer across the capillary wall, this will cause a change and will also make your curve steeper. But at the same time, the brain does not just contain a fixed space where diffusion in extracellular space takes place. We know from tissue culture that there is actually considerable movement of cells in life. We know that there are pressure pulses from the blood vessels. There is a constant streaming of the spinal fluid, and, therefore, there is undoubtedly movement of fluid back and forth within the extracellular space, quite apart from any diffusion. The net effect of this kind of fluid movement will tend to make this curve less steep. Thus, we have convection currents making this curve less steep. We have a loss across the capillaries (or into cells as by pinocytosis) plus the effect of diffusion in a sphere, having the opposite effect, so that these things might tend to cancel out and give the apparent good results that you had in matching your curve to the diffusion constant of inulin. I think these things are very difficult to sort out.

ADAMS: Thank you very much, Dr. Katzman. I believe that many of the points which have been raised can be dealt with in the discussions.

We still have several subjects to consider. We have heard a great deal about the electron microscopy of the different forms of experimental brain swelling. There have been certain inconsistencies in the reports. Doubtless some of these result from the fact that different species were being studied, and different models of edema produced. Also there was a distressing lack fo quantitative data concerning the various experimental models. Of course it is extremely difficult to create an experiment where one can follow a given lesion from its inception to its end and to obtain some measure of all of the different tissue components. Dr. Henry Webster and Dr. Adelbert Ames have been struggling with this for 2 or 3 years. Simple experiments in hypoxia and hypoglycemia require a measurement of the function of the living tissue which one can control continuously and a capacity to sample the tissue for biochemical and histopathological analyses as the conditions are produced and corrected. Volumetric data on size of organelles, whole cells and intercellular space are needed. This is a very large order, but we hope that this kind of study will be forthcoming from many of the fine laboratories that were reporting work here.

It would be regrettable if we parted company without those of you who know so much about experimental edemas telling us how they can be modified or controlled by some of the currently used therapeutic agents. We have before us almost every day cases of tumor where the symptomatology can be reduced in hours by the use of massive doses of corticosteroid, by a change in the osmolarity of the circulating blood, or possibly by changing the temperature of the body and the level of systolic blood pressure. Already reference has been made to the fact that it is almost impossible to withdraw the sodium and chloride from certain experimental lesions. I wonder if it would be worthwhile for us to discuss in the concluding section of our report what is known about the control of each of the four forms of edema that Dr. Katzman mentioned. Dr. Evans probably has as much experience with the clinical problems and their therapy as anyone. Will you please summarize or persuade others to do so?

EVANS: I shall be very brief. Prevention is clearly the best form of therapy, but man being what he is and not having advanced very far over the aeons, we presumably shall have to continue to face the problem of the immediate care of the head-injured patient. Our colleagues in anesthesiology have added to our understanding of the value of an adequate airway, the usefulness of tracheostomy, and the need of ensuing adequate gaseous exchange. Gaseous exchange is, however, only a fraction of the metabolic process, and it may be that the value of the cortical steroids, attested to by many, rests in its metabolic effect. There was not time in our oral presentation to discuss the role of the lipids in membrane function, but reference may be had to our detailed paper dealing with the importance of a continuous supply of metabolically produced energy in order to maintain normal glial structure and to support proper cellular hydration through the active transport of water and ions. Furthermore, I believe it should be emphasized again that the parameter of time has a great deal to do with the state of the intracranial contents at any particular moment, a fact which plagues the clinician who must always consider the changing physiological state of his patient. I do not believe I should close without expressing again some concern over the fact that many of the experimental models which have been cited during the symposium do not simulate those with which we are dealing clinically. Though the use of tetraethyl tin, freezing and other techniques broaden our knowledge of the reaction of the brain to noxious agents, I would make the plea for more studies with models that simulate clinical conditions.

ADAMS: Apparently you have not seen many frost-bitten or sun-burned brains among your patients. Would any of the investigators who have been studying these different types of experimental edema like to say something about the use of corticosteroids, urea, mannitol or other hypertonic solutions in the control of these lesions?

KATZMAN: In the form of edema that is least applicable to human disease, namely triethyl tin edema, there is a very marked effect of corticosteroids in preventing the development of this edema as has been reported by Taylor, et al. (Neurology, 15:667, 1965).

QUADBECK: We were successful in our experiments on animals with cold injury edema using urea, glucose, osmotic therapy, drugs which seal the blood-brain barrier, and with compounds which increase the glucose transport into the brain. We also treated several patients in our hospital in this way and were successful, even where the neurosurgeons had not been successful.

ADAMS: Dr. Klatzo, have you any experience in the control of the cold-injured brain?

KLATZO: Unfortunately, we have not done much in this direction. The only measure which definitely reduced the spreading of edema due to cold lesion is lowering of the systolic blood pressure, which I have reported at this symposium. In this respect, I wonder to what extent the beneficial effect of hypothermia, so widely reported in the literature, may be related to concurrent hypotension.

BEKS: In our work, about which I told you this morning, we experimented with cats. After they had symptoms of brainstem compression, we gave them intravenously urea, mannitol and lasix in equivalent doses. After urea the intraventricular pressure fell to a low level within a short period. After mannitol a much slower and smaller decrease in this pressure occurred. Lasix had little, if any, influence. The period of low intraventricular pressure after urea was much longer than that after mannitol.

CLASEN: We have used quite a few things to try to treat the edema associated with freezing lesions. Intravenous hypertonic glucose, dextran, and albumin had no demonstrable effect (Surg. Gyne. Obs. 104: 591-606, 1957). The results with urea were the same as those reported by Dr. Pappius (Arch. Neurol. 12: 424-434, 1965). We were unable to demonstrate an effect with steroids given one hour after injury with sacrifice 11 hours later (Arch. Neurol., in press). We have also used reserpine, following Dr. Levine's lead in this area that implantation of serotonin into the brain produces a periodic acid-Schiff positive type of edema (Amer. J. Path., 42: 97-110.) Again, the results were negative. The administration of the diuretic Furosemide (Lasex) was also without demonstrable effect. Positive results have been obtained with systemic hypothermia. Dr. H. L. Rosomoff has published several papers on this (Arch. Neurol., 13: 337-345) and we have reported a decreased mortality in rabbits treated with hypothermia combined with prednisolone (Surg. Gyne. Obs., 108: 333-338, 1959). There seems to be no question that if the animal is hypothermic and is maintained in a hypothermic state the edema is decreased, but whether or not this remains when the animal is rewarmed is an open question.

ADAMS: Thank you. I think you would agree, Dr. Pappius, that in water intoxication the correction of the hypo-osmolarity of the blood can bring about, at least in a certain phase of the lesion, a rather rapid restitution of function. This has been witnessed in the hospital wards quite regularly.

PAPPIUS: We had a series of cats with freezing lesions which were pretreated for 3 or 4 days with cortisone before the lesion was made. We could not demonstrate any effect on the water content or the sodium and potassium content of the edematous tissues of the pretreated animals. We concluded that in our model the cortisone pretreatment for three days before the lesion was made does not affect the parameters we are measuring.

OPPELT: I would like to answer Dr. Katzman's comments regarding our method of measuring extracellular space. The prime purpose of these experiments was to establish that there is sufficient extracellular space present in the in vivo brain, and that this decreases at least 50% when the tissue dies. We were not interested in establishing very precise figures, or in delineating small differences in extracellular space between various brain regions. Should the mathematical objections be justified, only a very small change in our values would result. The fact that our brain diffusion coefficients closely agree with those reported in the literature and with those we obtained in agar argues for correct mathematics having been used in our calculations. Secondly, as to capillary wall permeability to inulin, some inulin will cross the capillary wall. This would tend to make us underestimate the true brain extracellular space. Analysis of the diffusion profile in the brain suggests that this capillary wall permeability is not an important factor. Thirdly, as to bulk flow in the brain affecting the diffusion kinetics, an extensive mathematical analysis of our findings by Dr. C. S. Patlak (to be published) indicates that this does not occur to a significant extent.

ADAMS: Dr. Cumings, would you like to make any concluding remarks on the general biochemical approach to this problem of experimental edema? Where are the obvious gaps and what steps should be taken in the future?

CUMINGS: Since it is already so late, I feel that I should perhaps only make one or two comments. I largely agree with Dr. Tower when he talks about the attempts that have been made to make too many separate compartments. I think that in our group we have tried to avoid this as much as we can. We have experimented only with tin and distilled water. Both of these give rise to generalized lesions thus allowing no normal control in the same animal. This is an error, if you like, but we have no choice. I think I should say that in tin, Aldridge and his group have shown quite clearly that perhaps the main effect is an enzymic action on mitochondria and probably other enzymes associated with the cell. Distilled water in monkeys produces well-marked edema with an increase in protein, whereas in the case of tin there is no such increase in protein, and no apparent gross abnormality of protein pattern. In man, Dr. Lowenthal, who has unfortunately left us, showed an altered protein distribution, but he was using cellulose acetate or agar, so it is a little difficult to get an exact distinction as to which actual protein was involved. The proteins we have shown to be increased, particularly albumin as well as possibly some globulins might be derived from blood, tumor or brain. This is something we have got to look into further. I think there is little doubt from the work of both Lowenthal's group and ours that the fluid is in fact obtained from blood or from plasma, and as was said earlier, is derived from the breakdown in blood vessels, capillaries or the blood-brain barrier. I might perhaps add that in our experience in brains in very young children suffering from burns and who develop swelling of the brain do in fact always have a raised water content. We usually find no change in enzymes or electrolytes but this is again difficult because the entire brain is affected and the only normal you have is by comparing other brains of the same age, and this is not really reliable at this age of a child. Albumin is almost invariably absent; in fact it is very like tin edema in many respects. I think that's all I would wish to say except that Dr. Davson, who is still not here, has always claimed—and I hope he won't complain that I am misquoting him—that about a 15% extracellular space has been determined by biochemical techniques, so I don't think we need to consider as much as 30%, for 15% is more than adequate to answer all our worries biochemically.

ADAMS: Ladies and gentlemen, we are all becoming weary of this discussion. It falls to the lot of Dr. Seitelberger and his colleagues to try to record this entire three-day meeting and to draw some sensible deductions from it. Certainly our presence here indicates that all of us are convinced that brain swelling is one of the important problems in neurology and neuropathology and that certain forms of it underlie many lesions. The experimental study of these states has added tremendously to our understanding of them. You have heard excellent summaries of the problems by Dr. Katzman and Dr. Zimmerman and are now in a better position to see how some of these experimental models might apply to man. There is certainly a tremendous amount of work to be done, but the tools by which one can approach these problems are now in our hands, and I think it is just a matter of time until many refinements of experimental technique will enable us to obtain definitive answers to the questions that we have been asking today. I am sure Dr. Seitelberger and all other members of the colloquium hope that those of you who have come here and spent your time so generously in participating in these discussions will leave here even more challenged by these problems and will approach them with renewed effort. Thank you very much.

MIX
Papier aus verantwortungsvollen Quellen
Paper from responsible sources
FSC® C105338

If you have any concerns about our products,
you can contact us on
ProductSafety@springernature.com

In case Publisher is established outside the EU,
the EU authorized representative is:
Springer Nature Customer Service Center GmbH
Europaplatz 3, 69115 Heidelberg, Germany

Printed by Libri Plureos GmbH
in Hamburg, Germany